Principles of Behavioral
and Cognitive Neurology

Principles of Behavioral and Cognitive Neurology

SECOND EDITION

M.-Marsel Mesulam

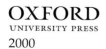

OXFORD
UNIVERSITY PRESS
2000

OXFORD
UNIVERSITY PRESS

Oxford   New York
Athens   Auckland   Bangkok   Bogotá   Buenos Aires   Calcutta
Cape Town   Chennai   Dar es Salaam   Delhi   Florence   Hong Kong   Istanbul
Karachi   Kuala Lumpur   Madrid   Melbourne   Mexico City   Mumbai
Nairobi   Paris   São Paulo   Singapore   Taipei   Tokyo   Toronto   Warsaw

and associated companies in
Berlin   Ibadan

Library of Congress Cataloging-in-Publication Data
Principles of behavioral and cognitive neurology /
[edited by] M-Marsel Mesulam.— 2nd ed.
p.   cm.
Rev. ed. of: Principles of behavioral neurology /
[edited by] M-Marsel Mesulam. c1985.
Includes bibliographical references and index.
ISBN 0-19-513475-3
1. Mental Illness—Etiology.   2. Neuropsychology.
3. Brain—Diseases—Complications.
I. Mesulam, M-Marsel.   II. Principles of behavioral neurology.
[DNLM: 1. Neuropsychology.   2. Cognition—psychology.
WL 103.5 P957 2000]   RC454.4.P73   2000   616.89—dc21
DNLM/DLC   for Library of Congress   99-15581

9 8 7 6 5 4 3 2

Printed in the United States of America
on acid-free paper

Dedicated to the memories of

Frank Benson
Norman Geschwind
Jean-Louis Signoret

who contributed to
the first edition of this book
and whose inspiration
remains alive
in the second.

Preface

The contributors to the first edition of this book were encouraged to emphasize principles rather than details. They were so successful that the book went through eight printings without appearing to become obsolete. Eventually, however, it became clear that new facts needed to be incorporated into a second edition. The magnitude of this venture was not fully realized until after the current project was initiated. Even authors whose task appeared to be as simple as updating an already excellent chapter decided to undertake an extensive and often complete rewriting. The second edition retains the spirit and philosophy of the first, but with an almost completely new content.

The first edition was published in 1985, at a time when basic neuroscience was undergoing several crucial developments: The connections of the monkey brain were being charted with axonally transported tracers, details of chemical neuroanatomy were being revealed with immunohistochemistry, neuronal physiology was being explored with single-unit recordings in behaving animals, and primate models of human neuropsychological syndromes were being established with the help of targeted ablations. These advances were incorporated into the first edition of this book and lent a new sophistication to the traditional interpretation of brain–behavior relationships. Functional imaging remained somewhat peripheral in the first edition. Although the methodology had been introduced a decade earlier, it had not yet started to yield truly novel information beyond what had been established by traditional behavioral neurology.

This second edition was written during another period of self-renewal for behavioral neurology, this time driven predominantly by developments in functional magnetic resonance imaging (fMRI). In the past, functional imaging was almost entirely confined to positron emisson tomography. This expensive technology was available to very few centers, which became the privileged gatekeepers of research in this area. The advent of fMRI led to the radical democratization of this field. In many parts of the world, qualified investigators working in the vicinity of a research-friendly clinical radiology department can now access modern functional imaging technology. Although fMRI is not perfect, its widespread availability, flexibility, and anatomical resolution have fueled much of the recent excitement in this field.

Research in behavioral neurology and neuropsychology had traditionally focused on patients with focal brain lesions. Paradigmatic patients such as Hughlings Jackson's Dr. Z., Paul Broca's Tan-tan, John Harlow's Phineas Gage, and Brenda Milner's H.M. provided lasting insights into the behavioral neuroanatomy of emotion, language, comportment, and memory. Despite these achievements, however, the epistemological limitations inherent in determining the function of an area on the basis of the dysfunction caused by its destruction are widely acknowledged. These limitations can be overcome by combining the clinical approach with functional imaging. Within the context of such a dual approach, focal lesions help to infer the location of areas that are critical for a given cognitive skill. The functional imaging of neurologically intact subjects performing the same cognitive task helps to assess the validity of these inferences and reveals the additional areas that participate in the neural coordination of that cognitive operation. The integration of these two complementary approaches leads to the identification of the large-scale neural networks that subserve individual cognitive domains.

There was a time when the cognitive scientists did not know much about the brain and the behavioral neurologist knew even less about cognitive neuroscience. The availability of functional imaging has changed this situation and has encouraged collaborative interactions between these two disciplines. The behavioral neurologist, who is now in a position to perform imaging studies on neurologically intact subjects, needs the expertise of the cognitive scientist for hypothesis-driven research and paradigm design. In turn, the cognitive scientist looks to the clinician for access to patients with focal lesions and for clinically based constraints (reality checks) to keep the interpretation of functional imaging experiments within the bounds of plausibility. This new and flourishing alliance of behavioral neurology/neurospychology/neuropsychiatry with cognitive science has played a pivotal role in the further modernization of this field. Through this alliance, the cognitive scientist has become a bit of a behavioral neurologist, and the behavioral neurologist a bit of a cognitive scientist. The addition of the word "cognitive" to the title of this edition reflects this trend.

In contrast to the spectacular advances that have taken place in revealing the functional landscape of the human brain, little progress has been made in understanding its connectivity. Two levels of neural connectivity contribute to the functional organization of the brain. First, genetically determined axonal connections specify the type of information that a given area will process. Second, experience-induced modifications in the synaptic strengths of these connections enable the gradual accumulation of a knowledge base that is unique for each individual. Although corticocortical and corticosubcortical connections are very well delineated in the monkey brain, there is almost no corresponding information for the human brain. The literature tends to ignore this major gap and gives the misleading impression that the human brain is like a large monkey brain with similar, if not identical, connections. Anatomical, electrophysiological, imaging-based, and computational methods are currently being developed to explore the connectivity of the human brain. These approaches are at embryonic but promising stages. This is an area that will almost undoubtedly witness very significant advances in the next decade.

Experience-induced modifications of synaptic strengths are particularly difficult to identify. We tend to think of plasticity as a phenomenon confined to early life. In fact, dendritic and synaptic remodeling occurs throughout the life span and helps us learn new associations, adapt to new situations, and compensate for the wear and tear of everyday life. These dynamic aspects of brain structure are very poorly understood, even in simple animal models. A deep understanding of exactly how a new face or new word alters the synaptology of the human brain is unlikely to become available for decades to come. Major technological and conceptual leaps in the basic neurosciences will be required to initiate progress in this aspect of human neurobiology.

In these cost-conscious times, clinicians are asked to justify their existence by the value they add to patient care. The behavioral neurologist has traditionally been consulted to localize brain lesions, determine whether symptoms which seem to defy plausibility (such as those of temporolimbic epilepsy or Capgras's syndrome) are neurological (organic) or psychiatric, and chart a course for treatment and re-habilitation. The remarkable advances in neuroimaging may initially seem to have marginalized the contributions of the clinician to lesion localization. It is worth considering, however, that a specialized understanding of brain–behavior relation-ships is often necessary to assess the relevance of neuroimaging results. In the dementias, furthermore, early diagnosis depends on the neuropsychological detec-tion of abnormalities at a time when imaging studies can be entirely normal. In-sights into the intricacies of neurobehavioral syndromes and into their modes of recovery also fall within the expertise of clinicians in this field. This specialized knowledge improves the quality of differential diagnosis, prognosis, and rehabili-tation planning. The behavioral neurologist and neuropsychiatrist provide addi-tional expert guidance for the pharmacological treatment of cognitive and behav-ioral impairments. Considering the large number of medical and neurological diseases that impair mental function, it would seem that the services of the behav-ioral neurologist, neuropsychologist, and neuropsychiatrist will continue to attract considerable demand.

This second edition maintains the general structure and objectives of the first. The chapters are comprehensive and authoritative. The purpose is to provide a clinically inspired but scientifically guided approach to behavioral and cognitive neurology. Chapter 1 provides a broad overview of behavioral neuroanatomy as a background for all the other chapters. This chapter also includes a review of frontal syndromes, the limbic system, hemispheric asymmetry, and large-scale distributed networks. Chapter 2 offers a systematic approach to formal and bedside neuro-psychological testing. Chapters 3–7 contain detailed reviews of confusional states, neglect syndromes, memory disorders, aphasia-alexia-agraphia, aprosodia, and complex visual deficits. They link clinical observations to the neurobiology of the relevant syndromes. The chapters on language and memory have new authorship in this edition. Chapters 8–10 focus on diseases of great interest to behavioral and cognitive neurology, namely temporolimbic epilepsy, major psychiatric syndromes, and the dementias. The last two of these chapters, those on the psychiatric syndromes and dementia, are new and address areas that were not covered in the first edition.

I want to thank Fred Plum who asked me to edit the first edition and Fiona Stevens, Susan Hannan, and Nancy Wolitzer who have skillfully guided the transformation of this second edition from manuscript to finished book.

Chicago, Ill.   M.-M. M.
May 1999

Preface to the First Edition

One factor that has contributed prominently to the rapid growth and evolution of contemporary behavioral neurology is the distinctly multi-disciplinary approach to patient care and research. The phenomenal progress in the basic neurosciences, for example, has provided a source of new direction and enthusiasm for the clinician. In turn, clinical observations are once again beginning to guide basic experimentation, as they had done so fruitfully during the earlier days of both disciplines. Many of the recent developments in the areas of attention, emotion, memory, and dementia owe their impetus to this fertile interaction.

Since the single most fundamental aspect of behavioral neurology is the systematic assessment of mental state, the neuropsychologist has played one of the most important roles in the development of the entire field. The relationship between psychiatry and neurology is also central to behavioral neurology. Although this interaction is not new, it is undergoing a welcome revival. For example, temporolimbic epilepsy is now regularly included in the differential diagnosis of atypical psychiatric problems; some cases of shyness and childhood depression have been linked to a developmental right hemisphere dysfunction; and it is now generally accepted that substantial alterations of mood, personality, and comportment may arise as the sole manifestation of focal injury not only in the frontal lobes but also in various parts of the right hemisphere. These are only some of the developments that have fueled the intensity of the interchange between psychiatry and neurology.

This is not to say that there is an inexorable movement toward reclassifying all psychiatric diseases within the neurologic nosology. In fact, for the vast majority of patients who seek outpatient psychiatric help, a neurologic approach is no more useful (or desirable) than a chemical analysis of the ink would be for deciphering the meaning of a message. However, new discoveries on the cerebral organization of emotion and personality are prompting the inclusion of neurologic causes into the differential diagnosis of many conditions that have traditionally been attributed to idiopathic psychiatric disorders.

Attitudes that once considered the organic approach as the insensitive sledgehammer of psychiatry and the area of behavior as the soft underbelly of neurology are rapidly changing. Behavioral neurology is now firmly established as a *bona fide* specialty that includes, among other fields of interest, the borderland area between neurology and psychiatry. It also provides an outlook that focuses on the behavioral consequences of almost all neurologic diseases and of many medical conditions that influence brain physiology. The clinical mandate of behavioral neurology is vast and its future is bright. The growth of this field promises to be of major benefit to a large group of patients, who can hope to receive a new understanding for conditions that have not been of central interest to the mainstream of modern medical, neurologic, and psychiatric practices. These developments are also likely to have a considerable impact on the scientific investigation of brain-behavior relationships.

This book aims to provide a background for some of the major areas in behavioral neurology. Chapter 1 contains a survey of anatomic and physiologic principles that guide the interpretation of brain-behavior interactions. Chapter 2 gives an overview of the mental state assessment and its correlations with cerebral damage. This chapter also places a special emphasis on the examination of elderly and demented patients. Chapters 3 through 7 contain in-depth analyses of major behavioral areas: attention, memory, language, affect, and complex perceptual processing. Chapter 8 is somewhat unique in dealing with a single disease process. This appeared justified in view of the remarkable spectrum of psychiatric and endocrinologic conditions that are seen in conjunction with temporolimbic epilepsy. Chapters 9 through 11 survey recent advances in the behavioral application of evoked potentials, regional metabolic scanning, and quantitative computerized tomography.

Each chapter in this book contains a broad range of information, which can provide not only an introductory background for clinicians who are new to the field but also an update for the expert. However, this book will not accomplish its full purpose unless it also proves useful to the basic neuroscientist who is interested in bridging the gap between the experimental laboratory and the human brain.

During the preparation of this book, it has been a pleasure to work with Fred Plum, M.D., Editor-in-Chief of the Contemporary Neurology Series, Sylvia K. Fields, Ed.D., Senior Medical Editor at F.A. Davis, Ann Huehnergarth, Production Editor, and the other F.A. Davis staff members who have directed the production process. I also want to thank my secretary, Leah Christie, who diligently participated in the preparation and editing of almost every chapter in this book.

M.-M. M.

Contents

Contributors

DAVID BEAR, M.D.
Director of Telepsychiatry
Acadia Hospital
Professor of Psychiatry
University of Massachusetts
Worcester, Massachusetts, USA

ANTONIO DAMASIO, M.D., PH.D.
M.W. Van Allen Professor and Head
Department of Neurology
University of Iowa College of Medicine
Iowa City, Iowa, USA

HANNA DAMASIO, M.D.
Professor and Director
Human Neuroanatomy and Neuroimaging
   Laboratory
Department of Neurology
University of Iowa College of Medicine
Iowa City, Iowa, USA

HANS J. MARKOWITSCH
Professor
Abteilungssprecher
Facultät für Psychologie und
   Sportwissenschaft
Abteilung für Psychologie
Universität Bielefeld
Bielefeld, Germany

M.-MARSEL MESULAM, M.D.
(EDITOR)
Ruth and Evelyn Dunbar Professor of
   Neurology and Psychiatry
Director, Cognitive Neurology and
   Alzheimer's Disease Center
Northwestern University Medical School
Chicago, Illinois, USA

MARGARET G. O'CONNOR, PH.D.
Director of Neuropsychology
Behavioral Neurology Unit
Beth Israel Deaconess Medical Center
Assistant Professor of Neurology
Harvard Medical School
Boston, Massachusetts, USA

ROBERT POST, M.D.
Chief of Biological Psychiatry Branch
National Institute of Mental Health
Bethesda, Maryland, USA

MATTHEW RIZZO, M.D.
Professor, Department of Neurology
Division of Behavioral Neurology &
   Cognitive Neuroscience
University of Iowa College of Medicine
Iowa City, Iowa, USA

ELLIOTT D. ROSS, M.D.
Professor, Department of Neurology
University of Oklahoma Health Science
  Center
Director, Center for Alzheimer's and
  Neurodegenerative Disorders
Department of Veterans Affairs Medical
  Center
Oklahoma City, Oklahoma, USA

DONALD L. SCHOMER, M.D.
Chief, Division of Clinical
  Neurophysiology and the
  Comprehensive Epilepsy Program
Associate Professor of Neurology
Department of Neurology
Beth Israel Deaconess Medical Center
Boston, Massachusetts, USA

MARGITTA SEECK, M.D.
Department of Neurology
University Hospital of Geneva
Geneva, Switzerland

PAUL SPIERS, PH.D.
Visiting Scientist
Clinical Research Center
Massachusetts Institute of Technology
Boston, Massachusetts, USA

DANIEL TRANEL, PH.D.
Professor and Chief, Benton
  Neuropsychology Laboratory
Department of Neurology
Division of Behavioral Neurology &
  Cognitive Neuroscience
University of Iowa College of Medicine
Iowa City, Iowa, USA

SANDRA WEINTRAUB, PH.D.
Associate Professor and
Head of Neuropsychology, Northwestern
  University Medical School
Department of Psychiatry and Behavioral
  Sciences
Cognitive Neurology and Alzheimer's
  Disease Center
Northwestern University
Chicago, Illinois, USA

Principles of Behavioral
and Cognitive Neurology

1

Behavioral Neuroanatomy
Large-Scale Networks, Association Cortex, Frontal Syndromes, the Limbic System, and Hemispheric Specializations

M.-Marsel Mesulam

Faced with an anatomical fact proven beyond doubt, any physiological result that stands in contradiction to it loses all its meaning.... So, first anatomy and then physiology; but if first physiology, then not without anatomy.
—Bernhard von Gudden (1824–1886), quoted by Korbinian Brodmann, in Laurence Garey's translation

I. Introduction

The human brain displays marked regional variations in architecture, connectivity, neurochemistry, and physiology. This chapter explores the relevance of these regional variations to cognition and behavior. Some topics have been included mostly for the sake of completeness and continuity. Their coverage is brief, either because the available information is limited or because its relevance to behavior and cognition is tangential. Other subjects, such as the processing of visual information, are reviewed in extensive detail, both because a lot is known and also because the information helps to articulate general principles relevant to all other domains of behavior.

Experiments on laboratory primates will receive considerable emphasis, especially in those areas of cerebral connectivity and physiology where relevant information is not yet available in the human. Structural homologies across species are always incomplete, and many complex behaviors, particularly those that are of greatest interest to the clinician and cognitive neuroscientist, are either rudimentary or absent in other animals. Nonetheless, the reliance on animal data in this chapter is unlikely to be too misleading since the focus will be on principles rather than specifics and since principles of organization are likely to remain relatively stable across closely related species.

The nature of the relationship between brain structure and behavior is a central theme for all chapters in this book. Neuroscience texts tend to highlight the relatively invariant relationships between anatomy and function. Damage to the optic tract or striate cortex, for example, always leads to a contralateral homonymous hemianopia and a thoracic cord transection always leads to paraplegia and incontinence. The approach to cognition and comportment was initially based on the expectation that analogous relationships would be uncovered and that it would be possible to identify centers for "hearing words," "perceiving space," or "storing memories." These expectations need to be modified to accommodate modern observations which show that the structural foundations of cognitive and behavioral domains take the form of partially overlapping large-scale networks organized around reciprocally interconnected cortical epicenters.[329,334,339] The components of these networks can be divided into *critical* versus *participating* areas. Lesions which irreversibly impair performance in a cognitive domain help to identify network components that are *critical* for its integrity, whereas activations obtained by functional imaging when subjects are performing tasks related to the same domain also reveal the areas that *participate* in its coordination. The traditional approach based on the investigation of patients with focal brain disease can thus be integrated with functional imaging experiments in order to obtain a more complete picture of the relationships between brain structure and behavior.

At least five large-scale networks can be identified in the human brain: (*1*) a right hemisphere-dominant spatial attention network with epicenters in dorsal posterior parietal cortex, the frontal eye fields, and the cingulate gyrus; (*2*) a left hemisphere-dominant language network with epicenters in Wernicke's and Broca's areas; (*3*) a memory-emotion network with epicenters in the hippocampo–entorhinal regions and the amygdaloid complex; (*4*) an executive function–comportment network with epicenters in lateral prefrontal cortex, orbitofrontal cortex, and posterior parietal cortex; and (*5*) a face-and-object identification network with epicenters in lateral temporal and temporopolar cortices. The neuroanatomical building blocks and overall organizational principles of these networks are reviewed in this chapter. The purpose is to provide a broad perspective which can serve as a background for the more detailed discussions in Chapter 3 (spatial attention), Chapters 4, 8, and 9 (memory and emotion), Chapters 5 and 6 (language), and Chapter 7 (face and object recognition).

II. PARTS OF THE CEREBRAL CORTEX

The human cerebral cortex contains approximately 20 billion neurons spread over nearly 2000 square centimeters of surface area.[394,520] The study of the cerebral cortex can be quite challenging. There is no universal agreement on terminology, no distinct boundaries that demarcate one region from another, and, in most instances, no clear correspondence among lobar designations, traditional topographic landmarks, cytoarchitectonic boundaries, and behavioral specializations. Furthermore, one part of the brain can have more than one descriptive name, and cytoarchitectonic (striate cortex), functional (primary visual cortex), topographic (calcarine cortex), and eponymic (Brodmann's area [BA] 17) terms can be used interchangeably to designate the same area.

Cytoarchitectonic maps, such as the one by Brodmann,[56] show that the cerebral hemispheres can be subdivided into numerous regions based on *microscopically* identified variations in neuronal architecture. In contemporary usage, however, a statement such as "activation was seen in area 9" is based on a *topographically* identified match between the target region and the region labeled as area 9 on Brodmann's map. This usage can lead to potential inaccuracies since some brains have topographical landmarks which differ from those of the brain illustrated by Brodmann, and since there may be substantial interindividual differences in the distribution of cytoarchitectonic areas, even when sulcal and gyral landmarks are identical. For these reasons, a descriptive neuroanatomical designation such as the "middle temporal gyrus," based on an easily identifiable topographic landmark, may be potentially more accurate than a cytoarchitectonic designation such as "area 21," which requires microscopic examination for verification. Brodmann's map is also quite uninformative when it comes to the cytoarchitectonic parcellation of the cortex within the banks of the cortical sulci. This is a major problem since much of the cerebral cortex lies buried within sulcal banks. Although there are no immediate means for resolving these challenges, it is important to recognize their existence in order to avoid potentially misleading conclusions. Since the anatomical information in this chapter is highly condensed, the reader may want to consult more comprehensive texts by Brodmann[57] (now available in English translation), Duvernoy,[128] Mai,[309] and Nieuwenhuys and associates.[386]

The absence of clear anatomical boundaries has encouraged the development of numerous approaches to the subdivision of the cerebral cortex. The resultant maps can be divided into two groups: those based primarily on *structural* (architectonic) features and those based primarily on *functional* affiliations. Proponents of the first school have constructed a variety of cortical maps, ranging in complexity from the map of Exner,[137] which boasted hundreds of sharply delineated subdivisions, to the more modest and also more widely accepted ones of Brodmann,[56] the Vogts,[537] von Economo,[539] and Flechsig.[147] The second school is more difficult to identify since few of its proponents have produced systematic surveys of the entire brain. Members of this second school include theoreticians of brain function such as Campbell,[69] Broca,[55] Filimonoff,[145] Yakovlev,[565] and Sanides.[465] The thinking of this second school has led to the subdivision of the cerebral cortex into the five major functional subtypes which are reviewed below: *limbic, paralimbic, heteromodal association, unimodal association, and primary sensory–motor.*[335] The principal factual base for this parcellation is derived from anatomical, physiological, and behavioral experiments in macaque monkeys. The homologies to the human brain have been inferred from comparative cytoarchitectonics, electrophysiological recordings, functional imaging, and the behavioral effects of focal lesions (Figs. 1–1 through 1–7).

The Limbic Zone (Corticoid and Allocortical Formations)

The basal forebrain is usually considered a subcortical structure. However, some of its constituents can be included within the boundaries of the cerebral cortex because they are situated directly on the ventral and medial surfaces of the cerebral hemi-

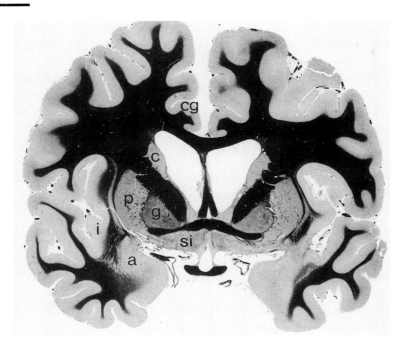

FIGURE 1–1. Coronal section through the basal forebrain of 25-year-old human brain stained for myelin. The substantia innominata (si) and the amygdaloid complex (a) are located on the surface of the brain. They represent "corticoid" components of the cerebral hemispheres. Other abbreviations: c=head of the caudate nucleus; cg=cingulate gyrus; g=globus pallidus; i=insula. Magnification ×1.6.

spheres. These basal forebrain structures include the septal region, the substantia innominata, the amygdaloid complex, and perhaps also the anterior olfactory nucleus (Fig. 1–1). Because of their simplified cytoarchitecture, these structures can be designated "corticoid," or cortex-like. In some corticoid areas such as the septal region and the substantia innominata, the organization of neurons is so rudimentary that no consistent lamination can be discerned and the orientation of dendrites is haphazard (Fig. 1–2a). All corticoid areas have architectonic features which are in part cortical and in part nuclear. This duality is particularly conspicuous in the amygdala (Fig. 1–3a).

The next stage of cortical organization carries the designation of "allocortex." This type of cortex contains one or two bands of neurons arranged into moderately well-differentiated layers (Figs. 1–2b, and 1–3b). The apical dendrites of the constituent neurons are well developed and display orderly patterns of orientation. There are two allocortical formations in the mammalian brain: (1) the hippocampal complex (that is, the dentate gyrus, the CA1–4 fields, and the subicular areas), which also carries the designation of "archicortex;" and (2) the piriform or primary olfactory cortex, which is also known as "paleocortex." The corticoid and allocortical formations collectively make up the limbic zone of the cerebral cortex.

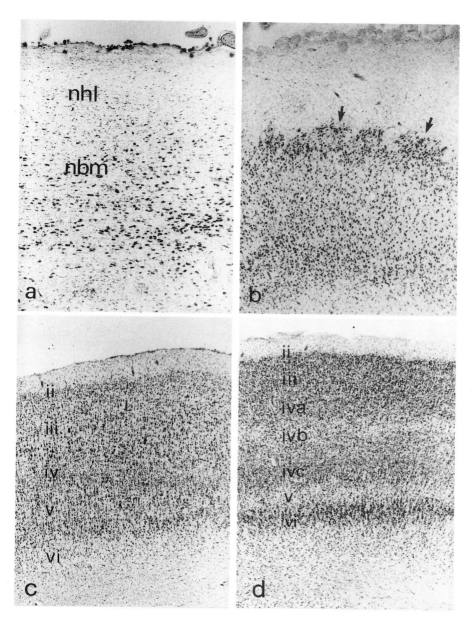

FIGURE 1–2. Four types of cortex in the human brain as shown with cresyl violet staining. In order to facilitate comparison, the pial surface is toward the top in all four photomicrographs. a. An example of corticoid cytoarchitecture. This is a photomicrograph of the substantia innominata showing the nucleus basalis of Meynert (nbm) and the more superficial horizontal limb nucleus of the diagonal band (nhl). The lamination is incomplete and there is no uniformity in the orientation of neurons. b. An example of allocortex from the subicular portion of the hippocampal formation. Two layers can be identified: an external pyramidal layer (arrows) and an internal pyramidal layer. Dendrites within each layer have a relatively uniform orientation. c. An example of homotypical isocortex from prefrontal heteromodal cortex. There are six distinct layers including two granular bands in layers ii and iv. d. An example of idiotypic cortex from the striate visual area. There are at least seven layers, many strongly granular. From corticoid to idiotypic cortex there is a gradual increase of cell density and laminar differentiation. Magnification ×10.

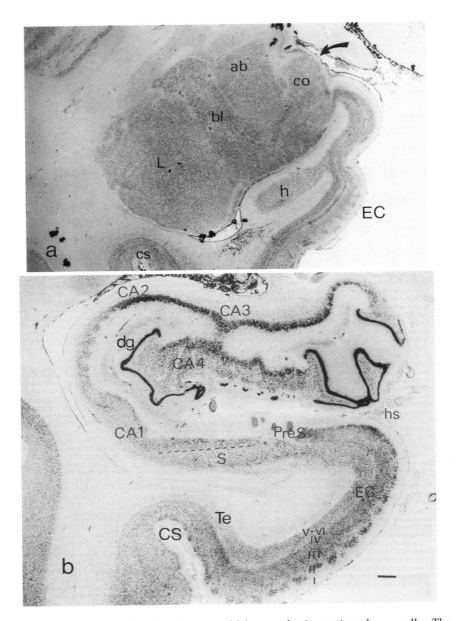

FIGURE 1–3. Amygdala in a 25-year-old human brain sectioned coronally. The cortical nucleus (co) extends to the surface of the brain (curved arrow). As in the case of other corticoid areas, the amygdala has a cytoarchitecture that is partly cortical partly nuclear. There is direct continuity with entorhinal cortex (EC). There is also direct continuity between EC and the hippocampus (h). Other abbreviations: ab=accessory basal nucleus of the amygdala; bl=basolateral nucleus of the amygdala; cs=collateral sulcus; L=lateral nucleus of the amygdala. Magnification ×6. b. Hippocampal complex in a 28-year-old human brain sectioned coronally. Through the CA1 and subiculum (S), the hippocampal complex merges into parahippocampal paralimbic areas such as the presubiculum (PreS), entorhinal cortex (EC), and transentorhinal (perirhinal) cortex (Te). The allocortical architecture of the CA1–4 and subicular sectors undergoes a gradual transition into the multilayered architecture of EC. In contrast to isocortical areas which contain a band of granular neurons in layer II, layer II of EC contains an agranular band of stellate cell islands. Other abbreviations: CS=collateral sulcus; dg=dentate gyrus; hs=hippocampal sulcus. The scale bar in the lower right represents 1 mm. Both a and b were stained with cresyl violet.

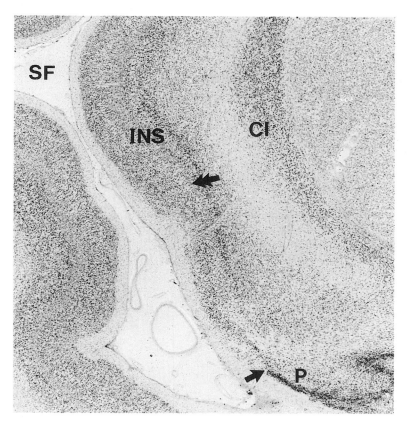

FIGURE 1–4. Insula of the rhesus monkey. The single arrowhead points to the direct continuity between piriform allocortex (P) and the insular paralimbic cortex. Adjacent to piriform allocortex, the insula has two or three agranular layers. More dorsally, a granular layer IV begins to appear (double arrowhead). There is further differentiation of insular cortex in the dorsal direction toward parietal isocortex. Abbreviations: Cl=claustrum; INS=insula; P=piriform cortex; SF=sylvian fissure. Magnification ×30.

The Paralimbic Zone (Mesocortex)

The next level of structural complexity is encountered in the paralimbic regions of the brain, also known as "mesocortex." These areas are intercalated between allocortex and isocortex so as to provide a gradual transition from one to the other. Allocortical cell layers often extend into paralimbic areas (Figs. 1–3b, and 1–4). The sectors of paralimbic areas which abut upon allocortex are also known as "periallocortical" or "juxtaallocortical" whereas the sectors which abut upon isocortex can be designated "proisocortical" or "periisocortical." The demarcations among these sectors are never sharp and always include zones of gradual transition. In most paralimbic areas, the transitional changes from periallocortex to periisocortex include:

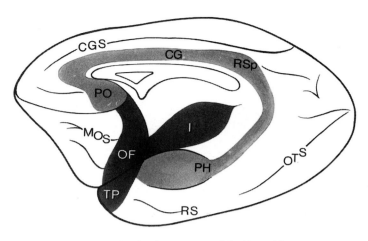

FIGURE 1–5. The belt of olfactocentric (black) and hippocampocentric (gray) paralimbic areas in the brain of the rhesus monkey. Abbreviations: CG=cingulate cortex; CGS=cingulate sulcus; I=insula; MOS=medial orbitofrontal sulcus; OF=posterior orbitofrontal cortex; OTS=occipitotemporal sulcus; PH=parahippocampal region; PO=parolfactory area; RS=rhinal sulcus; RSp=retrosplenial area; TP=temporopolar cortex.

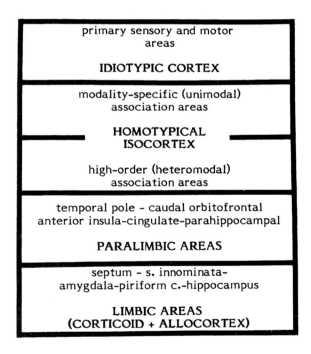

FIGURE 1–6. Cortical zones of the human brain.

1. Progressively greater accumulation of small granular neurons (star pyramids) first in layer IV and then in layer II
2. Sublamination and columnarization of layer III
3. Differentiation of layer V from layer VI and of layer VI from the underlying white matter,
4. An increase of intracortical myelin, especially along the outer layer of Baillarger (layer IV).

In general, the emergence of relatively well-differentiated granular cell bands in layers IV and II, the sublamination of layer III, and the differentiation of layer V from layer VI mark the end of the paralimbic zone and the onset of six-layered homotypical isocortex.

There are five major paralimbic formations in the human brain: (*1*) the orbitofrontal cortex (posterior parts of Brodmann's area [BA]11–12 and all of BA13); (*2*) the insula (BA14–16); (*3*) the temporal pole (BA38); (*4*) the parahippocampal cortices (including the presubiculum and parasubiculum, the entorhinal area, the prorhinal area, and the perirhinal (transentorhinal) area, corresponding to BA27–28 and 35); and (*5*) the cingulate complex (including the retrosplenial, ventral cingulate, and parolfactory areas, corresponding at least in part to BA23–26, 29–33).

These five paralimbic regions form an uninterrupted girdle surrounding the medial and basal aspects of the cerebral hemispheres. The paralimbic belt can be divided into two major groups: the olfactocentric and the hippocampocentric (Fig. 1–5). The olfactory piriform cortex provides the allocortical nidus for the orbitofrontal, insular, and temporopolar paralimbic areas (Fig. 1–4), whereas the hippocampus and its supracallosal rudiment (known as the induseum griseum) provide the allocortical nidus for the cingulate and parahippocampal components of the paralimbic brain (Fig. 1–3b).[343] The olfactocentric and hippocampocentric sectors of the paralimbic belt merge into each other within the orbitofrontal and anterior parahippocampal cortices.[369]

Homotypical Association Isocortex (the Heteromodal and Unimodal Zones)

By far the greatest area of the cerebral cortex in the human brain is devoted to six-layered homotypical isocortex (or neocortex), also known as "association isocortex" (Fig. 1–2c). Association isocortex can be subdivided into two major zones: modality-specific (unimodal) and high-order (heteromodal) (Fig. 1–6). Unimodal sensory association areas are further divided into "upstream" and "downstream" components: Upstream areas are only one synapse away from the relevant primary sensory area whereas downstream areas are at a distance of two or more synapses from the corresponding primary area. Unimodal sensory association isocortex is defined by three essential characteristics:

1. The constituent neurons respond predominantly, if not exclusively, to stimulation in only a single sensory modality.

2. The predominant sensory information comes from the primary sensory cortex and other unimodal regions of that same modality.
3. Lesions yield deficits only in tasks guided by that modality.

Unimodal visual association cortex can be divided into an upstream peristriate component which includes areas BA18–19, and a downstream temporal component which includes inferotemporal cortex (BA21–20) in the monkey and the fusiform, inferior temporal and probably parts of the middle temporal gyri in the human.[339] Unimodal auditory association cortex covers the superior temporal gyrus (BA22) and perhaps also parts of the middle temporal gyrus (BA21) in the human.[98] The connectivity of the monkey brain would suggest that the posterior part of the superior temporal cortex (BA22) displays the properties of upstream auditory association cortex whereas the more anterior part of this gyrus and the dorsal banks of the superior temporal sulcus may fit the designation of downstream auditory association cortex.[398]

In the monkey brain, BA5 in the superior parietal lobule represents an upstream component of somatosensory unimodal association cortex whereas parts of BA7b in the inferior parietal lobule and the posterior insula may represent its downstream components.[343,398] In the human, unimodal somatosensory association cortex may include parts of BA5 and BA7 in the superior parietal lobule and perhaps parts of BA40 in the anterior parts of the inferior parietal lobule (Fig. 1–7). The subdivision of unimodal auditory and somatosensory association cortices into upstream and downstream areas in the human remains to be elucidated. Unimodal association areas for olfaction, taste, and vestibular sensation have not been fully characterized. Premotor regions (anterior BA6 and posterior BA8) fulfill the role of motor "association" areas because they provide the principal cortical input into primary motor cortex.

The heteromodal component of association isocortex is identified by the following characteristics:

1. Neuronal responses are not confined to any single sensory modality.
2. The predominant sensory inputs come from unimodal areas in multiple modalities and from other heteromodal areas.
3. Deficits resulting from lesions in these areas are always multimodal, and never confined to tasks under the guidance of a single modality.

Some neurons in heteromodal association areas respond to stimulation in more than one modality, indicating the presence of direct multimodal convergence.[34,46] More commonly, however, there is an admixture of neurons with different preferred modalities.[232,237] Many neurons have sensory as well as motor contingencies.[233,374] Others change firing in ways that are responsive to motivational relevance.[305] Defined in this fashion, heteromodal cortex includes the types of regions which have been designated as high order association cortex, polymodal cortex, multimodal cortex, polysensory areas, and supramodal cortex.[350] The monkey brain contains heteromodal areas in prefrontal cortex (BA9, 10, 45, 46, anterior BA8, an-

1. Progressively greater accumulation of small granular neurons (star pyramids) first in layer IV and then in layer II
2. Sublamination and columnarization of layer III
3. Differentiation of layer V from layer VI and of layer VI from the underlying white matter,
4. An increase of intracortical myelin, especially along the outer layer of Baillarger (layer IV).

In general, the emergence of relatively well-differentiated granular cell bands in layers IV and II, the sublamination of layer III, and the differentiation of layer V from layer VI mark the end of the paralimbic zone and the onset of six-layered homotypical isocortex.

There are five major paralimbic formations in the human brain: (*1*) the orbitofrontal cortex (posterior parts of Brodmann's area [BA]11–12 and all of BA13); (*2*) the insula (BA14–16); (*3*) the temporal pole (BA38); (*4*) the parahippocampal cortices (including the presubiculum and parasubiculum, the entorhinal area, the prorhinal area, and the perirhinal (transentorhinal) area, corresponding to BA27–28 and 35); and (*5*) the cingulate complex (including the retrosplenial, ventral cingulate, and parolfactory areas, corresponding at least in part to BA23–26, 29–33).

These five paralimbic regions form an uninterrupted girdle surrounding the medial and basal aspects of the cerebral hemispheres. The paralimbic belt can be divided into two major groups: the olfactocentric and the hippocampocentric (Fig. 1–5). The olfactory piriform cortex provides the allocortical nidus for the orbitofrontal, insular, and temporopolar paralimbic areas (Fig. 1–4), whereas the hippocampus and its supracallosal rudiment (known as the induseum griseum) provide the allocortical nidus for the cingulate and parahippocampal components of the paralimbic brain (Fig. 1–3b).[343] The olfactocentric and hippocampocentric sectors of the paralimbic belt merge into each other within the orbitofrontal and anterior parahippocampal cortices.[369]

Homotypical Association Isocortex (the Heteromodal and Unimodal Zones)

By far the greatest area of the cerebral cortex in the human brain is devoted to six-layered homotypical isocortex (or neocortex), also known as "association isocortex" (Fig. 1–2c). Association isocortex can be subdivided into two major zones: modality-specific (unimodal) and high-order (heteromodal) (Fig. 1–6). Unimodal sensory association areas are further divided into "upstream" and "downstream" components: Upstream areas are only one synapse away from the relevant primary sensory area whereas downstream areas are at a distance of two or more synapses from the corresponding primary area. Unimodal sensory association isocortex is defined by three essential characteristics:

1. The constituent neurons respond predominantly, if not exclusively, to stimulation in only a single sensory modality.

terior BA11–12), the inferior parietal lobule (parts of BA7), lateral temporal cortex within the banks of the superior temporal sulcus (junction of BA22 with BA21), and the parahippocampal region.[398] In the human brain the analogous zones of heteromodal cortex are located in prefrontal cortex (BA9–10, 45–47, anterior 11–12, anterior 8), posterior parietal cortex (posterior BA7, BA39–40), lateral temporal cortex (including parts of BA37 and BA21 in the middle temporal gyrus), and portions of the parahippocampal gyrus (parts of BA36–37).

Unimodal and heteromodal areas are characterized by a six-layered homotypical architecture. There are some relatively subtle architectonic differences between unimodal and heteromodal areas. In general, the unimodal areas have a more differentiated organization, especially with respect to sublamination in layers III and V, columnarization in layer III, and more extensive granularization in layer IV and layer II. On these architectonic grounds, it would appear that heteromodal cortex is closer in structure to paralimbic cortex and that it provides a stage of cytoarchitectonic differentiation intercalated between paralimbic and unimodal areas.

Idiotypic Cortex (the Primary Sensory-Motor Zones)

Primary visual, auditory, somatosensory, and motor cortices are easily delineated on cytoarchitectonic and functional grounds. Primary visual cortex (also known as V1, striate cortex, calcarine cortex or BA17) covers the banks of the calcarine fissure; primary auditory cortex (also known as A1, or BA41–42) covers Heschl's gyrus on the floor of the Sylvian cistern; primary somatosensory cortex (also known as S1, usually meant to include BA3a, 3b, 1, and 2) is located in the postcentral gyrus; and primary motor cortex (also known as M1) includes BA4 and probably also a posterior rim of BA6 in the precentral gyrus.

There are two divergent opinions about these primary areas. One is to consider them as the most elementary (even rudimentary) component of the cerebral cortex; the other is to consider them as its most advanced and highly differentiated component.[465] The latter point of view can be supported from the vantage point of cytoarchitectonics. Thus, the primary visual, somatosensory, and auditory cortices display a "koniocortical" architecture representing the highest level of development with respect to granularization and lamination (Fig. 1–2d), whereas primary motor cortex displays a unique "macropyramidal" architecture characterized by highly specialized giant pyramidal neurons known as Betz cells.

The visual, auditory, and somatosensory systems provide the major channels of communication with the extrapersonal world. The information transmitted by these channels plays a critical role in shaping all aspects of cognition and comportment. The primary and unimodal areas related to these modalities are cytoarchitectonically highly differentiated and quite large. The vestibular, gustatory, and olfactory sensations do not have the same type of prominence in the primate brain. The corresponding primary areas are cytoarchitectonically less differentiated, smaller, and closer to limbic structures. Primary gustatory cortex is located at the in BA43; the primary vestibular area lies within the posterior Sylvian fissure, where the temporal lobe joins the insula and parietal lobe; and the primary olfactory cortex is a core limbic region located at the confluence of the insular, orbitofrontal, and temporopolar areas.[195,341,407]

III. CORTICAL ORGANIZATION, CONNECTIVITY, AND TRANSMODAL AREAS

As shown above, the cerebral hemispheres can be subdivided into five essential types of cortex which collectively display a spectrum of cytoarchitectonic differentiation ranging from the simplest to the most complex (Fig. 1–6). The corticoid and allocortical areas, collectively designated core "limbic" structures, are extensively interconnected with the hypothalamus. Through neural and also humoral mechanisms, the hypothalamus is in a position to control electrolyte balance, glucose levels, basal temperature, metabolic rate, autonomic tone, hormonal state, sexual phase, circadian oscillations, and immunoregulation, and to modulate the experience and expression of hunger, aggression, fear, flight, thirst, and libido.[42,58,365,463,515,559] In keeping with these functions of the hypothalamus, the cortical areas of the limbic zone assume pivotal roles in the regulation of memory, emotion, motivation, hormonal balance, and autonomic function. These specializations of limbic structures are related to the upkeep of the internal milieu (homeostasis) and the associated operations necessary for the preservation of the self and the species.

The opposite pole of Figure 1–6 is occupied by the architectonically highly differentiated and functionally highly specialized primary sensory and motor areas. These parts of the cerebral cortex are most closely related to the extrapersonal space: Primary sensory cortex provides an obligatory portal for the entry of information from the environment into cortical circuitry, and primary motor cortex provides a final common pathway for coordinating the motor acts which allow us to manipulate the environment and alter our position within it. Unimodal, heteromodal, and paralimbic cortices are intercalated between the two poles of Figure 6. They provide neural bridges that mediate between the internal and the external worlds so that the needs of the internal milieu are discharged according to the opportunities and restrictions that prevail in the extrapersonal environment. These three intercalated zones enable the associative elaboration of sensory information, its linkage to motor strategies, and the integration of experience with drive, emotion, and autonomic states. Two of these zones, the unimodal and heteromodal, are most closely involved in perceptual elaboration and motor planning whereas the paralimbic zone plays a critical role in channeling emotion and motivation to behaviorally relevant motor acts, mental content, and extrapersonal events.

Connectivity of the Cerebral Cortex

Components of each zone in Figure 1–6 have *extramural* connections with components of other functional zones and *intramural* connections within the same zone. Experimental evidence, gathered mostly in the brain of the monkey, shows that the most intense extramural connectivity of an individual cortical area occurs with com-

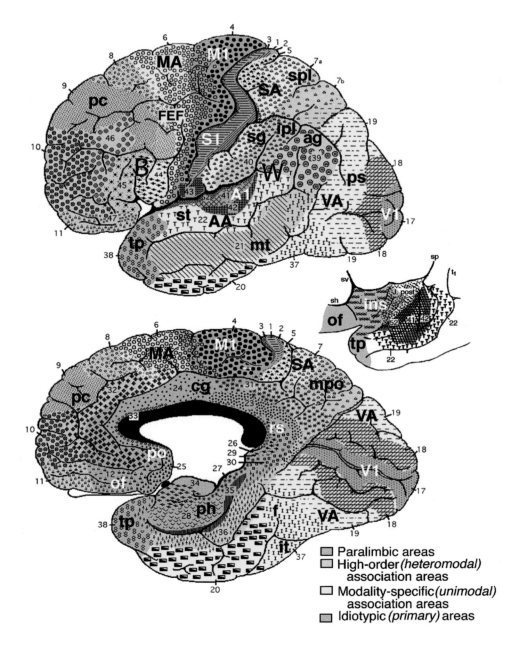

FIGURE 1–7. Distribution of functional zones in relationship to Brodmann's map of the human brain. The boundaries are not intended to be precise. Much of this information is based on experimental evidence obtained from laboratory animals and needs to be confirmed in the human brain. Abbreviations: AA = auditory association cortex; ag = angular gyrus; A1 = primary auditory cortex; B = Broca's area; cg = cingulate cortex; f = fusiform gyrus; FEF = frontal eye fields; ins = insula; ipl = inferior parietal lobule; it = inferior temporal gyrus; MA = motor association cortex; mpo = medial parietooccipital area; mt = middle temporal gyrus; M1 = primary motor area; of = orbitofrontal region; pc = prefrontal cortex; ph = parahippocampal region; po = parolfactory area; ps = peristriate cortex; rs = retrosplenial area; SA = somatosensory association cortex; sg = supramarginal gyrus; spl = superior parietal lobule; st = superior temporal gyrus; S1 = primary somatosensory area; tp = temporopolar cortex; VA = visual association cortex; V1 = primary visual cortex; W = Wernicke's area.

ponents of the two immediately adjacent functional zones in Figure 1–6. For example, although all types of cortical areas, including association isocortex, receive direct hypothalamic projections,[344] such connections reach their highest intensity within components of the limbic zone. The constituents of this zone, the septal area, the nucleus basalis of the substantia innominata, the amygdaloid complex, piriform cortex, and the hippocampus, are the parts of the cerebral cortex which have the most intense reciprocal connections with the hypothalamus.[11,342,562] In keeping with the organization shown in Figure 1–6, the second major source of extramural connections for limbic structures originates in the paralimbic zone. Thus, the amygdala receives one of its most extensive extramural cortical inputs from the insula; the hippocampus from the entorhinal sector of the parahippocampal region; and the piriform cortex as well as the nucleus basalis from the group of olfactocentric paralimbic areas.[342,343,533]

An analogous analysis can be extended to the other zones in Figure 1–6. Paralimbic areas, for example, have the most extensive extramural connections with limbic and heteromodal areas. This has been demonstrated experimentally in the case of the anterior insula, the parahippocampal formation, the temporal pole, the cingulate complex, and posterior orbitofrontal cortex.[343,367,369,397,533,534] Furthermore, the most extensive extramural interconnections of heteromodal areas are with components of the paralimbic zone, on one hand, and with those of the unimodal zone, on the other.[23,24,249,350,395,398] Finally, the major extramural connections of unimodal areas occur with primary areas, on one hand, and heteromodal areas, on the other, while primary areas derive their major inputs from unimodal areas and the external world.[249,395] Although some connections jump across the levels shown in Figure 1–6, they are not as prominent as those that link two immediately adjacent levels. Thus, the amygdala is known to have monosynaptic connections with unimodal association isocortex and even primary visual cortex, but these are not nearly as substantial as its connections with the hypothalamus and paralimbic regions.[3] The position of a cortical area in Figure 1–6 thus helps to specify its most salient connections with other cortical areas.

Within the context of this general plan of organization, Figure 1–8 summarizes the sensory–fugal pathways which sequentially convey sensory information from primary sensory to unimodal, heteromodal, paralimbic, limbic, and hypothalamic areas of the monkey brain.[3,343,367,369,397,398,530] This pattern of connectivity displays a polarization which fits the basic plan shown in Figure 1–6. The pathways in Figure 1–8 are based on the organization of visual and auditory pathways, two modalities that play a crucial role in shaping cognition and comportment. Although somatosensory pathways follow many of the same principles of organization, they also display unique properties such as the existence of monosynaptic connections between primary sensory and primary motor areas. Olfactory and gustatory pathways have a different plan of organization, reflecting their closer relationship to the internal rather than the external milieu.

Many cortical areas also have intramural cortical connections with other components of the same functional zone. These are extremely well developed within the limbic, paralimbic, and heteromodal zones. Of all the nonfrontal cortical neu-

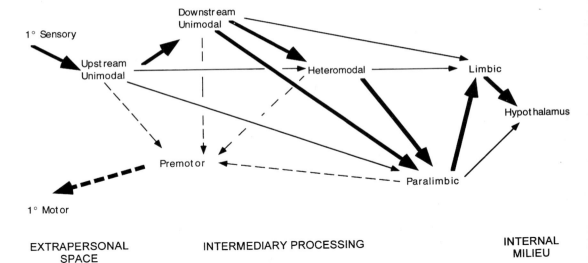

FIGURE 1–8. The straight arrows illustrate monosynaptic sensory–fugal neural connections in the visual and auditory modalities. Thick arrows represent more massive connections than thin arrows. The broken arrows illustrate motor output pathways.[339]

rons which projected to a subsector of prefrontal heteromodal cortex, for example, 37% were located within unimodal areas, 18% in paralimbic regions, and 44% in other heteromodal cortices.[23] Paralimbic formations such as the insula, posterior orbitofrontal cortex, the temporal pole, entorhinal cortex and cingulate cortex also have very prominent interconnections with each other.[343,367,369,397] In contrast, the intramural connections of primary sensory–motor and upstream unimodal sensory association areas have a particularly restricted distribution. Upstream unimodal association areas in different modalities, for example, have no interconnections with each other. Except for the connection from primary somatosensory to primary motor cortex, there are also no neural projections interconnecting primary areas in different modalities. It appears, therefore, that there is a premium on channel width within the limbic, paralimbic, and heteromodal regions of the cerebral cortex whereas the emphasis is on fidelity within the upstream unimodal and primary sensory–motor areas.

Intermediary Processing and Transmodal Areas

A fundamental characteristic of the primate brain is the insertion of obligatory synaptic relays between stimulus and response, and also between the representation of the internal milieu (at the level of the hypothalamus) and that of the external world (at the level of primary sensory–motor cortex). These intercalated synaptic relays collectively provide the substrates for "intermediary" or "integrative" processing (Fig. 1–8). The psychological outcomes of intermediary processing are known as "cognition," "consciousness," and "comportment" and include the diverse manifestations of memory, emotion, attention, language, planning, judgment, insight, and thought. Intermediary processing has a dual purpose. First, it protects channels of sensory input and motor output from the motivationally-driven influence of the internal milieu. Secondly, it enables identical stimuli to trigger different responses depending on situational context, past experience, present needs, and contemplated consequences. The neurons that support intermediary processing are located within the unimodal, heteromodal, paralimbic, and limbic zones of the cerebral cortex.

The synaptic architecture of intermediary processing shapes the nature of cognition and comportment.[339] In species with simpler brains, intermediary processing is shallow and does not allow much of a distinction to be made between appearance and significance.[339] The automatic linkage between stimulus and response in such species leads to the many manifestations of instinctual behaviors. A turkey hen with a newly hatched brood, for example, will treat every moving object within the nest as an enemy unless it utters the specific peep of its chicks.[471] If a hen is experimentally made deaf, it will invariably kill all its own newly hatched progeny. Furthermore, male sticklebacks (which are red on the ventral side) will automatically attack any stimulus with a "red below" pattern as if it were a rival.[300] In these behaviors, the physical dimensions of a stimulus trigger preprogrammed behavioral sequences which are relatively impervious to contextual peculiarities. A major role of intermediary processing is to transcend such rigid stimulus–response linkages and to enable behavior to be guided by contextual significance rather than appearance.

Unimodal areas contain the initial synaptic relays for intermediary processing. These areas are extremely well developed in the human brain. The absence of interconnections linking a unimodal area in one sensory modality with another in a different modality protects the sensory fidelity of experience and delays cross-modal contamination until further encoding has been accomplished. Unimodal areas are thus in a position to register the most accurate representation of sensory experience. These areas can encode the perceptual characteristics of specific sensory events, determine if the sensory features of complex entities such as words or faces are identical or not, and even store all the necessary information in stable memory traces. However, in the absence of access to information in other modalities, unimodal areas do not have the ability to lead from word to meaning, from physiognomy to facial recognition, or from isolated sensory events to coherent experiences. Such integration of sensation into cognition necessitates the participation of "transmodal" areas.[339]

The defining feature of a transmodal area is the ability to support cross-modal integration and, thus, the lack of specificity for any single modality of sensory processing. All components of heteromodal, paralimbic, and limbic zones are therefore also transmodal. A precise localization of transmodal areas became possible through the tracing of corticocortical connections in the monkey brain. The basic organization of these connections was first described in two classic papers, one by Pandya and Kuypers[395] and the other by Jones and Powell.[249] These papers revealed the existence of a hierarchically organized set of pathways for linking sensory cortices to primary, secondary, and sometimes even tertiary modality-specific association areas which, in turn, sent convergent projections to heteromodal sensory association zones.

The field of neuroscience had been primed to anticipate such a sequential organization through the work of Hubel and Wiesel, who had demonstrated a hierarchy of simple, complex, and hypercomplex neurons in primary visual cortex, each successive level encoding a more composite aspect of visual information.[230] The discoveries of Pandya and Kuypers and Jones and Powell seemed to be extending this serial and convergent organization from the realms of sensation to those of cognition. A great deal of emphasis was placed on the pivotal role of multimodal convergence in all aspects of mental function, including the storage of memories, the formation of concepts, and the acquisition of language.[169,249,331,395,396,533]

While the importance of serial processing and multimodal convergence to cognitive function was widely accepted, some potentially serious computational limitations of such an arrangement were also acknowledged.[178,334,456] Two of these objections are particularly relevant: (1) If knowledge of α is to be encoded in convergent form by a small number of neurons, the brain would have to resolve the cumbersome problem of conveying α-related information in all relevant modalities to the one highly specific address where this convergent synthesis is located. (2) The modality-specific attributes of α would succumb to cross-modal contamination during the process of convergence and the sensory fidelity of the experience would be lost. This second circumstance can be likened to the mixing of yellow and blue to obtain green, a process which precludes the subsequent extraction of the original hues from the resultant mixture.

The surfacing of these concerns coincided with the development of newer and more powerful neuroanatomical methods based on the intra-axonal transport of horseradish peroxidase and tritiated amino acids. Experiments based on these methods started to show that the sensory–fugal flow of information was more complicated than previously surmised: there was a central thread of serial processing from one synaptic level to another but there were also multiple parallel pathways, feedforward and feedback connections, and multiple sites for divergence and convergence. The synaptic templates based on this type of connectivity appeared to have much greater computational power. The objections to the convergent encoding of knowledge, for example, could be addressed by assuming that the principal role of transmodal areas is to create directories (or addresses, maps, look-up tables) for binding (rather than mixing) modality-specific fragments of information into coherent experiences, memories, and thoughts. This alternative process can be likened to obtaining green by superimposing a blue and a yellow lens which can then be separated from each other to yield back the original uncontaminated colors. Transmodal areas appeared to fulfill two functions: (1) the establishment of limited cross-modal associations related to the target event and (2) the formation of a directory pointing to the distributed components of the related information.[339] Transmodal areas could thus enable the binding of modality-specific information into multimodal representations that protect the fidelity of the initial encoding.

Transmodal areas are not centers for storing convergent knowledge but rather critical gateways for integrating and accessing the relevant distributed information.[336,339] They also provide "neural bottlenecks" in the sense that they constitute regions of maximum vulnerability for lesion-induced deficits in the pertinent cognitive domain. All transmodal areas receive similar sets of sensory information and mediate analogous neural computations. However, each transmodal area displays a distinctive profile of behavioral specializations which is determined by its overall pattern of neural connections and physiological characteristics. This chapter will review several illustrative examples of this organization, including the pivotal role of midtemporal cortex for face and object recognition, Wernicke's area for lexical labeling, the hippocampo–entorhinal complex for explicit memory, prefrontal cortex for working memory, the amygdala for emotion, and dorsal parietal cortex for spatial attention.

IV. FUNCTIONS OF INDIVIDUAL CORTICAL ZONES: PRIMARY SENSORY AND MOTOR AREAS

Primary Visual Cortex

Primary visual cortex (V1, BA17 in Fig. 1–7) covers the occipital pole and the banks of the calcarine fissure. This region is also known as striate cortex because of the conspicuous myelinated stripe of Gennari (or of Vicq d'Azyr) which is easily detected in layer IV even by the naked eye inspection of unstained specimens. Retinal input is relayed to striate cortex through the lateral geniculate nucleus. The importance of visual input to striate cortex is shown by the fact that fully 70% of all its neural input comes from the lateral geniculate nucleus.[124] The entire visual field is mapped onto striate cortex with great spatial precision. The striate cortex in each hemisphere receives input from the contralateral visual field. Dorsal parts of striate cortex contain a representation of the lower visual field while the ventral parts represent the upper visual field. The central (macular, foveal) part of the visual field is mapped onto the most posterior part of striate cortex and has the greatest magnification factor. More anterior parts of V1 along the calcarine fissure contain representations of progressively more peripheral parts of the visual field. Except for the representation of the vertical meridian, striate cortex in the monkey does not have callosal interhemispheric connections.[260]

The physiological exploration of neurons in primary visual cortex (V1) has led to one of the most exciting chapters in neuroscience. These neurons have an exquisite organization of connectivity which leads to the orderly encoding of information about the orientation, movement, binocular disparity, color, length, spatial frequency, and luminance of objects. Individual neurons preferentially sensitive to different aspects of visual information display a relative segregation into a multi-dimensional mosaic of columns, layers, and cytochemically differentiated patches.[298] In the rhesus monkey, extensive (but almost certainly incomplete) bilateral removals of striate cortex lead to a loss of fine visual discrimination of stationary objects. However, visuospatial orientation and the ability to reach toward moving peripheral targets may remain relatively intact.[114]

In humans, partial destruction of geniculostriate pathways leads to characteristic visual field deficits within which conscious form perception of still objects is lost. Some ability for reaching towards visual stimuli in the blind field may be retained even though the patient may deny awareness of the stimulus.[408,549] This residual capacity, known as "blindsight," may be subserved by retinocollicular projections which are subsequently relayed to the pulvinar nucleus of the thalamus and ultimately to visual association and parietal areas.[462] It appears that the retinogeniculocalcarine pathway is necessary for conscious visual experience whereas the parallel retinocolliculothalamic pathway may be sufficient to support visual reaching, even when the targets are not consciously perceived (also see Chapter 7).

Primary Auditory Cortex

The primary auditory koniocortex (BA41 and 42), also known as A1, is located on Heschl's gyrus within the posterior aspect of the superior temporal plane (Fig. 1–7). This area receives inputs from the part of the medial geniculate body which functions as the thalamic relay nucleus in the auditory modality. There is a tonotopic organization in A1 so that the low frequencies are represented more anteriorly than the higher frequencies.[328] In addition to A1, the superior temporal plane of the monkey also contains a second tonotopically organized area, R, which also receives input from the medial geniculate nucleus.[433] Both of these areas can be activated by pure tones.

Single unit recordings in monkeys show that A1 units are sensitive to the location of sound sources.[38] For example, some A1 units are much more active when the animal is required to identify the location of a sound source than when the task is merely the detection of the sound. Neurons in the A1 region of each hemisphere are likely to give a brisker response to sounds originating in the contralateral extrapersonal space. Furthermore, bilateral ablations of A1 (usually extending into adjacent association cortex) lead to deficits in a task that requires the monkey to walk toward the source of a sound.[213] However, the spatial map in A1 is not nearly as specific as the map in V1.

Primary auditory cortex does not display the type of strictly contralateral representation characteristic of primary visual and somatosensory cortices. Through multisynaptic pathways which have extensive decussations in the brainstem, the A1 of each hemisphere has access to information from both ears even though the influence of the contralateral ear appears to be stronger. Therefore, unilateral A1 lesions do not lead to contralateral deafness. In fact, such lesions would probably remain undetectable without the assistance of auditory evoked potentials or dichotic listening tasks. In the latter test, the simultaneous delivery of stimuli to both ears yields excessive suppression of the input into the ear contralateral to the A1 lesion. In contrast to the primary visual and somatosensory thalamic relay nuclei, which have no substantial connections with the pertinent unimodal association areas, the medial geniculate body has major projections not only to A1 but also to the unimodal auditory association areas in the adjacent superior temporal gyrus.[347]

Therefore, complete cortical deafness is unlikely to arise unless there is bilateral damage both to A1 and also to the adjacent auditory association areas.

Primary Somatosensory Cortex

The postcentral gyrus contains the primary somatosensory cortex, S1 (Fig. 1–7). This area is the major recipient of projections from the lateral, medial, and superior sectors of the ventroposterior lateral thalamic nucleus, which is the principal thalamic relay for the ascending somatosensory pathways. Some investigators have convincingly argued that only BA3b should be included in S1 since BA1 and especially BA2 have characteristics more consistent with those of upstream unimodal somatosensory association cortex.[256] The designation "S1" in the literature, however, usually refers collectively to BA3a, 3b, 1 and 2, a usage that will be followed here. The contralateral half of the body surface is somatotopically mapped onto S1 in each hemisphere. The mouth and face areas are represented most ventrally; the hand, arm, trunk, and thigh more dorsally, and the leg and foot medially.[406,445]

In the monkey brain, single unit recordings show that BA3a is preferentially activated by muscle spindle afferents; BA3b and 1 by cutaneous input, and BA2 by joint receptors. In the monkey, BA2 lesions impair size and curvature discrimination, BA1 lesions impair texture discrimination, and both types of deficits arise after BA3b lesions.[73,427] Neurons in S1 are particularly responsive to *active* tactile exploration. Thus, in one study tactile stimulation of the finger led to the activation of 13 of 76 S1 neurons only when the monkey's finger was moving but not when it was at rest.[107] In humans, S1 damage (usually encroaching on BA3, 1 and 2) tends to be associated with a selective impairment of the so-called "cortical" sensations such as two-point discrimination, touch localization, graphesthesia, position sense, and stereognosis, whereas touch, pain, and temperature detection may remain relatively preserved (Fig. 1–9A).[95,444]

Primary Motor Cortex

The primary motor cortex (M1) is located in front of the central sulcus (Fig. 1–7). The M1 contains a body representation which closely parallels that of S1.[406] The M1 region can be identified on the basis of three characteristics:

1. The cytoarchitecture is dominated by the presence of large pyramidal neurons which reach their greatest size in BA4 (Betz cells).
2. The threshold for eliciting movement upon stimulation is lower in M1 than in any other cortical area.
3. The M1 region contains the greatest density of neurons giving rise to corticospinal and corticobulbar fibers.

The literature is not always clear about the distinction between M1 and premotor cortex. Some have argued that only BA4 (the Betz cell zone) deserves to be included

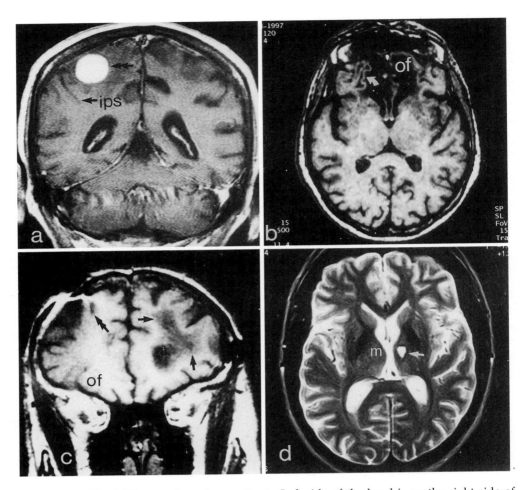

FIGURE 1–9. The MRI scans from four patients. Left side of the head is on the right side of each scan. a. A 91-year-old woman with an anaplastic neoplasm confined to the postcentral gyrus of the right hemisphere (double arrows), probably involving mostly BA2. Touch and temperature sensations were preserved but two-point discrimination and graphesthesia were impaired in the upper left extremity. In keeping with the sparing of more posterior parts of parietal cortex, reaching, grasping, and manual exploration were intact. b. A 63-year-old woman after the removal of an olfactory groove meningioma. There is almost no brain tissue left in the region that should have contained orbitofrontal cortex (of). The remaining orbitofrontal cortex is reduced to a sclerotic ribbon (curved arrow). The dorsolateral prefrontal cortex was completely spared. The patient displayed severe disinhibition and other comportmental abnormalities despite relatively intact cognitive functions. c. A 47-year-old man after the removal of a left prefrontal glioma. The area of encephalomalacia in the left dorsolateral prefrontal cortex is shown by the single arrows. A shunt was introduced through the right dorsolateral prefrontal cortex and caused tissue injury (double arrow). The additional signal void on that side is probably an artifact due to the shunt. Orbitofrontal cortex (of) was spared. The patient displayed the abulic type of frontal lobe syndrome as well as attentional deficits. d. A 41-year-old man suffered an acute stroke which involved the mediodorsal nucleus (m) of the thalamus on the left (arrow). He displayed a clinical picture which contained elements of amnesia and a frontal lobe syndrome.

in M1, others that M1 should include not only BA4 but also the posterior half of BA6.[543,560] Many neurons in M1 fire in conjunction with reaching movements. Single cells display a coarse directional tuning but populations of neurons can encode vectors pointing in the direction of the upcoming reaching movement.[167] Experiments in monkeys show that the M1 output is especially important in controlling the early recruited portion of the motoneuron pool involved in precise fine movements.[136] In keeping with these physiological characteristics, extensive M1 removals in monkeys lead to relatively subtle deficits, mostly confined to individual finger movements, while other movements and especially posture and gait remain relatively intact.[277]

The clinical consequences of lesions confined to M1 in humans are poorly understood. Some would argue that such lesions may only impair fractionated distal limb movements while leaving muscle tone and strength of proximal muscles intact. Others argue that M1 lesions lead to increased tendon reflexes and to widespread paralysis of entire limbs.[284] Experiments based on transcranial magnetic stimulation suggest that the human M1 plays a greater role in the performance of complex than simple finger movements.[168] "Idiomotor apraxia" refers to an inability to convert verbal commands into skilled movements which require the fractionated control of distal limb musculature (Chapter 2). This type of apraxia may result from lesions which interrupt the multisynaptic pathways leading from posterior association areas to M1 via intermediary relays in premotor and supplementary motor areas. The execution of commands aimed at the axial musculature may remain preserved in these patients since such movements may not depend on the integrity of pyramidal pathways.[169] As in S1, the hand and foot representations of M1 have no callosal connectivity.[260] Since this arrangement is likely to promote hemispheric independence of hand control, it may provide at least one essential anatomical substrate for the development of handedness.

V. FUNCTIONS OF MODALITY-SPECIFIC (UNIMODAL) SENSORY ASSOCIATION AREAS

The sensory–fugal streams of information processing enter their first "associative" stage within modality-specific (unimodal) association areas. Each group of unimodal areas conveys modality-specific information to the limbic system (for memory and emotion), prefrontal cortex (for working memory and other executive functions), perisylvian cortex (for language functions), temporal cortex (for object recognition), dorsal parietal cortex (for spatial attention) and premotor cortex (for the sensory guidance of movement and praxis). Lesions that damage unimodal sensory association cortex or its connections may give rise to two major types of behavioral deficits.

1. Selective perceptual deficits (such as "achromatopsia" and "akinetopsia") even when other functions in that sensory modality remain intact.

2. Modality-specific "agnosias" and "disconnection syndromes" (such as "prosopagnosia" and "pure word deafness."

Visual Unimodal Association Areas—Color, Motion, Shape, Objects, Faces, Words and Spatial Targets

The unimodal visual association areas in the human brain occupy peristriate cortex (BA18–19), and parts of the fusiform, inferior temporal, and middle temporal gyri (BA37, 20, 21). In the monkey, primary visual cortex (V1) projects to V2 (BA18) in a topographically well-ordered fashion. Areas V1 and V2 then give rise to multiple parallel pathways that project to numerous specialized peristriate visual association areas, located mostly within BA19 and designated V3, V4, V5 (MT), VP, V6 (PO), V7, and V8. The further occipitofugal flow of visual information takes the form of two divergent multisynaptic pathways, a dorsal one (also known as the "where" pathway) directed toward parietal and frontal cortex, and a ventral one (also known as the "what" pathway) directed toward downstream temporal visual association areas and the limbic system.[526] A similar organization is likely to exist in the human brain (Figs. 1–10 and 1–11a, b).

Figure 1–11a summarizes the cortical connectivity of the visual system of the monkey brain based on the review by Felleman and Van Essen.[141] Virtually all of these connections are reciprocal. They are represented on a template of concentric circles where each circle is separated from the next by at least one unit of synaptic distance. V1 occupies the first synaptic level. The subsequent synaptic levels follow

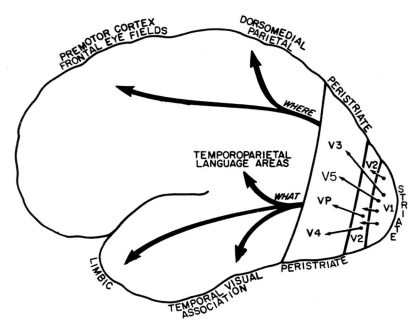

FIGURE 1–10. Organization of visuofugal pathways in the human brain.

a "downstream," "feedforward," "sensory–fugal," or "bottom-up" direction with respect to the visual modality, whereas descending levels can be described as following a "feedback," "sensory–petal," or "top–down" direction.

In the monkey, areas V2, V3, V4, and V5 (MT) are monosynaptically connected with V1 and therefore constitute "upstream" visual association areas whereas MST (medial superior temporal area), LIP (lateral intraparietal sulcus), posterior and anterior inferotemporal cortex (PIT and AIT in BA20–21), temporal area TF (BA 20), and the posterior inferior parietal lobule (BA7a) constitute some of the "downstream" visual association areas at the third and fourth synaptic levels. Although areas LIP, TF, and 7a also display features of heteromodal cortex, they appear to have subregions (such as Opt in the inferior parietal lobule and the posterior part of area TF) that may be engaged predominantly in the processing of visual information.[13,350,398] The LIP, TF, 7a nodes in Figure 1–11a represent these relatively modality-specific subregions.

The primary dimension of visual mapping is retinotopic and is achieved by finely tuned neurons which provide an exquisitely ordered spatial representation of the visual fields in V1. Other dimensions of visual experience such as color and motion are mapped in V1 and V2 by coarsely tuned neurons and become more fully characterized at further synaptic stages, including V4 and perhaps V8 (corresponding in part to area PIT or TEO) for color and V5 (MT) and MST for motion. The gradual increase of response latency, visual field size, and response complexity in the progression from V1 to V2, V4, PIT, and AIT confirms the existence of a synaptic hierarchy in the organization of visuofugal pathways. Although a visual event activates nodes at higher levels of this hierarchy with increasing latencies (11 ms between V1 and V2 and 9 ms between V1 and V5, but 40 ms from V1 to PIT-AIT), all areas eventually become concurrently active in the course of visual processing.[123,424] It seems as if each node is continuously passing on information to the others rather than fulfilling its part of the processing and then transmitting a completed product to the next station.[518]

COLOR AND MOVEMENT

The specialization of V4 (and perhaps V8) for color and of V5 (MT) and MST for movement have been documented in the monkey and human.[198,221,530] Studies based on functional imaging for example, have shown that the posterior parts of the lingual and, to a lesser extent, fusiform gyri in the human brain are sensitive to color stimulation.[80,303] The unilateral destruction of these areas in patients is usually associated with a contralateral loss of color perception ("hemi-achromatopsia") without equivalent impairments of visual acuity, movement perception, or object identification.[103,335] Lesions which interrupt the output of these areas to language cortex can lead to "color anomia," an inability to name colors despite intact color perception.

Other functional activation studies have shown that a laterally situated area in the middle temporal gyrus, at the confluence of BA19 and 37, displays selective activation in response to visual motion.[545] This region appears to represent the human homologue of area V5 (MT) and perhaps also MST in the monkey. Its bilateral destruction causes a state known as "akinetopsia" where the patient cannot perceive visual motion although acuity and color perception may be relatively preserved.[335,577,578] The clinical dissociation of achromatopsia from akinetopsia proves that the V1 projections to color-sensitive and motion-sensitive areas are organized in parallel rather than in series. The presence of such parallel pathways would be expected to increase processing efficiency by allowing the simultaneous analysis of multiple attributes associated with a visual event.

FORM AND COMPLEX PATTERNS

The elementary sensory features encoded at the first two synaptic levels are used by more downstream areas along the ventral visuofugal pathway for the discrimination of form and complex patterns. In the monkey, a posterolateral inferotemporal region (area TEO or PIT, at the junction of lateral BA19 with BA20–21) plays a critical role in form and pattern discrimination.[564] A homologous area in the human brain includes parts of the fusiform gyrus, just anterior to V4, and probably extends into the adjacent lingual and inferior occipital gyri.[199,259] This region appears to be involved in the construction of shape from simpler visual features since it becomes activated by tasks that require attention to both simple and complex shapes and does not give differential responses to upright versus inverted faces,

---

FIGURE 1–11. a, b. Each concentric ring represents a different synaptic level. Any two consecutive levels are separated by at least one unit of synaptic distance. Level 1 is occupied by the primary sensory cortex. Small empty circles represent macroscopic cortical areas or "nodes," one to several centimeters in diameter. Nodes at the same synaptic level are reciprocally interconnected by the black arcs of the concentric rings. Colored lines represent reciprocal monosynaptic connections from one synaptic level to another. a. Visual pathways as demonstrated by experimental neuroanatomical methods in the macaque brain. b. Visual (green), auditory (blue), and transmodal (red) pathways in the human brain. Individual pathways are inferred from the experimental work in the monkey. The anatomical identity of many of the nodes is not specified because their exact anatomical location is not critical. The assumption is that these *types* of anatomical interconnections and functionally specialized nodes exist in the human brain even though their exact location has not yet been determined. The terms "dorsal" and "ventral" refer to the separation of visuofugal pathways, especially at the fourth synaptic level, into dorsal and ventral streams of processing. The gaps in the circles at the first four levels indicate the absence of monosynaptic connections between modality-specific components of auditory and visual pathways. Abbreviations: A1=primary auditory cortex; AIT=anterior inferotemporal cortex; f=area specialized for face encoding; L=the hippocampal–entorhinal or amygdaloid components of the limbic system; LIP=lateral intraparietal cortex; MST=medial superior temporal cortex; P=heteromodal posterior parietal cortex; Pf=lateral prefrontal cortex; s=area specialized for encoding spatial location; PIT=posterior inferotemporal cortex; T=heteromodal lateral temporal cortex; TF=part of medial inferotemporal cortex; v=area specialized for identifying individual voice patterns, V1=primary visual cortex, V2, V3, V4, V5=additional visual areas; W=Wernicke's area; wr=area specialized for encoding word forms; 7a(Opt)=part of dorsal parieto-occipital cortex. c. Disconnection syndromes that arise when unimodal sensory–fugal pathways in the visual (green), auditory (blue), and somatosensoty (purple) modalities become disconnected from motor–premotor cortex, the language network, the limbic system, and the heteromodal cortices involved in face and object recognition. Question marks indicate that the proposed syndromes have not yet been identified.

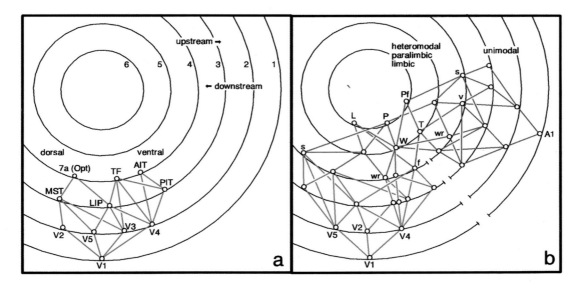

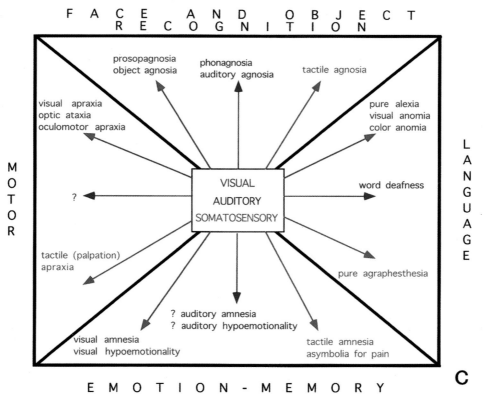

real versus nonsense objects, or novel versus familiar stimuli.[86,93,198,208,209,259,313] In comparison to the brain of the macaque monkey, the components of the ventral visuofugal pathway in the human appear to have been tucked ventromedially, probably in response to the expansion of the lateral temporal and posterior parietal cortices.

VENTRAL PATHWAY: FACES, OBJECTS, AND WORDS

If the identification of complex visual events and objects had to be based on a sequential compilation of the orientation, contour, color, form, and motion data encoded at the first three synaptic levels, perception would probably take an inordinately long time and might not allow the rapid recognition of frequently encountered and behaviorally significant patterns. This potential limitation is overcome at the fourth synaptic level of the ventral visuofugal pathways where neuronal groups selectively tuned to specific visual categories promote the rapid identification of entities such as faces, objects, and words. In the monkey, the anterior inferotemporal area (AIT or anterior BA20–21) contains neuronal ensembles specialized for face and object identification.[115,190] In the human brain, functional imaging studies, electrophysiological evoked responses, and the location of lesions in patients with the syndrome of prosopagnosia indicate that the homologous areas specialized for face and object identification are located predominantly within the midportion of the fusiform gyrus (BA37 and BA20).[10,103,423,485]

The "face" area in the human brain ("f" in Fig. 1–11b) is more strongly activated by faces than by other objects.[258] It is also more strongly activated by upright and intact faces than by inverted or scrambled ones but does not show a differential response to familiar versus novel faces.[183,209] This area therefore appears to encode faces at a categorical or generic level prior to the stage of individual recognition. The fourth synaptic level of the human brain contains additional regions specialized for the identification of other common objects such as chairs and houses.[235] An area specialized for the encoding of word forms and word-like letter strings ("wr" in Fig. 1–11b) has also been identified in this region, at a location perhaps slightly more lateral to that of the fusiform face area.[388,423] A second potential visual word-form identification area may be located in a more lateral occipitotemporal region, at the confluence of BA19 with BA37.[409] Considering the extremely recent emergence of written language in human phylogeny, the word-form area is almost certainly not genetically programmed. A more likely possibility is that it represents an experiential modification of neuronal subgroups within populations specialized for the encoding of faces and objects. The visual word-form areas could thus mediate a sort of processing where written words are handled as objects rather than as symbols.

Neurological lesions which damage these face, object, and word areas (or their outputs to transmodal object recognition and language areas) lead to the syndromes of "prosopagnosia" (face recognition deficit), "associative visual object agnosia" (object recognition deficit), and "pure alexia" (visual word recognition deficit) (Fig. 1–11c). These conditions are described in greater detail in Chapters 5 and 7. In other patients, lesions which interrupt the connections from the visual association cortices to the limbic system give rise to states of "visual hypoemotionality" (where visual experiences no longer elicit the appropriate emotional response) and "visual amnesia" (where new memories cannot be formed when the input is in the visual modality) (Fig. 11c).[26,454] In one patient, damage to visuoamygdaloid pathways prompted a cancellation of a *Playboy* subscription, apparently because the visual evocation of erotic feelings had become blunted.[26]

DORSAL PATHWAY AND SPATIAL ORIENTATION

The fourth synaptic level in Figure 1–11b also contains components of the dorsal visuofugal pathways ("s" in Fig. 1–11b). This part of visual association cortex encodes visual information in the form of spatial vectors which can be used to guide attentional behaviors (Chapter 3). Neurons in parts of area 7a of the macaque, for example, can compute the spatial coordinates of extrapersonal visual events by combining retinotopic location with information about eye position.[579] Some of these neurons display a tuning for visual events in head-centered or even world-centered coordinates so that relevant events can become targets of visual or manual grasp (Chapter 3). Functional imaging experiments based on tasks of spatial localization indicate that the analogous region in the human brain may be located in the dorsal occipitoparietal region, at the junction of BA19 with BA7, probably including the banks of the posterior intraparietal sulcus.[208] Damage to these dorsal visual areas or to their connections contributes to the emergence of visuospatial disorientation syndromes such as "hemispatial visual neglect," "dressing apraxia" (inability to align body axis with garment), "simultanagnosia" (inability to integrate visual detail into a coherent whole), "optic ataxia" (deficits of reaching toward visual targets), and "optic apraxia" (oculomotor exploration deficits). The latter three manifestations are collectively known as "Bálint's syndrome." These visuospatial syndromes are described in greater detail in Chapters 3 and 7.

GROUP ENCODING AND DISTRIBUTED PROCESSING

Neuronal ensembles within downstream visual association areas provide representations of objects and faces through a process of group encoding. The tuning is broad and coarse: One neuron may be activated by several faces and the same face may excite several neurons.[447] The face neurons in inferotemporal cortex are selectively responsive to category-specific canonical features such as intereye distance, style of hair, expression, and direction of gaze.[568] Neurons sensitive to similar types of canonical features form vertical columns measuring approximately 0.4 mm in diameter. Several adjacent columns responsive to similar features may be linked to form larger "patches" or modules measuring several millimeters.[204,513] Groups of such patches may form interconnected but distributed ensembles collectively tuned to the entire set of canonical features that define an object class. The tangential interpatch connections that are necessary for establishing such an organization could be stabilized during the period of cortical development and subsequently strengthened by experience through the mediation of temporally correlated multifocal activity.[301]

    Although neurons in a given column respond preferentially to similar canonical features of an object or face, optimal tuning properties vary among constituent cells so that columnar activation may encode generic properties whereas the activities of individual cells within the column may help to encode distinguishing (subordinate) features of unique exemplars.[157] In response to an object, a small subset of neurons in a given column can fire maximally and set constraints to guide the interpretation of less active neurons within the same ensemble.[166] Identification can thus start by matching the coarse (or generic) features and then focusing on finer (subordinate) detail. A visual entity may be represented by a small number of modules, each broadly selective for some reference object or face, which collectively measure the *similarity* of the target stimulus to the reference entities. This type of encoding, also known as "second-order isomorphism," is thought to be computationally more parsimonious than representations based on a more direct isomorphic mapping of the target shape.[130]

The processing parsimony offered by this organization is substantial.[134] A very large number of faces can be encoded by a small number of neurons, recognition can be graded (rather than all or none) and based on partial information, the same information can be probed through multiple associations, generalizations based on few common features (or analysis based on differences) can be achieved rapidly, the progression from categorical to subordinate identification can proceed smoothly, and damage or refractory states in a subset of neurons within the ensemble can lead to a graceful, partial degradation of function. These neurons can achieve a rapid detection of behaviorally relevant, recurrent, and composite visual events, obviating the need for a cumbersome sequential compilation of the more elementary sensory features. The face-responsive ensembles also display considerable plasticity, so some neurons alter their firing rate to a given face when it becomes more familiar or when a new one is added to the set,[448] suggesting that the identity of an individual face is not encoded by fixed rates of firing but by the *relative* firing frequencies (and perhaps interneuronal correlation patterns) across the entire ensemble. The general principles that guide the visual identification of faces probably also apply to the encoding of other classes of objects, words, and spatial targets.

The downstream unimodal association areas of the cerebral cortex display prominent learning effects. Following the pairing of pattern α to pattern β in a paired-associates task, for example, an anterior inferotemporal (AIT) neuron responsive to β but not to α increases its firing in anticipation of β toward the end of the delay period following stimulation by α, showing that it has learned the arbitrary association between the two stimuli.[384] Neurons in AIT also display a familiarity response to faces encountered as long as 24 hours ago, indicating that the initial exposure had been stored in long-term memory.[138] These observations have led to the suggestion that the downstream visual association cortices in the temporal lobe act as a "memory storehouse" for object vision.[358,384] Modifications of synaptic efficacy, such as those necessary for long-term potentiation and depression, have been obtained in the human middle and inferior temporal gyri and could mediate similar long-term encoding.[82] The downstream components of unimodal visual association areas can thus not only identify but also record visual events.

The anatomical areas that play crucial roles in the identification of color, movement, faces, words, objects and spatial targets display *relative* rather that *absolute* specializations. For example, V4 participates not only in color perception but also in selective attention, the identification of salience, and the encoding of form.[92,366,470] In turn, the identification of color information may involve not only V4 and V8 but also a part of lateral peristriate cortex.[94] Furthermore, neuronal ensembles selectively tuned to canonical features of faces participate, although to a lesser extent, in encoding other visual entities.[447] Any visual input can probably activate all of the nodes along the visual pathways shown in Figure 11b. However, stimuli with canonical features of faces are likely to cause optimal activation in the face area, those with the canonical features of words in the word area, and so on. Thus, the neural representation of a face could be conceptualized as a plane that has its highest peak over the face area but which also has lesser peaks over numerous other nodes of visual association cortex. This organization has been designated "selectively distributed processing"[336,480] to set it apart from other models based on equipotentiality[285] and modularity.[150]

Auditory Unimodal Association Areas

Primary auditory areas A1 and R receive their thalamic input from the medial geniculate nucleus and are responsive to pure tones. Another auditory area, CM, depends on inputs from A1 and R for its pure-tone responses. Area CM is more responsive to complex broad-band stimuli and to the high frequencies used for sound localization.[433] It appears, therefore, that the primate brain may contain multiple auditory areas just as it contains multiple visual areas (Fig. 1–11b).

In the monkey, pitch and pure tone discrimination are accomplished at the level of A1 and closely related upstream auditory association areas of the posterior superior temporal gyrus. The identification of complex auditory sequences, the discrimination of species-specific calls, and the localization of sounds, however, engage more downstream auditory association areas of the superior temporal gyrus.[91,214] The role of the superior temporal gyrus in the identification of species-specific calls appears analogous to the role of downstream visual association cortex in face identification, both processes serving crucial functions in social communication.

In keeping with the organization of visuofugal pathways, the auditory pathways of the monkey brain may also be divided into dorsal and ventral components. Area Tpt of the posterior superior temporal gyrus, for example, may belong to the dorsal audiofugal stream of processing and may be specialized for detecting the spatial localization of sound sources, whereas the more anterior and ventral parts of the superior temporal gyrus may be specialized for identifying complex auditory sequences and species-specific vocalizations.[91,214,289] As in the case of visual pathways, unimodal auditory cortex can also store modality-specific memories. Thus, lesions that destroy auditory unimodal association areas impair the retention of auditory sequences.[239]

A similar organization may exist in the human brain. Neurons in A1 of the human brain are sensitive to pure tones and pitch whereas those of the mid- to anterior parts of the superior temporal gyrus are relatively unresponsive to pure tones and nonlinguistic noises but respond to specific phonetic parameters of spoken language.[113,409,576] The superior temporal gyrus neurons are broadly tuned to the segmentation and sequencing of phonemes as well as to their coherence within polysyllabic and compound words.[98] They encode speech at a presemantic level since they respond to spoken real words as readily as to distorted backward speech.[98] These neurons may be analogous to the visual word-form neurons of the fusiform and adjacent inferotemporal areas where words and letter strings are processed as perceptual patterns rather than symbols. Approximately half of the neurons in parts of the middle temporal gyrus (BA21) give highly selective responses, mostly in the form of suppression, to understandable speech but not to distorted speech.[98]

Although the evidence is not as easily interpreted as in the case of visual pathways, it appears that upstream auditory areas in the human brain tend to encode more elementary features of sound such as frequency and pitch, whereas downstream areas may contain neuronal groups that encode more composite features related to the identification of words ("wr" in Fig. 1–11B), the localization of sound sources for attentional targeting ("s" in Fig. 1–11B), the categorization of object-specific sounds, and perhaps also the characterization of individual voice patterns (area "v" in Fig. 1–11B). Lesions of unimodal auditory association cortex or of its connections give rise to complex "auditory perceptual impairments" (such as the inability to identify variations in timber or sound sequences), "cortical deafness" (inability to recognize meaningful verbal and nonverbal auditory patterns despite normal brainstem auditory potentials), "pure word deafness" (inability to understand or repeat spoken language despite good recognition of environmental sounds and no other language deficit), "auditory agnosia for environmental sounds" (inability to identify sounds characteristic of objects despite good speech comprehension), and "phonagnosia" (inability to recognize the identity of familiar voices despite preserved recognition of spoken words and environmental sounds).[317,417] The first two deficits are caused by damage to upstream unimodal auditory association cortex (usually in the presence of variable A1 involvement) whereas the latter three may reflect damage to downstream auditory association cortex or functional disconnections of auditory association areas from transmodal cortices related to language comprehension and object recognition (Fig. 1–11c).

Pure word deafness and auditory agnosia can have "apperceptive" as well as "associative" subtypes (or components). In the apperceptive form, the clinical deficit can be attributed to a degradation of the auditory percept, whereas in the associative form it is caused by the inability of an otherwise intact auditory percept to activate transmodal areas related to language comprehension and object recognition. The exact anatomical correlates underlying these clinical subtypes have not yet been identified. Conceivably, the apperceptive component becomes prominent when the lesion encroaches on A1 and upstream unimodal association cortex whereas the apperceptive component dominates when the lesion is confined to the downstream auditory association cortex and its outputs.

The traditional literature gives the impression that Wernicke's area is confined to auditory association cortex in the posterior third of the superior temporal gyrus. This is quite unlikely since the deficit in Wernicke's aphasia is multimodal and impairs language comprehension in all modalities of input. A more likely possibility is that Wernicke's area extends into heteromodal cortical areas and that the posterior third of the superior temporal gyrus constitutes only one of its components. Damage to this component is likely to be responsible for the auditory aspects (such as word deafness) of Wernicke's aphasia.

Somatosensory Association Areas and Secondary Somatosensory Cortex

As mentioned in the section on primary somatosensory cortex, BA1 and 2 have characteristics of upstream unimodal association cortex although they are traditionally included within S1. In the monkey, the superior parietal lobule (BA5) is the major recipient of S1 projections (mostly from BA2) and displays the properties of an upstream unimodal somatosensory association area. The sensory responses of approximately 98% of the neurons in BA 5 are confined to the somatosensory modality. However, the firing patterns show an intramodal convergence among deep and superficial sensations, thus indicating a higher order neuronal processing than in S1.[374] The superior parietal lobule is a major source of projections to dorsal premotor cortex and therefore plays an important role in the coordination of complex movements.[556] For example, neurons in BA5 have somatosensory receptive fields with directionally tuned responses coded in arm- or body-centered coordinates. Neurons in BA5 give responses that are more closely related to the significance of the stimulus and the motor planning that it elicits than the actual execution of the movement.[67] Anterior parts of the inferior parietal lobule (BA7b) and parts of the insula may contain the downstream somatosensory association areas of the monkey brain.[343,398] Some BA7b neurons are activated when the monkey attempts to grasp an object of interest, even in the absence of visual input, but not when the arm is moved passively.[233]

A Secondary Somatosensory area (S2) has been identified within the sylvian fissure of the monkey brain at the junction of the insula with the parietal operculum. It contains a somatotopic representation which is somewhat coarser than the one in S1. The S2 area receives inputs from the inferior ventroposterior nucleus (VPI) of the thalamus, from all components of S1, and from the anterior part of the inferior parietal lobule (BA7b). It is a major source of somatosensory projections to the posterior insula which relays this information to the limbic system via the amygdala.[343] Damage to S2 can impair tactile learning in the monkey, probably because it induces a somatosensory–limbic disconnection.[378] These observations suggest that S2 has mixed characteristics of primary somatosensory cortex as well as of unimodal somatosensory association cortex.

In the rhesus monkey, the entire superior parietal lobule has been designated as area 5 by Brodmann. In the human, BA5 is confined to an anterior rim of the superior parietal lobule. The rest of the human superior parietal lobule is designated BA7 (Fig. 1–7). In the monkey, however, BA7 was used by Brodmann to designate the cortex of the inferior parietal lobule. For the purposes of this chapter, BA5, the anterior part of BA7 in the superior parietal lobule, parts of the posterior insula, and an anterior segment of the supramarginal gyrus (BA40) will be included within the group of unimodal somatosensory association areas in the human brain (Fig. 1–7). Based on topographic similarities, BA5 and anterior BA7 of the human brain may be homologous to BA5 in the monkey whereas anterior BA40 and the anterior intraparietal sulcus may be homologous to BA7b.

In the human, an S2 area has been located in a region of the parietal operculum adjacent to the dorsal insula.[401] Functional imaging suggests that S2 may participate in pain perception.[88] In some patients, lesions in the region of S2 give rise to a loss of pain perception without impairing other discriminative somatosensory modalities. This is the only lesion site which gives rise to such a dissociation: Thalamic lesions impair all modalities and S1 lesions cause the reverse dissociation (Fig 1–9a). In other patients, lesions in the region of S2 (but also involving the insula and parietal operculum) can give rise to painful contralesional disesthesias of the type seen in the thalamic Dejerine-Roussy syndrome.[474] Similar lesions can also lead to "pain asymbolia," a condition where the patient fails to display the expected aversive and emotional response to pain anywhere in the body although the ability to discriminate sharp from dull may be intact.[44] The syndrome of pain asymbolia (and the tactile amnesia which has been described in monkeys with S2 lesions) would appear to represent somatosensory–limbic disconnection syndromes (Fig. 1–11c). Pain asymbolia can be conceptualized as a somatosensory analogue of visual hypoemotionality.

The somatosensory association areas (BA5, 7, and perhaps also anterior BA40 and the posterior insula) in the human brain are likely to play essential roles in the finer aspects of touch localization, active manual exploration, the somatosensory coordination of reaching and grasping, and the encoding of complex somatosensory memories. The anterior bank of the intraparietal sulcus (corresponding mostly to BA40) has, in fact, been shown to play a critical role in coordinating the prehensile movements required for object grasping.[47] In Braille readers, unimodal somatosensory areas may encode word forms in a manner that is similar to the modality-specific encoding of word forms in visual and auditory association cortices.

Neural outputs of somatosensory association cortex in the human brain are likely to have the same types of targets as those of visual and auditory association cortices. They would therefore be expected to follow a posterior pathway directed to heteromodal association areas of the parietal lobe, an anterior pathway directed toward premotor and prefrontal cortices, and ventral pathways directed toward the language areas, the limbic system, and temporoparietal heteromodal cortex. The projections directed to the limbic system are likely to originate predominantly from S2 and the insula whereas the others are likely to arise also from BA5, anterior BA7, and perhaps anterior BA40.

Interrupting the projections from somatosensory cortex to parietal heteromodal areas may disrupt spatial orientation, tactile search, and the ability to align the body axis with other solid objects during the process of dressing, sitting in a chair, or getting into bed. These types of lesions may therefore give rise to the somatosensory integration deficits associated with dressing apraxia, hemispatial neglect, and other aspects of spatial disorientation.[261] Other types of posterior parietal or insular lesions may interrupt somatosensory projections to temporoparietal transmodal areas and may be responsible for the emergence of a somatosensory object recognition deficit known as "tactile agnosia" (inability to recognize an object by palpation alone in a patient who can draw the palpated object and has no other somatosensory deficit).[75] Lesions which disconnect somatosensory areas from the language network could conceivably give rise to "pure agraphesthesia" (or pure somesthetic alexia), a syndrome which could be considered the somatosensory analogue of pure word deafness and pure alexia (Fig. 1–11c).[158] The interruption of the pathway from somatosensory cortex to premotor and supplementary motor areas may be responsible for the emergence of a modality-specific "tactile apraxia" wherein objects cannot be handled without visual guidance.[110] Functional imaging experiments suggest that this pathway is likely to originate from the anterior intraparietal sulcus.[47]

VI. MOTOR ASSOCIATION AREAS (PREMOTOR CORTEX, SUPPLEMENTARY MOTOR AREA, FRONTAL EYE FIELDS)

The motor association areas anterior to M1 constitute the principal, if not exclusive, source of cortical projections into M1. Premotor cortex contributes a substantial number of descending corticospinal and corticobulbar fibers but at a lower density than M1.[519] Microstimulation of this region elicits movement but the threshold for this is higher than in M1.[547] Furthermore, the movement patterns that are elicited upon stimulation of motor association cortex are much more intricate than those elicited by M1 stimulation and often involve both sides of the body. Lesions in motor association areas yield complex deficits of movement in the absence of weakness, dystonia, dysmetria, or hyperreflexia. In the human brain, motor association cortex includes the premotor cortex (anterolateral BA6), the frontal eye fields in BA6, the supplementary motor area in the medial wall of the cerebral hemisphere (mostly BA6), the supplementary eye fields, the posterior parts of Broca's area (BA44), and perhaps parts of BA8.

Investigations of motor association areas in the monkey are revealing an organization with a level of complexity that rivals that of visual pathways. Several premotor areas have been identified within the traditional boundaries of BA6, each with a potentially different specialization.[314,440,556] According to one nomenclature, these areas have been designated F2–F7.[440] Premotor areas receive input from numerous unimodal and heteromodal areas of the brain so that they have access to complex information in all major sensory modalities.[547] Although premotor neurons respond to sensory stimuli, the responses usually vary according to the movement that will follow. For example, visually responsive neurons in premotor cortex show one response to a visual cue that triggers a movement and a different response when the same cue requires the animal to withhold movement.[557]

In the monkey, the interconnections between posterior parietal cortex and the premotor areas of BA6 are organized with exquisite anatomical and functional specificity. The projection from anterior intraparietal cortex (AIP) to frontal premotor area F5, for example, is part of a visuomotor circuit for preshaping the hand as it prepares to grasp a three dimensional tool (see Fig. 3–14). Neurons in F5 fire not only during grasping but also while viewing a graspable object even when no motor response is required, perhaps reflecting the stage at which a visually elicited motor program is unfolding.[376] A similar organization may exist in the human brain, where the lateral bank of the anterior intraparietal sulcus may provide the source of projections that allow premotor and supplementary motor cortices to coordinate object grasping and other aspects of prehension.[47] As in the monkey, the visual observation of tools leads to the activation of the human dorsal premotor cortex even when no movement is emitted,[186] suggesting that this area may play an important role in the visually triggered programming of movements related to tool usage.

In monkeys which were taught to elevate a lever to obtain reward, a surface-negative slow potential appears over premotor cortex about 1 second prior to the movement and gradually increases until about 100 ms before the movement.[206] This slow potential may reflect the neural mechanisms which subserve motor intention and initiation. The proportion of neurons showing activity only during such preparatory phases of a movement is much higher in the supplementary motor area than in M1.[7] Furthermore, neurons that can store information related to an entire sequence of goal-directed movements are frequently found in the supplementary motor area but not in M1, suggesting that the supplementary motor area plays an important role in coordinating multistep movement strategies and perhaps also in the encoding of procedural learning.[514]

In keeping with these observations, finger movements lead to the activation of M1 as well as the supplementary motor area whereas imagined movements activate predominantly the latter.[446,505] Furthermore, experiments based on transcranial magnetic stimulation show that premotor cortex plays a critical role in the early stages of movement selection when choices among competing alternatives need to be made.[472] The supplementary motor cortex and premotor cortex may therefore play important roles in motor planning and response selection. These areas may also play a critical role in the initiation of motor responses and the ability to sustain motor output. The paucity of speech output in "transcortical motor aphasia" (a nonfluent aphasia with intact repetition and comprehension) and "aphemia" (a nonaphasic, nondysarthric impairment of fluency) may thus result from a disconnection of the premotor and supplementary motor cortices from Broca's area.[154]

Components of motor association cortex modulate the sensory guidance, initiation, inhibition, planning, and perhaps also learning of complex movements.[53] Damage to these areas results in category-specific (or conditional) disturbances of movement. Monkeys with lesions in area 6, for example, have no primary weakness but are no longer able to change the nature of a motor act in response to differential sensory cues.[202,362] In the human, lesions in the frontal eye fields lead to impaired exploratory eye movements even when spontaneous eye movements remain intact; lesions in the premotor part of Broca's area lead to dysarthria for speech but do not interfere with singing; and damage to the supplementary motor cortex may interfere with motor initiation but not with the other phases of the movement.[177,361]

The frontal epicenter of the language network is known as Broca's area. It includes premotor cortex in BA44 and also adjacent heteromodal cortex (Fig. 1–7).[334] The examination of patients with focal lesions indicates that Broca's area is likely to play a critical role in translating neural word forms into their articulatory sequences and also in sequencing words and their endings into utterances that have a meaning-appropriate syntactic structure. This sequencing role attributed to Broca's area is consistent with the other specializations of premotor and prefrontal cortex. In keeping with these functional characteristics, inferred on the basis of clinical observations, Broca's area shows preferential metabolic activation in tasks that require neurologically intact subjects to decipher the meaning of a syntactically complex sentence and also in tasks that entail grapheme-to-phoneme transformations, even when the articulatory output is imaginary.[70,173]

Lesions that disconnect BA6 from the posterior components of the language network may cause multimodal "ideomotor apraxia" (inability to pantomime the use of an object upon verbal command) although the patient may have no difficulty making the same movement upon being handed or shown the actual object.[169] Two types of "modality-specific apraxias" have also been reported: Some patients cannot pantomime the use of an object presented visually although they can perform the movement correctly when asked to do so verbally; others cannot perform the correct movements if asked to handle an object in the absence of visual guidance.[110,566] These deficits, respectively designated "visual apraxia" and "tactile (or palpatory) apraxia," appear to be caused by lesions which interrupt visual or somatosensory projections to premotor and supplementary motor areas (Fig. 1–11c). The movement deficits caused by damage to motor association areas reflect a disconnection between cognition and action rather than an impairment of strength or mobility.

VII. TEMPORAL HETEROMODAL CORTEX AND AGNOSIAS— TRANSMODAL GATEWAYS FOR THE RECOGNITION OF FACES, OBJECTS, AND VOICES

As discussed above, downstream visual association cortices (such as "f" in Fig. 1–11b) are essential for the perceptual encoding of faces and objects. By itself, this information would provide an isolated percept devoid of meaning or context. The ability of this modality-specific information to activate the relevant multimodal associations that lead to recognition requires the mediation of transmodal cortical areas. In the monkey, for example, unimodal anterior inferotemporal cortex (AIT) neurons are sensitive to the visual properties of faces whereas more downstream transmodal neurons of the superior temporal sulcus also encode their familiarity.[573] In humans, exposure to unfamiliar faces activates unimodal visual association areas in the fusiform face region, whereas familiar faces also activate transmodal nodes, including those in lateral midtemporal cortex.[183] Heteromodal cortices in the middle temporal gyrus (represented by area T in Fig. 1–11b) may therefore act as transmodal gateways for linking the visual representation of faces with the additional associations (such as the name, voice, and personal recollections) that collectively lead to recognition.

Some neurological lesions lead to a specific face recognition deficit known as "associative prosopagnosia." This syndrome is most commonly caused by bilateral lesions in the mid-to-anterior parts of the lingual and fusiform gyri (Chapter 7). As noted earlier, these are the parts of the brain that contain the unimodal visual association areas specialized for the encoding of faces and other complex objects. According to Fig. 1–11b, prosopagnosia can potentially arise as a consequence of at least three types of lesions: (1) those that damage area "f," (2) those that interrupt the connections between upstream visual association areas and area "f," and (3) those that interrupt the connections between area "f" and transmodal node T. Relatively simpler aspects of perception (for example, the ability to tell if two faces have an identical shape or not) can be preserved in these patients, presumably because more upstream visual association areas remain intact. Face recognition and identification can also be impaired in patients who have the simultanagnosia of Bálint's syndrome. This is known as an "apperceptive prosopagnosia" because it reflects a deficit in the spatial integration of the visual percept itself. In contrast to associative prosopagnosia, the patient with apperceptive prosopagnosia is usually unable to determine if two faces are perceptually identical or not.

Although patients with associative prosopagnosia cannot recognize familiar faces by visual inspection, recognition becomes possible when information in a nonvisual modality, for example, the voice pattern characteristic of that person, becomes available. This auditory information can presumably access transmodal area T through area "v" of unimodal auditory cortex in Fig. 1–11b, leading to the activation of the other distributed associations that lead to recognition. Furthermore, a face that is not consciously recognized can occasionally still elicit a physiological emotional response,[27,521] presumably because the damage is located downstream to "f" and interrupts its connections to area T but not to limbic areas such as those represented by area L in Fig. 1–11b.

As described in Chapter 7, patients with prosopagnosia may have no difficulty in the generic recognition and naming of object classes (for example, they may recognize and name a car as a car or a face as a face) but may not be able to determine the make of a particular car, recognize a favorite pet, or identify a personal object from among other examples of the same category.[103] This additional feature of prosopagnosia, a generalized impairment in recognizing unique members of a larger object group, raises the possibility that area "f" may also participate in the identification of objects other than faces or, alternatively, that the lesion sites may involve adjacent regions that encode additional object categories.

If prosopagnosia represents an inability to recognize unique exemplars of visually encoded object categories, "associative visual object agnosia" represents an impairment that extends to the level of categorical recognition. The patient with this syndrome can neither name a familiar object nor describe its nature and use. While a prosopagnosic patient can tell that a face is a face and a pencil is a pencil, a patient with object agnosia is unable to perform this task but retains the ability to determine if two objects are perceptually identical or not. Since the encoding of proprietary features may require more information than the encoding of generic features, prosopagnosia may represent the outcome of a smaller or more downstream lesion than that associated with object agnosia. Although clinical reports show that the lesions in object agnosia appear very similar to those in prosopagnosia, minor differences in lesion size or location could easily escape detection in case studies.

A second potential distinction between prosopagnosia and object agnosia may be based on the memory systems that support the recognition of generic versus proprietary information. The generic recognition of familiar objects is part of semantic knowledge, whereas the recognition of familiar faces and objects is more closely related to personal experience. Although prosopagnosia and object agnosia are usually seen after bilateral lesions, these syndromes do occasionally arise after unilateral lesions, in which case prosopagnosia tends to result from lesions in the right hemisphere and object agnosia from lesions in the left.[140] This dissociation is interesting since the right hemisphere appears to have a greater role in the activation of autobiographical memories.[146]

Associative agnosias have also been identified in the auditory and tactile modalities. Patients with a condition known as "auditory (object) agnosia" fail to associate the ringing of a telephone or the siren of an ambulance with the corresponding object although more elementary auditory perceptual abilities remain relatively preserved. This syndrome may reflect a disconnection of unimodal auditory areas specialized for encoding the auditory properties of familiar objects from transmodal nodes (such as T in Fig. 1–11b) that coordinate their multimodal recognition. The lesions that give rise to auditory agnosia typically involve auditory association cortex, usually in the right hemisphere, but the more detailed anatomical correlates of this relatively rare syndrome remain to be elucidated.[500] The auditory analog of prosopagnosia is known as "phonagnosia." It reflects an inability to recognize the identity of familiar voices, potentially in the absence of other major auditory deficits.[417,535] This rare syndrome may reflect a disconnection of area "v" in unimodal auditory association cortex from transmodal node T.

"Tactile agnosia," the inability to recognize objects by palpation, in the absence of any other somatosensory or aphasic deficits, is a much less frequently encountered condition.[75] It can theoretically be differentiated from astereognosis by showing that patients with tactile agnosia (as opposed to those with astereognosis) can draw the objects they palpate, even when the palpation fails to elicit recognition. Stereognosis is an apperceptive deficit whereas tactile agnosia is an associative deficit of somatosensory object recognition. The responsible lesion, usually located in the insula or posterior parietal cortex, would be expected to interrupt the projections from downstream somatosensory association cortex to a transmodal node equivalent to T in Figure 11b.

The modality-specific agnosias highlight the importance of sensory–fugal pathways to the process of recognition and offer a neuroanatomical basis for distinguishing perception from recognition. Associative agnosias arise when unimodal areas specialized for the perceptual encoding of objects are damaged or when they fail to access pivotal transmodal gateways that enable multimodal integration. More elementary perceptual processes, subserved by more upstream unimodal areas, remain relatively intact in patients with associative agnosias. The relevant transmodal areas, such as the heteromodal cortices of the middle temporal gyrus, are not centers for the convergent storage of knowledge related to faces and objects, but optimal conduits for accessing the relevant distributed associations that collectively lead to accurate recognition. Other cognitive domains, such as language, spatial awareness, explicit memory, and emotion, display analogous principles of organization but revolve around transmodal gateways located in different parts of the brain.

VIII. Wernicke's Area as a Temporoparietal Transmodal Gateway for Language

Language allows the elaboration and communication of experiences and thoughts through the mediation of arbitrary symbols known as words. Broca's and Wernicke's areas constitute the two epicenters of a distributed language network. Broca's area, located in BA44 and adjacent heteromodal prefrontal cortices, occupies the syntactic/articulatory pole of the language network whereas Wernicke's area occupies its lexical/semantic pole.[334] Wernicke's area has no universally accepted boundary. It is usually defined as "the region which causes Wernicke's aphasia when damaged." Some investigators would confine Wernicke's area to auditory association cortex in the posterior third of the superior temporal gyrus (BA22). As noted above, the multimodal nature of Wernicke's aphasia argues against this possibility. There are numerous reasons for concluding that Wernicke's area includes not only the posterior third of BA22 but also the immediately adjacent parts of heteromodal cortex in BA39–40 and perhaps also parts of the middle temporal gyrus.[334]

As described in Chapter 5, damage to almost any component of the language network can give rise to naming and word-finding deficits. However, Wernicke's area is one of the very few lesion sites that elicits two-way naming deficits where the patient can neither retrieve the name for an object nor point to the appropriate object when the name is supplied by the examiner. Such observations may give the impression that Wernicke's area is a storage site for word representations. However, clinical research shows that Wernicke's area is as unlikely to be the repository of a mental lexicon as the middle temporal cortex is to be the repository of the knowledge of faces and objects. Instead, the role of Wernicke's area might be conceptualized as that of a transmodal gateway which coordinates reciprocal interactions between the sensory representations of word forms and the arbitrary (second-order or symbolic) associations that give them meaning. According to this formulation, damage to Wernicke's area does not necessarily obliterate word representations but makes it impossible to understand (decode) words in any modality of input or to link (encode) percepts and concepts into corresponding word forms. This is why Wernicke's aphasia entails not only a deficit in comprehending language in all modalities of input but also a deficit in expressing thoughts in meaning-appropriate words.

Experiments based on functional imaging show that naming (lexical access) is a highly distributed function mediated by "prelexical" areas adjacent to those that support the perceptual encoding of the object or feature to be named.[80,106,312,313] Lexical labeling is thus anchored to the perceptual mapping of the corresponding experience. These category-specific prelexical areas are located outside of Wernicke's area. They are necessary but not sufficient for naming since damage to Wernicke's area causes severe naming deficits even when these prelexical areas are intact. The prelexical areas provide *implicit* lexical representations that need to be made explicit through the mediation of Wernicke's area and other components of the language network.[339]

Although its spontaneous development only in humans endows language with a sense of uniqueness, its neurological foundations are quite analogous to those of other cognitive domains.[389] Word forms, for example, are likely to be encoded within unimodal auditory and visual areas according to the principles that also guide the encoding of faces and objects. Lexical labeling, furthermore, can be conceptualized as a component of object recognition in the sense that a name is as much an attribute of an object as its color, location, or past associations. Word comprehension is also an object recognition task where the perceptual features first lead to the categorical identification of a word as a word, then to a subordinate-level identification of the individual word, and finally to the establishment of the multiple arbitrary associations that define its meaning through the mediation of transmodal nodes in Wernicke's area and adjacent perisylvian language areas. Word recognition and retrieval thus proceed according to principles that also guide object recognition, except that the critical transmodal gateways are located in perisylvian cortex rather than in midtemporal cortex.

The analogy between the neural organization of language and object recognition is further emphasized by the existence of two types of verbal associative agnosias known as pure alexia and pure word deafness. In contrast to prosopagnosia and object agnosia, which emerge when visual information cannot access area T in Fig. 1–11b, pure alexia (word blindness) emerges when areas that encode visual word forms ("wr" in Fig. 1–11b) are disconnected from visual input or when they cannot communicate with Wernicke's area and related components of the left hemisphere language network (W in Fig. 1–11b). This usually happens when a lesion of area V1 in the left hemisphere (which, by itself, yields a right homonymous hemianopia) occurs in conjunction with a lesion of the splenium, a region of the corpus callosum which conveys visual information from one hemisphere to the other. The splenial lesion interferes with the transcallosal transfer of visual information from the intact visual areas of the right hemisphere to the visual word-form areas ("wr" in Fig. 1–11b) and transmodal language areas (area W) of the left hemisphere. These areas thus become completely disconnected from ipsilateral as well as contralateral visual input. The patient with pure alexia is not blind since objects and faces presented to the left hemifield can be recognized with no difficulty as they activate area T. There is no aphasia either since Wernicke's area and other core language areas are intact and can receive word-form information in the auditory modality. However, upon being asked to read, the patient appears illiterate since language-related transmodal nodes such as area W in Fig. 1–11b can no longer receive word-form information in the visual modality.

A similar analysis applies to pure word deafness which arises when area "wr" in unimodal auditory cortex is cut off from auditory input or when it cannot communicate with relevant transmodal nodes in area W (Fig. 1–11b). Pure word deafness can be seen after bilateral lesions or after unilateral temporal lobe lesions in the language-dominant hemisphere (usually left) which disconnect ipsilateral as well as transcallosal auditory inputs from components of the language network. The patient with pure word deafness is not deaf and can readily interpret most environmental sounds since parts of primary auditory cortex and auditory association areas are usually intact. Such patients are not aphasic and show no impairment of reading, writing, or speaking since the language areas are mostly intact. When exposed to speech, however, the patient reacts to it as an alien tongue that cannot be deciphered since the auditory information cannot reach language-related transmodal nodes such as those in Wernicke's area. The term "pure" word deafness can be used in a strong sense, meaning that the only auditory deficit is for understanding spoken language, or in a weak sense, meaning that the only language deficit is for auditory comprehension.[417] This second definition encompasses a larger number of patients.

The somatosensory equivalent of pure alexia and pure word deafness can be designated "pure agraphesthesia" (or somesthetic alexia) (Fig. 1–11c). One patient with this syndrome could not identify letters presented in the tactile modality to either hand despite a preservation of other somatosensory functions including stereognosis (naming the object by palpation) and the ability to determine if two letters presented in the somatosensory modality were same or different.[158] The responsible lesion was located in the posterior parietal cortex of the left hemisphere and appears to have disconnected somatosensory association cortex from Wernicke's area and other components of the language network.

Domains as different as object recognition and language can thus share common principles of organization. In each case, specialized transmodal nodes act as critical gateways for looking up and binding distributed multimodal information upon being queried by relevant unimodal inputs. Each of these processes entails multimodal integration, but much of this integration is based on knowing where to look up the information rather than on the presence of a privileged site where an ultimate convergent synthesis becomes stored.

IX. Functions and Syndromes of Posterior Parietal Heteromodal Cortex

The posterior parietal heteromodal cortices (BA7, 39, 40) of the human brain provide sites for multimodal interactions related to praxis, language, visuomotor integration, generation of motor plans, and spatial attention.[9,29,90,390,505] Clinical observations have led to the suggestion that the inferior parietal lobule of the language-dominant (usually left) hemisphere may contain spatiotemporal representations of learned skilled movements ("praxicons") which are then translated into the appropriate motor output through the mediation of premotor cortex.[215] Damage to this part of the brain gives rise to a type of ideomotor apraxia where the patient is unable either to pantomime the use of an object specified by the examiner or to infer the nature of the object when the examiner pantomimes its use.[215]

Lesions which spare Wernicke's area but which involve the adjacent heteromodal fields of the angular gyrus in the language-dominant hemisphere give rise to complex combinations of anomia, alexia, acalculia, dysgraphia, finger identification disturbances, and left–right naming difficulties in the absence of additional language deficits. This collection of impairments is collectively known as the "left angular gyrus (or left parietal) syndrome." When only the last four of these deficits emerge in isolation, the term "Gerstmann syndrome" is used to identify the clinical picture. Both syndromes indicate a breakdown in complex multimodal interactions related to verbal processing. In contrast to "pure alexia," which is a modality-specific disconnection syndrome, the alexia which arises in conjunction with angular gyrus damage is caused by a breakdown of multimodal associations related to language and is known as a "central alexia."

Damage to the heteromodal cortices of the inferior parietal lobule in the right hemisphere leads to deficits in tasks of spatial attention, visuospatial integration, and drawing (construction). This is known as the "right parietal lobe syndrome." Patients fail tasks of mental rotation and cannot identify objects viewed from uncommon perspectives. The posterior parietal cortex also plays a pivotal role in spatial attention and causes contralesional neglect when damaged (Chapter 3). Functional imaging experiments show that the part of posterior parietal cortex that is critical for spatial attention (area P in Fig. 1–11b) is centered around the intraparietal cortex.[172,390] Its proposed role in the attentional network is to integrate distributed spatial information (originating from "s" in multiple modalities as shown in Fig. 1–11b) in all relevant sensory modalities.[336] When this area is damaged, the modality-specific channels of information related to the extrapersonal space may remain intact but cannot be bound into the type of coherent and interactive representation that is necessary for the adaptive deployment of spatial attention. As in the relationship of transmodal nodes to other cognitive domains, posterior parietal cortex is not a dedicated center which contains a spatial map but a critical gateway for accessing and integrating information related to the attention-related representation and exploration of the extrapersonal space. This aspect of posterior parietal function is reviewed in greater detail in Chapter 3.

Other components of the right parietal syndrome include "anosognosia" (minimization or denial of illness), "dressing apraxia" (inability to align the body axis with the axis of the garment), "construction apraxia" (drawing difficulty), confusional states, route finding deficits, and disturbances in navigating the body with respect to solid objects such as beds and chairs. As noted above, Bálint's syndrome represents a breakdown of all visuospatial integration and usually arises after bilateral dorsal lesions in posterior parietal cortex. Such lesions interrupt the dorsal visuofugal pathway shown in Fig. 1–10, giving rise to optic apraxia, optic ataxia and simultanagnosia as described in Chapter 7.

In addition to these deficits, lesions in parietotemporal heteromodal cortices also yield perturbations of mood and motivation. The neglect which results from parietal lesions, for example, includes an aspect of motivational indifference for the contralateral hemispace, and anosognosia reflects a global impairment in the emotional response to disability. In other patients, lesions in the posterior parietotemporal regions of the right hemisphere lead to psychotic and affective disturbances.[192,422] Furthermore, patients with Wernicke's aphasia can show severe mood alterations ranging from anger to paranoia and indifference. These clinical manifestations might reflect a disruption of the complex sensory–limbic interactions which take place within heteromodal cortices.

In the brain of the monkey, anatomical and physiological evidence suggests the presence of an additional heteromodal field in the ventromedial parts of the temporal lobe, corresponding to the medial part of BA20.[117,484] An analogous area may also be present in the human brain, perhaps including parts of BA36, 20 and 37, along the banks of the collateral sulcus (Fig. 1–7). Cerebrovascular accidents that involve this heteromodal association area and adjacent paralimbic regions give rise to agitated confusional states (Chapter 3).

X. Prefrontal Heteromodal Cortex and Frontal Lobe Syndromes: Attention, Executive Functions, and Comportment

The frontal lobes undergo a striking expansion in the course of phylogenetic evolution. In the human brain, they occupy approximately one-third of the cerebral hemispheres. The frontal lobes can be divided into three functional sectors (Fig. 1–7).

1. A "motor–premotor" sector includes BA4 and 6, the supplementary motor area (medial aspect of BA6), the frontal eye fields (BA6 in the human, BA8 in the monkey), the supplementary eye fields (BA6), and parts of Broca's area (BA44). Depending on the exact location of the lesion, damage to this component of the frontal lobe results in weakness, alteration of muscle tone, release of grasp reflexes, incontinence, akinesia, mutism, aprosody, apraxia, and some motor components of unilateral neglect and Broca's aphasia.

2. A "paralimbic" sector is located in the ventral and medial part of the frontal lobe and contains the cortices of the anterior cingulate complex (BA23, 32), the parolfactory gyrus (gyrus rectus, BA25), and the posterior orbitofrontal regions (BA11–13).

3. An extensive "heteromodal" sector contains BA9–10, anterior BA11–12, and BA45–47. In the monkey, this region receives neural inputs from unimodal areas in all the major sensory modalities, from all the other heteromodal regions of the brain, and from many paralimbic areas.[23,24,78,343,369,398] As in the case of parietotemporal heteromodal cortices, some neurons respond to a single preferred modality but are intermixed with those which respond to another; others are truly multimodal and respond to several kinds of sensory input.[34,46,237]

The terms "prefrontal cortex" and "frontal lobe syndrome" generally refer only to the paralimbic and heteromodal sectors of the frontal lobe. Prefrontal cortex can be conceptualized as a site for the confluence of two functional axes: one for working memory–executive function–attention (with transmodal epicenters in prefrontal and posterior parietal cortex), and another for comportment (with transmodal epicenters in prefrontal cortex and orbitofrontal paralimbic cortex). The head of the caudate nucleus and the mediodorsal nucleus of the thalamus are critical subcortical components for both of these functional axes.

The Clinical Picture of Frontal Lobe Syndromes

Few subjects have engendered as much enigma, paradox and fascination as the behavioral affiliations of prefrontal cortex. While some authors have attributed the highest integrative faculties of the human mind to this part of the brain,[1,52,181] others have emphasized the surprising paucity of cognitive deficits in patients with substantial frontal lobe damage.[211,282] The case of Phineas Gage (also known as the Boston Crowbar Case), reported more than a century ago by Harlow,[203] remains paradigmatic for research on the frontal lobes. Gage was a reliable and upright foreman who became profane, irascible, and irresponsible following an accident during which a tamping rod was blown through his frontal lobes. The many reports that have been published since Harlow's paper have provided additional support for the conclusions derived from the case of Phineas Gage—namely, that frontal lobe damage can lead to dramatic alterations of strategic thinking, personality, emotional integration, and comportment (conduct) while leaving language, memory, and sensory–motor functions relatively intact. In an almost equally remarkable account, for example, Penfield recorded the effects of a right sided prefrontal lobectomy he had performed on his own sister.[404] Following the acute postoperative period, Penfield noted that his sister's judgment, insight, social graces, and cognitive abilities were quite preserved. When he visited her home as a dinner guest, however, he noticed a diminished capacity for the planned preparation and administration of the meal and a slowing of thinking.

The spectrum of behavioral changes observed in patients with prefrontal lesions is very broad. Some of these patients become puerile, profane, slovenly, facetious, grandiose, and irascible; others lose spontaneity, curiosity, and initiative and develop an apathetic blunting of feeling, drive, mentation, and behavior; others show an erosion of foresight, judgment, and insight, and lose the ability to delay gratification and often the capacity for remorse; still others show an impairment of abstract reasoning, creativity, problem solving, and mental flexibility, and become excessively concrete or stimulus-bound.[332,354] The orderly planning and sequencing of complex behaviors, strategic decision making based on the assessment of differential risks, the ability to heed several events simultaneously and flexibly shift the focus of concentration from one to the other, the capacity for grasping the context and gist of a complex situation, the resistance to distraction and interference, the ability to follow multistep instructions, the inhibition of immediate but inappropriate response tendencies, and the ability to sustain behavioral output without perseveration may each become markedly disrupted.[105,176,182,332]

Although the designation "frontal syndrome" is used as an umbrella term for the entire panoply of the behavioral changes noted above, each patient may have a different distribution of salient deficits. The specific pattern of the behavioral deficits in an individual patient is probably determined by the site, size, laterality, nature, and temporal course of the lesion and perhaps even by the past personality and age of the patient. In general, two types of frontal syndromes are seen. In one type, the loss of creativity, initiative and curiosity predominates and the patient shows apathy and emotional blunting. This can be designated as the "syndrome of frontal abulia." In a second type, the patient displays a dramatic impulsivity, together with a loss of judgment, insight, and foresight. This can be designated as the "syndrome of frontal disinhibition." In this second type of frontal syndrome, the dissociation between relatively intact "cognitive" functions and dramatically impaired comportment and emotional reactions can be quite striking.[135]

Following the surgical removal of an olfactory groove meningioma, for example, a 63-year-old administrator started to initiate intimate relations with total strangers, one of whom had just been released from jail. She agreed that her behavior was unwise and admitted that she "lacked brakes." However, neither the theft of personal belongings nor a bout of sexually transmitted disease could curb her poor judgment. In the office, her performance in so-called "frontal" tasks such as the *Luria motor sequences*, the *Stroop Interference Task*, the *Wisconsin Card Sorting Test*, and the *Tower of London* were all in the normal range. Her postsurgical scans indicated that the major area of damage involved the orbitofrontal cortex and that the dorsolateral prefrontal areas were relatively intact (Fig. 1–9b). A somewhat different clinical picture emerged in a 47-year-old attorney following the removal of a left prefrontal meningioma. Neuropsychological tests revealed some impairments of memory retrieval and reasoning abilities. The most dramatic changes, however, took the form of an amotivational state, emotional blunting, and a slowing of thinking. These impairments interfered with his professional activities and led to early retirement. The postsurgical scans showed a large left prefrontal lesion involving mostly the dorsolateral prefrontal cortex and sparing much of the orbitofrontal region (Fig. 1–9c). The lesion was predominantly unilateral but a shunt tube had been inserted through the dorsolateral prefrontal cortex of the contralateral hemisphere into the lateral ventricle and caused additional damage in the right hemisphere.

In keeping with these two examples, clinical experience suggests that lesions in orbitofrontal and medial frontal areas (that is, parts of the frontal lobe that contain paralimbic cortex) are more likely to trigger the disinhibition syndrome whereas lesions in the dorsolateral frontal lobe (the parts containing heteromodal cortex) are more likely to cause the abulic syndrome.[171,355] In chimpanzees and monkeys, dorsolateral prefrontal lesions elicit a predominantly abulic state whereas orbitofrontal lesions lead to emotional impulsivity.[64,241] The more dramatic manifestations of frontal lobe damage are seen after bilateral involvement. The deficits associated with unilateral lesions can be quite subtle and often elusive. The abulia of frontal lobe disease may be misinterpreted as a sign of depression whereas the disinhibition may occasionally lead to the mistaken diagnosis of mania.

Neuropsychology of Frontal Lobe Disease

As also noted in Chapter 3, prefrontal cortex plays a particularly critical role in attentional behaviors. The P300 response evoked by novel or deviant stimuli, for example, is critically dependent on the integrity of prefrontal cortex; an N2–P3 response over prefrontal cortex appears to determine the attentional resources that will be allocated to novel events; and the region of the frontal eye fields belongs to a distributed network for exploring the extrapersonal space and seeking motivationally relevant targets.[102,271,329] The abulic state resulting from frontal lobe lesions could thus represent the loss of neural mechanisms involved in novelty-seeking behaviors.

Frontal lobe lesions often impair "working memory," an attentional faculty which enables the mental manipulation and on-line holding of information for durations that fall between those of iconic memory and long-term "off-line" storage (Chapter 3). Such lesions also interfere with performance in tasks that require the inhibition of impulsive responses.[288] In keeping with these clinical correlations, single unit recordings in monkeys show that many prefrontal neurons alter their activity during the response inhibition phase of behavioral pradigms and that they emit responses related to the on-line holding of information during working memory tasks.[116,160] Furthermore, prefrontal neurons can also support the on-line *convergence* of information. In one experiment, for example, monkeys were given a task that required them to retain first the identity of an object and then its location. After participating in the on-line retention of object information in the initial working memory interval, many prefrontal neurons switched modes and maintained the on-line representation of spatial information during the second interval.[428]

As shown in Chapter 3, each part of unimodal association cortex seems to participate in the maintenance of working memory in its own area of specialization. Lateral prefrontal cortex, however, plays a critical supramodal role in orchestrating working memory in all domains of processing.[116] As a transmodal zone at the fifth and sixth synaptic levels in Figure 1–11b, prefrontal cortex (area Pf in Figure 1–11b) is interconnected with numerous transmodal and downstream unimodal areas and can exert a top–down influence upon the working memory activity of neurons in all of these areas.[116,161] Prefrontal cortex may thus play the role of a critical transmodal gateway for coordinating working memory in a manner analogous to the role of temporal transmodal cortex in object recognition, and of Wernicke's area in language.

Working memory is usually divided into two groups of processes: the attentional on-line maintenance of information and its volitional manipulation. The latter aspect is attributed to the function of a "central executive" agency. In human subjects, tasks emphasizing the executive aspects of working memory elicit the activation of prefrontal dorsolateral cortex,[101,271a] whereas tasks emphasizing the on-line maintenance of information elicit the activation of both prefrontal cortex and posterior parietal cortex.[90,279] These two interconnected heteromodal areas may thus function as the epicenters of a distributed network for the on-line holding aspect of working memory. In fact, working memory tasks enhance the electrophysiological coherence between the prefrontal and posterior parietal regions of the human brain.[466] Furthermore, clinical experience indicates that working memory deficits can arise after lesions in prefrontal as well as in posterior parietal cortex. In the latter instance, however, the clinical picture tends to be overshadowed by the other components of the parietal lobe syndrome. In contrast, working memory deficits may dominate the clinical presentation of many patients with prefrontal lesions.

Neuropsychological test results in patients with frontal lobe disease are consistent with the critical role of this area in working memory, executive function, and the inhibition of inappropriate impulses. Thus, concentration (as assessed by digit span), the ability to resist interference, hypothesis testing (as assessed by the *Wisconsin Card Sorting Test*), the ability to maintain a coherent stream of thought, the ability to scan mental content (as assessed by verbal fluency and memory retrieval tasks), the ability to resist immediate but inappropriate response tendencies (as assessed by the go–no go task), and the ability to internally program, select and sequence responses are usually impaired after prefrontal lesions. Cognitive flexibility, especially when behavior needs to be modified to fit novel contexts, is also vulnerable to frontal lobe damage.[175] During reasoning tasks, patients with frontal lobe disease tend to reach closure prematurely, jump to conclusions on the basis of incomplete information, perseverate, and find it difficult to explore alternative solutions to the same problem. Many of these cognitive deficits are attributed to a loss of "executive" functions because they reflect a failure to manipulate existing information rather than a failure to perceive, recognize, name, or remember. In keeping with these correlations, prefrontal activation is seen during the performance of verbal fluency and go–no-go tasks and during the initial exposure to a reasoning test but not during its second presentation.[76,144,304,412,438,439]

Frontal lobe disease leads to the emergence of stimulus-bound and concrete behaviors. Some patients display a remarkable tendency to imitate the examiner's gestures and behaviors even when no instruction has been given to do so; others feel compelled to use objects that they encounter even when the context is inappropriate.[293,294] These tendencies, descriptively labeled "imitation" and "utilization" behaviors, reflect slavish and reflex responses to the environment. Many cognitive functions coordinated by prefrontal cortex, including working memory, require rapid and reversible shifts of the attentional focus between external sensory events and internal mental representations. In a very general sense, prefrontal cortex can be said to orient the attentional focus toward internal mental processes whereas posterior parietal cortex orients it toward extrapersonal events.[332] When the brain is intact, these two tendencies balance each other and provide a setting where flexible transitions from one realm to the other can unfold without fixed bias. Prefrontal lesions disrupt this balance by tilting the emphasis away from internal mental processes toward stimulus-bound utilization behaviors, whereas posterior parietal lesions may tilt the emphasis away from external sensory events and promote sensory neglect.

The connectivity pattern in Figure 1–12 indicates that the frontal lobe provides a site where association cortices and the limbic system interact. The limbic connections may allow the frontal lobes, especially their paralimbic components, to link the sensorial aspects of external events with the visceral and emotional states they elicit. The establishment of such linkages would allow the original visceral state to

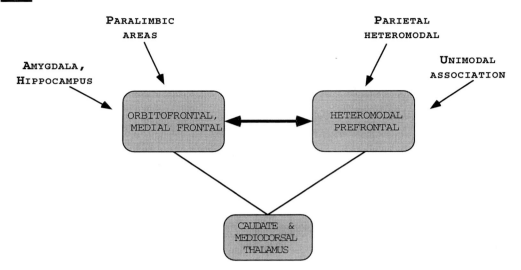

FIGURE 1–12. Major connections of prefrontal cortex.

be reactivated upon the recurrence or even anticipation of a similar event.[105] The anticipatory induction of such a visceral state could then generate a positive or negative valence that biases the choice of subsequent behaviors. In neurologically intact individuals, such visceral states can play important roles in the covert guidance of decision making, especially when the decisions require an instantaneous assessment of relative risk.[32]

Damage to the orbitofrontal or medial components of the frontal lobes can interfere with the interactions between behavior and visceral state and may provide a physiological substrate for poor judgment and foresight.[105] As opposed to normal subjects who emitted anticipatory changes of skin conductance when pondering risky choices, for example, patients with ventral and medial prefrontal lesions failed to generate such responses, appeared unresponsive to the consequences of their actions, and failed to acquire a successful strategy for making advantageous decisions.[32] This disengagement of behavior from emotional guidance may underlie the failure of these patients to learn from experience and their inability to inhibit behaviors which consistently have disastrous consequences. Prefrontal disease acquired early in life may thus interfere with the development of social restraint, leading to a syndrome of "comportmental" learning disabilities.[421]

Frontal lobe damage may also lead to a "task difficulty effect," whereby performance in virtually all areas begins to decline rapidly when the effort required of the patient exceeds a certain level. This indicates a motivational deficit rather than impairment of additional cognitive skills. Explicit memory is usually preserved except when there is major damage to the paralimbic components of the frontal lobes or when the lesions extend into the basal forebrain and hypothalamus.[351,359,492] Secondary memory disturbances emerge quite frequently as a consequence of the inattention, poor motivation, perseveration, and especially inefficient retrieval

(Chapter 4). Performance in most tests of perception, construction, language, and directed spatial attention can be quite intact even after massive damage to the anterior and ventromedial parts of prefrontal cortex.

Some patients with sizable frontal lobe lesions may have routine neurological and neuropsychological examinations that are quite unremarkable. This paucity of "objective" findings is sometimes responsible for overlooking the possibility of brain damage in some of these patients. Patients with known frontal lobe lesions and a history of major behavioral difficulties may behave impeccably in the office. This is in keeping with the notion that these patients are most impaired under circumstances with minimal external control, when self-guidance becomes critical. The office setting may introduce sufficient external structure to suppress some of these behavioral tendencies. The same patient who gives perfect answers to questions about hypothetical social or moral dilemmas in the office may also act with a total lack of judgment when faced with the real situation. The clinical adage that judgment and complex comportment cannot be tested in the office is particularly pertinent to the evaluation of patients with frontal lobe damage. It is also important to realize that the great majority of patients with frontal lobe disease do not have "frontal release signs" such as grasping, rooting, or sucking. These primitive reflexes emerge only if the lesion extends into the motor–premotor sectors of the frontal lobe.

Metaphysiology of Prefrontal Cortex

Frontal cortex is so heterogeneous with respect to structure, connectivity, and physiology that no single descriptive formulation can account for its multiple behavioral affiliations. There are, however, at least six key themes that help to provide a metaphysiological basis for the behavioral specializations of prefrontal cortex:

1. Even massive damage to prefrontal cortex leaves all sensation, perception, movement, and homeostatic functions intact. The heteromodal sector of the frontal lobe is probably the only nonlimbic part of the cerebral cortex entirely devoted to complex mental integration.

2. Prefrontal cortex has a high density of interconnections with almost all other heteromodal, unimodal, paralimbic, and limbic sectors of the cerebral cortex. Through these widespread connections, prefrontal cortex would be in a position to activate a given network, suppress another, and orchestrate network interactions.

3. As noted above, some prefrontal neurons display preferential activity during the response inhibition phase of go–no-go and delayed alteration tasks.[160] Prefrontal cortex may thus play an important role in inhibiting impulses that are not appropriate for the context and in disengaging stimuli from their customary responses so that alternative scenarios can be played out internally in a way that promotes flexibility, foresight, and planning.

4. Many of the visually responsive neurons in prefrontal cortex have far less specificity for color, size, orientation, or movement than for the behavioral relevance of the stimulus.[275,353] A neuron which responds briskly to a stimulus when it is associated with reward, for example, may drastically alter its response when the same stimulus becomes associated with an aversive or neutral outcome.[272,461] These response contingencies suggest that the neurons of prefrontal cortex can help to establish a subjective reality which is sensitive to significance rather than surface properties.

5. Its relationship to working memory suggests that prefrontal cortex can transform information access from a sequential process, where only one item can be heeded at any given time, to a conjunctive pattern where multiple items become concurrently accessible.[339] Through the mediation of working memory, representations of multiple external events and internal phenomena can unfold concurrently and interactively so that the focus of attention can move from one to the other. The resultant increase in the number of factors and variables that can be apprehended simultaneously would seem essential for dissociating appearance from significance, grasping changes of context, shifting from one mental set to another, assuming multiple perspectives, and comparing potential outcomes of contemplated actions. Disruptions in these aspects of mental function could lead to impairments of foresight, strategic thinking, and risk management.[176,182,354]

6. The orbitofrontal cortex and other paralimbic components of the frontal lobe provide transmodal nodes for binding thoughts, memories, and experiences with corresponding visceral and emotional states. Damage to this component interferes with the ability of emotion and visceral state to guide behavior, especially in complex and ambiguous situations.

Despite considerable advances in this area of research, it is difficult to dismiss the sense of uniqueness associated with frontal lobe function. It is quite remarkable, for example, that sizable frontal lobe lesions can remain clinically silent for many years. Even after massive bifrontal lesions in monkeys, chimpanzees, and humans, change can often be detected only in comparison with the previous personality of that individual rather than in reference to any set of absolute behavioral standards. In fact, many of the alterations associated with prefrontal lesions appear to overlap with the range of normal human behavior: There is a vast number of improvident, imprudent, irresponsible, inappropriate, and facetious individuals who have no evidence of demonstrable brain damage. In contrast, the lack of visible damage to the pertinent cerebral area is a rare occurrence in individuals with aphasia, amnesia, apraxia, or unilateral neglect. Perhaps this means that the prefrontal cortex underlies functions that are much less "hard wired" and that it acts predominantly as an orchestrator for integrating other cortical areas and for calling up behavior programs that are appropriate for context. Damage to this part of the brain would thus result in behavioral deficits that are context-dependent rather than absolute.

Frontal Lobe Versus Frontal Network Syndromes

The major cortical connections of the head of the caudate nucleus and the mediodorsal nucleus of the thalamus come from prefrontal cortex. These two structures can therefore be considered as subcortical components of the prefrontal network. In fact, clinical deficits identical to the frontal lobe syndromes can also be seen in patients with lesions in the head of the caudate nucleus or in the mediodorsal nucleus of the thalamus.[327,436,464,508] This may explain why so many extrapyramidal diseases tend to be associated with behavioral and cognitive changes that display at least some characteristic of the frontal syndrome.

Frontal syndromes can also emerge as common manifestations of multifocal white matter diseases or even metabolic encephalopathy.[558] Assuming that at least one physiological function of the frontal lobe is to integrate networks for combined action, multifocal partial lesions (none of which is individually severe enough to disrupt specific cognitive domains such as language or memory) could collectively undermine internetwork coordination and therefore lead to the manifestations of a frontal lobe syndrome. In fact, clinical experience suggests that subcortical lesions (as in cerebrovascular or demyelinating diseases) and toxic–metabolic encephalopathies are more frequent causes of the frontal syndrome than lesions which involve prefrontal cortex directly. In order to avoid the embarrassment of diagnosing frontal lobe disease in patients with no frontal pathology, it is preferable to use the term "frontal network syndrome" and to emphasize that the responsible lesion can be anywhere within the cortical or subcortical components of a distributed prefrontal network.

XI. Paralimbic (Mesocortical) Areas

A belt of paralimbic areas encircles the basal and medial aspects of the cerebral hemispheres (Figs. 1–5 and 1–7). The olfactocentric paralimbic formations include the temporal pole, the insula, and posterior orbitofrontal cortex. The hippocampocentric paralimbic formations include the parahippocampal "rhinal" cortices, the retrosplenial area, the cingulate gyrus, and the subcallosal (parolfactory) regions. Paralimbic areas provide zones of architectonic transitions from allocortical limbic areas to isocortical association cortex (Figs. 1–3B and 1–4). The peri-allocortical sectors of individual paralimbic areas are most heavily interconnected with the peri-allocortical sectors of other paralimbic areas and with core limbic areas, whereas the peri-isocortical sectors are more heavily interconnected with the peri-isocortical sectors of the other paralimbic areas and with sensory association cortices.[343,367,369] Reciprocal hypothalamic projections of medium density are found in all paralimbic areas and tend to be directed mostly to their peri-allocortical sectors. In keeping with this pattern of connectivity, the peri-allocortical sectors of paralimbic areas have more "limbic" behavioral specializations whereas the peri-isocortical sectors have specializations more similar to those of adjacent unimodal and heteromodal association cortices.

Paralimbic areas play an important role in linking cognition with visceral states and emotion. Even to a greater extent than heteromodal areas, paralimbic cortices are in a position to emphasize the behavioral relevance of a stimulus over its physical aspects. Paralimbic cortices make critical contributions to at least four types of behavior: (*1*) memory and learning, (*2*) the channeling of emotion and affiliative behaviors, (*3*) the linkage of visceral state, immune responses, and endocrine balance to mental state, (*4*) and the perception of pain, smell, and taste. The relationship of paralimbic areas to memory and emotion is discussed in subsequent sections on the hippocampus and amygdala (section XIII and XIV). The relationship to autonomic function, immune system, endocrine control, pain, smell and taste is reviewed in this section.

The Insula

The human insula contains up to seven sulci and could be considered as a separate lobe of the brain. The region where the insula becomes joined to the anterior part of the temporal lobe contains the piriform cortex and the agranular peri-allocortical sector of the insula (Fig. 1–4). Cytoarchitectonic differentiation emanates radially from this agranular peri-allocortical sector and establishes a gradual transition into the peri-isocortical sectors. The insula abuts upon the frontal and parietal opercula dorsally and the supratemporal plane ventrally. The peri-insular part of the frontoparietal operculum contains the gustatory cortex anteriorly and area SII posteriorly. The peri-insular parts of the temporal lobe contain piriform olfactory cortex anteriorly and the auditory and vestibular areas posteriorly. In the monkey, the more peri-allocortical anterior and ventral parts of the insula tend to be associated with autonomic, olfactory, gustatory, and other "limbic" functions whereas the peri-isocortical posterior insula displays many characteristics of somatosensory association cortex dorsally, auditory cortex ventrally, and vestibular cortex posteriorly.[16,195,343]

The limbic inputs into the insula come from primary olfactory cortex, the amygdala, and the nucleus basalis. The amygdaloid connections are reciprocal and directed predominantly to the peri-allocortical sectors of the insula. Through these pathways, the insula can relay somatosensory and other types of sensory information into the amygdala and can play an important role in mediating tactile learning and the reaction to pain. Insular lesions may thus contribute to the emergence of pain asymbolia and tactile learning impairments. Connectivity patterns suggest that the insula may provide a synaptic relay between Wernicke's and Broca's areas.[343] In keeping with these anatomical relationships, insular lesions can lead to aphasias and articulatory deficits.[127] These heterogeneous anatomical relationships and behavioral affiliations help to explain why so many functional imaging studies, based on so many different paradigms, include the insula in the list of cortical areas activated by the experimental task.

Orbitofrontal Cortex

The term "orbitofrontal cortex" is used to designate the entire ventral surface of the frontal lobes. The posterior part of orbitofrontal cortex abuts upon the parolfactory component of the cingulate complex, piriform olfactory cortex, the anterior olfactory nucleus, and the insula. This part of orbitofrontal cortex is architectonically more primitive and behaviorally more "limbic" in character. It has reciprocal hypothalamic projections of intermediate intensity. The limbic inputs into orbitofrontal cortex, directed predominantly to its posterior part, come from primary olfactory cortex, the nucleus basalis, the hippocampus, and the amygdala. The hippocampal projections are directed predominantly to the medial part of posterior orbitofrontal cortex.[369,450] Anterior orbitofrontal cortex has the appearance of granular isocortex and blends into the dorsolateral heteromodal components of prefrontal cortex. Its behavioral affiliations are likely to have many similarities with those of dorsolateral heteromodal prefrontal cortex. Orbitofrontal cortex is likely to play a critical role in the integration of visceral and emotional states with cognition and comportment. The most florid comportmental deficits associated with frontal lobe lesions can probably be attributed to the involvement of the orbitofrontal and adjacent medial frontal areas.

The Temporal Pole

The temporopolar cortex caps the anterior tip of the temporal lobe. Its junction with the insula occurs through piriform cortex. This junctional area also contains the peri-allocortical part of temporopolar cortex. Gradual cytoarchitectonic differentiation emanates radially from this sector and leads to the emergence of the peri-isocortical sectors dorsally and ventrally.[367] In addition to inputs from primary olfactory cortex, limbic connections are also established with the nucleus basalis, hippocampus, and especially the amygdala. The principal behavioral affiliations of temporopolar cortex include olfactory–gustatory–visceral function medially, auditory function dorsally, visual function ventrally, and multimodal integration laterally. The medial, dorsal and ventral parts of temporopolar cortex mediate sensory–limbic interactions whereas its lateral part may fulfill the role of a transmodal epicenter for face recognition.[165]

The Cingulate Complex and the Medial Frontal Area

The cingulate complex belongs to the hippocampocentric group of paralimbic areas. It includes the retrosplenial region, the cingulate gyrus, and the parolfactory area (Fig. 1–7). The peri-allocortical parts of the parolfactory and cingulate cortices abut upon the hippocampal rudiment (induseum griseum), display a distinctively non-isocortical architecture, and have the most prominent "limbic" affiliations. The more dorsal peri-isocortical part of the cingulate gyrus has characteristics of sensory association cortex posteriorly where it borders medial parietal cortex and of premotor cortex anteriorly where it borders the supplementary motor area.

The cingulate complex can be conceptualized as a supracallosal extension of the hippocampal–parahippocampal region: The induseum griseum is a dorsal extension of the hippocampus, the retrosplenial cortex of the presubiculum, and the cingulate gyrus of the parahippocampal gyrus. The parolfactory component (BA25) of the cingulate complex is in direct continuity with the gyrus rectus of orbitofrontal cortex and has reciprocal hypothalamic connections similar in intensity to those of orbitofrontal cortex. The major limbic connections of the cingulate complex come from the hippocampus and the amygdala. The hippocampal projections reach mostly the posterior parts of the cingulate complex whereas the amygdaloid projections are directed mostly to its anterior parts. In keeping with the characteristic pattern of paralimbic areas, the behavioral affiliations are heterogeneous and include attention, memory, learning, motivation, emotion, pain perception, and visceral function.[76,118,234] The role of the cingulate cortex in attention is discussed in Chapter 3.

There is often a tendency to refer to "medial frontal cortex" as if it represented a distinct and uniform entity. This region represents a confluence of the cingulate complex (BA32 and BA25), orbitofrontal cortex (posterior parts of BA11–13), and dorsolateral heteromodal prefrontal cortex (BA9–10). Neurological lesions in this part of the brain can thus give rise to complex combinations of comportmental, cognitive, attentional, and emotional disturbances.[288]

The "Rhinal" Cortices and the Parahippocampal Region

The parahippocampal component of the paralimbic belt contains the "rhinal" cortices (entorhinal, prorhinal, and perirhinal (transentorhinal) areas), the presubiculum, and the parasubiculum. Each of these components has a distinctly nonisocortical architecture. The entorhinal area is in direct anatomical continuity with the hippocampal complex and can be conceptualized as the peri-allocortical sector of the parahippocampal paralimbic region. (Fig. 1–3b). In the monkey, the prorhinal and perirhinal components are separated from each other by a prominent rhinal sulcus. The prorhinal cortex and the rhinal sulcus are both quite inconspicuous in the human brain. Instead, the collateral sulcus emerges as the dominant sulcal landmark and contains the perirhinal cortex in its medial bank. The banks of the collateral sulcus contain the transitional and peri-isocortical sectors of the parahippocampal paralimbic region (Fig. 3a, b).

The entorhinal and perirhinal (transentorhinal) areas are very prominent in the human brain. The entorhinal cortex reaches the crest of the collateral sulcus and blends into the transentorhinal (perirhinal) cortex on the medial bank of the sulcus. The rhinal cortices receive limbic connections from olfactory cortex, the nucleus basalis, the amygdala, and especially the hippocampus. Additional inputs come from multiple unimodal and heteromodal areas. The entorhinal and transentorhinal cortices collectively provide the single most critical relay for transmitting information from heteromodal and unimodal association areas into the hippocampal formation.[531] These projections travel within the perforant pathway. Reciprocal hippocampo–entorhinal projections originate from the subiculum and CA1 sector of the hippocampus. The two-way interconnections between the entorhinal–transentorhinal cortex and the hippocampus are so massive that the two structures could be conceptualized as forming a unified hippocampo–entorhinal complex. Although the rhinal cortices also have olfactory, emotional, and visceral functions, their major behavioral affiliations are in the areas of memory and learning (Section XIV).

Visceral, Immune, and Endocrine Regulation in Paralimbic and Limbic Areas

The intimate association of limbic and paralimbic areas with autonomic function has led to their collective characterization as the "visceral brain."[306] This characterization is supported by numerous experiments which show that electrical stimulations in the amygdala, hippocampus, anterior insula, anterior cingulate gyrus, posterior orbitofrontal cortex, and the temporal pole yield marked and consistent autonomic responses.[81,224,254,255,393,405,418,490,509,541] This is why autonomic discharges and visceral sensations are so common in patients with temporolimbic epilepsy (Chapter 8). The efferent limb of these autonomic responses in based on projections from limbic and paralimbic areas to the hypothalamus and brainstem whereas the afferent limb is based on multisynaptic visceral inputs from the brainstem and thalamus.[19,553]

Insular stimulation is most likely to yield gastrointestinal responses whereas stimulation in the each of the other areas (including the insula) yields cardiovascular and respiratory changes. Some autonomic effects of paralimbic stimulation can be quite dramatic and include inhibition of gastric peristalsis, respiratory arrest, and blood pressure changes of as much as 100 mm of mercury. Even multifocal cardiac necrosis can be obtained when monkeys with no intrinsic cardiovascular disease receive electrical stimulation to orbitofrontal cortex. Furthermore, cingulate lesions and amygdaloid stimulation can lead to the development of gastric ulcers in rats.[201,219,220]

Normal human emotions are associated with distinctive changes of heart rate, blood pressure, gastrointestinal motility, salivation, and sweating. These visceral correlates influence the way in which the emotion is expressed and experienced. On the maladaptive side, psychological stress increases blood pressure, promotes the formation of ulcers, leads to abnormalities of esophageal motility and can even induce potentially lethal cardiac arrythmias in the absence of cardiovascular predisposing factors.[87,302] Cognitive processes ranging from mental arithmetic to decision making can also elicit specific patterns of autonomic activity. Such autonomic responses vary according to the difficulty of the task, the type of ongoing information processing, the anticipated consequences of the contemplated response, and the significance of the task to the individual.[17,105,142,257,281,348] These autonomic concomitants can influence the performance of the cognitive task and its emotional coloring.[105,281] Paralimbic cortices are likely to play important roles in these linkages of visceral patterns to mood and cognition. Dysfunction of limbic or paralimbic areas may thus perturb the adaptive interactions between mental activity and visceral state, distort the experience of emotion, undermine the visceral guidance of comportment (as described in section X, on the frontal lobes), and perhaps even lead to the maladaptive (psychosomatic) autonomic manifestations of stress and anxiety.

Limbic and paralimbic areas also influence the function of the immune and endocrine systems. Associating a taste with an immunosuppressive drug causes rats to show an inhibition of immune responses when subsequently exposed to the same taste. This conditioned immunosuppression is severely impaired after insular (but not parietal) lesions.[426] Furthermore, lesions of the amygdala (as well as of the hippocampus and hypothalamus) lead to marked alterations in lymphoid cell number and lymphocyte activation.[58] Limbic and paralimbic areas may thus provide potential anatomical substrates for the putative influence of mental state upon immune responses and autoimmune disorders.[443] Through hypothalamic connections, limbic and paralimbic areas can influence the secretion of releasing factors which regulate the adrenal, thyroid, and gonadal endocrine systems. The reciprocal influence between limbic dysfunction and gonadal steroids is reviewed in Chapter 8.

Taste, Smell, and Pain in Paralimbic Areas

In contrast to the auditory, visual, and somatosensory sensations which are processed predominantly within association isocortex, olfaction, gustation, and pain are closely related to paralimbic and limbic zones of the brain. The primary olfactory cortex is itself an allocortical limbic structure, whereas the primary gustatory cortex is situated in the frontal operculum, immediately adjacent to the anterior insula.[465] In monkeys, cortical responses to olfactory and gustatory stimulation are readily obtained in the orbitofrontal and insular paralimbic areas.[511,512,516] Damage to temporopolar, anterior insular, or posterior orbitofrontal cortex in monkeys impairs behaviors that depend on olfactory and gustatory discrimination.[20,511,512]

In humans, anterior temporal lobectomy disrupts olfactory learning and discrimination whereas olfactory stimulation activates orbitofrontal, anterior insular, and amygdaloid regions.[131,264,432,575] In one experiment, exposure to a salty taste led to the activation of the insula, anterior cingulate, and parahippocampal gyrus, emphasizing the sensitivity of the entire paralimbic zone to gustatory stimulation.[268] In one of our patients, the appreciation of flavor was impaired by a stroke which involved the insula of the right hemisphere. A former gourmet with a penchant for French food and fine wine, the patient reported that he was no longer able to appreciate subtle flavors and that he had started to crave highly spiced foods he would have shunned in the past. This change occurred despite a preservation of the patient's ability to discriminate basic gustatory stimuli.

The close anatomical linkage between paralimbic regions and olfactory–gustatory sensation explains why olfactory and gustatory hallucinations are so common in temporolimbic epilepsy. Olfactory and gustatory sensations may have a close affiliation with the limbic and paralimbic zones of the brain because they have evolved from chemical senses closely related to the monitoring of the internal milieu. The limbic affiliations of these two modalities are consistent with the critical roles they play in the guidance of apetitive behaviors, the identification of territorial markers, and the regulation of sexual behaviors.

Another sensation closely linked to emotion and visceral state is pain. Paralimbic areas contain a particularly high density of endogenous opiates.[291] Functional imaging experiments have detected anterior insular and cingulate activation in response to noxious stimuli applied either to the viscera or to the periphery.[19,77] The relay of pain-related somatosensory information into limbic areas may be mediated by SII and the posterior insula. As described earlier, damage to these areas can cause an emotional indifference to noxious stimuli known as "pain asymbolia" (section V).

XII. LIMBIC STRUCTURES OF THE SEPTAL AREA, NUCLEUS BASALIS, AND PIRIFORM CORTEX

The constituents of the limbic zone include the septal area, the substantia innominata, the amygdala, the piriform cortex, and the hippocampal formation. These are the parts of the cerebral cortex which have the most intense reciprocal interconnections with the hypothalamus. The behavioral specializations of these limbic structures are similar to those of paralimbic regions but are even more closely related to memory, drive, and emotion.

Septal Nuclei and the Nucleus Basalis of the Substantia Innominata

The basal forebrain contains several interdigitated cell groups. Four of these cell groups (the medial septal nucleus, the vertical and horizontal nuclei of Broca's diagonal band, and the nucleus basalis of Meynert) contain neurons which provide the major cholinergic innervation for the cortical surface (Figs. 1–1 and 1–2a). In addition to cholinergic neurons, many of these cell groups also contain GABAergic neurons which project to the cerebral cortex.[188] The cholinergic cell bodies within the medial septal nucleus (also designated as Ch1) and those within the vertical limb nucleus of the diagonal band (Ch2) provide the major cholinergic input of the hippocampus, those of the horizontal limb nucleus (Ch3) provide the major cholinergic input into olfactory structures, and the cholinergic neurons of the nucleus basalis (Ch4) give rise to the major cholinergic innervation for all the other cortical zones and for the amygdala.[344] These cholinergic nuclei receive substantial neural inputs from the hypothalamus and from components of the limbic and paralimbic zones of the cerebral cortex.[342] In keeping with the organization illustrated in Figure 1–6, the Ch1–Ch4 cell groups send more massive projections to limbic and paralimbic areas than to other parts of the cerebral cortex.[340]

The septohippocampal pathway plays a critical role in the generation of the arousal-related θ rhythm in the hippocampus. Septal lesions in rats result in pathologically exaggerated emotional reactivity hyperdipsia, transient hyperphagia, and alterations in taste preferences.[191] Electrical spike activity has been reported in the septal area of patients with schizophrenia and electrical stimulation of this area has apparently lead to pleasurable sensations of an erotic nature.[210] From the vantage point of neuroanatomy, the nucleus basalis belongs to the limbic zone of the cerebral cortex and is also a telencephalic extension of the brainstem reticular core. In keeping with this dual nature, the cholinergic pathways from the nucleus basalis to the cerebral cortex play critical roles in both memory and attentional functions.[338] In rats, lesions of Ch4 neurons interfere with spatial memory.[43] In humans, the amnestic state in patients with anterior communicating artery aneurysms and septal tumors may be caused, at least in part, by the destruction of the Ch1–Ch4 cholinergic nuclei. In Alzheimer's disease, where memory loss is the single most salient aspect of the clinical picture, there is profound neurofibrillary degeneration of Ch4 neurons and loss of cortical cholinergic innervation (Chapter 10). However, in the presence of so many additional neuropathological lesions, the exact relationship between the cortical cholinergic depletion and the amnesia of Alzheimer's disease is difficult to determine. In the monkey, single unit recordings show that neurons of the nucleus basalis are sensitive to the motivational valence and novelty of sensory stimuli. These neurons alter their activity when the animal detects an edible object, especially if it is hungry and if the object happens to be a favorite food item.[112,449] This pattern of activity indicates that neurons of the nucleus basalis establish complex associations between sensory events and their motivational valence. The relevance of these cholinergic pathways to attentional tone, memory, and Alzheimer's disease is discussed further in section XVIII of this chapter and also in Chapters 3 and 10.

The Piriform Cortex

Piriform cortex (primary olfactory cortex) receives inputs from the olfactory bulb and is interconnected with the hypothalamus. In contrast to the other sensory modalities, olfactory information does not have to be relayed through the thalamus to reach the cerebral cortex since piriform cortex is directly interconnected with nearly all paralimbic and limbic areas of the brain.[11,343] The unique importance of olfactory sensation to sexual, territorial, and feeding behaviors is consistent with the location of piriform cortex within the limbic zone of cortical areas. Anosmic cetaceans such as whales and dolphins have a well-developed piriform cortex, raising the possibility that this region might have nonolfactory functions.[240] In the cat, for example, piriform cortex lesions induce hypersexuality whereas stimulation of this region alters the trigeminal receptive fields which elicit attack behavior upon stimulation.[49,187]

XIII. THE AMYGDALA, EMOTION, AND AFFILIATIVE BEHAVIORS: GATEWAY INTO THE NEUROLOGY OF VALUE

The primate amygdala contains more than a dozen nuclei, each with a different set of connections and physiological properties (Fig. 1–3a). Many of these nuclei have extensive reciprocal connections with the hypothalamus, the hippocampus and with the other components of the limbic and paralimbic zones. The amygdala receives olfactory information from piriform cortex, gustatory and somatosensory information through a relay in the insula, and auditory and visual information through relays in unimodal areas of the temporal lobe.[3, 343] Piriform and hypothalamic connections are more prominent in the medially situated nuclei whereas connections with unimodal and heteromodal association areas are more prominent in the lateral nucleus.

The critical role of the amygdala in the channeling of drive and emotion was highlighted by Downer's experiments in monkeys.[125] In these experiments, the forebrain commissures, including the optic chiasm, were sectioned and the amygdala on one side was ablated. As a consequence of these surgical manipulations, each eye could convey visual information only to the ipsilateral hemisphere and only one eye could convey visual information to an intact amygdala. In the preoperative period, monkeys reacted to human onlookers with characteristic aggressive displays. Following surgery, the animals remained quite placid when they viewed the onlookers through the eye ipsilateral to the amygdalectomy. When the eye ipsilateral to the intact amygdala was uncovered, however, the customary aggressive response was triggered. These experiments suggest that naturalistic visual experiences trigger the appropriate emotional response only if they have access to an intact amygdala.

The Downer experiments can be said to have created a state of monocular visual hypoemotionality by disconnecting one eye from the amygdala. A more extensive visuolimbic disconnection leads to the "Klüver-Bucy syndrome," which is seen in monkeys after bilateral lesions of the anterior temporal lobe, including the amygdala.[169,227] These animals show three salient behavioral changes: (1) They indiscriminately initiate sexual activity without regard to the appropriateness of the object. (2) They no longer show the customary aggressive–aversive reaction to their human keepers. (3) They seem to have lost the ability for visually distinguishing edible from inedible objects and keep mouthing all kinds of objects, discarding inedible ones only after buccal inspection. The one common denominator for these behaviors is a breakdown in the channeling of drive to the appropriate visual target in the extrapersonal space. It is not the drive that is necessarily altered, but its association with the proper object. Despite excessive mouthing, for example, monkeys with the Klüver-Bucy syndrome do not become obese.

The emotional valence of a sensory stimulus is based on its intrinsic hedonic properties, its acquired associations with other primary reinforcers and the current motivational state of the individual. The human amygdala plays a crucial role in modulating the neural impact of sensory stimuli according to each of these three factors. Thus, the amygdala is selectively activated by aversive (but not neutral) olfactory stimuli and fearful (but not neutral) facial expressions.[370,575] The amygdala also plays an important role in emotional conditioning, so neutral auditory stimuli which do not initially elicit amygdaloid activation start to do so after they are associated with conditioned fear.[280,287] Furthermore, the amygdala can give differential responses to identical sensory events when the state of the relevant motivation changes. Thus, the amygdala was activated by pictures of food when the subject was hungry but not when satiated; no such differential effect was elicited by pictures of tools.[278] Amygdaloid lesions can cause states of hypoemotionality in humans and can interfere with the acquisition of conditioned emotional responses to previously neutral stimuli.[3,33] In analogy to the organization of the other transmodal nodes in the cerebral cortex, the amygdala (represented by node L in Fig. 1–11b) may thus act as a transmodal gateway for linking the sensory representations of primary and secondary reinforcers with each other and with the mental and autonomic correlates of emotional and motivational valence. Through these processes, the amygdala can modulate the impact of a sensory event in a manner that reflects its intrinsic value and acquired significance.

Spontaneous discharges and electrical stimulations in the amygdala frequently trigger emotional experiences and other emotionally charged experiential phenomena in patients with temporolimbic epilepsy.[174] This relationship suggests that the amygdala may play an important role in linking drive and emotion not only to extrapersonal events but also to mental contents. A balanced mental life is built on congruous and relatively predictable interactions among experience and emotion so that pleasurable experiences and thoughts lead to positive emotions whereas painful ones trigger negative emotions. Severe disruptions in these fundamental relationships may arise as a consequence of disease in limbic and paralimbic regions of the brain, especially the amygdala. This may lead to an unpredictable and incongruous mapping of emotion onto experience in a way that may distort the entire texture of psychological reality.[330] Such disruptions may account for the wide spectrum of acute and chronic psychiatric syndromes ranging from panic attacks to dissociative states, depression, and schizophreniform conditions which have been described in patients with temporolimbic epilepsy (Chapters 8 and 9).

The participation of the amygdala in memory and learning is somewhat controversial (Chapter 4). In humans, bilateral amygdalectomy does not cause a major amnesia.[382,494] However, the amnesia resulting from hippocampal damage in monkeys becomes more severe if there is additional involvement of the amygdala.[358] In humans, amygdaloid lesions attenuate the facilitatory effects of emotional valence on memory processes, and functional imaging shows that amygdaloid activation mediates the influence of emotional valence upon learning.[322] The amygdala thus appears to have a dual role related to both attention and memory. Its role in attention is to selectively enhance the processing resources allocated to events with high emotional value, whereas its role in memory is to mediate the impact of emotional valence on memorability and also to encode the emotional valence of experience. The roles of the hippocampus and of the amygdala in memory can be dissociated from each other. Hippocampal lesions interfere with the explicit recall of specific events but not with the autonomic responses they elicit on the basis of their emotional significance, whereas amygdaloid lesions leave explicit recall intact but abolish the associated autonomic responses.[33]

The amygdala also participates in a wide range of behaviors related to conspecific affiliative behaviors, social emotions, and their communication. In monkeys, for example, amygdalectomy interferes with emotional vocalizations.[251] Radiotelemetered activity in freely moving monkeys shows intense amygdaloid activity during sexual and aggressive encounters.[270] In fact, amygdalectomy in monkeys alters conspecific aggressive behaviors and reverses the individual's position within dominance hierarchies.[455] Free-ranging rhesus monkeys with bilateral ablations in the amygdala and adjacent cortex fail to display appropriate aggressive and submissive gestures to the point where they become expelled from their social group.[120] In general, amygdaloid hyperactivity appears to enhance aggressive behaviors whereas hypoactivity appears to promote docility. Aggressive outbursts in temporolimbic epilepsy and in patients with episodic dyscontrol are occasionally time-locked to amygdaloid seizure activity and stereotaxic amygdalectomy has been performed to control intractable aggressive behaviors in some of these patients.[310,382,552]

In addition to the amygdala, paralimbic areas, especially those that receive their major limbic input from the amygdala, also play similar roles in modulating emotional responses, particularly those related to complex social situations and affiliative behaviors. In monkeys, for example, lesions which involve paralimbic parts of orbitofrontal cortex dramatically alter the emotional response to novel or threatening stimuli. These animals show enhanced aversive responses to relatively novel objects but a lowered aggressive reaction to humans and to a model snake.[64] Furthermore, bilateral ablations in the anterior cingulate region are associated with enhanced startle responses and a greater resilience to handling.[497] The olfactocentric component of the paralimbic belt plays an important role in the coordination of conspecific affiliative behaviors. Thus, orbitofrontal and temporopolar damage in monkeys decreases the effectiveness of aggressive encounters and results in a reduction of positive affiliative behaviors (such as grooming), eventually leading to the ostracism of the lesioned animal.[153,269,425] In keeping with these behavioral specializations, neurons in the amygdala and surrounding paralimbic areas are selectively responsive to eye contact with conspecifics.[59]

As in the monkey, the paralimbic areas of the human brain have also been implicated in behaviors related to emotion and motivation. Electrical stimulations of the anterior cingulate, insula and parahippocampal regions, for example, elicit mood alterations, dreamlike states, feelings of familiarity, and memory flashbacks.[22,174,552] Selective and persistent impairments in the ability to express emotion through modulations in the intonation of speech have been attributed to lesions in the cingulate area.[252] This area also plays an essential role in the motivational guidance of attentional functions.[266] Bilateral anterior cingulate lesions can lead to severe apathy and personality changes, occasionally reaching the severity of akinetic mutism.[12] Cingulotomy has helped some patients with intractable depression and obsessive compulsive disorders,[21] perhaps because it relieves states of rigid hyperattentiveness to pathological thoughts and emotions.

XIV. THE HIPPOCAMPUS AND THE BINDING OF DISTRIBUTED INFORMATION INTO EXPLICIT MEMORY: GATEWAY INTO THE NEUROLOGY OF RECOLLECTION

The encoding of distance, color, movement, and form displays considerable species-specific invariance and is relatively unaffected by peculiarities of individual experience. Much of mental content, however, is based on idiosyncratic associations which endow percepts and events with contextual anchors and personal significance. Components of the limbic and paralimbic zones of the cerebral cortex, especially the hippocampus and entorhinal cortex, play critical roles in the long-term storage and explicit recall of such arbitrary associations.

In monkeys, lesions of orbitofrontal and parolfactory cortex impair visual recognition and the ability to form associations between objects and reward;[351,359] insular damage yields modality-specific learning deficits in tasks of tactile discrimination;[379] temporopolar damage impairs visual memory;[381] and bilateral damage to the cingulate gyrus impairs performance in tasks that require the retention of spatial information.[377,420] In humans, orbitofrontal lesions have been associated with amnesias; and memory impairments of variable severity have been reported after damage to the cingulate region and retrosplenial cortex.[68,529,551] Despite the involvement of these paralimbic areas in memory and learning, however, the most severe amnestic states in monkeys and humans occur only when the hippocampo–entorhinal complex and its diencephalic connections are damaged (Chapter 4).

Through relays in entorhinal and transentorhinal (perirhinal) cortex, the hippocampus receives inputs from numerous paralimbic, heteromodal, and downstream unimodal association areas.[510,531] These multisynaptic pathways allow the hippocampus to receive information in all sensory modalities. As mentioned above, the reciprocal interconnections between the entorhinal–transentorhinal cortex and the hippocampus are so strong that the two may be conceptualized as forming a unified hippocampo–entorhinal complex. The hippocampal formation is also interconnected with the mammillary body of the hypothalamus, the limbic nuclei of the thalamus, and with other components of the limbic zone such as the amygdala and the septal area.[344,453] Although the hippocampo–entorhinal complex also participates in the neural regulation of emotion, autonomic activity, endocrine control, and immunoregulation, its principal behavioral affiliation is in the realms of memory and learning. In monkeys, selective hippocampal lesions yield only modest deficits in the retrieval phase of learning but the memory disturbance becomes much more severe when the entorhinal cortex is also damaged.[308,358] On occasion, apparently isolated hippocampal damage in humans can lead severe memory deficits.[581] However, the most severe human amnesias result when bilateral lesions involve both the hippocampus and the rhinal cortices.

In accessing established knowledge, such as the name of a color, the meaning of a word, or the identity of a familiar face, recall is based on stable associations that have been consolidated for many years. The recall of such consolidated semantic knowledge is coordinated by transmodal nodes (such as those in Wernicke's area and other parts of the temporal lobe) located outside of the limbic and paralimbic zones of the cerebral cortex. In order to encode and access *new* facts and experiences, however, fragile and initially sparse linkages have to be established, nurtured, and inserted into the matrix of existing knowledge.[339] This kind of learning, which is necessary for sustaining explicit, declarative, and episodic memory, is critically dependent on transmodal gateways within the limbic system, especially those of the hippocampo-entorhinal complex (represented by L in Fig. 1–11B).

As described in Chapter 4, the amnestic state caused by lesions of the hippocampo–entorhinal complex is characterized by a dissociation between the *explicit learning* of new experience, which is severely impaired, and the *implicit–procedural learning* of motor tasks and perceptual associations, which is relatively preserved. An amnestic patient, for example, may develop new motor skills, improve performance in priming and stem completion tasks, and learn to avoid situations that have recently been associated with aversive consequences, even when he or she has no conscious memories of the experiences that have led to this learning.[85,357,468] In addition to the impairment of new learning ("anterograde amnesia"), these patients also display a "retrograde amnesia" for events that occurred before the onset of the limbic lesion. The retrograde amnesia tends to be more severe for recent than for remote events, a temporal gradient known as "Ribot's law."

During the recovery stage of the retrograde amnesia, some patients display a gradual shrinkage of the time period encompassed by the retrograde memory loss, indicating that at least some of the retrograde amnesia had been due to a retrieval block rather than an obliteration of memory traces.[39] This set of circumstances raises the possibility that the limbic system may play its critical role in memory and learning by acting as a neural gateway for encoding and retrieval, without necessarily constituting the site where the memories (or engrams) are stored. According to this model, facts and events are initially recorded at multiple sites with an anatomical distribution that reflects the modality and category specificity of their constituent components. This information is relayed, through reciprocal multisynaptic pathways, to limbic transmodal nodes including the hippocampo–entorhinal complex (L in Fig. 1–11B). These limbic transmodal nodes are not storage sites of individual experiences. Instead, they enable the construction of directories (or address books) which can be used to look up and bind the distributed fragments of the relevant experience.[104,319,334,358,380,504]

The major role of limbic–paralimbic areas, especially the hippocampo–entorhinal complex, may thus be to orchestrate the coherent storage and reactivation of this distributed information. As a consequence of this organization, the fidelity of the original information is not corrupted by convergence, and the same memory can be probed through numerous associative approaches. In addition to mediating multifocal binding, the hippocampo–entorhinal complex also enhances the robustness with which other association areas encode the relevant components of information.[132,200,222] The role of the hippocampo–entorhinal complex in explicit memory is thus analogous to the role of Wernicke's area in language, prefrontal cortex in working memory, temporal cortex in face and object recognition, and posterior parietal cortex in spatial attention. Although some convergence may occur in limbic and paralimbic areas, the most detailed information related to recent experiences remains distributed in neocortical areas.

When a critical volume of the hippocampo–entorhinal complex is destroyed, the encoding of new information becomes less reliable, the binding of components becomes jeopardized, and retrieval loses its effectiveness. Consequently, fragments of new events cannot be integrated with the type of coherence that is necessary for supporting explicit–declarative–episodic memory, leading to the emergence of an amnestic state. However, at least some of the information related to new events continues to be encoded in nonlimbic association cortex in a manner that supports implicit learning. The unlinked form of this information helps to explain why implicit learning tasks such as priming are so sensitive to the surface (rather than associative) properties of the stimuli and why they are resistant to transmodal generalization.[468] There is probably no fundamental difference in the type of encoding that is involved in implicit versus explicit memory. In implicit memory, the information remains sequestered, within unimodal and heteromodal association areas; in explicit memory, it becomes incorporated into a coherent context through the binding function of limbic nodes, especially those within the hippocampo–entorhinal complex. In keeping with this formulation, tasks of explicit memory lead to the activation of medial temporolimbic as well as neocortical areas whereas tasks of implicit memory lead to the activation predominantly of neocortical areas.[207,479,503]

The hippocampo–entorhinal complex and association neocortex are involved in continuing processes of reconstruction, updating, and associative elaboration which collectively lead to the consolidation of new memories. At the initial stage of encoding, a new fact or event has few associations and depends on the limbic system for maintenance and coherent retrieval. In time, as additional linkages become established through reciprocal connections with other transmodal and unimodal areas, the relevant information becomes less dependent on the limbic system and can be accessed through numerous associative approaches, some of which may entirely bypass the hippocampo–entorhinal complex. The role of the hippocampo–entorhinal complex is likely to be most critical for the most recently acquired memories, for those that have limited resonance with other mental contents, for those that have been registered casually rather than intentionally, for those with relatively weak emotional valence, for those that require extensive cross-modal integration, for those that have been recalled rarely and have therefore failed to establish associative elaboration, and for those that require the reactivation of idiosyncratic contextual anchors related to temporal and spatial circumstances. The existence of such multiple factors helps to explain why the vulnerability of a memory to retrograde amnesia is not always a simple function of its time of acquisition and why clear temporal gradients are not universally found in amnestic patients.[339]

Why is new learning so dependent on the limbic structures of the medial temporal lobe? A tentative answer may be based on the constraints that the CNS faces: The number of neurons is fixed with little hope of obtaining many new ones, every existing neuron is already occupied by previously stored information, new information needs to be written on top of existing items, and the amount of new information is boundless. The CNS may therefore need to be protected from learning too rapidly and indiscriminately since this could jeopardize the stability of existing knowledge.[319] An initial filtering is provided by attentional systems which select subsets of behaviorally relevant events for further consideration. The limbic system appears to erect a second line of defense. It provides a mechanism that allows the rapid learning of behaviorally relevant relationships but in an initially transient (limbic-dependent) form that may induce a relatively small amount of permanent change in association cortex. This transitional period may allow new memories to enter associative readjustments before being assimilated in a more permanent form and also to compete with each other, allowing only the fittest to solidify their hold on precious synaptic space. Through these processes, the limbic system simultaneously satisfies the need to limit the indiscriminate influx of new learning and the need to adapt to a rapidly changing environment.[318]

The question may also be asked, why a function as vital as explicit memory displays a critical dependency on a phylogenetically primitive part of the brain such as the limbic system. One explanation is that explicit and declarative memory could have developed to recall contingencies associated with food and danger. In the course of phylogenetic development, the scope of explicit memory could have expanded beyond the confines of apetitive and defensive behaviors while maintaining its anatomical dependency on the limbic system. The obligatory involvement of the limbic system in memory and learning also insures that sensory events with high emotional and motivational valence will enjoy a competitive advantage. Furthermore, the limbic system is particularly prone to long-term potentiation effects and is also one of the few areas that continue to display axonal sprouting during adulthood.[37,48] These properties make the limbic system highly suitable for serving a critical role in the organization of new learning.

The way in which the hippocampo–entorhinal complex constructs a directory (or look-up table) for binding and looking up distributed information remains poorly understood. At least one mechanism may be based on the Hebbian rule of covariance according to which the temporal coherence of neural activity within a set of simultaneously active and reciprocally interconnected neurons produces a record that can be used for the subsequent reactivation of the entire set in response to the activation of one of its components.[99,339] The orderly connections which lead from the entorhinal cortex to the dentate gyrus of the hippocampus (via the perforant path), from the dentate gyrus to CA4 and CA3 (via the mossy fibers), from CA3 to CA1 (via the Shaffer collaterals), from CA1 to the subiculum, from the subiculum back to the entorhinal cortex, and the pathways which interconnect the hippocampo–entorhinal complex with nearly all components of heteromodal and unimodal areas contain the synaptic architecture that could use Hebbian processes for binding and reactivating the distributed components of explicit memory.

The registration, storage, and recall of recent experience involves a great deal of sorting, associative search, recombination, selection, and on-line reintegration, processes that are generally attributed to working memory and the related executive functions of prefrontal heteromodal cortex as reviewed in section X of this chapter. In fact, prefrontal cortex does participate in numerous memory-related functions, including the reconstruction of context and temporal order, the on-line manipulation of encoding and retrieval, and the associative search of internal data stores. It also provides contextual constraints to keep the reconstructed memories within the bounds of plausibility. Damage to prefrontal cortex undermines the effectiveness of encoding and retrieval, causes an impoverishment of associative linkages that are necessary for reconstructing context and temporal order, decreases the speed with which internal data stores are searched, and also increases the tendency to confabulate.[100,337,372] In keeping with these clinical observations, almost all tasks of explicit memory yield consistent activation in heteromodal association cortices, especially in prefrontal areas.[524] Although they share a common nomenclature, it is important to emphasize that working memory and explicit memory are behaviorally and neurologically distinct phenomena. Lateral prefrontal cortex lesions interfere with working memory and occasionally impair the efficiency of encoding and retrieval but never give rise to severe amnesias. Conversely, limbic lesions which give rise to severe amnesias usually leave working memory abilities quite intact.

The process of explicit memory allows each person to construct a unique record of experience and knowledge based on events of personal significance. The encoding and retrieval of a memory can involve almost all parts of the cerebral cortex, but with an orderly anatomical distribution of component processes: relevant uni-modal and transmodal areas encode the sensory aspects; the limbic system, especially the hippocampo–entorhinal complex, binds this information into a coherent whole; and prefrontal areas guide the orderliness of storage and retrieval.

XV. THE LIMBIC SYSTEM

The boundaries of the "limbic system" have ebbed and welled to fit the whims of individual investigators. Some have even denied the existence of a limbic system, mostly because of uncertainties in defining its boundaries. There are, however, many sound anatomical and functional reasons for postulating the existence of such a neural system. The following components are usually included within the limbic system. Collectively, they define what is probably its most extensive boundaries:

1. The hypothalamus
2. The limbic (allocortical and corticoid) components of cortex
3. The paralimbic cortical belt
4. The limbic striatum (olfactory tubercle and the nucleus accumbens), the limbic pallidum, the ventral tegmental area of Tsai, and the habenula
5. The limbic and paralimbic thalamic nuclei (anterior dorsal [AD], anterior ventral [AV], anterior medial [AM], laterodorsal [LD], mediodorsal [MD], medial pulvinar [PM] and other midline nuclei)

One justification for lumping these five groups of structures into a unified system is based on the fact that they are tightly interconnected (Fig. 1–13). These connections form many distinct circuits. One of these, based on synaptic relays that lead from the hippocampus sequentially to the mammillary body (via the fornix), to the anterior thalamic nuclei (via the mammillothalamic tract), to the cingulate gyrus, to the presubiculum, to the entorhinal cortex, and back to the hippocampus (via the perforant pathway), is known as the Papez circuit. Components of this circuit play crucial roles in memory and learning.[399] Some of the connections shown in Figure 1–13 are so strong that damage to their sites of origin or termination tends to trigger retrograde or transsynaptic degeneration in the areas with which they are interconnected.[517]

Components of the limbic system also have common neurochemical, physiological, and perhaps even immunological properties. Dopaminergic, cholinergic, and endogenous opiate markers, for example, are more concentrated within the cortical components of the limbic system than in other parts of the cerebral cortex.[291,349] Furthermore, as discussed in Chapter 9, topical anesthetics such as lidocaine, procaine, and cocaine are powerful activators of limbic and paralimbic areas whereas they tend to depress the activity of other cortical regions.[419] Components of the limbic system also have a greater capacity for synaptic plasticity than other parts of the cerebral cortex. They are therefore highly suited to the encoding of new associations but also highly vulnerable to pathological processes such as kindling and epilepsy (Chapter 8). The preferential affinity of the herpes simplex virus for

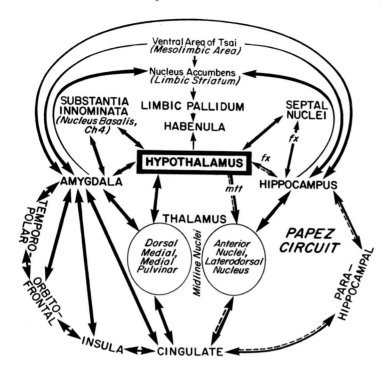

FIGURE 1–13. Major connections of the limbic system. Abbreviations: fx=fornix; mtt=mammillothalamic tract.

almost all cortical components of the limbic system suggests that these cortical areas may even share antigenically common sites recognized by the virus.

The single most important feature which unifies the constituents of the limbic system is the presence of shared behavioral specializations. These can be summarized under five categories:

1. The binding of distributed information related to recent events and experiences in a manner that supports declarative/episodic/explicit memory
2. The channeling of emotion and drives (such as hunger, thirst, libido) to extrapersonal events and mental content
3. The linking of mental activity with autonomic, hormonal, and immunological states
4. The coordination of affiliative behaviors related to social cohesion
5. Perception of smell, taste, and pain

Each of these behavioral realms has been discussed earlier in the course of reviewing the behavioral neuroanatomy of individual limbic and paralimbic structures. Damage to any of the structures shown in Figure 1–13 can cause impairments in one or more of these behavioral categories. However, the limbic system can also be divided into amygdaloid and hippocampal spheres of influence. The olfactocentric paralimbic areas tend to fall within the amygdaloid sphere of influence whereas the components of the Papez circuit fall within the hippocampal sphere of influence. The former are more closely associated with emotion, motivation, affiliative behaviors, and autonomic–hormonal–immunological function, whereas the latter are more involved in learning and memory.

The clinical diagnosis of a persistent global amnestic state always indicates the presence of bilateral limbic lesions, usually within the hippocampal sphere of influence. The most common damage sites associated with severe amnesia are the hippocampo–entorhinal complex, the limbic thalamus, the hypothalamus (especially the mammillary bodies), the fornix, and the basal forebrain (Chapter 4). The concept of a unified network gains further support from the observation that the amnesias resulting from hippocampo–entorhinal lesions and those resulting from thalamic or hypothalamic lesions display clinical features that are nearly indistinguishable. Limbic lesions almost always give rise to multimodal impairments. In contrast, lesions that interrupt connections between unimodal areas and the limbic system give rise to modality-specific disconnection syndromes such as asymbolia for pain, visual hypoemotionality, visual amnesia, and tactile learning deficits (Fig. 1–11c).

Considering its behavioral affiliations, the limbic system would also appear to constitute the most likely site of dysfunction for those psychiatric diseases that might turn out to have identifiable biological causes. Schizophrenia, major depression, post-traumatic stress syndromes, and panic states have each been associated with variable sorts of structural and metabolic dysfunction within components of the limbic system (Chapter 9).[109,315,324,345,431] Conversely, known lesions within the limbic system can commonly induce a great variety of "psychiatric" symptomatology. Examples include the experiential phenomena, panic attacks, dissociative states, fugues, and schizophreniform states of temporolimbic epilepsy; the agitated confusional states of parahippocampal infarctions; the sexual and apetitive dysfunctions of septal–hypothalamic lesions; and the comportmental abnormalities of the medial and basal frontal lobe syndromes.

XVI. BASAL GANGLIA AND CEREBELLUM

The importance of the basal ganglia (striatum and globus pallidus) and cerebellum to motor function is well known. The basal ganglia play a critical role in the automatic execution of learned motor plans, and the cerebellum regulates the rate, range, and force of movement.[225,311] Several lines of investigation indicate that these areas may also influence the neural control of cognition and comportment.

The Striatum (Caudate, Putamen, Nucleus Accumbens, Olfactory Tubercle)

The striatum receives neural inputs from the substantia nigra and cerebral cortex but does not send reciprocal projections back to the cerebral cortex. The inputs from the cerebral cortex are glutamatergic and those from the substantia nigra are dopaminergic. The output of the striatum is directed predominantly to the globus pallidus and uses GABA, enkephalin, and substance P as the transmitter substances. The globus pallidus projects to the ventrolateral and ventral anterior nuclei of the thalamus which, in turn, project to the frontal lobe, giving rise to a multisynaptic striatopallidothalamocorticostriatal loop. Some of these connections are organized to form relatively distinct skeletomotor, oculomotor, prefrontal, and limbic circuits.[8]

The striatum contains four components: the caudate, the putamen, the olfactory tubercle, and the nucleus accumbens. The caudate and putamen receive cortical inputs predominantly from association cortex and primary sensory–motor areas. The dopaminergic input to these striatal components originates in the pars compacta of the substantia nigra. The olfactory tubercle and nucleus accumbens receive cortical inputs from limbic and paralimbic parts of the brain, including the insula, amygdala, and hippocampus.[84,189,385,532] The dopaminergic innervation of these two striatal components originates in the ventral tegmental area of Tsai, which is just medial to the substantia nigra.[196] On the basis of this connectivity pattern, the nucleus accumbens and olfactory tubercle can be designated the "limbic striatum" whereas the caudate and putamen are usually designated the "dorsal striatum" or "neostriatum."

Dopamine turnover is higher in the limbic striatum than in the neostriatum.[542] The limbic striatum also has behavioral specializations which are different from those of the dorsal striatum. For example, disrupting the dopaminergic pathways from the ventral tegmental area to the limbic striatum of the rat results in locomotor hyperactivity and deficits in passive avoidance learning whereas interrupting the nigrostriatal pathway to the dorsal striatum yields hypoactivity and bradykinesia.[286] In the cat, activation of the nucleus accumbens reduces the receptive field for the hypothalamic biting reflex and therefore modulates the channeling of aggression to extrapersonal targets.[180] The human limbic striatum is involved in the neuropathology of Parkinson's disease, Alzheimer's disease, and perhaps also Huntington's disease.[30,244,481] However, its behavioral specializations remain poorly understood. Although the nucleus accumbens has been implicated in the pathogenesis of schizophrenia, the evidence remains circumstantial at best.[507]

The projections from the cerebral cortex to the dorsal striatum display a complex topographic arrangement. Projections from each cortical area form multiple patches of terminals within the striatum. Patches of projections from separate areas of association cortex are more likely to show partial overlap or interdigitation if the relevant cortical areas are interconnected with each other.[483,570] This organization implies that there may be some mirroring of corticocortical interaction patterns within the striatum. Although this arrangement may largely subserve motor control, it may also reflect the role of the striatum in nonmotor integrative functions. In the monkey, for example, a subgroup of caudate and putamen neurons responds during the visual presentation of primary reward but not necessarily during the motor act of pressing the bar which leads to the reward.[14,387] Damage to the basal ganglia causes selective learning deficits in tasks which require the switching between response strategies, suggesting that the caudate and putamen may play a critical role in the acquisition and retention of procedural knowledge.[414] This functional affiliation may help to explain why procedural learning can remain relatively preserved in patients who develop severe amnestic states as a consequence of cortical lesions.

The head of the caudate nucleus receives most of its input from dorsolateral prefrontal cortex. In monkeys, lesions in this sector of the caudate yield deficits which are essentially identical to those that emerge upon ablating prefrontal cortex,[238] supporting the view that striatal regions have behavioral specializations which are similar to those of the cortical areas from which they receive their major cortical input. In keeping with this formulation, patients with caudate lesions can develop the abulic form of the frontal network syndrome and display a severe loss of self-motivation.[197]

Mental-state impairments with features of the frontal lobe syndrome emerge in almost all basal ganglia diseases. In Parkinson's disease, for example, prominent cognitive changes, especially related to "executive" functions, arise quite frequently.[228] In Huntington's disease, cognitive and comportmental changes reminiscent of the frontal lobe syndrome may precede the motor symptoms and may emerge at a time when the pathological changes appear confined to the caudate nucleus.

In some patients, lesions in the caudate and putamen have also been associated with the emergence of agitation, aphasia, and unilateral neglect.[72] In almost all such cases, the adjacent white matter is also involved, making it difficult to determine whether these deficits reflect damage to the striatum or to the adjacent fibers. Experiments based on functional imaging show that the human neostriatum is frequently activated by tasks which require the shifting of spatial attention (Chapter 3).

Lesions and metabolic hyperactivity in the striatum have both been described in obsessive-compulsive disorders as well as in patients with Tourette's syndrome, a condition characterized by tics and obsessive-compulsive symptoms.[133,546] Although the relationship to motor function is considered a general property of the entire neostriatum, motor cortex sends projections only to the putamen, not to the caudate.[276] The motor deficits in extrapyramidal diseases may thus have a closer correlation with pathological changes in the putamen whereas the cognitive deficits may have a closer correlation with pathology in the caudate and limbic striatum.

The Globus Pallidus

The globus pallidus receives striatal outflow and projects to the ventrolateral and anterior ventral thalamic nuclei, the habenula, and the subthalamic nucleus. The primate globus pallidus has four easily identifiable components: (1) the outer (lateral) segment, (2) the inner (medial) segment, (3) the ventral pallidum located under the anterior commissure, and (4) the pars reticulata of the substantia nigra.

There is essentially no disagreement about the crucial role of the globus pallidus in motor control. In the monkey, approximately 50% of the neurons of the lateral and internal globus pallidus fire in relationship to the direction of movement.[360] The reversible inactivation of the globus pallidus in monkeys yields a severe and reversible breakdown of a learned flexion–extension movement but only when the animal is blindfolded.[226] In humans, lesions of the globus pallidus (caused by anoxia, carbon monoxide or cyanide poisoning, cerebrovascular accidents, wasp stings, Wilson's disease, or Hallervorden-Spatz disease) are frequently associated with severe rigidity and bradykinesia.

The lateral pallidum and the dorsal parts of the medial pallidum receive their striatal input predominantly from the caudate and putamen. The ventral pallidum, however, receives a major striatal projections from the nucleus accumbens.[217] Many neurons of the ventral pallidum respond to amygdaloid stimulation, and this response is probably mediated through the nucleus accumbens.[571] In the monkey, the core of the internal pallidal segment projects to the motor thalamus. However, a medial crescent of this pallidal segment projects predominantly to the lateral habenula, which is generally considered a structure closely related to the limbic system.[400] Damage to the medial globus pallidus of monkeys severely disrupts species-specific sexual display patterns.[307] Furthermore, only very few neurons of the ventral pallidum fire in relationship to movements.[360]

These observations have led to the inclusion of the ventral and medial parts of the pallidum within the limbic system and to the suggestion that these pallidal components may have predominantly nonmotor behavioral affiliations. In the human, pallidal lesions can be associated with severe deficits of motivation, judgment, and insight. Some of these patients may display a profound abulia and occasionally obsessive-compulsive symptomatology.[283] As in the case of striatal lesions, pallidal lesions also lead to a clinical picture that has many features of the frontal lobe syndrome. The pars reticulata of the substantia nigra is a posterior extension of the globus pallidus and may participate in the programming of saccadic eye movements toward actual or remembered targets.[223] Its behavioral correlates in the human brain are not understood.

The Cerebellum

The cerebellum receives inputs through the inferior cerebellar peduncle (carrying fibers from the ipsilateral spinal cord, inferior olive, vestibular nuclei) and the middle cerebellar peduncle (carrying information from the contralateral pontine nuclei). It sends its major projection, through the superior cerebellar peduncle, to the ventrolateral nucleus of the contralateral thalamus. The ventrolateral nucleus then projects predominantly to the motor–premotor areas of the frontal lobe which, in turn, project to the pontine nuclei, completing the multisynaptic cerebellothalamocorticopontocerebellar loop. Each cerebellar hemisphere receives input from the ipsilateral side of the body and is interconnected with the contralateral cerebral hemisphere. Cerebellar lesions thus give rise to ipsilesional motor symptoms. As in the case of limbic pathways, cerebellar connections are remarkably robust and create linkages that exert transsynaptic trophic influences. Thus, through a mechanism known as "diaschisis," frontal infarctions cause acute contralateral cerebellar hypometabolism, and cerebellar lesions can cause widespread contralateral cortical inactivation.[50,473] Eventually, frontal lobe lesions can even lead to a severe transsynaptic atrophy of the contralateral cerebellum.

Neuroanatomical experiments in monkeys have shown that the inputs to the pontine nuclei come not only from motor–premotor cortex but also from multiple association cortices in the occipital, parietal, temporal, and frontal lobes and also from components of the limbic system.[475] Through these connections, cortical areas related to nearly every cognitive and comportmental domain have potential access to the cerebellar hemispheres via a synaptic relay in the pontine nuclei. The reciprocal cerebellofugal projections appear to have a more restricted distribution since cerebellar projections (relayed via the dentate nucleus and other deep cerebellar nuclei) are directed predominantly to the ventrolateral nucleus of the thalamus, which projects mostly to premotor cortex. Although the ventrolateral nucleus may also project to cortical areas beyond motor–premotor cortex, such projections are likely to be relatively minor or multisynaptic.

Traditional neurological textbooks tend to confine the discussion of the cerebellum to its motor functions. However, the clinical examination of patients with cerebellar damage and the functional imaging of neurologically intact subjects have raised the possibility that the cerebellum may have nonmotor behavioral affiliations. Even unilateral cerebellar lesions, for example, can impair performance in tasks of attention (as assessed by digit span), verbal fluency, and reasoning and can lead to a flattening of affect and to the emergence of disinhibited behaviors.[50,475] These cognitive and behavioral deficits can be quite prominent in some patients.

Reports of visuospatial deficits after cerebellar lesions are difficult to interpret because they have usually been based on poor performance in construction tasks which require motor coordination. Difficulties of articulation have been recorded but true aphasic disorders are rare. Deficits of explicit–declarative memory have also been detected but can probably be attributed to the underlying attentional impairments. It is interesting to note that the cerebellar activation seen during word generation tasks in neurologically intact subjects tends to disappear with practice and there is no evidence that cerebellar lesions interfere with spatial attention.[143,567] It is therefore unlikely that the cerebellum plays a major role in the control of explicit memory, spatial attention, or language. The nonmotor symptomatology (of attention, reasoning and comportment) in patients with cerebellar damage seems to display many features of the frontal lobe syndrome, a relationship which is consistent with the preferential funneling of the cerebellothalamic outflow pathways into the frontal lobes.

Although the cerebellum is unlikely to play a major role in explicit memory, cerebellar lesions impair the acquisition of eyeblink conditioning.[321] Furthermore, the major output nucleus of the cerebellum (the dentate) shows much greater activation during attempts at solving a pegboard puzzle than during the execution of comparable movements not related to problem solving.[265] These observations suggest that the cerebellum, together with the basal ganglia, may play an important role in motor (procedural) learning. Cerebellar neuronal loss has been reported in infantile autism but does not appear to be a consistent feature of this mysterious condition.[28,416]

In contrast to basal ganglia lesions which frequently lead to severe and easily observable cognitive and comportmental deficits, cerebellar lesions do so less frequently and less prominently. Considering its neural connectivity, however, it is quite likely that the cerebellum influences the function of many, if not all, cognitive domains. This relationship could take the form of a global influence upon the state of information processing (perhaps similar to the role of ascending cholinergic and noradrenergic pathways) or it could display regional variations that link specific parts of the cerebellum to specific behavioral domains (as in the relationship of the basal ganglia and thalamus to behavior). The striatopallidothalamocorticostriatal as well as the cerebellothalamocorticopontocerebellar loops are both organized so as to receive afferents from nearly all cortical areas (through the mediation of the striatum and pontine nuclei) but confine the outputs (through the mediation of the thalamus) preferentially into the frontal lobes. This funneling of projections into the frontal lobes may help to explain why patients with either basal ganglia or cerebellar lesions display clinical pictures reminiscent of the frontal lobe syndrome.

XVII. The Thalamus

Almost all thalamic nuclei have extensive reciprocal connections with the cerebral cortex. The one exception is the reticular nucleus, which receives cortical input but does not project back to cortex.[246] Except for the reticular and perhaps intralaminar nuclei, thalamic nuclei have very few, if any, interconnections with each other. Each thalamic nucleus, with the possible exception of the primary sensory relay nuclei, projects to multiple cortical areas and each cortical area is interconnected with many thalamic nuclei. However, most thalamic nuclei have preferred cortical targets and each cortical area has a principal source of thalamic input. Single thalamic neurons projecting to multiple cortical areas through axonal collaterals are rare.[40,368] In general, primary sensory and motor areas have the most restricted thalamic connectivity whereas heteromodal and paralimbic areas have the most heterogeneous connections. The principal thalamic nucleus of a cortical area tends to project predominantly to layer IV whereas the less specific thalamic inputs also reach the more superficial cortical layers. Thalamic nuclei can be subdivided on the basis of the specializations of their preferred cortical targets (Fig. 1–14). Boundaries of thalamic nuclei are rarely sharp and the nomenclature is subject to variation. In the following account, the nomenclature will follow that of the Carpenter and Sutin[74] and will be supplemented, wherever necessary, by the nomenclature of Olszewski[392] and Jones.[247]

Thalamic Nuclei of Primary Sensory and Motor Areas

The sensory relay nuclei are the easiest to identify. The posterior part of the ventroposterior lateral nucleus (VPLp), the principal division of the ventroposterior medial nucleus (VPM), the posterior part of the ventromedial nucleus (VMp), and the ventroposterior inferior nucleus (VPI) are the major sensory relay nuclei of the somatosensory modality: They receive fibers from the medial lemniscus, trigeminothalamic tract, and the spinothalamic tract and project to primary somatosensory cortex (S1) and S2. The VMp nucleus receives input predominantly from the spinothalamic tract and may relay pain sensation to the insula and perhaps S2.[96] The

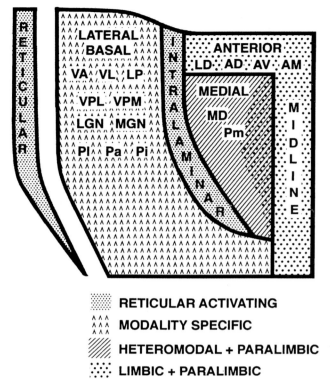

RETICULAR ACTIVATING

MODALITY SPECIFIC

HETEROMODAL + PARALIMBIC

LIMBIC + PARALIMBIC

FIGURE 1–14. A schematic diagram of the four major groups of thalamic nuclei. Abbreviations: AD=anterior dorsal; AM=anterior medial; AV=anterior ventral; LD=laterodorsal; LGN=lateral geniculate; LP=lateroposterior; MD=mediodorsal; MGN=medial geniculate; Pi=inferior pulvinar; Pl=lateral pulvinar; Pm=medial pulvinar; Pa=anterior pulvinar; VA=ventral anterior; VL=ventral lateral; VPL=ventroposterior lateral; VPM=ventroposterior medial.

VPM nucleus also receives input from the nucleus of the tractus solitarius and relays taste information to the primary gustatory area and the anterior insula.[375] The lateral geniculate nucleus (LGN) is the sensory relay nucleus for the visual modality: It receives input from the eye and projects to primary visual cortex (V1). The medial geniculate nucleus (MGN) is the sensory relay nucleus for the auditory modality: It receives input from the inferior colliculus and projects to primary auditory cortex (A1).

Damage to the VPLp or to the LGN gives rise to contralateral hemihypesthesia and hemianopia, respectively. In contrast to S1 lesions, which do not abolish pain sensation (probably because the thalamic projections to S2 are spared), VPLp lesions generally lead to a loss of pain sensation as well. Since inputs from both ears reach the MGN in each hemisphere, unilateral damage to this thalamic nucleus does not lead to contralateral ear deafness. In fact, unilateral MGN lesions may be extremely difficult to detect clinically and may only cause contralateral suppression during dichotic auditory stimulation. The major thalamic input into primary motor cortex

(M1) comes from the ventrolateral nucleus (VL) and the anterior ventroposterior lateral nucleus (VPLa).[250,469] Lesions involving these motor nuclei of the thalamus may give rise to contralateral clumsiness and dysmetria.

Thalamic Nuclei of Modality-Specific (Unimodal) Association Cortex

In the rhesus monkey, the major thalamic projections to the somatosensory association cortex of the superior parietal lobule (BA5) come from the lateroposterior nucleus (LP) and perhaps also from the anterior subdivision of the pulvinar nucleus (Pa).[250] The nuclei which provide the major projection to visual unimodal association areas include the inferior (Pi) and lateral (Pl) subdivisions of the pulvinar nucleus.[35,63,527] The Pi receives inputs from the superior colliculus and may mediate "blindsight" in patients with V1 lesions. In the monkey, Pi and Pl neurons give retinotopically mapped responses to visual stimuli and lesions of the inferior pulvinar disrupt visual discrimination behaviors.[79,410] The unimodal auditory association cortex receives its major thalamic input from the MGN and probably also from an adjacent rim of the pulvinar.[63,347] Thus, the MGN is the source of thalamic projections not only to A1 but also to the auditory association cortex. The motor association cortex receives its major thalamic input from the ventrolateral nucleus (VL) and perhaps from parts of the ventral anterior nucleus (VA).[469,489] The VL nucleus receives pallidal and cerebellar output and is the principal nucleus through which the basal ganglia and cerebellum influence the cerebral cortex.

Transmodal Nuclei of the Thalamus: Nuclei of Heteromodal, Paralimbic, and Limbic Cortex

The lateral part of the medial dorsal nucleus (MD) is the major thalamic nucleus for prefrontal heteromodal cortex. In keeping with this connectivity pattern, bilateral MD lesions in the monkey reproduce deficits in spatial delayed alternation similar to those associated with prefrontal ablations.[236] The medial pulvinar nucleus (Pm) and parts of the adjacent lateral posterior nucleus (LP) are the major nuclei for the heteromodal cortices of the inferior parietal lobule, the banks of the superior temporal sulcus and the parahippocampal region.[350,522,569] In contrast to Pi and Pl, which give retinotopically organized responses to simple visual stimuli, Pm neurons respond to the attentional salience of stimuli and may play a role in the focusing of selective attention.[441]

The close interconnectivity between the heteromodal and paralimbic zones of the cerebral cortex is also reflected in the arrangement of thalamic connections. Thus, the MD and Pm are major thalamic nuclei not only for prefrontal and posterior parietal heteromodal cortices but also for the entire paralimbic belt. The medial parts of MD (including the magnocellular component), for example, give rise to the major thalamic projections of the orbitofrontal and anterior cingulate regions whereas the Pm has prominent reciprocal projections with the insula, temporal pole, orbitofrontal cortex, parolfactory gyrus, posterior cingulate, parahippocampal gyrus, and temporopolar cortex.[184,185,367,375,451,569] The MD and Pm also have direct limbic connections. Thus, the medial and magnocellular parts of MD have connections with the amygdala, piriform cortex, and the septal region whereas Pm has connections with the amygdala and the hippocampal complex.[4,194,216,248,383] In addition to sharing many common connections, the MD and Pm nuclei blend into each other without distinct boundaries.

Another group of nuclei are collectively known as the nuclei of the "anterior tubercle." These nuclei include the anterior thalamic nucleus (its dorsal [AD], ventral [AV], and medial [AM] components) and the laterodorsal nucleus (LD). They provide the major thalamic connections for the posterior cingulate cortex, the retrosplenial area, entorhinal cortex, and the hippocampal complex.[4,299,569] The anterior thalamic nucleus receives direct hypothalamic input through the mammillothalamic tract and is therefore an important component of the Papez circuit. Nuclei situated close to the thalamic midline are collectively designated midline or paramedian nuclei. These include the paratenial, paraventricular, subfascicular, central, and reuniens nuclei. They have extensive projections with paralimbic areas such as the temporal pole and anterior cingulate gyrus and also with the hippocampal formation.[184,563,569]

On the basis of these connectivity patterns, the midline, anterior, MD, and Pm nuclei have been included within the limbic system. The paraventricular and MD nuclei in the monkey contain neurons that are sensitive to the previous occurrence of stimuli, suggesting that they could play important roles in recognition memory.[139] In monkeys, lesions which involve the medial parts of the MD nucleus and adjacent midline nuclei lead to visual object recognition deficits similar to those obtained after the ablation of limbic and paralimbic cortex in the medial temporal lobe.[5]

In patients, the clinical consequences of lesions in the MD nucleus reflect its frontal and limbic connections (Figs. 1–9d and 1–15). Thus, cerebrovascular lesions that involve the medial part of MD bilaterally can give rise to amnestic states that are almost indistinguishable from those associated with hippocampo–entorhinal lesions, the one difference being that confabulations appear to be more likely after the thalamic lesions.[352,492,502] However, the lesions in many of these cases also extend into the anterior and midline nuclei and into the mammillothalamic tract, so the exact role of the MD lesion in the genesis of human "thalamic amnesia" is not entirely clear. In the Wernicke-Korsakoff encephalopathy, severe amnestic states are associated with MD and Pm lesions, but almost always in conjunction with additional lesions of the mammillary bodies.[536]

A rather frequent clinical consequence of a unilateral left MD lesion is characterized by the triad of a frontal lobe syndrome, verbal memory loss, and anomia. In such patients, the MD lesion may induce a remote EEG slowing and hypoperfusion within dorsolateral prefrontal cortex,[464] and, less frequently, within the temporal lobe. Loss of judgment and insight is the predominant finding in some patients with unilateral MD lesions, and amnesia in others. The anomia is rarely severe. Lesions of the right pulvinar nucleus, including its medial component, have been associated with contralateral neglect for the left extrapersonal space, and electrical stimulation of the left medial pulvinar has been reported to induce transient anomia.[66,391] Bilateral MD thalamotomies are also said to reduce schizophrenic agitation and intractable anxiety.[498]

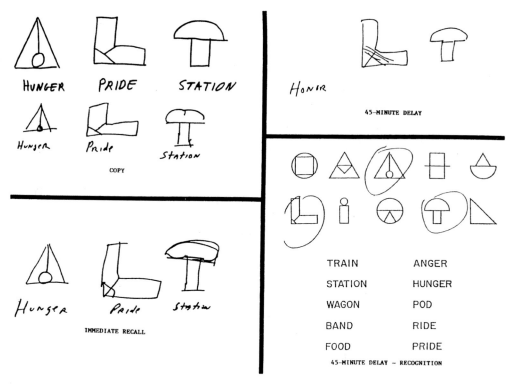

FIGURE 1–15. Performance of the patient whose lesion is shown in Figure 1–9d. The patient can copy all items and can hold them in working memory for immediate recall. However, recall in 45 minutes is very poor, especially for the verbal items. Recognition (tested by asking the patient to circle the items he was given to memorize) improves nonverbal memory but not verbal memory. This pattern is consistent with a material-specific amnesia for verbal material.

These observations show that the transmodal thalamic nuclei display behavioral affiliations that are similar to those of their principal cortical targets. While it is easy to understand how thalamic sensory relay nuclei influence the function of their cortical projection sites, it is much more difficult to surmise the role of the transmodal nuclei. Corticothalamocortical loops involving heteromodal, paralimbic, and limbic areas could conceivably help to imprint local associative linkages, reactivate them under specific behavioral conditions, and, as will be described below, maintain coactivation boundaries for large-scale neurocognitive networks.

The Reticular and Intralaminar Nuclei of the Thalamus

The reticular nucleus of the thalamus as well as the intralaminar nuclei (e.g., the limitans, paracentralis, centralis lateralis, centromedian, and parafascicularis) have strong associations with the ascending reticular activating pathways. The putative role of these thalamic nuclei in the control of arousal and attention is discussed in Chapter 3.

XVIII. CHANNEL FUNCTIONS AND STATE FUNCTIONS

Many axonal pathways that interconnect one cortical area with another (or with specific sectors of the basal ganglia and thalamus) are organized in the form of reciprocal point-to-point channels where the principal sites of origin and the major fields of termination are of approximately equivalent size. This point-to-point connectivity provides the basic anatomical substrate of specific channel functions. Damage to channels such as the splenium of the corpus callosum, the frontotemporal uncinate fasciculus, or the insulo–amygdaloid pathway leads to specific impairments such as pure alexia, memory retrieval deficits, and asymbolia for pain. In addition to these point-to-point channels, each cortical area also receives widespread modulatory connections which arise from small groups of neurons and which innervate the entire cerebral cortex either directly or through thalamic relays. These pathways employ small amines and GABA as transmitters and determine the overall *state* of information processing rather than the contents of the information that is being transmitted along the point-to-point channels. These modulatory pathways play important roles in coordinating behavioral states related to arousal, attention, mood, and motivation. At least six such pathways can be identified in the primate brain (Fig. 1–16). Five of these reach the cerebral cortex directly without a thalamic relay whereas the sixth is relayed through the thalamus.

1. Cholinergic and GABAergic projections from the basal forebrain to the cerebral cortex[344]
2. Histaminergic projections from the lateral and medial hypothalamus to the cerebral cortex[344,434,540]
3. Serotonergic projections from the brainstem raphe nuclei to the cerebral cortex[371]
4. Noradrenergic projections from the nucleus locus coeruleus to the cerebral cortex[364]
5. Dopaminergic projections from the substantia nigra and the ventral tegmental area of Tsai to the cerebral cortex[60]
6. Cholinergic projections from the brainstem reticular formation to the thalamus[212,243,346]

Each of these modulatory pathways is organized in such a way that a relatively small group of neurons can induce rapid modulations in the information processing state of the entire cerebral cortex. The cholinergic projection from the brainstem to the thalamus, for example, promotes arousal by facilitating the transthalamic passage of sensory information toward the cerebral cortex. The other five modulatory pathways have direct access to the cerebral cortex without any thalamic relay. Each of these pathways displays a slightly different pattern of cortical distribution and physiological specialization. Thus, cortical cholinergic innervation is most intense within limbic areas whereas the noradrenergic projections tend to favor primary sensory areas. Furthermore, cholinergic projections tend to synapse onto cortical

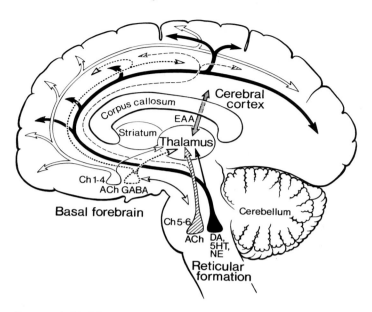

FIGURE 1–16. Neuroanatomy of modulatory pathways in the human brain. Abbreviations: ACh=acetylcholine; Ch1–4=the cholinergic neurons of the septum, diagonal band nuclei, and the nucleus basalis; Ch5–6=the cholinergic neurons of the brainstem, DA=dopamine; EAA=excitatory amino acids; NE=norepinephrine; 5HT=serotonin. The dashed and dotted lines indicate pathways which have not yet been documented in the human brain.

pyramidal neurons whereas the serotonergic projections synapse onto inhibitory interneurons.[164,338,495,496]

The cholinergic innervation of the cerebral cortex arises predominantly from the nucleus basalis of the substantia innominata. The neurons of this nucleus are particularly responsive to novel and motivationally relevant sensory events.[555] The major effect of acetylcholine upon neurons of the cerebral cortex is mediated through the m1 subtype of muscarinic receptors and causes a prolonged reduction of potassium conductance so as to make cortical neurons more receptive to other excitatory inputs.[320,467] Cortical cholinergic pathways also promote EEG desynchronization, long term potentiation (LTP), and experience-induced synaptic remodeling.[25,99,231] The ascending cholinergic pathway from the basal forebrain is therefore in a position to enhance the immediate neural impact and long-term memorability of motivationally relevant events. The nucleus basalis also gives rise to a GABAergic projection directed to the cerebral cortex.[155] At least in the rat, this pathway innervates inhibitory cortical interneurons but its functional specializations remain poorly understood.

The noradrenergic innervation of the cerebral cortex arises from the nucleus locus coeruleus. The neurons of this nucleus are more responsive to the motivational relevance (or meaning) of a stimulus than to its sensorial properties.[15] Neocortical norepinephrine increases the signal-to-noise ratio and timing precision of cortical neurons in a way that enhances the specificity of neural responses to sensory events.[151,274,290,371] The cortical response to the stimulation of a single vibrissa in rats, for example, loses some of its discrete localization when the norepinephrine innervation to cortex is interrupted.[97] At the behavioral level, noradrenergic transmission modulates novelty-seeking behaviors, the focusing of attention and also resistance to distraction.[54,430,482]

The dopaminergic projections of the cerebral cortex arise from the substantia nigra and ventral tegmental area of Tsai. These dopaminergic cells are selectively responsive to motivationally relevant stimuli and to cues that signal their existence.[476] They appear to encode discrepancies between the prediction and occurrence of reward and may therefore convey teaching signals for learning apetitive behaviors.[476] In keeping with these characteristics, the dopaminergic projections from the ventral tegmental area to the cerebral cortex and nucleus accumbens appear to play an important role in mediating the neural processes related to substance addiction.[415] Furthermore, both dopamine and acetylcholine promote cortical responses related to working memory.[119,159,179]

The serotonergic projection to the cerebral cortex arises from the brainstem raphe nuclei. The electrical stimulation of these neurons can induce an arousal-related pattern of low voltage fast activity in the cerebral cortex.[126] Serotonergic agonists reduce distractibility in a two-choice runway task, suggesting that serotonin may modulate the sensory gating of behaviorally relevant cues in the environment.[51] Ascending serotonergic pathways can also influence the state of hunger and aggressivity and may mediate the subjective effects of alcohol.[292] The hypothalamus is the source of a relatively light histaminergic projections to the cerebral cortex. Histamine receptors are widely distributed throughout the cerebral cortex and have been implicated in the regulation of cortical arousal, energy metabolism, autonomic function, and sensitivity to pain.[540]

One anatomical feature common to all of these modulatory corticopetal projections is the absence of equally well-developed reciprocal projections from the cerebral cortex.[333] The nucleus basalis, for example, projects to all parts of the cerebral cortex but receives cortical projections from only a handful of limbic and paralimbic areas. The other cortically projecting cell groups shown in Figure 1–16 also receive sparse cortical projections, most of which come from limbic and paralimbic areas.[245,413] This asymmetry of corticofugal versus corticopetal connections allows the neurons of the basal forebrain, substantia nigra–ventral tegmental area, brainstem raphe, and nucleus locus coeruleus to rapidly shift information processing states throughout the cerebral cortex in a way that is responsive primarily to the demands of the limbic system and internal milieu with relatively little intervention from feedback loops emanating from heteromodal, unimodal, and primary cortices.

Many psychiatric diseases, including mania, depression, paranoia, obsessive-compulsive disorders, and chronic anxiety, are characterized by pathological biases in the interpretation of events and experiences. When compared to control subjects, for example, patients with generalized anxiety disorder show greater metabolic activation of temporal and frontal cortex during the passive viewing of neutral stimuli.[561] Such altered responses, even to neutral stimuli, may indicate the existence of a fundamental processing state abnormality which biases the impact of all experience. Indirect evidence based on the pharmacological treatment of depression and anxiety with noradrenergic and serotonergic agents and of paranoia with dopamine blockers suggests that the modulatory pathways of the cerebral cortex may play important roles in setting such fixed attitudinal biases in the processing of sensory experience.

It is unlikely that there will be a one-to-one relationship between any of these modulatory pathways and specific cognitive or comportmental domains. In general, however, the activation of these modulatory pathways provides a mechanism for augmenting the neural responses to motivationally relevant events, facilitating their storage in memory, enhancing their access to on-line processing resources, sharpening the attentional focusing they elicit, and increasing their impact on consciousness. These projections are in a position to alter the tone, coloring, and interpretation of experience rather than its content. In addition to cholinergic and monoaminergic receptors, many areas of the cerebral cortex, but especially components of the limbic system, also contain receptors for estrogen, testosterone, and other steroids.[493] Alterations in the circulating level of these hormones, as in puberty or menopause, could influence behavioral states in a manner analogous to the effect of the modulatory projection systems.

The modulatory projections reviewed in this section are part of the ascending reticular activating system, which is discussed in greater detail in Chapter 3. These pathways highlight the multiple factors that contribute to the neural control of cognition and comportment. Language, spatial orientation, attention, memory, and emotion are each subserved by large-scale networks which contain multiple point-to-point channels. These pathways encode the perceptual, motor, visceral, and affective components of the relevant behavior and the way in which these components are interlinked. The modulatory pathways influence the processing states within which these domain-specific channels function. In the course of remembering, for example, the content of what is recalled is determined primarily by the information that flows along the point-to-point sensory–limbic interconnections. The speed and efficiency of the recall, and perhaps the perspective from which the information is interpreted, however, may be regulated by the activity of the modulatory pathways that innervate the relevant regions of limbic and association cortex. In the realm of emotion, the point-to-point projections of the amygdala and related limbic structures may determine the linkage of a specific thought or event with a specific feeling and visceral state whereas the modulatory pathways may introduce an intrinsic bias favoring one mood over another and may determine the intensity of the emotion and its influence on other aspects of mental activity. Among all the complex factors involved in the neural control of comportment and cognition, those that represent the contributions of these modulatory pathways are the most accessible to therapeutic manipulation by existing pharmacological agents. This is why the pathways shown in Figure 1–16 represent the major targets of modern psychopharmacology.

XIX. HEMISPHERIC SPECIALIZATION AND ASYMMETRY

The functional organization of the human brain is characterized by multiple hemispheric asymmetries. Asymmetry of structure and function is not unique to the human brain. The frog's habenula has two subnuclei on the left but only one in the right, the chimpanzee's temporal plane is larger on the left, and the hypoglossal nerve displays an asymmetrical influence on bird song.[163,193,554] The purpose of asymmetry is unknown but may reflect the biological advantage of concentrating the controlling components of a network within a single hemisphere in order to minimize transcallosal conduction delays.[437]

Left Hemisphere Specializations: Praxis and Language

One aspect of hemispheric asymmetry that is accessible to everyday experience is handedness. Ninety percent of the population is said to be right handed. In this vast majority of the population, the right hand can easily master complex movements, especially those associated with the usage of tools, whereas the left hand tends to be remarkably clumsy when asked to perform the same task. The words dexterity (from Latin, *dexter*, right) and adroitness (from French, *droit*, right) are used as synonyms for skillfulness, and the word gauche (from French, *gauche*, left) as a synonym for all that is awkward. Since the two hands are mirror images of each other and have an identical musculature and innervation, handedness is clearly based on an asymmetrical CNS control of movement rather than on a physical peculiarity of the left hand.

The prevalence of right-handedness has led to the assumption that the contralateral left hemisphere of the human brain is more highly specialized for skilled movements (praxis). Support for this hypothesis has come from several directions. First, apraxias are more commonly seen after damage to the left hemisphere. Secondly, functional imaging experiments in right handers show that the right motor cortex displays substantial activation only when complex finger movements are performed by the contralateral left hand whereas the left hemisphere displays substantial activation during the performance of these movements by either hand.[429] The execution of simple movements is not associated with such asymmetry. Furthermore, transcranial magnetic stimulation of left premotor cortex impairs response selection in both hands whereas stimulation in the right premotor cortex cause a disruption only in the contralateral hand.[472] The left hemisphere thus controls complex movements in both sides of the body whereas the influence of the right hemisphere is confined to the contralateral side.

The absence of direct callosal connections in the hand representation of M1 may promote the independent control of each hand and may make handedness possible. The influence of the left motor cortex upon the ipsilateral limbs may be exerted through the uncrossed contingent of the pyramidal tract or through callosal connections. There is apparently no anatomical asymmetry in either M1 or S1 of the human brain, but the putamen and globus pallidus may be approximately 10%

larger on the left than on the right, and the left pyramidal tract may be the first to cross in the medulla.[263,411,550]

The conclusion that the left hemisphere is also specialized for language function has been based on clinical observations showing that approximately 90% or right handers and 60% of left handers develop aphasia only after damage to the left hemisphere. The fact that more than half of left handers develop aphasia after left hemisphere lesions also shows that the specialization for language and handedness can have dissociable anatomical substrates. Only a few right handers become aphasic after right hemisphere lesions (a condition which is usually designated "crossed aphasia"). Non-right-handers have a better chance of recovery from aphasia caused by left hemisphere damage, presumably because the intact right hemisphere has a greater potential for mediating language functions.

Experiments on split-brain patients have shown that the left hemisphere in most right handers contains all the machinery for language function, whereas the right hemisphere cannot produce spoken or written language but has a rudimentary capacity for understanding the meaning of some words. In keeping with these observations, experiments based on dichotic listening and on the tachistoscopic presentation of visual stimuli show a right ear and visual field (and therefore left hemisphere) advantage for all language-mediated tasks in neurologically intact subjects.[501] In functional imaging experiments, language tasks elicit prominent left hemisphere activation whereas the contralateral right hemisphere activation can be quite negligible.[29] Clinical observations have shown that acalculia is more common after damage to the left hemisphere, suggesting that the left hemisphere is also specialized for the verbal manipulation of numbers.

The supratemporal plane, a region which is generally included in Wernicke's area, is frequently larger on the left side of the human brain.[152,170] This anatomical asymmetry is noticeable even during embryonic development.[83] In one study, nearly 90% of chimpanzee brains that were investigated also displayed a larger supratemporal plane on the left.[163] Since this asymmetry seems to be almost as frequent in the chimpanzee as in humans, since the absence of supratemporal plane asymmetry does not prevent humans from acquiring language, and since chimpanzees have shown little enthusiasm for developing language during the past several million years, it appears that the anatomical asymmetry of the supratemporal plane is neither necessary nor sufficient for the emergence of language function.

Right Hemisphere Specialization for Complex Non-Linguistic Perceptual Skills, including Face Identification

The specialized functions of the left hemisphere have been appreciated for more than a hundred years. In contrast, the specializations of the right hemisphere did not gain widespread acceptance until much later, leading to its initial characterization as the "minor" or "silent" hemisphere. A great deal of clinical and experimental evidence gathered since then has now led to the conclusion that the right hemisphere has numerous behavioral specializations and that these can be divided into at least four realms of function: (1) Complex and nonlinguistic perceptual tasks, including face identification, (2) Spatial distribution of attention, (3) emotion and affect, (4) and paralinguistic aspects of communication.

Experiments based on dichotic listening show a left ear (and therefore right hemisphere) advantage for pitch and melody identification; and tachistoscopic experiments show a left visual-field (and therefore right hemisphere) superiority for depth perception, spatial localization, and the identification of complex geometric shapes.[267,491,501] Furthermore, the left hand is usually more accurate in judging the orientation of a rod by palpation.[41] In keeping with these observations, experiments based on functional imaging and event-related potentials have reported a greater activation of the right hemisphere during the performance of nonverbal complex perceptual tasks, including those that require mental rotation.[316,402]

A left visual-field superiority can also be demonstrated in the processing of perceptual information related to unfamiliar faces. If subjects who are briefly exposed to a new face are subsequently presented with two photographic composites, one consisting of the two left sides and the other of the two right sides of the face, they tend to conclude that the composite made of the right side (which had been viewed through the left visual field) more closely resembles the original face. Thus, the information in the left visual field (coming from the right side of the other person's face) plays the more important role in determining the way in which the face is remembered. This phenomenon can acquire potential behavioral relevance during everyday life since most faces are distinctly asymmetrical. Despite this apparent superiority of the right hemisphere in the processing of information related to faces, severe prosopagnosia is usually seen in the context of bilateral lesions, suggesting that both hemispheres take part in the *recognition* of faces (Chapter 7).

In keeping with these functional asymmetries shown in neurologically intact subjects, a voluminous and continuously expanding literature shows that right hemisphere lesions, especially those located in the posterior aspects of the hemisphere, lead to a much greater impairment of complex visuospatial tasks.[501] Thus, the judgment of line orientation, visually guided stylus maze performance, the *Block Design Test* of the *Wechsler Adult Intelligence Scale*, the tactile judgment of rod orientation, the ability to identify objects presented from an unusual visual perspective, and the ability to detect variations in a familiar melody are more impaired after right hemisphere lesions when compared to left hemisphere lesions.[41,111,262,326,487,544] Constructional tasks, especially those that require the reproduction of three-dimensional perspective, are also more severely impaired after by in the right hemisphere. Even memory processes show hemispheric asymmetry (Fig. 1–15). Thus, patients with left temporal lobectomy are more impaired in learning verbal material whereas patients with right temporal lobectomies are more impaired in the memorization of nonlinguistic complex perceptual material, especially those that involve spatial relationships.[356]

The right hemisphere specialization for complex perceptual function becomes more pronounced if the task is made especially difficult and also if some memorization is required for successful performance.[525] Prior experience with the task, individual skills, and peculiarities in the mode of information processing may also influence the extent of hemispheric asymmetry. While naïve listeners show a right hemisphere superiority in recognizing melodies and tone sequences, for example, musically experienced individuals as well as those who use a more analytical style of information processing may show a greater activation of the left hemisphere.[45,316] However, during the processing of particularly complex musical material, such as the recognition of fugue themes, even professional musicians showed greater right hemisphere activation.[538] There are also gender differences: For example, the left hemisphere superiority for language and the right hemisphere superiority for complex perceptual tasks may both be more pronounced in males than in females.[121,323,488] In women, hemispheric asymmetry in cognitive tasks may vary according to the stage of the menstrual cycle.[550] It seems, therefore, that the most consistent right hemisphere specializations for complex perceptual tasks are likely to be obtained in right-handed male subjects who are performing unfamiliar and difficult perceptual tasks. It also appears advisable to specify the menstrual state of female subjects participating in such experiments.

Right Hemisphere Specialization for Spatial Attention

Numerous observations lead to the conclusion that the right hemisphere is specialized for distributing attention within the extrapersonal space. According to a model that is described in Chapter 3, the right hemisphere contains the neural machinery for shifting attention symmetrically to both sides of space whereas the left hemisphere contains the machinery for shifting attention almost exclusively in the contralateral hemispace and in a contraversive direction. This leads to the emergence of marked contralateral neglect after right hemisphere injury but not after equivalent left hemisphere injury. This pattern of right hemisphere specialization is seen even in left handers and even in those with documented right hemisphere dominance for language.[499] It appears, therefore, that the right hemisphere specialization for spatial attention may be more tightly conserved than the left hemisphere specialization for language. Preliminary morphometric investigations show that parts of the posterior parietal cortex may be larger in the right hemisphere, especially in right handed males.[242] The relevance of this anatomical asymmetry to the hemispheric specialization for spatial attention remains poorly understood.

Right Hemisphere, Emotion, and Affect

Inappropriate jocularity in response to hemiplegia (also known as "anosognosia") is seen almost exclusively in patients right hemisphere infarcts. In contrast, deep dejection and dysphoria (sometimes leading to what is known as the "catastrophic reaction") are more common in patients with left hemisphere infarcts.[162,442] This clinical observation has led to the inference that the right hemisphere may normally introduce a negative (dysphoric) emotional bias to experience whereas the left hemisphere may introduce a more positive (euphoric) bias.[122,435,459,477] According to this hypothesis, normal mood reflects a balance between these two tendencies. Right hemisphere lesions would tilt the balance toward inappropriate jocularity whereas left hemisphere lesions would tilt it toward despondency and depression.[229,442] Such hemispheric asymmetries may originate quite early in life. For example, there is greater EEG activation over the left hemisphere when 10-month-old infants are shown happy faces.[108]

The inferences derived from the nature of the emotional reactions to hemiplegia are based on the assumption that the despondency in response to right hemiplegia is comparable to the jocularity which emerges after right hemiplegia, except that it is of the opposite valence. However, one could also argue that the despondency of right hemiplegics is an entirely appropriate reaction to a devastating event whereas the jocularity of left hemiplegics is always inappropriate. The phenomenon of anosognosia may thus show that the right hemisphere plays a more essential role in promoting appropriate emotional reactions to life experiences.

In keeping with this last inference, numerous observations suggest that the right hemisphere is more highly specialized for coordinating nearly all aspects of emotional expression (affect) and experience (mood). For example, the ability to *express* emotional tone through speech prosody, facial expression, or gesture and also the ability to *identify* the nature of the emotion expressed through prosody and facial expression are both more impaired after lesions in the right side of the brain.[2,6,36,273,523] Furthermore, experiments in neurologically intact subjects show that the right hemisphere is better equipped for encoding (expressing) and decoding (identifying) affect. Thus, emotional expressions are more accentuated on the left side of the face and there is a left visual field advantage in the identification of emotional expressions.[218,373,460]

Additional evidence favors a right hemisphere specialization also for the *experience* of emotions. For example, experiments which used the electrodermal response as an index of emotional experience found that patients with right hemisphere lesions were markedly impaired in their visceral responses to emotional stimuli whereas those with left hemisphere injury were not.[580] Furthermore, emotionally loaded questions elicited a larger number of leftward eye movements, a finding which some would interpret as an indication of greater right hemispheric activation in response to the induced emotional state.[478] In a rather remarkable study, neurologically intact subjects were asked to stimulate themselves into sexual climax while their EEGs were being monitored. The results showed that the EEG amplitude during orgasm was greater over the right hemisphere.[89]

There are also indications that affective disease may be more closely associated with right hemisphere dysfunction. It has been suggested, for example, that left-sided temporolimbic seizure foci are more likely to be associated with ideational disorders whereas right-sided foci are more likely to be associated with mood disturbances.[31] Mood disorders are also more common in conjunction with right- than left sided brain damage.[297] Even in patients with otherwise typical manic-depressive disturbances, the EEG power spectra tend to show greater disturbances over the right hemisphere.[149] In fact, when patients with manic-depressive disease were given a dichotic listening task, their performance was similar to the performance of individuals with right temporal lobectomy.[574] Furthermore, neurological signs indicative of right hemisphere dysfunction may be seen during depression and may disappear when the depression is treated.[61] The relationship between unconscious mental content and the motor system also shows a more intimate linkage in the right hemisphere. Thus, the left side of the body appears more responsive to hypnotic suggestion.[148,458] Furthermore, unilateral hysterical paralysis is more frequently encountered in the left side of the body, even in left-handers.[506] In view of the close interrelation between emotion and autonomic tone, it is also interesting to note that the right hemisphere may have a greater influence on determining heart rate.[452,572]

In summary, while each hemisphere may impart an emotional perspective of opposite polarity to the interpretation of experience, this asymmetry seems to be embedded within a greater right hemisphere specialization for all processes related to mood and affect. The modulation of mood and affect is coordinated by limbic and nonlimbic components of the cerebral hemispheres: the nonlimbic neocortical components may play important roles in integrating, interpreting, and communicating emotions, whereas the limbic components may play a more fundamental role in generating emotions, linking them to visceral responses, and channeling them to appropriate targets. Functional asymmetry related to mood and affect is probably much more pronounced in the non-limbic than limbic areas which participate in these realms of behavior.

Paralinguistic Aspects of Communication, Communicative Competence, and the Right Hemisphere

Phoneme production, word choice, syntax, and grammar constitute the linguistic aspects of speech. They are under the dominant control of the left hemisphere in the vast majority of the population. As shown in Chapter 6, however, there is much more to communication, and even to speech, than these formal linguistic features. For want of better terminology, such additional components can be designated the "paralinguistic" aspects of communication. They collectively contribute to the emergence of communicative competence. The encoding and decoding of mood through variations of emotional prosody, facial expression and gestures are some of the paralinguistic aspects of communication. As noted above and in Chapter 6, these channels of communication are under the influence of the right hemisphere.

In addition to mood, speech prosody is also used to denote emphasis and attitude. The same word choice and word order, for example, could convey completely different messages depending of the distribution of stress and inflection in the utterance. These attitudinal aspects of prosody are also controlled by the right hemisphere.[486,548] Another aspect of paralinguistic communication is the ability to comprehend situational context through nonlinguistic cues. Patients with right hemisphere injury are impaired in this very important area of communicative competence.[36] Furthermore, neurologically intact individuals show a left ear (right hemisphere) advantage in the ability to infer context and intent during the dichotic presentation of sentences which have been altered to render the verbal material indecipherable while keeping the melodic structure intact.[129]

The modulation of verbal output (how much to say and when to yield the floor), the choice of appropriate address (*tu* versus *vous*), and the choice of proper pitch (using a higher frequency and simpler language when speaking to a child) constitute additional paralinguistic functions which could conceivably also fall under the preferential control of the right hemisphere. In fact, right hemisphere lesions, especially those that involve the superior temporal gyrus, promote excessive language output and the use of unnecessarily complicated technical vocabulary.[273] One of our patients with a right temporal lesion, for example, became uncharacteristically brazen and abrasive following a right temporal infarction.[331] From his hospital room he would keep calling the physician's office and use forms of address and a conversational style which reflected inappropriate familiarity. The same patient also talked excessively would not take the cue to "yield the floor" during conversation. The inappropriate conduct of patients with right hemisphere injury may reflect, at least in part, an inability to decipher nonlinguistic channels of communication and to adjust behavior to fit the demands of the prevailing context.

XX. DISTRIBUTED LARGE-SCALE NETWORKS AND THEIR CORTICAL EPICENTERS

Transmodal nodes in midtemporal cortex, Wernicke's area, posterior parietal cortex, prefrontal cortex, amygdala, and the hippocampo–entorhinal complex link distribute information into coherent multimodal assemblies necessary for face and object recognition, naming, working memory, spatial attention, emotional channeling, and explicit memory. These transmodal areas provide the cortical epicenters of large-scale distributed networks.

The domain of spatial attention was used to explore the internal organization of such networks. As shown in Chapter 3, the distribution of attention within the extrapersonal space is coordinated by a large-scale network built around three epicenters: one in the region of the frontal eye fields, another in the region of the intraparietal sulcus, and a third in the cingulate gyrus. The architecture of connectivity among the components of this network was investigated in an experiment where the regions of the frontal eye fields and posterior parietal cortex were each injected with a different retrogradely transported tracer. The resultant pattern of retrograde labeling showed that these two epicenters of the attentional network were interconnected not only with each other and the cingulate gyrus but also with an identical set of 12 additional cortical areas. Furthermore, both injection sites received common projections from the mediodorsal and medial pulvinar nuclei of the thalamus and sent interdigitating and partially overlapping projections to the striatum.[368,570]

This pattern of connectivity, summarized in Figure 1–17, may reflect an organization that is common to all large-scale networks.[334] In this figure, A and B represent two interconnected epicenters of any large-scale neural network. They could represent the frontal eye fields and posterior parietal cortex in the network for spatial attention, midtemporal and temporopolar cortices in the network for face and object recognition, the amygdala and the hippocampo–entorhinal complex in

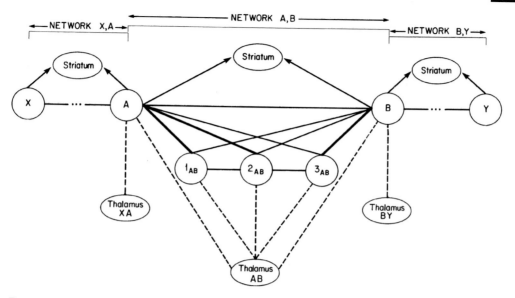

FIGURE 1–17. General architecture of large-scale distributed networks.

the emotion–memory network, Wernicke's area and Broca's area in the language network, and prefrontal cortex and posterior parietal cortex in the working memory–executive function network. The axonal transport experiments mentioned above indicate that if one member of such a pair, say A, is interconnected with additional cortical areas such as 1, 2, and 3, then B is also interconnected with the same three cortical areas. Consequently, if A transmits a message, B will receive it directly, but also through the alternative vantage points provided by areas 1, 2, and 3. This arrangement enables parallel processing and contains multiple nodes where seamless transitions between parallel and serial processing can occur. In resolving a complex cognitive problem such as reconstructing a past memory, selecting words to express a thought, or figuring out the identity of a face, a set of cortical areas interconnected in this fashion can execute an extremely rapid survey of a vast informational landscape while considering numerous goals, constraints, scenarios, and hypotheses until the entire system settles into a state of least conflict which becomes identified as the solution to the cognitive problem.

Because cortical areas tend to have very extensive corticocortical projections, individual sectors of association cortex are likely to belong to multiple intersecting networks. With rare exceptions, however, thalamic subnuclei have almost no connections among each other. As shown in the anatomical experiments mentioned earlier, some thalamic subnuclei can project to both epicenters of an individual large scale neural network. Thalamic subnuclei can thus fulfill the very important role of setting coactivation boundaries for separating the activity of one network from the activity of others.[334] A similar view was expressed by Penfield, who suggested that thalamic nuclei could act as integrators of the cortical areas involved in speech and language.[403] As noted earlier, interconnected cortical areas are likely to send interdigitating projections to the striatum. Since the striatum receives cortical inputs but does not project back to the cerebral cortex, it could serve the role of an efference synchronizer (or filter) for coordinating the outputs of cortical areas in a given network. The human brain contains at least five large-scale neurocognitive networks that are organized in this fashion.

Dorsal Parietofrontal Network for Spatial Orientation

The cortex around the intraparietal sulcus, the frontal eye fields, and the cingulate gyrus constitute the three interconnected epicenters. The parietal component displays a relative specialization for the perceptual representation of behaviorally relevant locations and their transformation into targets for attentional actions; the frontal component displays a relative specialization for choosing and sequencing exploratory and orienting movements; and the cingulate gyrus displays a relative specialization for the distribution of effort and motivation. Additional critical components are located in the striatum and thalamus. Damage to this network yields deficits of spatial attention and exploration such as contralesional hemispatial neglect, simultanagnosia, and the other components of Bálint's syndrome. For reasons that have been reviewed, contralesional neglect occurs almost exclusively after right-sided damage to this network whereas Bálint's syndrome tends to arise after bilateral lesions. (See Chapters 3 and 7 for further detail.)

Limbic Network for Memory and Emotion

The hippocampo–entorhinal complex and the amygdala constitute the two interconnected epicenters. The former displays a relative specialization for memory and learning, and the latter for drive, emotion, and visceral tone. Additional critical components are located in the paralimbic cortices, the hypothalamus, the limbic thalamus, and the limbic striatum. Damage to this network yields deficits of memory, emotion, affiliative behaviors, and autonomic regulation. Severe deficits usually occur only after bilateral lesions. On occasion, unilateral left sided lesions give rise to a multimodal amnesia but this is transient. More frequently, unilateral lesions in the left give rise to prominent deficits of verbal memory whereas unilateral lesions on the right give rise to nonverbal memory deficits which are usually quite mild. (See Chapter 4 for further detail.)

Perisylvian Network for Language

The two epicenters of this network are known as Broca's area and Wernicke's area. According to the opinions expressed in this chapter, Broca's area includes the premotor region BA44 and the adjacent heteromodal fields of BA45–47; Wernicke's area includes the posterior part of auditory association cortex in BA22 and also adjacent heteromodal fields in BA39–40 and perhaps BA21. Broca's area displays a relative specialization for the articulatory, syntactic, and grammatical aspects of language whereas Wernicke's area displays a specialization for the lexical and semantic aspects. Additional components of this network are located in the striatum, thalamus and the association areas of the frontal, temporal, and parietal lobes. Damage to this network yields aphasia, alexia, and agraphia. Such deficits are seen only after damage to the left hemisphere in the majority of the population. (See Chapters 5 and 6 for further detail.)

Ventral Occipitotemporal Network for Face and Object Recognition

The middle temporal gyrus and the temporal pole appear to contain the transmodal epicenters for this network. Additional critical components are located in the fusiform gyrus and inferior temporal gyrus. Damage to this network yields recognition deficits such as object agnosia and prosopagnosia. The lesions that cause such deficits are almost always bilateral. The fusiform gyrus is the most common site of lesions, probably because it is the only part of this network with a vascular supply that makes bilateral damage likely. On occasion, unilateral left-sided lesions can lead to object agnosia, and unilateral right-sided lesions to prosopagnosia. (See Chapter 7 for further detail.)

Prefrontal Network for Executive Function and Comportment

Prefrontal heteromodal cortex and orbitofrontal cortex are the major cortical epicenters involved in the coordination of "comportment," whereas prefrontal heteromodal cortex and posterior parietal cortex provide epicenters for a network involved in working memory and related executive functions. The head of the caudate nucleus and the mediodorsal nucleus of the thalamus are additional critical components. Deficits of comportment are more frequently associated with lesions of orbitofrontal and adjacent medial frontal cortex whereas deficits of executive function and working memory are more frequently associated with damage to dorsolateral prefrontal cortex. Clinically significant deficits are usually seen only after bilateral lesions. On occasion, unilateral left-sided lesions give rise to a syndrome of abulia whereas unilateral right-sided lesions give rise to behavioral disinhibition. The network for working memory displays a partial overlap with the network for spatial attention (Chapter 3).

Neuroanatomical experiments in the homologous regions of the monkey brain have shown that the components of these five networks are interconnected according to the pattern shown in Figure 1–17.[334,483] All of these networks receive their sensory information from the common set of unimodal cortical areas shown in Figure 1–11b. The differences in the resultant cognitive functions are determined by the anatomical location and specializations of the relevant transmodal epicenters. The large-scale network approach predicts that many, if not all, network components will be activated in concert during the performance of any task in a given cognitive domain. In keeping with this prediction, tasks related to spatial awareness, language, working memory, explicit memory, and object identification in human subjects have each led to the collective activation of the relevant epicenters noted earlier.[29,62,207,253,325,390,412,457] Functional imaging experiments cannot yet determine whether all network components are activated simultaneously or if the temporal sequence of activation varies according to the nature of the task. Such questions can be addressed by combining functional imaging with event-related potentials.[402]

Selectively Distributed Processing and Shifts of Network Affiliations

As noted in section V, unimodal association areas display regional specializations which follow the principles of selectively distributed processing. A similar organization can be discerned in large-scale neural networks. For example, Wernicke's area occupies the lexical–semantic pole of the language network but also participates in articulation and syntax whereas Broca's area occupies the articulatory–syntactic pole of the network but also participates in phonological discrimination and lexical access.[71,334] In the case of spatial attention, the frontal eye fields occupy the motor–exploratory pole of the relevant network but also participate in the compilation of perceptual representations whereas posterior parietal cortex occupies the sensory–representational pole but also participates in the programming of exploratory movements.[329] In the limbic network, the hippocampal complex is most closely related to explicit memory but also plays a role in emotional modulation whereas the amygdaloid complex is most closely related to emotional modulation but also participates in the encoding of emotionally salient memories.[65,363]

The nature of selectively distributed processing was probed experimentally in subjects undergoing depth electrode recordings as they were being investigated for the surgical treatment of epilepsy. The subjects were shown a large number of faces and common objects and were asked to engage in one of four tasks: detection of familiarity, perceptual matching, perceptual categorization, and working memory. Recording sites were located in the hippocampus, amygdala, inferotemporal cortex, and lateral prefrontal cortex. A recording site was noted to be engaged by a given task if the averaged evoked potentials to two contrasting stimuli (e.g., familiar versus unfamiliar faces) differed significantly.[480]

The results showed that all four recording sites were engaged by multiple tasks, but each with a distinct profile of selectivity. The hippocampus was the one area that did not seem to show a definite preference for one task over another, probably because none of the tasks required long-term explicit memory. The probability of activation was highest in the amygdala when the goal of the task was the detection of familiarity and emotional relevance; in the inferotemporal cortex when the goal was perceptual categorization or perceptual matching; and in prefrontal cortex when the goal was to hold information in working memory. These results show that there are no object or face "centers" in the brain but that activation is selectively distributed according to a probabilistic function determined by the goal of the task.

According to the plan of organization shown in Figure 1–17, cortical nodes are likely to participate in the function of more than one network. How (or whether) a cortical area can be recruited differentially into one network versus another remains poorly understood. Top-down connections could conceivably play a role in this process. For example, Friston showed that a region of inferotemporal cortex was able to yield differential activation to faces versus other objects only when there was a high level of activation in a region of posterior parietal cortex.[156] In another experiment, the same set of subjects were given two tasks, one of face identification, the other of spatial attention.[325] A region that corresponds to the parietal component of the attentional network (BA7), a region of prefrontal cortex (BA46) related to the frontal component of the same network, and a part of inferotemporal cortex (BA21) involved in face and object identification were activated by both tasks. However, the activation of BA7 in the task of object identification was much more strongly correlated with the activation of BA21 than with that of BA46, whereas the converse relationship was observed during the task of spatial attention. These results suggest that individual cortical areas can dynamically shift affiliation from one network to another depending on the overall goal of the task.

The mechanisms underlying these shifts of network affiliation have not been elucidated. Changes in behavioral context can alter the way in which the activity of a neuron is temporally correlated with the activity of another in the same area of the cerebral cortex.[528] Such effects could allow a rapid association and dissociation of local clusters into distinct functional subgroups, each favoring a different network linkage. These types of dynamic network reconfigurations occur in the stomatogastric ganglion of decapod crustacea, where they appear to be controlled by monoaminergic inputs.[205] Furthermore, in the lamprey, the same group of neurons mediates swimming, burrowing, and crawling and can be reoriented from one task-specific network to the other by serotonin through the modulation of a calcium-activated potassium current.[18] Conceivably, network realignments in the primate brain could also be influenced by the modulatory monoaminergic and cholinergic synapses of the cerebral cortex.

XXI. Overview and Conclusions

The evidence reviewed in this chapter shows that the cerebral cortex of the human brain can be divided into five functional zones which collectively provide a spectrum of architectonic differentiation and functional specialization. The zone with the least differentiated architecture and the strongest hypothalamic connectivity is designated "limbic." Its behavioral affiliations are polarized toward the coordination of visceral state, endocrine balance, immunoregulation, drive, emotion and memory. These neural functions emphasize homeostasis, the internal milieu, self preservation, and the propagation of the species. At the other end of the spectrum, the zone of primary sensory–motor cortex displays the most differentiated architecture and has the most immediate contact with the extrapersonal world. Its constituents coordinate skilled movements and encode accurate representations of sensory events. The intervening zones of unimodal, heteromodal, and paralimbic cortex enable the associative elaboration of incoming information and its linkage to action, drive, visceral state and emotion. These intervening zones support the type of integrative processes that are necessary for consciousness and cognition.

Multisynaptic streams of processing mediate the incorporation of sensory information into cognition and consciousness. At the first synaptic level, sensation is mapped by finely tuned neurons into a primary dimension—retinotopic for vision and tonotopic for audition. The second synaptic level mediates the more differentiated extraction of specific attributes such as color and motion. The third and fourth synaptic levels play critical roles in the perceptual encoding of faces, objects, words, and extrapersonal targets by ensembles of coarsely tuned neurons. Motivational, emotional, and attentional modulations are relatively weak at the first two synaptic levels but become increasingly more influential at higher synaptic levels where they help to depict a version of the world based on significance rather than appearance.

The fifth and sixth synaptic levels contain the heteromodal, paralimbic and limbic regions of the cerebral cortex, collectively known as *transmodal* areas. Transmodal areas enable the coherent binding of distributed multimodal information. They are critical for transforming perception into recognition, words into meaning, scenes and events into experiences, and spatial locations into targets for exploration. They also constitute epicenters for large-scale distributed networks. Cortical components of networks are interconnected with an architecture that enables rapid transitions from parallel to serial processing. Their functional organization follows the principles of selectively distributed processing. Each cortical node of a network can potentially belong to several intersecting networks and can dynamically shift allegiance from one to the other depending on the goal of the task.

One of the most important functions of the CNS is to convert the product of neural activity into stable memories. Facts and events that are destined to be registered in memory are composed of modality-specific sensory components. The initial encoding of these components occurs within unimodal areas and provides the perceptual information that can mediate implicit memory. The construction of consciously accessible memories necessitates a transformation of these isolated fragments into coherent multimodal representations. The multimodal binding that subserves this process is coordinated by the hippocampo–entorhinal complex and related limbic structures. Since behaviorally relevant events are more likely to elicit limbic activation, this arrangement promotes the preferential learning of behaviorally relevant experiences. Newly encoded memories remain more heavily dependent on the integrity of limbic connections for months to years as they gradually become consolidated through extensive associative linkages. Once memories are consolidated, the binding of their constituents becomes more dependent on transmodal areas outside of the limbic system and they become less vulnerable to limbic lesions. Thus, recently acquired facts, experiences, and associations are vulnerable to limbic lesions whereas memories of early childhood, the names of objects, and general facts about the world are not.

Since the nature, purpose, and consequences of environmental incidents are relatively unpredictable, any new event is likely to activate many, if not all, networks, at least initially. The steps of perceptual identification, deployment of spatial attention, lexical labeling, association with past experiences, linkage to emotional and visceral patterns, assessment of present context, planning of options, and prediction of consequences are likely to proceed simultaneously and iteratively as a rapid succession of scripts, scenarios, and hypotheses. The most relevant ensembles and networks are gradually expected to dominate the landscape of neural activity as they become more and more resonant with current goals and constraints. The solution to a cognitive problem or task could be defined as the settling of the entire system into a state of best fit. This would not constitute the final product of a hierarchical assembly line but rather a complex surface with many peaks and valleys spread over much of the cerebral cortex. There would be both localization (phrenology) and equipotentiality in the course of this process but the localization would be distributed and the equipotentiality would display regional selectivity.

From a strictly behavioral point of view, the existence of consciousness might be inferred when a living organism responds to environmental events in an adaptive way that is not entirely automatic. According to such a definition, consciousness is a property shared by numerous species. There are, however, differences of detail. The path from sensation to cognition in simpler brains with less intermediary processing is straight and narrow, leading to an equally modest texture of consciousness. In the human brain, the multiple paths inserted between the first and sixth synaptic levels of Figure 1–11b introduce a vast spatial expansion of the neural landscape that links sensation to cognition. Each node in Figure 1–11b provides a nexus for the convergence of afferents and the divergence of efferents. The resulting template allows the emergence of a large number of alternative trajectories as sensation becomes transformed into cognition. In the course of this process, obligatory one-to-one linkages between stimulus and response become transcended in a manner that greatly increases cognitive and behavioral flexibility. Working memory further expands the horizon of consciousness by stretching the temporal influence of internally or externally generated events and by increasing the number of processing channels that can be accommodated simultaneously.

Not all sensory events that activate the nodes in Figure 1–11b are necessarily accessible to consciousness. Some facts and events can be encoded in ways that covertly influence subsequent behavior even when the subject appears to have no conscious awareness of the relevant information. The phenomena of blindsight in hemianopic patients, implicit memory in amnesic patients, and autonomic responsivity to familiar faces in prosopagnosic patients have been reviewed earlier and provide examples of dissociations between neural encoding and conscious awareness. Furthermore, the conscious awareness of some sensory experiences may be delayed by up to 500 ms beyond the time of the initial cortical response, during which the incoming impulses appear to acquire "neuronal adequacy."[295,296] It appears, therefore, that the accessibility of an event to explicit consciousness and introspective commentary is the byproduct of a special type of cortical activity and not an automatic consequence of sensory encoding. Access to the level of explicit consciousness would appear to be most likely for components of experience that can elicit coherent binding and multimodal associative elaboration through the intercession of transmodal nodes.

Considering this remarkably complex organization, it is hardly surprising that the diseases of the human brain cause equally complex symptom clusters, some of which may appear to defy plausibility. One purpose of this chapter has been to show that basic facts related to the anatomy and physiology of the human brain can help to elucidate the relationship between the site of disease and the nature of the behavioral impairment. An equally important purpose has been to show that these facts may also guide the exploration of neurobiological principles which link brain structure to cognition and comportment.

This work was supported in part by NS 30863 and NS 20285 from the National Institute for Neurological Disorders and Stroke and AG 13854 from the National Institute on Aging.

REFERENCES

1. Ackerly, S: Instinctive, emotional and mental changes following prefrontal lobe extirpation. Am J Psychiatry 92:717–729, 1935.
2. Adolphs, R: Cortical systems for the recognition of emotion in facial expressions. J Neurosci 16:7678–7687, 1996.
3. Aggleton, J P: The contribution of the amygdala to normal and abnormal emotional states. Trends Neurosci 16:328–333, 1993.
4. Aggleton, J P, Desimore, R and Mishkin, M: The origin, course and termination of the hippocampothalamic projections in the macaque. J Comp Neurol 243:409–421, 1986.
5. Aggleton, J P and Mishkin, M: Visual recognition impairment following medial thalamic lesions in monkeys. Neuropsychologia 21:189–197, 1983.
6. Ahern, G L, Schomer, D L, Kleefield, J, Blume, H, Cosgrove, G R, Weintraub, S and Mesulam, M-M: Right hemisphere advantage for evaluating emotional facial expressions. Cortex 27:193–202, 1991.
7. Alexander, G E and Crutcher, M D: Preparation for movement: neural representations of intended direction in three motor areas of the monkey. J Neurophysiol 64:133–150, 1990.
8. Alexander, G E, Crutcher, M D and DeLong, M R: Basal ganglia-thalamocortical circuits: parallel substrates for motor, oculomotor, "prefrontal" and "limbic" functions. Prog Brain Res 85:119–146, 1990.
9. Alivisatos, B and Petrides, M: Functional activation of the human brain during mental rotation. Neuropsychologia 35:111–118, 1997.
10. Allison, T, McCarthy, G, Nobre, A, Puce, A and Belger, A: Human extrastriate visual cortex and the perception of faces, words, numbers, and colors. Cereb Cortex 5:544–554, 1994.
11. Amaral, D G, Veazey, R B and Cowan, W M: Some observations on hypothalamo-amygdaloid connections in the monkey. Brain Res 252:13–27, 1982.
12. Amyes, E W and Nielsen, J M: Clinicopathologic study of vascular lesions of the anterior cingulate region. Bull Los Angeles Neurol Soc 20:112–130, 1955.
13. Andersen, R A, Asanuma, C, Essick, C and Siegel, R M: Corticocortical connections of anatomically and physiologically defined subdivisions within the inferior parietal lobule. J Comp Neurol 113:65–113, 1990.
14. Apicella, P, Legallet, E and Trouche, E: Responses of tonically discharging neurons in the monkey striatum to primary rewards delivered during different behavioral states. Exp Brain Res 116:456–466, 1997.
15. Aston-Jones, G, Rajkowski, J and Kubiak, P: Conditioned responses of monkey locus coeruleus neurons anticipate acquisition of discriminative behavior in a vigilance task. Neuroscience 80:697–715, 1997.
16. Augustine, J R: Circuitry and functional aspects of the insular lobe in primates including humans. Brain Res Rev 22:229–244, 1996.

17. Ax, A F: The physiological differentiation between fear and anger in humans. Psychosom Med 15:433–442, 1953.
18. Ayers, J A, Carpenter, G A, Currie, S and Kinch, J: Which behavior does the lamprey central motor program mediate? Science 221:1312–1314, 1983.
19. Aziz, Q, Andersson, J L, Valind, S, Sundin, A, Hamdy, S, Jones, A K, Foster, E R, Langstrom, B and Thompson, D G: Identification of human brain loci processing esophageal sensation using positron emission tomography. Gastroenterology 113:50–59, 1997.
20. Bagshaw, M H and Pribram, K H: Cortical organization in gustation (*Macaca mulatta*). J Neurophysiol 16:499–508, 1953.
21. Ballentine, H T Jr, Levey, B A, Dagi, T F and Diriunas, I B: Cingulotomy for psychiatric illness: report of 13 years experience. In Sweet, W H, Obrador, S and Martin-Rodriques, J G (Eds.): Neurosurgical Treatment in Psychiatry, Pain and Epilepsy. University Park Press, Baltimore, 1977, pp. 333–353.
22. Bancaud, J, Talairach, J, Geier, S, Bonis, A, Trottier, S and Manrique, M: Manifestation comportementales induites par la stimulation eléctrique du gyrus cingulaire antérieur chez l'homme. Rev Neurol (Paris) 132:705–724, 1976.
23. Barbas, H and Mesulam, M-M: Organization of afferent input to subdivisions of area 8 in the rhesus monkey. J Comp Neurol 200:407–431, 1981.
24. Barbas, H and Mesulam, M M: Cortical afferent input to the principalis region of the rhesus monkey. Neuroscience 15:619–637, 1985.
25. Baskerville, K A, Schweitzer, J B and Herron, P: Effects of cholinergic depletion on experience-dependent plasticity in the cortex of the rat. Neuroscience 80:1159–1169, 1997.
26. Bauer, R M: Visual hypoemotionality as a symptom of visual-limbic disconnection in man. Arch Neurol 39:702–708, 1982.
27. Bauer, R M: Autonomic recognition of names and faces in prosopagnosia. Neuropsychologia 22:457–469, 1984.
28. Bauman, M and Kemper, T L: Histoanatomic observations of the brain in early infantile autism. Neurology 35:866–874, 1985.
29. Bavelier, D, Corina, D, Jezzard, P, Padmanabhan, S, Clark, V P, Karni, A, Prihster, A, Braun, A, Lalwani, A, Rauschecker, J P, Turner, R and Neville, H: Sentence reading: a functional MRI study at 4 tesla. J Cog Neurosci 9:664–689, 1997.
30. Beal, M F, Bird, E D, Langlais, P J and Martin, J B: Somatostatin is increased in the nucleus accumbens in Huntington's disease. Neurology 34:663–666, 1984.
31. Bear, D and Fedio, P: Quantitative analysis of interictal behavior in temporal lobe epilepsy. Arch Neurol 34:454–467, 1977.
32. Bechara, A, Damasio, H, Tranel, D and Damasio, A R: Deciding advantageously before knowing the advantageous strategy. Science 275:1293–1295, 1997.
33. Bechara, A, Tranel, D, Damasio, H, Adolphs, R, Rockland, C and Damasio, A R: Double dissociation of conditioning and declarative knowledge relative to the amygdala and hippocampus in humans. Science 269:1115–1118, 1995.
34. Benevento, L A, Fallon, J, Davis, B J and Rezak, M: Auditory-visual interaction in single cells in the cortex of the superior temporal sulcus and the orbital frontal cortex of the macaque monkey. Exp Neurol 57:849–872, 1977.
35. Benevento, L A and Rezak, M: The cortical projections of the inferior pulvinar and adjacent lateral pulvinar in the rhesus monkey (*Macaca mulatta*): an autoradiographic study. Brain Res 108:1–24, 1976.
36. Benowitz, L I, Bear, D M, Rosenthal, R, Mesulam, M M, Zaidel, E and Sperry, R W: Hemispheric specialization in nonverbal communication. Cortex 19:5–11, 1983.
37. Benowitz, L I, Perrone-Bizzozero, N I, Filkelstein, S P and Bird, E D: Localization of the growth-associated phosphoprotein GAP-43 (B-50, F1) in the human cerebral cortex. J Neurosci 9:990–995, 1989.
38. Benson, D A, Hienz, R D and Goldstein, M H Jr: Single-unit activity in the auditory cortex

of monkeys actively localizing sound sources: Spatial tuning and behavioral dependency. Brain Res 219:249–267, 1981.

39. Benson, D F and Geschwind, N: Shrinking retrograde amnesia. J Neurol Neurosurg Psychiatry 30:539–544, 1967.

40. Bentivoglio, M, Molinari, M, Minciacchi, D and Macchi, G: Organization of the cortical projections of the posterior complex and intralaminar nuclei of the thalamus as studied by means of retrograde tracers. In Macchi, G, Rustioni, A and Spreafico, R (Eds.): Somatosensory Intergation in the Thalamus. Elsevier, Amsterdam, 1983, pp. 338–363.

41. Benton, A L, Varney, N R and Hamsher, K D S: Lateral differences in tactile directional perception. Neuropsychologia 16:109–114, 1978.

42. Benzo, C A: The hypothalamus and blood glucose regulation. Life Sci 32:2509–2515, 1983.

43. Berger-Sweeney, J, Heckers, S, Mesulam, M-M, Wiley, R G, Lappi, D A and Sharma, M: Differential effects upon spatial navigation of immunotoxin-induced cholinergic lesions of the medial septal area and nucleus basalis magnocellularis. J Neurosci 14:4507–4519, 1994.

44. Berthier, M, Starkstein, S and Leiguarda, R: Asymbolia for pain: a sensory-limbic disconnection syndrome. Ann Neurol 24:41–49, 1988.

45. Bever, T G and Chiarello, R J: Cerebral dominance in musicians and nonmusicians. Science 185:537–539, 1974.

46. Bignall, K E and Imbert, M: Polysensory and cortico-cortical projections to frontal lobe of squirrel and rhesus monkeys. Electroencephalogr Clin Neurophysiol 26:206–215, 1969.

47. Binkofski, F, Dohle, C, Posse, S, Stephan, K M, Hefter, H, Seitz, R J and Freund, H-J: Human anterior intraparietal area subserves prehension. Neurology 50:1253–1259, 1998.

48. Bliss, T V and Collinridge, G L: A synaptic model of memory: long-term potentiation in the hippocampus. Nature 361:31–39, 1993.

49. Block, C H, Siegel, A and Edinger, H: Effects of amygdaloid stimulation upon trigeminal sensory fields of the lip that are established during hypothamically-elicited quiet biting attack in the cat. Brain Res 197:39–55, 1980.

50. Botez, M I: The neuropsychology of the cerebellum: an emerging concept. Arch Neurol 49:1229–1230, 1992.

51. Boulenguez, P, Foreman, N, Chauveau, J, Segu, L and Buhot, M-C: Distractability and locomotor activity in rat following intracollicular injection of a serotonin 1B-1D agonist. Behav Brain Res 67:229–239, 1995.

52. Brickner, R M: An interpretation of frontal lobe function based upon the study of a case of partial bilateral frontal lobectomy. Assoc Res Nerv Ment Dis Proc 13:259–351, 1934.

53. Brinkman, C and Porter, R: Supplementary motor area and premotor area of monkey cerebral cortex: functional organization and activities of single neurons during performance of a learned movement. In Desmedt, J E (Ed.): Motor Control Mechanisms in Health and Disease. Raven Press, New York, 1983,

54. Britton, D R, Ksir, C, Britton, K T, Young, D and Koob, G F: Brain norepinephrine depleting lesions selectively enhance behavioral responsiveness to novelty. Physiol Behav 33:473–478, 1984.

55. Broca, P: Anatomie comparée des circomvolutions cérébrales: le grand lobe limbique dans la série des mammifères. Revue Anthropologique 1:384–498, 1878.

56. Brodmann, K: Vergleichende Lokalisationlehre der Grosshirnrinde in ihren Prinzipien dargestellt auf Grund des Zellenbaues. J A Barth, Leipzig 1909.

57. Brodmann, K: Localisation in the Cerebral Cortex. Translated by L. J. Garey Smith-Gordon, London, 1994.

58. Brooks, W H, Cross, R J, Roszman, T L and Markesberg, W R: Neuroimmunomodulation: neural anatomical basis for impairment and facilitation. Ann Neurol 12:56–61, 1982.

59. Brothers, L and Ring, B: Mesial temporal neurons in the macaque monkey with responses selective for aspects of social stimuli. Behav Brain Res 57:53–61, 1993.

60. Brown, R M, Crane, A M and Goldman, P S: Regional distribution of monamines in the cerebral cortex and subcortical structures of the rhesus monkey: concentrations and in vivo synthesis rates. Brain Res 168:133–150, 1979.

61. Brumback, R A, Stanton, R D and Wilson, H: Right cerebral hemispheric dysfunction. Arch Neurol 41:248–249, 1984.

62. Bullmore, E T, Rabe-Hesketh, S, Morris, R G, Williams, S C R, Gregory, L, Gray, J A and Brammer, M J: Functional magnetic resonance image analysis of a large-scale neurocognitive network. Neuroimage 4:16–33, 1996.

63. Burton, H and Jones, E G: The posterior thalamic region and its cortical projection in New World monkeys. J Comp Neurol 168:249–301, 1976.

64. Butter, C M and Snyder, D R: Alterations in aversive and aggressive behaviors following orbital frontal lesions in rhesus monkeys. Acta Neurobiol Exp 32:525–565, 1972.

65. Cahill, L, Babinsky, R, Markowitsch, H and McGaugh, J L: The amygdala and emotional memory. Nature 377:295–296, 1995.

66. Cambier, J, Elghozi, D and Strube, E: Lésion du thalamus droit avec syndrome de l'hémisphere mineur. Discussion du concept de négligence thalamique. Rev Neurol (Paris) 136:105–116, 1980.

67. Caminiti, R, Ferraina, S and Johnson, P B: The sources of visual information to the primate frontal lobe: a novel role for the superior parietal lobule. Cortex 32:319–328, 1996.

68. Cammalleri, R, Gangitano, M, D'Amelio, M, Raieli, V, Raimondo, D and Camarda, R: Transient topographical amnesia and cingulate cortex damage: a case report. Neuropsychologia 34:321–326, 1996.

69. Campbell, A W: Histological Studies on the Localization of Cerebral Function. University Press, Cambridge, 1905.

70. Caplan, D, Alpert, N and Waters, G: Effects of syntactic structure and propositional number on patterns of regional cerebral blood flow. J Cog Neurosci 10:541–552, 1998.

71. Caplan, D, Hildebrandt, N and Makris, N: Location of lesions in stroke patients with deficits in synactic processing in sentence comprehension. Brain 119:933–949, 1996.

72. Caplan, L R, Schmahmann, J D, Kase, C S, Feldmann, E, Baquis, G, Greenberg, J P, Gorelick, P B, Helgason, C and Hier, D B: Caudate infarcts. Arch Neurol 47:133–143, 1990.

73. Carlson, M: Characteristics of sensory deficits following lesions of Brodmann's areas 1 and 2 in the postcentral gyrus of *Macaca mulatta*. Brain Res 204:424–430, 1981.

74. Carpenter, M B and Sutin, J: Human Neuroanatomy. Williams & Wilkins, Baltimore, 1983.

75. Caselli, R J: Tactile agnosia and disorders of tactile perception. In Feinberg, T E and Farah, M J (Eds.): Behavioral Neurology and Neuropsychology. McGraw-Hill, New York, 1997, pp. 277–288.

76. Casey, B J, Trainor, R J, Orrendi, J L, Schubert, A B, Nystrom, L E, Giedd, J N, Castellanos, F X, Haxley, J V, Noll, D C, Cohen, J D, Forman, S D, Dahl, R E and Rapoport, J L: A developmental functional MRI study of prefrontal activation during performance of a go-no-go task. J Cog Neurosci 9:835–847, 1997.

77. Casey, K L, Minoshima, S, Berger, K L, Koeppe, R A, Morrow, T J and Frey, K A: Positron emission tomographic analysis of cerebral structures activated specifically by repetitive noxious heat stimuli. J Neurophysiol 71:802–807, 1994.

78. Cavada, C and Goldman-Rakic, P S: Posterior parietal cortex in rhesus monkey. II. Evidence for segregated corticocortical networks linking sensory and limbic areas with the frontal lobe. J Comp Neurol 287:422–445, 1989.

79. Chalupa, L M, Coyle, R S and Lindsley, D B: Effect of pulvinar lesions on visual pattern discrimination in monkeys. J Neurophysiol 39:354–369, 1976.

80. Chao, L L, Weisberg, J A, Wiggs, C L, Haxby, J V, Ungerleider, L G and Martin, A: Cortical regions associated with perception, naming and knowledge of color. Neuroimage 5: S54, 1997.

81. Chapman, W P, Livingston, K E and Poppen, J L: Effect upon blood pressure of electrical stimulation of tips of temporal lobes in man. J Neurophysiol 13:65–71, 1950.

82. Chen, W R, Lee, S, Kato, K, Spencer, D D, Shepherd, G M and Williamson, A: Long-term modifications of synaptic efficacy in the human inferior and middle temporal cortex. Proc Natl Acad Sci USA 93:8011–8015, 1996.

83. Chi, J G, Dooling, E C and Gilles, F H: Gyral development of the human brain. Ann Neurol 1:86–93, 1977.

84. Chikama, M, McFarland, N R, Amaral, D G and Haber, S N: Insular cortical projections to functional regions of the striatum correlate with cortical cytoarchitectonic organization in the primate. J Neurosci 17:9686–9705, 1997.

85. Claparède, M: Récognition et moiité. Arch Psychol 11:79–90, 1911.

86. Clark, V P, Maisog, J M and Haxby, J V: FMRI studies of face memory using random stimulus sequences. Neuroimage 5:S50, 1997.

87. Clause, R E and Lustman, P J: Psychiatric illness and contraction abnormalities of the esophagus. N Engl J Med 309:1337–1342, 1983.

88. Coghill, R C, Talbot, J D, Evans, A C, Meyer, E, Gjedde, A, Bushnell, M C and Duncan, G H: Distributed processing of pain and vibration by the human brain. J Neurosci 14:4095–4108, 1994.

89. Cohen, H D, Rosen, R C and Goldstein, L: Electroencephalographic laterality changes during human sexual orgasm. Arch Sex Behav 5:189–199, 1976.

90. Cohen, J D, Peristein, W M, Braver, T S, Nystrom, L E, Noll, D C, Jonides, J and Smith, E E: Temporal dynamics of brain activation during a working memory task. Nature 386:604–606, 1997.

91. Colombo, M, Rodman, H R and Gross, C G: The effects of superior temporal cortex lesions on the processing and retention of auditory information in monkeys (*Cebus apella*). J Neurosci 16:4501–4517, 1996.

92. Connor, C E, Gallant, J L, Preddie, D C and Van Essen, D C: Responses in area V4 depend on the spatial relationship between stimulus and attention. J Neurophysiol 75:1306–1308, 1996.

93. Corbetta, M, Miezin, F M, Dobmeyer, S, Shulman, G L and Petersen, S: Selective and divided attention during visual discriminations of shape, color, and speed: functional anatomy by positron emission tomography. J Neurosci 11:2383–2402, 1991.

94. Corbetta, M, Miezin, F M, Dobmeyer, S, Shulman, G M and Petersen, S E: Attentional modulation of neural processing of shape, color and velocity in humans. Science 248:1556–1559, 1990.

95. Corkin, S, Milner, B and Rasmussen, T: Somatosensory thresholds. Arch Neurol 23:41–58, 1970.

96. Craig, A D, Bushnell, M C, Zhang, E-T and Blomqvist, A: A thalamic nucleus specific for pain and temperature sensation. Nature 372:770–773, 1994.

97. Craik, R L, Hand, P J and Levin, B E: *Locus coeruleus* input affects glucose metabolism in activated rat barrel cortex. Brain Res Bull 19:495–499, 1987.

98. Creutzfeldt, O, Ojemann, G and Lettich, E: Neuronal activity in the human lateral temporal lobe. I. Responses to speech. Brain Res 77:451–475, 1989.

99. Cruikshank, S J and Weinberger, N M: Evidence for the Hebbian hypothesis in experience-dependent physiological plasticity of neocortex: a critical review. Brain Res Rev 22:191–228, 1996.

100. Curran, T, Schacter, D L, Norman, K A and Galluccio, L: False recognition after a right frontal lobe infarction: memory for general and specific information. Neuropsychologia 35:1035–1049, 1997.

101. D'Esposito, M, Detre, J A, Alsop, D C, Shin, R K, Atlas, S and Grossman, M: The neural basis of the central executive system of working memory. Nature 378:279–281, 1995.

102. Daffner, K R, Mesulam, M-M, Scinto, L F M, Cohen, L G, Kennedy, B F, West, W C and Holcomb, P J: Regulation of attention to novel stimuli by frontal lobes: an event-related potential study. Neuroreport 9:787–791, 1998.

103. Damasio, A R: Disorders of complex visual processing: agnosias, achromatopsia, Balint's syndrome, and related difficulties of orientation and construction. In Mesulam, M-M (Ed.): Principles of Behavioral Neurology. F. A. Davis, Philadelphia, 1985, pp. 259–288.

104. Damasio, A R: The brain binds entities and events by multiregional activation from convergence zones. Neur Comp 1:123–132, 1989.

105. Damasio, A R: On some functions of the human prefrontal cortex. Ann NY Acad Sci 769:241–251, 1995.

106. Damasio, H, Grabowski, T J, Tranel, D, Hichwa, R D and Damasio, A R: A neural basis for lexical retrieval. Nature 380:499–505, 1996.

107. Darian-Smith, I, Sugitani, M, Heywood, J, Korita, K and Goodwin, A: Touching textured surfaces: cells in somatosensory cortex respond both to finger movement and to surface features. Science 218:906–909, 1982.

108. Davidson, R J and Fox, N A: Asymmetrical brain activity discriminates between positive and negative affective stimuli in human infants. Science 218:1235–1247, 1982.

109. De Cristofaro, M T, Sessarego, A, Pupi, A, Biondi, F and Faravelli, C: Brain perfusion abnormalities in drug-naive, lactate-sensitive panic patients: a SPECT study. Biol Psychiatry 33:505–512, 1993.

110. De Renzi, E, Faglioni, P and Sorgato, P: Modality-specific and supramodal mechanisms of apraxia. Brain 105:301–312, 1982.

111. De Renzi, E, Faglioni, P and Villa, P: Topographical amnesia. J Neurol Neurosurg Psychiatry 40:498–505, 1977.

112. DeLong, M R: Activity of pallidal neurons during movement. J Neurophysiol 34:414–427, 1971.

113. Démonet, J-F, Chollet, F, Ramsay, S, Cardebat, D, Nespoulous, J-L, Wise, R, Rascol, A and Frackowiak, R: The anatomy of phonological and semantic processing in normal subjects. Brain 115:1992.

114. Denny-Brown, D and Chambers, R A: Physiological aspects of visual perception. I. Functional aspects of visual cortex. Arch Neurol 33:219–227, 1976.

115. Desimone, R: Face-selective cells in the temporal cortex of monkeys. J Cog Neurosci 3: 1–8, 1991.

116. Desimone, R: Neural mechanisms for visual memory and their role in attention. Proc Natl Acad Sci USA 93:13494–13499, 1996.

117. Desimone, R and Gross, C G: Visual areas in the temporal cortex of the macaque. Brain Res 178:363–380, 1979.

118. Devinsky, O, Morrell, M J and Vogt, B A: Contributions of anterior cingulate cortex to behaviour. Brain 118:279–306, 1995.

119. Dias, E C, Compaan, D M, Mesulam, M-M and Segraves, M A: Selective disruption of memory-guided saccades with injecton of a cholinergic antagonist in the frontal eye field of monkey. Soc Neurosci Abstr 22:418, 1996.

120. Dicks, D, Myers, R E and Kling, A: Uncus and amygdala lesions: effects on social behavior in the free-ranging rhesus monkey. Science 165:71, 1969.

121. Dimond, S J: Sex differences in brain organization. Behav Brain Sci 3:215–263, 1980.

122. Dimond, S J, Farrington, L and Johnson, P: Differing emotional response from right and left hemisphere. Nature 261:690–692, 1976.

123. Dinse, H R and Kruger, K: The timing of processing along the visual pathway in the cat. Neuroreport 5:893–897, 1994.

124. Doty, R W: Nongeniculate afferents to striate cortex in macaques. J Comp Neurol 218: 159–173, 1983.

125. Downer, C L J: Interhemispheric integration in the visual system. In Mountcastle, V B

(Ed.): Interhemispheric Relations and Cerebral Dominance. Johns Hopkins University Press, Baltimore, 1962, pp. 87–100.

126. Dringenberg, H C and Vanderwolf, C H: Neocortical activation: modulation by multiple pathways acting on central cholinergic and serotonergic systems. Exp Brain Res 116:160–174, 1997.

127. Dronkers, N F: A new brain region for coordinating speech articulation. Nature 384:159–161, 1996.

128. Duvernoy, H: The Human Brain. Springer-Verlag, Wien, 1991.

129. Dwyer, J H I and Rinn, W E: The role of the right hemisphere in contextual inference. Neuropsychologia 19:479–482, 1981.

130. Edelman, S: Representation is representation of similarities. Behav Brain Sci 21:449–467, 1998.

131. Eichenbaum, H, Morton, T H, Potter, H and Corkin, S: Selective olfactory deficits in case H.M. Brain 106:459–472, 1983.

132. Eichenbaum, H, Schoenbaum, G, Young, B and Bunsey, M: Functional organization of the hippocampal memory system. Proc Natl Acad Sci USA 93:13500–13507, 1996.

133. Eidelberg, D, Moeller, J R, Antonini, A, Kazumata, K, Dhawan, V, Budman, C and Feigin, A: The metabolic anatomy of Tourette's syndrome. Neurology 48:927–934, 1997.

134. Erickson, R P: The across-fiber pattern theory: an organizing principle for molar neural function. Contrib Sensory Physiol 6:79–110, 1982.

135. Eslinger, P J and Damasio, A R: Severe disturbance of higher cognition after bilateral frontal lobe ablation: patient EVR. Neurology 35:1731–1741, 1985.

136. Evarts, E V, Fromm, C, Kroller, J and Jennings, V A: Motor cortex control of finely graded forces. J Neurophysiol 49:1199–1215, 1983.

137. Exner, S: Untersuchungen über Localisation der Functionen in der Grosshirnrinde des Menschen. W. Braumuller, Vienna, 1881.

138. Fahy, F L, Riches, I P and Brown, M W: Neuronal activity related to visual recognition memory: long-term memory and the encoding of recency and familiarity information in the primate anterior and medial inferior temporal and rhinal cortex. Exp Brain Res 96:457–472, 1993.

139. Fahy, F L, Riches, I P and Brown, M W: Neuronal signals of importance to the performance of visual recognition memory tasks: evidence from recordings of single neurones in the medial thalamus of primates. Prog Brain Res 95:401–416, 1993.

140. Farah, M J and Feinberg, T E: Visual object agnosia. In Feinberg, T E and Farah, M J (Eds.): Behavioral Neurology and Neuropsychology. McGraw-Hill, New York, 1997, pp. 239–244.

141. Felleman, D J and Van Essen, D C: Distributed hierarchical processing in the primate cerebral cortex. Cereb Cortex 1:1–47, 1991.

142. Fenz, W D and Epstein, S: Gradients of physiological arousal in parachutists as a functon of an approaching jump. Psychosom Med 29:33–51, 1967.

143. Fiez, J A: Cerebellar contributions to cognition. Neuron 16:13–15, 1996.

144. Fiez, J A, Raife, E A, Balota, D A, Schwarz, J P and Raichle, M E: A positron emission tomography study of the short-term maintenance of verbal information. J Neurosci 16:808–822, 1996.

145. Filimonoff, I N: A rational subdivision of the cerebral cortex. Arch Neurol Psychiatry 58:296–311, 1947.

146. Fink, G R, Markowitsch, H J, Reinkemeier, M, Bruckbauer, T, Kessler, J and Heiss, W-D: Cerebral representation of one's own past: neural networks involved in autobiographical memory. J Neurosci 16:4275–4282, 1996.

147. Flechsig, P: Anatomie des menschlichen Gehirns und Rückenmarks. Verlag von Georg Thieme, Leipzig, 1920.

148. Fleminger, J J, McClure, G M and Dalton, R: Lateral response to suggestion in relation to handedness and the side of psychogenic symptoms. Br J Psychiatry 136:562–566, 1980.

149. Flor-Henry, P: On certain aspects of the localization of the cerebral systems regulating and determining emotion. Biol Psychiatry 14:677–698, 1979.

150. Fodor, J A: The Modularity of Mind. MIT Press, Cambridge, Massachusetts, 1983.

151. Foote, S L, Bloom, F E and Aston-Jones, G: Nucleus locus coeruleus: new evidence of anatomical and physiological specificity. Physiol Rev 63:844–914, 1983.

152. Foundas, A L, Leonard, C M, Gilmore, R, Fennell, E and Heilman, K M: Planum temporale asymmetry and language dominance. Neuropsychology 32:1225–1231, 1994.

153. Franzen, E A and Myers, R E: Neural control of social behavior: prefrontal and anterior temporal cortex. Neuropsychologia 11:141–157, 1973.

154. Freedman, M, Alexander, M P and Naeser, M A: Anatomical basis of transcortical motor aphasia. Neurology 34:409–417, 1984.

155. Freund, T F and Meskenaite, V: γ-Amynobutyric acid-containing basal forebrain neurons innervate inhibitory interneurons in the neocortex. Proc Natl Acad Sci USA 89:738–742, 1992.

156. Friston, K J: Imaging cognitive anatomy. TICS 1:21–27, 1997.

157. Fujita, I, Tanaka, K, Ito, M and Cheng, K: Columns for visual features of objects in monkey inferotemporal cortex. Nature 360:343–346, 1992.

158. Fukatsu, R, Fujii, T and Yamadori, A: Pure somaesthetic alexia: somaesthetic-verbal disconnection for letters. Brain 121:843–850, 1998.

159. Furey, M L, Pietrini, P, Haxby, J V, Alexander, G E, Lee, H C, VanMeter, J, Grady, C L, Shetty, U, Rapoport, S I, Schapiro, M B and Freo, U: Cholinergic stimulation alters performance and task-specific regional cerebral blood flow during working memory. Proc Natl Acad Sci USA 94:6512–6516, 1997.

160. Fuster, J, Bauer, R H and Jervey, J P: Cellular discharge in the dorsolateral prefrontal cortex of the monkey in cognitive tasks. Exp Neurol 77:679–694, 1982.

161. Fuster, J M, Bauer, R H and Jervey, J P: Functional interactions between inferotemporal and prefrontal cortex in a cognitive task. Brain Res 330:299–307, 1985.

162. Gainotti, G: The relationships between emotions and cerebral dominance: a review of clinical and experimental evidence. In Gruzelier, J and Flor-Henry, P (Eds.): Hemisphere Asymmetries of Function in Psychopathology. Elsevier, North-Holland, 1979, pp. 21–34.

163. Gannon, P J, Holloway, R L, Broadfield, D C and Braun, A R: Asymmetry of chimpanzee planum temporale: humanlike pattern of Wernicke's brain language area homolog. Science 279:220–222, 1998.

164. Gaspar, P, Berger, B, Febvert, A, Vigny, A and Henry, J P: Catecholamine innervation of the human cerebral cortex as revealed by comparative immunohistochemistry of tyrosine hydroxylase and dopamine-beta-hydroxylase. J Comp Neurol 279:249–271, 1989.

165. Gauthier, I, Anderson, A W, Tarr, M J, Skudlarski, P and Gore, J C: Levels of categorization in visual recognition studied using functional magnetic resonance imaging. Curr Biol 7:645–651, 1997.

166. Geisler, W S and Albrecht, D G: Bayesian analysis of identification performance in monkey visual cortex: nonlinear mechanisms and stimulus certainty. Vision Res 35:2723–2730, 1995.

167. Georgopoulos, A P: Motor cortex and cognitive processing. In Gazzaniga, M S (Ed.): The Cognitive Neurosciences. The MIT Press, Cambridge, MA, 1995, pp. 507–517.

168. Gerloff, C, Corwell, B, Chen, R, Hallett, M and Cohen, L G: The role of the human motor cortex in the control of complex and simple finger movement sequences. Brain 121: 1695–1709, 1998.

169. Geschwind, N: Disconnection syndromes in animals and man. Brain 88:237–294, 1965.

170. Geschwind, N and Levitsky, W: Human brain: left-right asymmetries in temporal speech region. Science 161:186–187, 1968.

171. Girgis, M: The orbital surface of the frontal lobe of the brain and mental disorders. Acta Psychiatr Scand Suppl 222:7–58, 1971.

172. Gitelman, D R, Nobre, A N, Parrish, T B, LaBar, K S, Kim, Y-H, Meyer, J R and Mesulam, M-M: A large-scale distributed network for spatial attention: an fMRI study with stringent behavioral controls. Brain 122: 1093–1106, 1999.

173. Gitelman, D R, Nobre, A C, Gupta, T, Parrish, T B, Thompson, C K, LaBar, K S, Kim, Y-H and Mesulam, M-M: Phonological and semantic functional activations: parallel studies using fMRI. Soc Neurosci Abstr 24:1173, 1998.

174. Gloor, P, Olivier, A, Quesney, A F, Andermann, F and Horowitz, S: The role of the limbic system in experiential phenomena of temporal lobe epilepsy. Ann Neurol 12:129–144, 1982.

175. Godefroy, O and Rousseaux, M: Novel decision making in patients with prefrontal or posterior brain damage. Neurology 49:695–701, 1997.

176. Goel, V, Grafman, J, Tajik, J, Gana, S and Danto, D: A study of the performance of patients with frontal lobe lesions in a financial planning task. Brain 120:1805–1822, 1997.

177. Goldberg, M E and Segraves, M A: Visuospatial and motor attention in the monkey. Neuropsychologia 25:107–118, 1987.

178. Goldman-Rakic, P S: Topography of cognition: parallel distributed networks in primate association cortex. Annu Rev Neurosci 11:137–156, 1988.

179. Goldman-Rakic, P S and Friedman, H S: The circuitry of working memory revealed by anatomy and metabolic imaging. In Levin, H S, Eisenberg, H M and Benton, A L (Eds.): Frontal Lobe Function and Dysfunction. Oxford University Press, New York, 1991, pp. 72–91.

180. Goldstein, J M and Siegal, J: Stimulation of ventral tegmental area and nucleus accumbens reduce receptive fields for hypothalamic biting reflex in cats. Exp Neurol 72:239–246, 1981.

181. Goldstein, K: The significance of the frontal lobes for mental performances. J Neurol Psychopathol 17:27–40, 1936.

182. Goldstein, L H, Bernard, S, Fenwick, P B, Burgess, P W and McNeil, J: Unilateral frontal lobectomy can produce strategy application disorder. J Neurol Neurosurg Psychiatry 56: 274–276, 1993.

183. Gorno Tempini, M L, Price, C, Vandenberghe, R, Josephs, O, Kapur, N, Cappa, S F and Frackowiak, R S J: Functional anatomy of a common semantic system for names and faces. Neuroimage 5:S560, 1997.

184. Gower, E C and Mesulam, M M: Some paralimbic connections of the medial pulvinar nucleus in the macaque. Soc Neurosci Abstr 4:75, 1978.

185. Gower, E C and Mesulam, M M: Thalamic connections of paralimbic cortex in the temporal pole of the macaque. Soc Neurosci Abstr 5:75, 1979.

186. Grafton, S T, Fadiga, L, Arbib, M A and Rizzolatti, G: Premotor cortex activation during observation and naming of familiar tools. Neuroimage 6:231–236, 1997.

187. Green, J D, Clemente, C D and DeGroot, J: Rhinencephalic lesions and behavior in cats. J Comp Neurol 108:505–536, 1957.

188. Gritti, I, Mainville, L and Jones, B E: Codistribution of GABA with acetylcholine-synthesizing neurons in the basal forebrain of the rat. J Comp Neurol 329:438–457, 1993.

189. Groenewegen, H J, Becker, N and Lohman, A: Subcortical afferents of the nucleus accumbens septi in the cat, studied with retrograde axonal transport of horseradish peroxidase and bisbenzimide. Neuroscience 5:1903–1916, 1980.

190. Gross, C G, Rocha-Miranda, C E and Bender, D B: Visual properties of neurons in inferotemporal cortex of the macaque. J Neurophysiol 35:96–111, 1972.

191. Grossman, S P: Behavioral functions of the septum: a re-analysis. In DeFrance, J F (Ed.): The Septal Nuclei. Plenum Press, New York, 1976, pp. 361–422.

192. Guard, O, Delpy, C, Richard, D and Dumas, R: Une cause mal connue de confusion mentale: le ramollissemant temporal droit. Rev Med 40:2115–2121, 1979.

193. Gugliemotti, V and Fiorino, L: Asymmetry in the left and right habenulo-interpeduncular tracts in the frog. Brain Res Bull 45:105–110, 1998.

194. Guillery, R W: Afferent fibers to the dorso-medial thalamic nucleus in the cat. J Anat 93:403–419, 1959.

195. Guldin, W O and Grüsser, O-J: Is there a vestibular cortex? Trends Neurosci 21:254–259, 1998.

196. Haber, S N and Fudge, J L: The primate substantia nigra and VTA: integrative circuitry and function. Crit Rev Neurobiol 11:323–342, 1997.

197. Habib, M and Poncet, M: Loss of vitality, of interest and of the affect (athymhormia syndrome) in lacunar lesions of the corpus striatum. Rev Neurol (Paris) 144:571–577, 1988.

198. Hadjikhani, N, Liu, A K, Dale, A M, Cavanagh, P and Tootell, R B H: Retinotopy and color sensitivity in human visual cortex area V8. Nat Neurosci 1:235–241, 1998.

199. Halgren, E, Dale, A M, Sereno, M I, Tootell, R B H, Marinkovic, K and Rosen, B R: Location of fMRI responses to faces anterior to retinotopic cortex. Neuroimage 5:S150, 1997.

200. Halgren, E, Wilson, C L and Stapleton, J M: Human medial temporal-lobe stimulation disrupts both formation and retrieval of recent memories. Brain Cogn 4:287–295, 1985.

201. Hall, R E and Cornish, K: Role of the orbital cortex in cardiac dysfunction in unesthe- tized rhesus monkey. Exp Neurol 56:289–297, 1977.

202. Halsband, U and Passingham, R: The role of premotor and parietal cortex in the direc- tion of action. Brain Res 240:368–372, 1982.

203. Harlow, J M: Recovery from the passage of an iron bar through the head. Mass Med Soc Publ 2:327–346, 1868.

204. Harries, M H and Perrett, D I: Visual processing of faces in temporal cortex: physiolog- ical evidence for a modular organization and possible anatomical correlates. J Cog Neu- rosci 3:9–24, 1991.

205. Harris-Warrick, R M and Marder, E: Modulation of neural networks for behavior. Annu Rev Neurosci 14:39–57, 1991.

206. Hashimoto, S, Gemba, H and Sasaki, K: Analysis of slow cortical potentials preceding self-paced hand movements in the monkey. Exp Neurol 65:218–229, 1979.

207. Haxby, J V, Clark, V P and Courtney, M: Distributed hierarchical neural systems for visual memory in human cortex. In Hyman, B T, Duyckaerts, C and Christen, Y (Eds.): Connections, Cognition and Alzheimer's Disease. Springer Verlag, Berlin, 1997, pp. 167– 180.

208. Haxby, J V, Horwitz, B, Ungerleider, L G, Maisong, J M, Pietrini, P and Grady, C L: The functional organization of human extrastriate cortex: a PET-rCBF study of selective atten- tion to faces and locations. J Neurosci 14:6336–6363, 1994.

209. Haxby, J V, Martin, A, Clark, V P, Hoffman, E A, Schouten, J L and Ungerleier, L G: The processing of faces, inverted faces and other objects in the ventral object vision pathway. Neuroimage 5:S4, 1997.

210. Heath, R G: Studies in Schizophrenia. University Press, Cambridge, MA, 1959.

211. Hebb, D D: Man's frontal lobes. Arch Neurol Psychiatry 54:10–24, 1945.

212. Heckers, S, Geula, C and Mesulam, M M: Cholinergic innervation of the human thala- mus: dual origin and differential nuclear distribution. J Comp Neurol 325:68–82, 1992.

213. Heffner, H and Masterton, B: Contribution of auditory cortex to sound localization in the monkey (*Macaca mulatta*). J Neurophysiol 38:1340–1358, 1975.

214. Heffner, H E and Heffner, R S: Temporal lobe lesions and perception of species-specific vocalizations by macaques. Science 226:75–76, 1984.

215. Heilman, K M, Watson, R T and Rothi, L G: Disorders of skilled movements: limb apraxia. In Feinberg, T E and Farah, M J (Eds.): Behavioral Neurology and Neuropsy- chology. McGraw-Hill, New York, 1997, pp. 227–235.

216. Heimer, L: The olfactory connections of the diencephalon in the rat. Brain Behav Evol 6:484–523, 1972.

217. Heimer, L and Wilson, R D: The subcortical projections of the allocortex: similarities in

the neural associations of the hippocampus, the piriform cortex and the neocortex. In Santini, M (Ed.): Golgi Centennial Symposium. Proceedings. Raven Press, New York, 1975, pp. 177–193.

218. Heller, W and Levy, J: Perception and expression of emotion in right-handers and left-handers. Neuropsychologia 19:263–272, 1981.

219. Henke, P G: The telencephalic limbic system and experimental gastric pathology. Neurosci Biobehav Rev 6:381–390, 1982.

220. Henke, P G: Stomach pathology and the amygdala. In Aggleton, J P (Ed.): The Amygdala. Wiley-Liss, New York, 1992, pp. 324–338.

221. Heywood, C and Cowey, A: With color in mind. Nat Neurosci 1:171–173, 1998.

222. Higuchi, S-I and Miyashita, Y: Formation of mnemonic neuronal responses to visual paired associates in inferotemporal cortex is impaired by perirhinal and entorhinal lesions. Proc Natl Acad Sci USA 93:739–743, 1996.

223. Hikosaka, O and Wurtz, R H: Visual and oculomotor functions of monkey substantia nigra pars reticulata: III. Memory-contingent visual and saccade responses. J Neurophysiol 49:1268–1284, 1983.

224. Hoffman, B L and Rasmussen, T: Stimulation studies of insular cortex of *Macaca mulatta*. J Neurophysiol 16:343–351, 1953.

225. Holmes, G: The cerebellum of man: Hughlings Jackson lecture. Brain 62:1–30, 1939.

226. Horel, J, Meyer-Lohmann, J and Brooks, V B: Basal ganglia cooling disables learned arm movements of monkeys in the absence of visual guidance. Science 195:584–586, 1977.

227. Horel, J A and Misantone, L J: The Klüver-Bucy syndrome produced by partial isolation of the temporal lobe. Exp Neurol 42:101–112, 1974.

228. Hornykiewicz, O and Kish, S J: Neurochemical basis of dementia in Parkinson's disease. Can J Neurol Sci 11:185–190, 1984.

229. House, A, Dennis, M, Warlow, C, Hawton, K and Molyneux, A: Mood disorders after stroke and their relation to lesion location. A CT scan study. Brain 113:1113–1129, 1990.

230. Hubel, D H and Wiesel, T N: Receptive fields and functional architecture in two non-striate visual areas (18 and 19) of the cat. J Neurophysiol 28:229–289, 1965.

231. Huerta, P T and Lisman, J E: Heightened synaptic plasticity of hippocampal CA1 neurons during a cholinergically induced rhythmic state. Nature 364:723–725, 1993.

232. Hyvärinen, J: Regional distribution of functions in parietal association area 7 of the monkey. Brain Res 206:287–303, 1981.

233. Hyvärinen, J and Poranen, A: Function of the parietal associative area 7 as revealed from cellular discharges in alert monkeys. Brain 97:673–692, 1974.

234. Ironside, R and Guttmacher, R: The corpus callosum and its tumours. Brain 52:442–483, 1929.

235. Ishai, A, Ungerleider, L G, Martin, A, Maisog, J M and Haxby, J V: fMRI reveals differential activation in the ventral object vision pathway during the perception of faces, houses, and chairs. Neuroimage 5:S149, 1997.

236. Isseroff, A, Rosvold, H E, Galkin, T W and Goldman-Rakic, P S: Spatial memory impairments following damage to the mediodorsal nucleus of the thalamus in rhesus monkeys. Brain Res 232:97–113, 1982.

237. Ito, S I: Prefrontal unit activity of macaque monkeys during auditory and visual reaction time tasks. Brain Res 247:39–47, 1982.

238. Iversen, S D: Behavior after neostriatal lesions in animals. In Divac, I and Oberg, R G E (Eds.): The Neostriatum. Pergamon Press, Oxford, 1979, pp. 195–210.

239. Iversen, S D and Mishkin, M: Comparison of superior temporal and inferior prefrontal lesions on auditory and non-auditory tasks in rhesus monkeys. Brain Res 55:355–367, 1973.

240. Jacobs, M D, Morgane, P J and McFarland, W L: The anatomy of the brain of the Bottlenose Dolphin (*Tursiops truncatus*). Rhinic lobe (Rhinencephalon) I. The paleocortex. J Comp Neurol 141:205–272, 1971.

241. Jacobsen, C: Studies of cerebral function in primates. I. The functions of the frontal association areas in monkeys. Comp Psychol Monogr 13:3–60, 1936.

242. Jäncke, L, Schlaug, G, Huang, Y and Steinmetz, H: Asymmetry of planum parietale. Neuroreport 5:1161–1163, 1994.

243. Jasper, H H: Functional properties of the thalamic reticular system. In Adrian, E D, Bremer, F, Jasper, H H and Delafresnaye, J F (Eds.): Brain Mechanisms and Consciousness. Charles C Thomas, Springfield, IL, 1954, pp. 374–401.

244. Javoy-Agid, F and Agid, Y: Is the mesocortical dopaminergic system involved in Parkinson disease? Neurology 30:1326–1330, 1980.

245. Jodo, E, Chiang, C and Aston-Jones, G: Potent excitatory influence of prefrontal cortex activity on noradrenergic Locus Coeruleus neurons. Neuroscience 83:63–79, 1998.

246. Jones, E G: Some aspects of the organization of the thalamic reticular complex. J Comp Neurol 162:285–308, 1975.

247. Jones, E G: The Thalamus. Plenum Press, New York, 1985.

248. Jones, E G and Burton, H: A projection from medial pulvinar to the amygdala in primates. Brain Res 104:142–147, 1976.

249. Jones, E G and Powell, T P S: An anatomical study of converging sensory pathways within the cerebral cortex of the monkey. Brain 93:37–56, 1970.

250. Jones, E G, Wise, S P and Coulter, J D: Differential thalamic relationships of sensory-motor and parietal cortical fields in monkeys. J Comp Neurol 183:833–881, 1979.

251. Jurgens, U: Amygdalar vocalization pathways in the squirrel monkey. Brain Res 241: 189–196, 1982.

252. Jurgens, W and Von Cramon, D: On the role of the anterior cingulate cortex in phonation: A case report. Brain Lang 15:234–248, 1982.

253. Just, M A, Carpenter, P A, Keller, T A, Eddy, W F and Thulborn, K R: Brain activation modulated by sentence comprehension. Science 274:114–116, 1996.

254. Kaada, B R: Cingulate, posterior orbital, anterior insular and temporal pole cortex. In Magoun, H W (Ed.): Neurophysiology. Waverly Press, Baltimore, 1960, pp. 1345–1372.

255. Kaada, B R, Pribram, K H and Epstein, J A: Respiratory and vascular responses in monkeys from temporal pole, insula, orbital surface and cingulate gyrus. J Neurophysiol 12: 348–356, 1949.

256. Kaas, J H: What, if anything, is SI? Organization of first somatosensory area of cortex. Physiol Rev 63:206–231, 1983.

257. Kahnemann, D, Tursky, B, Shapiro, D and Crider, A: Pupillary, heart rate and skin resistance changes during a mental task. J Exp Psychol 79:164–167, 1969.

258. Kanwisher, N, McDermott, J and Chun, M M: The fusiform face area: a module in human extrastriate cortex specialized for face perception. J Neurosci 17:4302–4311, 1997.

259. Kanwisher, N, Woods, R P, Iacobini, M and Mazziotta, J C: A locus in human extrastriate cortex for visual shape analysis. J Cog Neurosci 9:133–142, 1997.

260. Karol, E A and Pandya, D N: The distribution of the corpus callosum in the rhesus monkey. Brain 94:471–486, 1971.

261. Kase, C S, Troncoso, J F, Court, J E, Tapia, J F and Mohr, J P: Global spatial disorientation. J Neurol Sci 34:267–278, 1977.

262. Kertesz, A: Right hemisphere lesions in construction apraxia and visuospatial deficit. In Kertesz, A (Ed.): Localization in Neuropsychology. Academic Press, New York, 1983, pp. 455–470.

263. Kertesz, A and Geschwind, N: Patterns of pyramidal decussation and their relationship to handedness. Arch Neurol 24:326–332, 1971.

264. Kettenmann, B, Hummel, C, Stephan, H and Kobal, G: Multiple olfactory activity in the human neocortex identified by magnetic source imaging. Chem Senses 22:493–502, 1997.

265. Kim, S-G, Ugurbil, K and Strick, P L: Activation of a cerebellar output nucleus during cognitive processing. Science 265:949–951, 1994.

266. Kim, Y-H, Gitelman, D R, Parrish, T B, Nobre, A C, LaBar, K S and Mesulam, M-M:

Posterior cingulate activation varies according to the effectiveness of attentional engagement. Neuroimage 7:S67, 1998.

267. Kimura, D: The asymmetry of the human brain. Sci Am 228:70–78, 1973.

268. Kinomura, S, Kawashima, R, Yamada, K, Ono, S, Itoh, M, Yoshioka, S, Yamaguchi, T, Matsui, H, Miyazawa, H, Itoh, H, Goto, R, Fujiwara, T, Satoh, K and Fukuda, H: Functional anatomy of taste perception in the human brain studied with positron emission tomography. Brain Res 659:263–266, 1994.

269. Kling, A and Steklis, H D: A neural substrate for affiliative behavior in nonhuman primates. Brain Behav Evol 13:216–238, 1976.

270. Kling, A, Steklis, H D and Deutsch, S: Radiotelemetered activity from the amygdala during social interactions in the monkey. Exp Neurol 66:88–96, 1979.

271. Knight, R T: Decreased response to novel stimuli after prefrontal lesions in man. Electroencephalogr Clin Neurophysiol 59:9–20, 1984.

271a. Koechlin, A, Basso, G, Pietrini, P, Panzer, S, Grafman, J,: The role of the anterior prefrontal cortex in human cognition. Nature 399:148–151, 1999.

272. Kojima, S: Prefrontal unit activity in the monkey: relation to visual stimuli and movements. Exp Neurol 69:110–123, 1980.

273. Kolb, B and Taylor, L: Affective behavior in patients with localized cortical excisions: Role of lesion site and side. Science 214:89–91, 1981.

274. Kossi, M and Vater, M: Noradrenaline enhances temporal auditory contrast and neuronal timing precision in the cochlear nucleus of the mustached bat. J Neurosci 9:4169–4178, 1989.

275. Kubota, K, Tonoike, M and Mikami, A: Neuronal activity in the monkey dorsolateral prefrontal cortex during a discrimination task with delay. Brain Res 183:29–42, 1980.

276. Künzle, H: Bilateral projections from precentral motor cortex to the putamen and other parts of the basal ganglia: An autoradiographic study in Macaca fascicularis. Brain Res 88:195–209, 1975.

277. Kuypers, H: Anatomy of descending pathways. In Brooks, VB (Ed.): Handbook of Physiology-The Nervous System II. American Physiological Society, Bethesda, MD, 1981, pp. 597–666.

278. LaBar, K, Gitelman, D R, Parrish, T B, Kim, Y-H, Nobre, A C and Mesulam, M-M: Motivational state selectively modulates amygdala activation to apetitive visual stimuli. Neuroimage 9: S765, 1999.

279. LaBar, K, Gitelman, D R, Parrish, T B, Kim, Y H and Mesulam, M-M: Overlap of frontoparietal activations during covert spatial attention and verbal working memory in the same set of subjects: an fMRI study. Neuroimage, in press.

280. LaBar, K S, Gatenby, J C, Gore, J C, LeDoux, J E and Phelps, E A: Human amygdala activation during conditioned fear acquisition and extinction: a mixed trial fMRI study. Neuron 20:937–945, 1998.

281. Lacey, J I: Somatic response patterning and stress: some revisions of activation theory. In Appley, M H and Trumbull, R (Eds.): Psychological Stress. Appleton-Century-Crofts, New York, 1967, pp. 14–37.

282. Landis, C: Psychology. In Mettler, F A (Ed.): Selective Partial Ablation of the Frontal Cortex. Paul B. Hoeber, New York, 1949, pp. 492–496.

283. Laplane, D: Obsessive-compulsive disorders caused by basal ganglia diseases. Rev Neurol (Paris) 150:594–598, 1994.

284. Laplane, D, Talairach, J, Meininger, V, Bancaud, J and Bouchareine, A: Motor consequences of motor area ablations in man. J Neurol Sci 31:29–49, 1977.

285. Lashley, K S: Brain Mechanisms and Intelligence. University of Chicago Press, Chicago, 1929.

286. Le Moal, M, Galey, D and Cardo, B: Behavioral effects of local injection of 6-hydroxydopamine in the medial ventral tegmentum in the rat. Possible role of the mesolimbic dopaminergic system. Brain Res 88:190–194, 1975.

287. LeDoux, J E, Thompson, M E, Iadecola, C, Tucker, L W and Reis, D J: Local cerebral blood flow increases during emotional processing in the conscious rat. Science 221:576–578, 1983.
288. Leimkuhler, M E and Mesulam, M-M: Reversible go-no go deficits in a case of frontal lobe tumor. Ann Neurol 18:617–619, 1985.
289. Leinonen, L, Hyvärinen, J and Sovijarvi, A R A: Functional properties of neurons in the temporo-parietal association cortex of awake monkey. Exp Brain Res 39:203–215, 1980.
290. Levin, B E, Craik, R L and Hand, P J: The role of epinephrine in adult rat somatosensory (SmI) cortical metabolism and plasticity. Brain Res 443:261–271, 1988.
291. Lewis, M E, Mishkin, M, Bragin, E, Brown, R M, Pert, C B and Pert, A: Opiate receptor gradients in monkey cerebral cortex: correspondence with sensory processing hierarchies. Science 211:1166–1169, 1981.
292. Lewis, M J: Alcohol reinforcement and neuropharmacological therapeutics. Alcohol and Alcoholism Suppl 1:17–25, 1996.
293. Lhermitte, F: Human autonomy and the frontal lobes. II. Patient behavior in complex and social situations. The "environmental dependency syndrome." Ann Neurol 19:335–343, 1986.
294. Lhermitte, F, Pillon, B and Serdaru, M: Human autonomy and the frontal lobes. I. Imitation and utilization behavior: a neuro-psychological study of 75 patients. Ann Neurol 19:326–334, 1986.
295. Libet, B: Brain stimulation and the threshold of conscious experience. In Eccles, J C (Ed.): Brain and Conscious Experience. Springer Verlag, New York, 1966, pp. 165–181.
296. Libet, B: Brain stimulation in the study of neuronal functions for conscious sensory experiences. Hum Neurobiol 1:235–242, 1982.
297. Lishman, W A: Brain damage in relation to psychiatric disability after head injury. Br J Psychiatry 114:373–410, 1968.
298. Livingstone, M and Hubel, D: Segregation of form, color, movement, and depth: anatomy, physiology and perception. Science 240:740–749, 1988.
299. Locke, S and Kerr, C: The projection of nucleus lateralis dorsalis of monkey to basomedial temporal cortex. J Comp Neurol 149:29–42, 1973.
300. Lorenz, K: Evolution and Modification of Behavior. University of Chicago Press, Chicago, 1965.
301. Löwel, S and Singer, W: Selection of intrinsic horizontal connections in the visual cortex by correlated neuronal activity. Science 255:209–212, 1992.
302. Lown, B, Temte, J V, Reich, P, Gaughan, C, Regestein, Q and Hai, H: Basis for recurring ventricular fibrillation in the absence of coronary heart disease and its management. N Engl J Med 294:623–629, 1976.
303. Lueck, C J, Zeki, S, Friston, K J, Deiber, M-P, Cope, P, Cunningham, V J, Lammertsma, A A, Kennard, C and Frackowiak, R S J: The colour centre in the cerebral cortex of man. Nature 340:386–389, 1989.
304. Lurito, J C, Kareken, D A, Lowe, M J, Chen, S A and Mathews, V P: Comparison of rhyming and word generation with FMRI. Neuroimage 7:S139, 1998.
305. Lynch, J C: The functional organization of posterior parietal association cortex. Behav Brain Sci 3:485–499, 1980.
306. MacLean, P D: Psychosomatic disease and the visceral brain: recent developments bearing on the Papez theory of emotion. Psychosom Med 11:338–353, 1949.
307. MacLean, P D: Effects of lesions of globus pallidus on species-specific display behavior of squirrel monkey. Brain Res 149:175–196, 1978.
308. Mahut, H, Moss, M and Zola-Morgan, S: Retention deficits after combined amygdalo-hippocampal and selective hippocampal resections in the monkey. Neuropsychologia 19:201–225, 1981.
309. Mai, J K, Assheuer, J and Paxinos, G: Atlas of the Human Brain. Academic Press, San Diego, CA, 1997.

310. Mark, V H and Ervin, F R: Violence and the Brain. Harper & Row, New York, 1970.

311. Marsden, C D: The mysterious motor function of the basal ganglia: the Robert Wartenberg lecture. Neurology 32:514–539, 1982.

312. Martin, A, Haxby, J V, Lalonde, F M, Wiggs, C L and Ungerleider, L G: Discrete cortical regions associated with knowledge of color and knowledge of action. Science 270:102–105, 1995.

313. Martin, A, Wiggs, C L, Ungerleider, L G and Haxby, J V: Neural correlates of category-specific knowledge. Nature 379:649–652, 1996.

314. Matelli, M, Luppino, G and Rizzolatti, G: Patterns of cytochrome oxidase activity in the frontal agranular cortex of the macaque monkey. Behav Brain Res 18:125–136, 1985.

315. Mayberg, H S: Limbic-cortical dysregulation: a proposed model of depression. J Neuropsychiat Clin Neurosci 9:471–481, 1997.

316. Mazziotta, J C, Phelps, M E, Carson, R E and Kuhl, D E: Tomographic mapping of human cerebral metabolism: auditory stimulation. Neurology 32:921–937, 1982.

317. Mazzucchi, A, Marchini, C, Budai, R and Parma, M: A case of receptive amusia with prominent timbre perception defect. J Neurol Neurosurg Psychiatry 45:644–647, 1982.

318. McClelland, J L: The organization of memory. A Parallel distributed processing perspective. Rev Neurol (Paris) 150:570–579, 1994.

319. McClelland, J L: Constructive memory and memory distortions: a parallel-distributed processing approach. In Schacter, D L, Coyle, J T, Fischbach, G D, Mesulam, M-M and Sullivan, L E (eds.): Memory Distortion. Harvard University Press, Cambridge, MA, 1995, pp. 69–90.

320. McCormick, D A: Cellular mechanisms of cholinergic control of neocortical and thalamic neuronal excitability. In Steriade, M and Biesold, D (Eds.): Brain Cholinergic Systems. Oxford University Press, Oxford, 1990, pp. 236–264.

321. McCormick, D A and Thompson, R F: Cerebellum: essential involvement in the classically conditioned eyelid response. Science 223:296–299, 1984.

322. McGaugh, J L, Cahill, L and Roozendaal, B: Involvement of the amygdala in memory storage: Interaction with other brain systems. Proc Natl Acad Sci USA 93:13508–13514, 1996.

323. McGlone, J: Sex differences in human brain asymmetry: a critical survey. Behav Brain Sci 3:215–263, 1980.

324. McGuire, P K: The brain in obsessive-compulsive disorder. J Neurol Neurosurg Psychiatry 59:457–459, 1995.

325. McIntosh, A R, Grady, C L, Ungerleider, L G, Haxby, J V, Rapoport, S I and Horwitz, B: Network analysis of cortical visual pathways mapped with PET. J Neurosci 14:655–666, 1994.

326. Meerwaldt, J D and Van Harskamp, F: Spatial disorientation in right hemisphere infarction. J Neurol Neurosurg Psychiatry 45:586–590, 1982.

327. Mendez, M F, Adams, N L and Lewandowski, K S: Neurobehavioral changes associated with caudate lesions. Neurology 39:349–354, 1989.

328. Merzenich, M M and Brugge, J F: Representation of the cochlear partition on the superior temporal plane of the macaque monkey. Brain Res 50:275–296, 1973.

329. Mesulam, M-M: A cortical network for directed attention and unilateral neglect. Ann Neurol 10:309–325, 1981.

330. Mesulam, M-M: Dissociative states with abnormal temporal lobe EEG. Multiple personality and the illusion of possession. Arch Neurol 38:176–181, 1981.

331. Mesulam, M-M: Patterns in behavioral neuroanatomy; Association areas, the limbic system, and hemispheric specialization. In Mesulam, M-M (Ed.): Principles of Behavioral Neurology. F. A. Davis, Philadelphia, 1985, pp. 1–70.

332. Mesulam, M-M: Frontal cortex and behavior. Ann Neurol 19:320–325, 1986.

333. Mesulam, M-M: Asymmetry of neural feedback in the organization of behavioral states. Science 237:537–538, 1987.

334. Mesulam, M-M: Large-scale neurocognitive networks and distributed processing for attention, language, and memory. Ann Neurol 28:597–613, 1990.
335. Mesulam, M-M: Higher visual functions of the cerebral cortex and their disruption in clinical practice. In Albert, D M and Jakobiec, F A (Eds.): Principles and Practice of Ophthalmology, Vol. 4. Saunders, Philadelphia, 1994, pp. 2640–2653.
336. Mesulam, M-M: Neurocognitive networks and selectively distributed processing. Rev Neurol (Paris) 150:564–569, 1994.
337. Mesulam, M-M: Notes on the cerebral topography of memory and memory distortion: a neurologist's perspective. In Schacter, D L, Coyle, J T, Fischbach, G D, Mesulam, M-M and Sullivan, L E (Eds.): Memory Distortion. Harvard University Press, Cambridge, MA, 1995, pp. 379–385.
338. Mesulam, M-M: The systems-level organization of cholinergic innervation in the cerebral cortex and its alterations in Alzheimer's disease. Prog Brain Res 109:285–298, 1996.
339. Mesulam, M-M: From sensation to cognition. Brain 121:1013–1052, 1998.
340. Mesulam, M-M, Hersh, L B, Mash, D C and Geula, C: Differential cholinergic innervation within functional subdivisions of the human cerebral cortex: a choline acetyltransferase study. J Comp Neurol 318:316–328, 1992.
341. Mesulam, M-M and Mufson, E J: Insula of the old world monkey. I. Architectonics in the insulo- orbito-temporal component of the paralimbic brain. J Comp Neurol 212:1–22, 1982.
342. Mesulam, M-M and Mufson, E J: Neural inputs into the nucleus basalis of the substantia innominata (Ch4) in the rhesus monkey. Brain 107:253–274, 1984.
343. Mesulam, M-M and Mufson, E J: The insula of Reil in man and monkey. In Peters, A and Jones, E G (Eds.): Cerebral Cortex, Vol. 4. Plenum Press, New York, 1985, pp. 179–226.
344. Mesulam, M-M, Mufson, E J, Levey, A I and Wainer, B H: Cholinergic innervation of cortex by the basal forebrain: cytochemistry and cortical connections of the septal area, diagonal band nuclei, nucleus basalis (substantia innominata), and hypothalamus in the rhesus monkey. J Comp Neurol 214:170–197, 1983.
345. Mesulam, M-M: Schizophrenia and the brain (editorial). N Engl J Med 322:842–845, 1990.
346. Mesulam, M-M, Mufson, E J, Wainer, B H and Levey, A I: Central cholinergic pathways in the rat: an overview based on an alternative nomenclature (Ch1-Ch6). Neuroscience 10:1185–1201, 1983.
347. Mesulam, M-M and Pandya, D N: The projections of the medial geniculate complex within the sylvian fissure of the rhesus monkey. Brain Res 60:315–333, 1973.
348. Mesulam, M-M and Perry, J: The diagnosis of love-sickness: experimental psychophysiology without the polygraph. Psychophysiology 9:546–551, 1972.
349. Mesulam, M-M, Rosen, A D and Mufson, E J: Regional variations in cortical cholinergic innervation: chemoarchitectonics of acetylcholinesterase-containing fibers in the macaque brain. Brain Res 311:245–258, 1984.
350. Mesulam, M-M, Van Hoesen, G W, Pandya, D N and Geschwind, N: Limbic and sensory connections of the inferior parietal lobule (area PG) in the rhesus monkey: a study with a new method for horseradish peroxidase histochemistry. Brain Res 136:393–414, 1977.
351. Meunier, M, Bachevalier, J and Mishkin, M: Effects of orbital frontal and anterior cingulate lesions on object and spatial memory in rhesus monkeys. Neuropsychologia 35:999–1015, 1997.
352. Michel, D, Laurent, B, Foyatier, N, Blanc, A and Portafaix, M: Etude de la mémoire et du langage dans une observation tomodensitométrique d'infarctus thalamique paramedian gauche. Rev Neurol (Paris) 138:533–550, 1982.
353. Mikami, A, Ito, S and Kubota, K: Visual response properties of dorsolateral prefrontal neurons during visual fixation task. J Neurophysiol 47:593–605, 1982.
354. Miller, L and Milner, B: Cognitive risk-taking after frontal or temporal lobectomy—II. The synthesis of phonemic and semantic information. Neuropsychologia 23:371–379, 1985.

355. Milner, B: Effects of different brain lesions on card sorting. Arch Neurol 9:90–100, 1963.

356. Milner, B: Hemispheric specialization: scope and limits. In Schmitt, F O and Warden, F G (Eds.): The Neuroscience: Third Study Program. MIT Press, Cambridge, MA, 1974, pp. 75–89.

357. Milner, B, Corkin, S and Teuber, H L: Further analysis of the hippocampal amnesic syndrome: 14-year follow-up study of HM. Neuropsychologia 6:215–234, 1968.

358. Mishkin, M: A memory system in the monkey. Philos Trans R Soc Lond Biol 298:85–92, 1982.

359. Mishkin, M and Bachevalier, J: Object recognition impaired by ventromedial but not dorsolateral prefrontal cortical lesions in monkeys. Soc Neurosci Abstr 9:29, 1983.

360. Mitchell, S J, Richardson, R T, Baker, F H and DeLong, M R: The primate globus pallidus: neuronal activity related to direction of movement. Exp Brain Res 68:491–505, 1987.

361. Mohr, J R, Pessin, M S, Finkelstein, S, Funkenstein, H H, Duncan, G W and Davis, K R: Broca's aphasia: pathologic and clinical. Neurology 28:311–324, 1978.

362. Moll, L and Kuypers, H: Premotor cortical ablations in monkeys: contralateral changes in visually guided behavior. Science 198:317–320, 1977.

363. Mongeau, R, Blier, P and Montigny, C D: The serotonergic and noradrenergic systems of the hippocampus: their interactions and the effects of antidepressant treatments. Brain Res Rev 23:145–195, 1997.

364. Moore, R Y and Bloom, F E: Central catecholamine neuron systems: anatomy and physiology of the norepinephrine and epinephrine systems. Ann Rev Neurosci 2:113–168, 1979.

365. Moore-Ede, M C, Czeisler, C A and Richardson, G S: Circadian timekeeping in health and disease. N Engl J Med 309:469–476, 1983.

366. Moran, J and Desimone, R: Selective attention gates visual processing in the extrastriate cortex. Science 229:782–784, 1985.

367. Morán, M A, Mufson, E J and Mesulam, M-M: Neural inputs into the temporopolar cortex of the rhesus monkey. J Comp Neurol 256:88–103, 1987.

368. Morecraft, R J, Geula, C and Mesulam, M-M: Architecture of connectivity within a cingulo-fronto-parietal neurocognitive network for directed attention. Arch Neurol 50:279–284, 1993.

369. Morecraft, R J, Geula, C and Mesulam, M-M: Cytoarchitecture and neural afferents of orbitofrontal cortex in the brain of the monkey. J Comp Neurol 323:341–358, 1992.

370. Morris, J S, Friston, K J, Buchel, C, Frith, C D, Young, A W, Calder, A J and Dolan, R J: A neuromodulatory role for the human amygdala in processing emotional facial expressions. Brain 121:47–57, 1998.

371. Morrison, J H and Magistretti, P J: Monoamines and peptides in cerebral cortex. Trends Neurosci 6:146–151, 1983.

372. Moscovitch, M: Confabulation. In Schachter, D L, Coyle, J T, Fischbach, G D, Mesulam, M-M and Sullivan, L E (Eds.): Memory Distortion. Harvard University Press, Cambridge, MA, 1995, pp. 226–251.

373. Moscovitch, M and Olds, J: Asymmetries in spontaneous facial expressions and their possible relation to hemispheric specialization. Neuropsychologia 20:71–81, 1982.

374. Mountcastle, V B, Lynch, J C, Georgopoulous, A, Sakata, H and Acuna, A: Posterior parietal association cortex of the monkey: command functions for operations within extrapersonal space. J Neurophysiol 38:871–908, 1975.

375. Mufson, E J and Mesulam, M-M: Thalamic connections of the insula in the rhesus monkey and comments on the paralimbic connectivity of the medial pulvinar nucleus. J Comp Neurol 227:109–120, 1984.

376. Murata, A, Fadiga, L, Fogassi, L, Gallese, V, Raos, V and Rizzolatti, G: Object representation in the ventral premotor cortex (area F5) of the monkey. J Neurophysiol 78:2226–2230, 1997.

377. Murray, E A and Mishkin, M: A further examination of the medial temporal lobe structures involved in recognition memory in the monkey. Soc Neurosci Abstr 9:27, 1983.

378. Murray, E A and Mishkin, M: Relative contributions of SII and area 5 to tactile discrimination in monkeys. Behav Brain Res 11:67–83, 1984.

379. Murray, E A, Nakamura, R K and Mishkin, M: A possible cortical pathway for somatosensory processing in monkeys. Soc Neurosci Abstr 6:654, 1980.

380. Nadel, L and Moscovitch, M: Memory consoliation, retrograde amnesia and the hippocampal complex. Curr Opin Neurobiol 7:217–227, 1997.

381. Nakamura, K and Kubota, K: The primate temporal pole: its putative role in object recognition and memory. Behav Brain Res 77:53–77, 1996.

382. Narabayashi, H, Nagao, T, Saito, Y, Yoshida, M and Nagahata, M: Stereotaxic amygdalectomy for behavior disorders. Arch Neurol 9:1–16, 1963.

383. Nauta, W: Neural associations of the amygdaloid complex in the monkey. Brain 85:505–520, 1962.

384. Naya, Y, Sakai, K and Miyashita, Y: Activity of primate inferotemporal neurons related to sought-target in pair-association task. Proc Natl Acad Sci USA 93:2664–2669, 1996.

385. Newman, R and Winans, S S: An experimental study of the ventral striatum of the golden hamster: I. Neuronal connections of the nucleus accumbens. J Comp Neurol 191: 167–192, 1980.

386. Nieuwenhuys, R, Voogd, J and van Huijzen, C: The Human Central Nervous System. Springer Verlog Berlin. 1988.

387. Nishino, H, Ono, T, Fukuda, M, Sasaki, K and Muramoto, K I: Single-unit activity in monkey caudate nucleus during operant bar pressing feeding behavior. Neurosci Lett 21: 105–110, 1981.

388. Nobre, A C, Allison, T and McCarthy, G: Word recognition in the human inferior temporal lobe. Nature 372:260–263, 1994.

389. Nobre, A C and Plunkett, K: The neural system of language: structure and development. Curr Opin Neurobiol 7:262–268, 1997.

390. Nobre, A C, Sebestyen, G N, Gitelman, D R, Mesulam, M-M, Frackowiak, R S J and Frith, C D: Functional localization of the system for visuospatial attention using positron emission tomography. Brain 120:515–533, 1997.

391. Ojemann, G A, Fedio, P and VanBuren, J M: Anomia from pulvinar and subcortical parietal stimulation. Brain 91:99–116, 1968.

392. Olszewski, J: The Thalamus of the *Macaca Mulatta*. S Karger, Basel, 1952.

393. Oppenheimer, S M, Gelb, A, Girvin, J P and Hachinski, V C: Cardiovascular effects of human insular cortex stimulation. Neurology 42:1727–1732, 1992.

394. Pakkenberg, B and Gundersen, H J G: Neocortical neuron number in humans: effect of sex and age. J Comp Neurol 384:312–320, 1997.

395. Pandya, D N and Kuypers, H G J M: Cortico-cortical connections in the rhesus monkey. Brain Res 13:13–36, 1969.

396. Pandya, D N and Seltzer, B: Association areas of the cerebral cortex. Trends Neurosci 5:286–290, 1982.

397. Pandya, D N, Van Hoesen, G W and Mesulam, M-M: Efferent connections of the cingulate gyrus in the rhesus monkey. Exp Brain Res 42:319–330, 1981.

398. Pandya, D N and Yeterian, E H: Architecture and connections of cortical association areas. In Peters, A and Jones, E G (Eds.): Cerebral Cortex, Vol. 4. Plenum Press, New York, 1985, pp. 3–61.

399. Papez, J W: A proposed mechanism of emotion. Arch Neurol Psych 38:725–744, 1937.

400. Parent, A and de Bellefeuille, L: Organization of efferent projections from the internal segment of the globus pallidus in primate as revealed by fluorescence retrograde labeling method. Brain Res 245:201–213, 1982.

401. Paulesu, E, Frackowiak, R S J and Bopttini, G: Maps of somatosensory systems. In Frackowiak, R S J, Friston, K J, Frith, C D, Dolan, R J and Mazziotta, J C (Eds.): Human Brain Function. Academic Press, San Diego, CA, 1997, pp. 183–242.

402. Pegna, A J, Khateb, A, Spinelli, L, Seeck, M, Landis, T and Michel, C M: Unraveling the cerebral dynamics of mental imagery. Hum Brain Map 5:410–421, 1997.

403. Penfield, W: The Mystery of the Mind. Princeton University Press, Princeton, NJ, 1975.
404. Penfield, W and Evans, J: The frontal lobe in man: a clinical study of maximum removals. Brain 58:115–133, 1935.
405. Penfield, W and Faulk, M E: The insula. Further observations on its function. Brain 78:445–470, 1955.
406. Penfield, W and Jasper, H: Epilepsy and the Functional Anatomy of the Human Brain. Little, Brown, Boston, 1954.
407. Penfield, W J: Vestibular sensation and the cerebral cortex. Ann Otol Rhinol Laryngol 66:691–698, 1957.
408. Perenin, M T and Jeannerod, M: Visual function within the hemianopic field following early cerebral hemidecortication in man-I. Spatial localization. Neuropsychologia 16:1–13, 1978.
409. Petersen, S E, Fox, P T, Posner, M I, Mintun, M and Raichle, M E: Positron emission tomographic studies of the cortical anatomy of single word processing. Nature 331:585–589, 1988.
410. Petersen, S E, Robinson, D L and Keys, W: Pulvinar nuclei of the behaving rhesus monkey: visual responses and their modulation. J Neurophysiol 54:867–886, 1985.
411. Peterson, B, Riddle, M A, Cohen, D J, Katz, L D, Smith, J C, Hardin, M T and Leckman, J F: Reduced basal ganglia volumes in Tourette's syndrome using three-dimensional reconstruction techniques from magnetic resonance images. Neurology 43:941–949, 1993.
412. Petrides, M, Alivisatos, B, Meyer, E and Evans, A C: Functional activation of the human frontal cortex during the performance of verbal working memory tasks. Proc Natl Acad Sci USA 90:878–882, 1993.
413. Peyron, C, Petit, J-M, Rampon, C, Jouvet, M and Luppi, P-H: Forebrain afferents to the rat dorsal raphe nucleus demonstrated by retrograde and anterograde tracing methods. Neuroscience 82:443–468, 1998.
414. Phillips, A G and Carr, G D: Cognition and the basal ganglia: a possible substrate for procedural knowledge. Can J Neurol Sci 14(3 Suppl):381–385, 1987.
415. Pich, E M, Pagliusi, S R, Tessari, M, Talabot-Ayer, D, Huijsduijnen van, R H and Chiamulera, C: Common neural substrates for the addictive properties of nicotine and cocaine. Science 275:83–86, 1997.
416. Piven, J, Saliba, K, Bailey, J and Arndt, S: An MRI study of autism: the cerebellum revisited. Neurology 49:546–551, 1997.
417. Polster, M R and Rose, S B: Disorders of auditory processing: evidence for modularity in audition. Cortex 34:47–65, 1998.
418. Pool, J L and Ransohoff, J: Autonomic effects on stimulating rostral portion of cingulate gyri in man. J Neurophysiol 12:385–392, 1949.
419. Post, R M, Kennedy, C, Shinohara, M, Squillace, K, Miyaoka, M, Suda, S, Ingvar, D H and Sokoloff, L: Metabolic and behavioral consequences of lidocaine-kindled seizures. Brain Res 324:295–303, 1984.
420. Pribram, K H, Wilson, W A Jr and Connors, J: Effects of lesions of the medial forebrain on alternation behaviors of rhesus monkeys. Exp Neurol 6:36–47, 1962.
421. Price, B H, Daffner, K R, Stowe, R M and Mesulam, M-M: The comportmental learning disabilities of early frontal lobe damage. Brain 113:1383–1393, 1990.
422. Price, B H and Mesulam, M: Psychiatric manifestations of right hemisphere infarctions. J Nerv Ment Dis 173:610–614, 1985.
423. Puce, A, Allison, T, Asgari, M, Gore, J C and McCarthy, G: Differential sensitivity of human visual cortex to faces, letterstrings, and textures: a functional magnetic resonance imaging study. J Neurosci 16:5205–5215, 1996.
424. Raiguel, S E, Legae, L, Gulyas, B and Orban, G A: Response latencies of visual cells in macaque areas V1, V2 and V5. Brain Res 493:155–159, 1989.
425. Raleigh, M J, Steklis, H K, Ervin, F R, Kling, A S and McGuire, M T: The effects of or-

bitofrontal lesions on the aggressive behavior of vervet monkeys (*Cercopithecus aethiops sabaeus*). Exp Neurol 66:158–168, 1979.

426. Ramírez-Amaya, V, Alvarez-Borda, B, Ormsby, C E, Martínez, R D, Pérez-Montfort, R and Bermúdez-Rattoni, F: Insular cortex lesions impair the acquisition of conditioned immunosuppression. Brain Behav and Immun 10:103–114, 1996.

427. Randolph, M and Semmes, J H: Behavioral consequences of selective subtotal ablations in the postcentral gyrus of *Macaca mulatta*. Brain Res 70:55–70, 1974.

428. Rao, S C, Rainer, G and Miller, E K: Integration of what and where in the primate prefrontal cortex. Science 276:821–824, 1997.

429. Rao, S M, Binder, J R, Bandettini, P A, Hammeke, T A, Yetkin, F Z, Jesmanowicz, A, Lisk, L M, Morris, G L, Mueller, W M, Estkowski, L D, Wong, E C, Haughton, V M and Hyde, J S: Functional magnetic resonance imaging of complex human movements. Neurology 43:2311–2318, 1993.

430. Rapoport, J L, Buchsbaum, M S, Zahn, T P, Weingartner, H, Ludlow, C and Mikkelsen, E J: Dextroamphetamine: cognitive and behavioral effects in normal prepubertal boys. Science 199:560–563, 1978.

431. Rauch, S L, van der Kolk, B A, Fisler, R E, Alpert, N M, Orr, S P, Savage, C R, Fischman, A J, Jenicke, M A and Pitman, R K: A symptom provocation study of posttraumatic stress disorder using positron emission tomography and script-driven imagery. Arch Gen Psychiatry 53:380–387, 1996.

432. Rausch, R, Serafitinides, E A and Crandall, P H: Olfactory memory in patients with anterior temporal lobectomy. Cortex 13:445–452, 1977.

433. Rauschecker, J P, Tian, B, Pons, T and Mishkin, M: Serial and parallel processing in rhesus monkey auditory cortex. J Comp Neurol 382:89–103, 1997.

434. Reiner, P B and McGeer, E G: Electrophysiology of cortically projecting histamine neurons of the rat hypothalamus. Neurosci Lett 73:43–47, 1987.

435. Reuter-Lorenz, P and Davidson, R J: Differential contributions of the two cerebral hemispheres to the perception of happy and sad faces. Neuropsychologia 19:1981.

436. Richfield, E K, Rwyman, R and Berent, S: Neurological syndrome following bilateral damage to the head of the caudate nuclei. Ann Neurol 22:768–771, 1987.

437. Ringo, J L, Doty, R W, Demeter, S and Simard, P Y: Time is of the essence: a conjecture that hemispheric specialization arises from interhemispheric conduction delay. Cereb Cortex 4:331–343, 1994.

438. Risberg, J and Ingvar, D H: Patterns of activation in the grey matter of the dominant hemisphere during memorizing and reasoning-a study of regional cerebral blood flow changes during psychological testing in a group of neurologically normal patients. Brain 96:737–756, 1973.

439. Risberg, J, Maximilian, A and Prohovnik, I: Changes of cortical activity patterns during habituation to a reasoning test. Neuropsychologia 15:793–798, 1977.

440. Rizzolatti, G, Fogassi, L and Gallese, V: Parietal cortex: from sight to action. Curr Opin Neurobiol 7:562–567, 1997.

441. Robinson, DL: Functional contributions of the primate pulvinar. Prog Brain Res 95:371–380, 1993.

442. Robinson, R G, Kubos, KL, Starr, L B, Rao, K and Price, T R: Mood disorders in stroke patients. Importance of location of lesion. Brain 107:81–93, 1984.

443. Rogers, M P and Fozdar, M: Psychoneuroimmunology of autoimmune disorders. Adv Neuroimmunol 6:169–177, 1996.

444. Roland, P E: Astereognosis. Arch Neurol 33:543–558, 1976.

445. Roland, P E and Larsen, B: Focal increase of cerebral blood flow during stereognosis testing in man. Arch Neurol 33:551–558, 1976.

446. Roland, P E, Larsen, B, Lassen, N A and Skinhoj, E: Supplementary motor area and other cortical areas in organization of voluntary movements in man. J Neurophysiol 43:118, 1980.

447. Rolls, E T: Information representation, processing, and storage in the brain: analysis at the single neuron level. In Changeux, J-P and Konishi, M (Eds.): The Neural and Molecular Bases of Learning. John Wiley, New York, 1987, pp. 503–540.

448. Rolls, ET, Baylis, CG, Hasselmo, ME and Nalwa, V: The effect of learning on the face selective responses of neurons in the cortex in the superior temporal sulcus of the monkey. Exp Brain Res 76:153–164, 1989.

449. Rolls, ET, Sanghera, M, K and Roper-Hall, A: The latency of activation of neurones in the lateral hypothalamus and substantia innominata during feeding in the monkey. Brain Res 164:121–135, 1979.

450. Rolls, E T, Yaxley, S and Sienkiewicz, Z J: Gustatory responses of single neurons in the caudolateral orbitofrontal cortex of the macaque monkey. J Neurophysiol 64:1055–1066, 1990.

451. Romanski, L M, Giguere, M, Bates, J F and Goldman-Rakic, P S: Topographic organization of medial pulvinar connections with the prefrontal cortex in the rhesus monkey. J Comp Neurol 379:313–332, 1997.

452. Rosen, A D, Gur, R C, Sussman, N, Gur, R E and Hurtig, H: Hemispheric asymmetry in the control of heart rate. Soc Neurosci Abstr 8:917, 1982.

453. Rosene, D L and Van Hoesen, G W: Hippocampal efferents reach widespread areas of cerebral cortex and amygdala in the rhesus monkey. Science 198:315–317, 1977.

454. Ross, E D: Sensory-specific and fractional disorders of recent memory in man. Arch Neurol 37:193–200, 1980.

455. Rosvold, H E, Mirsky, A F and Pribram, K: Influence of amygdalectomy on social behavior in monkeys. J Comp Physiol Psychol 47:173–178, 1954.

456. Rumelhart, D E and McClelland, J L: Parallel Distributed Processing. The MIT Press, Cambridge, MA, 1986.

457. Rumsey, J M, Horwitz, B, Donohue, B C, Nace, K, Maisog, J M and Andreason, P: Phonological and orthographic components of word recognition A PET-rCBF study. Brain 120:739–759, 1997.

458. Sackeim, H A: Lateral asymmetry in bodily response to hypnotic suggestion. Biol Psychol 17:437–447, 1982.

459. Sackeim, H A, Greenberg, M S, Weiman, A L, Gur, R C, Hungerbuhler, J P and Geschwind, N: Hemispheric asymmetry in the expression of positive and negative emotions: neurological evidence. Arch Neurol 39:210–218, 1982.

460. Sackeim, H A, Gur, R C and Savey, M C: Emotions are expressed more intensely on the left side of the face. Science 202:434–436, 1978.

461. Sagakami, M and Niki, H: Encoding of behavioral significance of visual stimuli by primate prefrontal neurons: relation to relevant task conditions. Exp Brain Res 97:423–436, 1994.

462. Sahraie, A, Weiskrantz, L, Barbur, J L, Simmons, A, Williams, S C R and Brammer, M J: Pattern of neuronal activity associated with conscious and unconscious processing of visual signals. Proc Natl Acad Sci USA 94:9406–9411, 1997.

463. Sakurai, T, Amemiya, A, Ishii, M, Matsuzaki, I, Chemelli, R M, Tanaka, H, Williams, S C, Richardson, J A, Kozlowski, G P, Wilson, S, Arch, J R S, Buckingham, R E, Haynes, A C, Carr, S A, Annan, R S, McNulty, D E, Liu, W-S, Terrett, J A, Elshourbagy, N A, Bergsma, D J and Yanagisawa, M: Orexins and orexin receptors: a family of hypothalamic neuropeptides and G protein-coupled receptors that regulate feeding behavior. Cell 92: 573–585, 1998.

464. Sandson, T A, Daffner, K R, Carvalho, P A and Mesulam, M M: Frontal lobe dysfunction following infarction of the left-sided medial thalamus. Arch Neurol 48:1300–1303, 1991.

465. Sanides, F: Functional architecture of motor and sensory cortices in primates in the light

of a new concept of neocortex evolution. In Noback, C R and Montagna, W (Eds.): The Primate Brain. Appleton-Century-Crofts, New York, 1970, pp. 137–208.

466. Sarnthein, J, Petsche, H, Rappelsberger, P, Shaw, G L and von Stein, A: Synchronization between prefrontal and posterior association cortex during human working memory. Proc Natl Acad Sci USA 95:7092–7096, 1998.

467. Sato, H, Hata, V, Hagihara, K and Tsumoto, T: Effects of cholinergic depletion on neuron activities in the cat visual cortex. J Neurophysiol 58:781–794, 1987.

468. Schacter, D L: Implicit memory: a new frontier for cognitive neuroscience. In Gazzaniga, M S (Ed.): The Cognitive Neurosciences. MIT Press, Cambridge, MA, 1995, pp. 813–824.

469. Schell, G R and Strick, P L: The orgin of thalamic inputs to the arcuate premotor and supplementary motor areas. J Neurosci 4:539–560, 1984.

470. Schiller, P: Effect of lesions in visual cortical area V4 on the recognition of transformed objects. Nature 376:342–344, 1995.

471. Schleidt, W and Schleidt, M: Störung der Mutter-Kind-Beziehung bei Truthühnern durch Gehorverlust. Behaviour 16:3–4, 1960.

472. Schluter, N D, Rushworth, M F S, Passingham, R E and Mills, K R: Temporary interference in human lateral premotor cortex suggests dominance for the selection of movements. Brain 121:785–799, 1998.

473. Schmahmann, J: An emerging concept. The cerebellar contribution to higher function. Arch Neurol 48:1178–1187, 1991.

474. Schmahmann, J D and Leifer, D: Parietal pseudothalamic pain syndrome. Clinical features and anatomic correlates. Arch Neurol 49:1032–1037, 1992.

475. Schmahmann, J D and Sherman, J C: The cerebellar cognitive affective syndrome. Brain 121:561–579, 1998.

476. Schultz, W: Dopamine neurons and their role in reward mechanisms. Curr Opin Neurobiol 7:191–197, 1997.

477. Schwartz, G E, Ahern, G L and Brown, S L: Lateralized facial muscle response to positive and negative emotional stimuli. Psychophysiology 16:561–571, 1979.

478. Schwartz, G E, Davidson, R J and Maer, F: Right hemisphere lateralization for emotion in the human brain: interactions with cognition. Science 190:286–288, 1975.

479. Seeck, M, Mainwaring, N, Cosgrove, R, Blume, H, Dubuisson, D, Mesulam, M-M and Schomer, D L: Neurophysiologic correlates of implicit face memory in intracranial visual evoked potentials. Neurology 49:1312–1316, 1997.

480. Seeck, M, Schomer, D, Mainwaring, N, Ives, J, Dubuissson, D, Blume, H, Cosgrove, R, Ransil, B J and Mesulam, M-M: Selectively distributed processing of visual object recognition in the temporal and frontal lobes of the human brain. Ann Neurol 37:538–545, 1995.

481. Selden, N, Mesulam, M-M and Geula, C: Human striatum: the distribution of neurofibrillary tangles in Alzheimer's disease. Brain Res 648:327–331, 1994.

482. Selden, N R W, Robbins, T W and Everitt, B J: Enhanced behavioral conditioning to context and impaired behavioral and neuroendocrine responses to conditioned stimuli following ceruleocortical noradrenergic lesions: support for an attentional hypothesis of central noradrenergic function. J Neurosci 10:531–539, 1990.

483. Selemon, L D and Goldman-Rakic, P D: Common cortical and subcortical targets of the dorsolateral prefrontal and posterior parietal cortices in the rhesus monkey: evidence for a distributed neural network subserving spatially guided behavior. Neuroscience 8:4049–4068, 1988.

484. Seltzer, B and Pandya, D N: Some cortical projections to the hippocampal area in the rhesus monkey. Exp Neurol 50:146–160, 1976.

485. Sergent, J, Ohta, S and MacDonald, B: Functional neuroanatomy of face and object processing: a positron emission tomography study. Brain 115:15–36, 1992.

486. Shapiro, B E and Danly, M: The role of the right hemisphere in the control of speech prosody in propositional and affective contexts. Brain Lang 25:19–36, 1985.

487. Shapiro, B E, Grossman, M and Gardner, H: Selective musical processing deficits in brain damaged populations. Neuropsychologia 19:161–169, 1981.

488. Shaywitz, B A, Shaywitz, S E, Pugh, K R, Constable, R T, Skudlarsky, P, Fulbright, R K, Bronen, R A, Fletcher, J M, Shankweiler, D P and Gore, J C: Sex differences in the functional organization of the brain for language. Nature 373:607–609, 1995.

489. Shindo, K, Shima, K and Tanji, J: Spatial distribution of thalamic projections to the supplemenrtary motor area and the primary motor cortex: a retrograde multiple labeling study in the macaque monkey. J Comp Neurol 357:98–116, 1995.

490. Showers, M and Lauer, E W: Somatovisceral motor patterns in the insula. J Comp Neurol 117:107–116, 1961.

491. Sidtis, J J: Predicting brain organization from dichotic listening performance: Cortical and subcortical functional asymmetries contribute to perceptual asymmetries. Brain Lang 17:287–300, 1982.

492. Signoret, J-L: Memory and amnesias. In Mesulam, M-M (Ed.): Principles of Behavioral Neurology. F. A. Davis, Philadelphia, 1985, pp. 169–192.

493. Simerly, R B, Chang, C, Muramatsu, M and Swanson, L W: Distribution of androgen and estrogen receptor mRNA-containing cells in the rat brain: an in situ hybridization study. J Comp Neurol 294:76–95, 1990.

494. Small, I F, Hemiburger, R F, Small, J G, Milstein, V and Moore, D F: Follow-up of sterotaxic amygdalotomy for seizure and behavior disorders. Biol Psychiatry 12:401–411, 1977.

495. Smiley, J and Goldman-Rakic, P S: Serotonergic axons in monkey prefrontal cerebral cortex synapse predominantly on interneurons as demonstrated by serial section electron microscopy. J Comp Neurol 367:431–443, 1996.

496. Smiley, J F, Morrell, F and Mesulam, M-M: Cholinergic synapses in human cerebral cortex: an ultrastructural study in serial sections. Exp Neurol 144:361–368, 1997.

497. Smith, W K: The results of ablation of the cingular region of the cerebral cortex. Fed Proc 3:42–43, 1944.

498. Spiegel, E A, Wycis, H T, Freed, H and Orchinik, C: The central mechanism of emotions. Am J Psychiatry 108:426–432, 1953.

499. Spiers, P A, Schomer, D L, Blume, H W, Kleefield, J, O'Reilly, G, Weintraub, S, Osborne-Shaefer, P and Mesulam, M-M: Visual neglect during intracarotid amobarbital testing. Neurology 40:1600–1606, 1990.

500. Spreen, O, Benton, A L and Fincham, R W: Auditory agnosia without aphasia. Arch Neurol 13:84–92, 1965.

501. Springer, S P and Deutsch, G: Left Brain, Right Brain. Freeman, San Francisco, 1981.

502. Squire, L R and Moore, R Y: Dorsal thalamic lesion in a noted case of human memory dysfunction. Ann Neurol 6:503–506, 1979.

503. Squire, L R, Ojemann, J G, Miezin, F M, Peterson, S E, Videen, T O and Raichle, M E: Activation of the hippocampus in normal humans: a functional anatomical study of memory. Proc Natl Acad Sci USA 89:1837–1841, 1992.

504. Squire, L R and Zola, S M: Structure and function of declarative and nondeclarative memory systems. Proc Natl Acad Sci USA 93:13515–13522, 1996.

505. Stephan, K M, Fink, G R, Passingham, R E, Silbersweig, D, Ceballos-Baumann, A O, Frith, C D and Frackowiak, R S: Functional anatomy of the mental representation of upper extremity movements in healthy subjects. J Neurophysiol 73:373–386, 1995.

506. Stern, D B: Handedness and the lateral distribution of conversion reactions. J Nerv Ment Dis 164:122–128, 1977.

507. Stevens, J R: Psychomotor epilepsy and schizophrenia: a common anatomy? In Brazier, M A B (Ed.): Epilepsy: Its Phenomena in Man. Academic Press, New York, 1973, pp. 190–214.

508. Strub, R L: Frontal lobe syndrome in a patient with bilateral globus pallidus lesions. Arch Neurol 46:1024–1027, 1989.

509. Sugar, O, Chusid, J G and French, J D: A second motor cortex in the monkey (*Macaca mulatta*). J Neuropathol Exp Neurol 7:182–189, 1948.

510. Suzuki, W A and Amaral, D G: Perirhinal and parahippocampal cortices of the macaque monkey: cortical afferents. J Comp Neurol 350:497–533, 1994.

511. Tanabe, T, Iino, M and Takagi, S F: Discrimination of ordors in olfactory bulb, pyriform-amygdaloid areas and orbitofrontal cortex of the monkey. J Neurophysiol 38:1284–1296, 1975.

512. Tanabe, T, Yarita, H, Iino, M, Ooshima, Y and Takagi, S F: An olfactory projection area in orbitofrontal cortex of the monkey. J Neurophysiol 38:1269–1283, 1975.

513. Tanaka, K: Inferotemporal cortex and object vision. Ann Rev Neurosci 19:109–139, 1996.

514. Tanji, J and Shima, K: Role for supplementary motor area cells in planning several movements ahead. Nature 371:413–416, 1994.

515. Thompson, R F: Foundations of Physiological Psychology. Harper & Row, New York, 1967.

516. Thorpe, S J, Rolls, E T and Maddison, S: The orbitofrontal cortex: neuronal activity in the behaving monkey. Exp Brain Res 49:93–115, 1983.

517. Torch, W C, Hirano, A and Solomon, S: Anterograde transneuronal degeneration in the limbic system: clinico-anatomical correlation. Neurology 27:1157–1163, 1977.

518. Tovée, M J: How fast is the speed of thought? Curr Biol 4:1125–1127, 1994.

519. Toyoshima, K and Sakai, H: Exact cortical extent of the origin of the corticospinal tract (CST) and the quantitative contribution to the CST in different cytoarchitectonic areas. A study with horseradish peroxidase in the monkey. J Hirnforsch 23:257–269, 1982.

520. Tramo, M J, Loftus, W, Thomas, C E, Green, R L, Mott, L A and Gazzaniga, M S: Surface area of human cerebral cortex and its gross morphological subdivisions: in vivo measurements in monozygatic twins suggest differential hemisphere effects of genetic factors. J Cog Neurosci 7:292–301, 1995.

521. Tranel, D and Damasio, A R: Autonomic recognition of familiar faces by prosopagnosics: evidence for knowledge without awareness. Neurology 35:119–120, 1985.

522. Trojanowski, J Q and Jacobson, S: Areal and laminar distribution of some pulvinar cortical efferents in rhesus monkey. J Comp Neurol 169:371–392, 1976.

523. Tucker, D M, Watson, R T and Heilman, K M: Discrimination and evocation of affectively intoned speech in patients with right parietal disease. Neurology 27:947–950, 1977.

524. Tulving, E, Kapur, S, Craik, FIM, Moskovitch, M and Houle, S: Hemispheric encoding/retrieval asymmetry in episodic memory: positron emission tomography findings. Proc Natl Acad Sci USA 91:2016–2020, 1994.

525. Umilta, C, Bagnara, S and Simion, F: Laterality effects for simple and complex geometrical figures, and nonsense patterns. Neuropsychologia 16:43–49, 1978.

526. Ungerleider, L G and Mishkin, M: Two cortical visual systems. In Ingle, D J, Mansfield, R J W and Goodale, M D (Eds.): The Analysis of Visual Behavior. MIT Press, Cambridge, MA, 1982, pp. 549–586.

527. Ungerleider, L G and Pribram, K H: Inferotemporal versus combined pulvinar-peristriate lesions in the rhesus monkey: effects on color, object and pattern discrimination. Neuropsychologia 15:481–498, 1977.

528. Vaadia, E, Haalman, I, Abeles, M, Bergman, H, Prut, Y, Slovin, H and Aertsen, A: Dynamics of neuronal interactions in monkey cortex in relation to behavioral events. Nature 373:515–518, 1995.

529. Valenstein, E, Bowers, D, Verfaellie, M, Heilman, K M, Day, A and Watson, R T: Retrosplenial amnesia. Brain 110:631–646, 1987.

530. Van Essen, D C: Functional organization of primate visual cortex. In Peters, A and Jones, EG (Eds.): Cerebral Cortex, Vol. 3. Plenum Publishing, New York, 1985, pp. 259–329.

531. Van Hoesen, G W: The parahippocampal gyrus. Trends Neurosci 5:345–350, 1982.

532. Van Hoesen, G W, Mesulam, M M and Haaxma, R: Temporal cortical projections to the olfactory tubercle in the rhesus monkey. Brain Res 109:375–381, 1976.

533. Van Hoesen, G W, Pandya, D N and Butters, N: Cortical afferents to the entorhinal cortex of the rhesus monkey. Science 175:1471–1473, 1972.

534. Van Hoesen, G W, Rosene, D L and Mesulam, M M: Subicular input from temporal cortex in the rhesus monkey. Science 205:608–610, 1979.

535. Van Lanckner, D R and Canter, G J: Impairment of voice and face recognition in patients with hemispheric damage. Brain Cogn 1:185–195, 1982.

536. Victor, M, Adams, R D and Collins, G H: The Wernicke-Korsakoff Syndrome. F. A. Davis, Philadelphia, 1971.

537. Vogt, C and Vogt, O: Allgemeinere Ergebnisse unserer Hirnforschung. Journal für Psychologie und Neurologie 25:279–461, 1919.

538. Vollmer-Haase, J, Finke, K, Hartje, W and Bulla-Hellwig, M: Hemispheric dominance in the processing of J. S. Bach fugues: a transcranial Doppler sonography (TCD) study with musicians. Neuropsychologia 36:857–867, 1998.

539. von Economo, C and Koskinas, G N: Die Cytoarchitektonik der Hirnrinde es erwachsenen Menschen. Springer, Vienna, 1925.

540. Wada, H, Inagaki, N, Yamatodani, A and Watanabe, T: Is the histaminergic neuron system a regulatory center for whole-brain activity? Trends Neurosci 14:415–418, 1991.

541. Wall, P D and Davis, G D: Three cerebral cortical systems affecting autonomic function. J Neurophysiol 14:508–517, 1951.

542. Walsh, F X, Thomas, T J, Langlais, P J and Bird, E D: Dopamine and homovanillic acid concentrations in striatal and limbic regions of the human brain. Ann Neurol 12:52–55, 1982.

543. Walshe, F: On the "syndrome of the premotor cortex" (Fulton) and the definition of the terms "premotor" and "motor" with a consideration of Jackson's views on the cortical representation of movements. Brain 58:49–80, 1935.

544. Warrington, E K: Neuropsychological studies of object recognition. Philos Trans R Soc Lond Biol 298:15–33, 1982.

545. Watson, J D, Myers, R, Frackowiak, R S, Hajnal, J V, Woods, R P, Mazziotta, J C, Shipp, S and Zeki, S: Area V5 of the human brain: evidence from a combined study using positron emission tomography and magnetic resonance imaging. Cereb Cortex 3:79–94, 1993.

546. Weilburg, J B, Mesulam, M-M, Weintraub, S, Buonanno, F, Jenike, M and Stakes, J W: Focal striatal abnormalities in a patient with obsessive-compulsive disorder. Arch Neurol 46:233–235, 1989.

547. Weinrich, M and Wise, S P: The premotor cortex of the monkey. J Neurosci 2:1329–1345, 1982.

548. Weintraub, S, Mesulam, M-M and Kramer, L: Disturbances in prosody. A right hemisphere contribution to language. Arch Neurol 38:742–744, 1981.

549. Weiskrantz, L, Warrington, E K, Sanders, M D and Marshall, J: Visual capacity in the hemianopic field following a restricted cortical ablation. Brain 97:709–728, 1974.

550. White, L E, Andrews, T J, Hulette, C, Richards, A, Groelle, M, Paydarfar, J and Purves, D: Structure of the human sensorimotor system. II: lateral symmetry. Cereb Cortex 7:31–47, 1997.

551. Whitty, C and Lewin, W: A Korsakoff Syndrome in the post-cingulectomy confusional state. Brain 83:648–653, 1910.

552. Wieser, H G: Depth recorded limbic seizures and psychopathology. Neurosci Biobehav Rev 7:427–440, 1983.

553. Willett, C J, Gwyn, D G, Rutherford, J G and Leslie, R A: Cortical projections to the nucleus of the tractus solitarius: an HRP study in the cat. Brain Res Bull 16:497–505, 1986.

554. Williams, H, Crane, L A, Hale, T K, Esposito, M A and Nottebohm, F: Right-side dominance for song control in the zebra finch. J Neurobiol 23:1006–1020, 1992.

555. Wilson, FAW and Rolls, E T: Neuronal responses related to novelty and familiarity of visual stimuli in the substantia innominata, diagonal band of Broca and periventricular region of the primate basal forebrain. Exp Brain Res 80:104–120, 1990.

556. Wise, S P, Boussaoud, D, Johnson, P B and Caminiti, R: Premotor and parietal cortex: corticocortical connectivity and combinational computations. Ann Rev Neurosci 20:25–42, 1997.

557. Wise, S P, Weinrich, M and Mauritz, K H: Motor aspects of cue-related neuronal activity in premotor cortex of the rhesus monkey. Brain Res 260:301–305, 1983.

558. Wolfe, N, Linn, R, Babikian, V L, Knoefel, J E and Albert, M L: Frontal systems impairment following multiple lacunar infarcts. Arch Neurol 47:129–132, 1990.

559. Wong, M-L, Al-Sheklee, A, Gold, P W and Licinio, J: Cytokines in the brain. In Rothwell, NJ (Ed.): Cytokines in the Nervous System. R. G. Landes, 1996, pp. 3–20.

560. Woolsey, C N, Settlage, P H, Meyer, D R, Sencer, W, Pinto Hamuy, T and Travis, A M: Patterns of localization in precentral and "supplementary" motor areas and their relation to the concept of a premotor area. Assoc Res Nerv Ment Dis 30:238–264, 1950.

561. Wu, J C, Buchsbaum, M S, Hershey, T G, Hazlett, E, Sicotte, N and Johnson, J C: PET in generalized anxiety disorder. Biol Psychol 29:1181–1199, 1991.

562. Wyss, J M, Swanson, L W and Cowan, W M: Evidence for an input to the molecular layer and the stratum granulosum of the dentate gyrus from the supramammillary region of the hypothalamus. Anat Embryol (Berl) 156:165–176, 1979.

563. Wyss, J M, Swanson, L W and Cowan, W M: A study of subcortical afferents to the hippocampal formation in the rat. Neuroscience 4:463–476, 1979.

564. Yaginuma, S, Niihara, T and Iwai, E: Further evidence on elevated discrimination limens for reduced patterns in monkeys with inferotemporal lesions. Neuropsychologia 20:21–32, 1982.

565. Yakovlev, P I: Pathoarchitectonic studies of cerebral malformations. III. Arrhinencephalies (Holotelencephalies). J Neuropath Exp Neurol 18:22–55, 1959.

566. Yamadori, A: Palpatory apraxia. European Neurology 21:277–283, 1982.

567. Yamaguchi, S, Tsuchiya, H and Kobayashi, S: Visuospatial attention shift and motor responses in cerebellar disorders. J Cog Neurosci 10:95–107, 1998.

568. Yamane, S, Kaji, S and Kawano, K: What facial features activate face neurons of the inferotemporal cortex of the monkey? Exp Brain Res 73:209–214, 1988.

569. Yeterian, E H and Pandya, D N: Corticothalamic connections of paralimbic regions in the rhesus monkey. J Comp Neurol 269:130–146, 1988.

570. Yeterian, E H and Van Hoesen, G W: Cortico-striate projections in the rhesus monkey: The organization of certain cortico-caudate connections. Brain Res 139:43–63, 1978.

571. Yim, C Y and Mogenson, G J: Response of ventral pallidal neurons to amygdala stimulation and its modulation by dopamine projections to nucleus accumbens. J Neurophysiol 50:148–161, 1983.

572. Yoon, B-W, Morillo, C A, Cechetto, D F and Hachinski, V: Cerebral hemispheric lateralization in cardiac autonomic control. Arch Neurol 54:741–744, 1997.

573. Young, M P and Yamane, S: Sparse population coding of faces in the inferotemporal cortex. Science 256:1327–1331, 1992.

574. Yozawitz, A, Bruder, G, Sutton, S, Sharpe, L, Gurland, B, Fleiss, J and Costa, L: Dichotic perception: evidence for right hemisphere dysfunction in affective psychosis. Br J Psychiatry 135:224–237, 1979.

575. Zald, D H and Pardo, J V: Emotion, olfaction, and the human amygdala: amygdala activation during aversive olfactory stimulation. Proc Natl Acad Sci USA 94:4119–4124, 1997.

576. Zatorre, R J, Evans, A C and Meyer, E: Neural mechanisms underlying melodic perception and memory for pitch. J Neurosci 14:1908–1919, 1994.

577. Zeki, S: Cerebral akinetopsia (visual motion blindness). Brain 114:811–824, 1991.
578. Zihl, J, Cramon, D, Mai, N and Schmid, C: Disturbance of movement vision after bilateral posterior brain damage. Further evidence and follow up observations. Brain 114: 2235–2252, 1991.
579. Zipser, D and Andersen, R A: A back-propagation programmed network that simulates response properties of a subset of posterior parietal neurons. Nature 331:679–684, 1988.
580. Zoccolatti, P, Scabini, D and Violani, C: Electrodermal responses in patients with unilateral brain damage. J Clin Neuropsychol 4:143–150, 1982.
581. Zola-Morgan, S, Squire, L R and Amaral, D G: Human amnesia and the medial temporal lobe: Enduring memory impairment following a bilateral lesion limited to field CA1 of the hippocampus. J Neurosci 6:2950–2967, 1986.

2

Neuropsychological Assessment of Mental State

Sandra Weintraub

I. Introduction: General Principles

The study of brain-damaged patients has shown that the traditional categories around which the mental state examination is organized (e.g., memory, language, reasoning, etc.) are not unitary. For example, some patients could have preserved language comprehension for commands requiring whole body movements but not for those requiring only limb movements; some may learn a new motor skill without conscious memory of the experience (see Chapter 4); yet others may *experience* emotion but are not able to *convey* it via modulations of prosody and facial expression (see Chapter 6). Functional imaging studies in healthy adults have demonstrated that performing even a simple mental task activates distributed neuroanatomical networks and not a single, dedicated "center." Furthermore, domains of mental processes are highly interactive, so an impairment in one may influence performance of tests in another. For example, a task of mental calculation may be failed because of a primary defect of attention or language, or because of an inability to sequence a series of goal-directed actions. These considerations have shaped the neuropsychological approach to testing mental state described in this chapter.

There are several reasons why it is unrealistic to expect that an "all-purpose," standardized, battery could be designed to test all complex neurobehavioral disorders and generate specific diagnoses. First, it is an arduous task to collect normative data for all the variables that can affect performance (i.e., age, gender, education, cultural and language backgrounds, medications, and others). Second, it would be impossible to structure a test with a level of difficulty that would consistently avoid "floor" and "ceiling" effects. Third, no standardized tests exist for diagnosing relatively rare neurobehavioral syndromes such as prosopagnosia or tactile agnosia. Fourth, no test is entirely selective for assessing its target domain. For example, memory tests based on word lists also require attention, motivation, and language processes for performance. Moreover, it may be necessary to improvise tests for unusual symptoms. In order to assess a reported loss of the capacity for mental visualization, for example, the patient could be asked to imagine the object that would be created by mentally rotating a "D" 90° degrees leftwards and attaching the letter "J" at the midpoint of its straight side (i.e., yields the form of an umbrella). Fifth, the objective examination of mental state tends to exclude a vast realm of human behaviors, including judgment, insight, curiosity, strength of will, foresight, compassion, and many aspects of problem-solving ability. Finally, there is no one-to-one relationship between scores on mental state tests and specific neurological diagnoses. Instead, test results characterize *patterns* of impairment which then lead to hypotheses about the most likely anatomical location of the responsible lesion and its most likely etiology.

Not all test results are equally easy to interpret. For example, calling a toothbrush a "tweebspee" or failing to name objects by palpation only when they are placed in the left hand is abnormal from any frame of reference and does not need to be compared to normative standards for interpretation. However, failure to name items only at the upper levels of difficulty on the *Boston Naming Test (BNT)*[88] requires normative comparison since a certain percentage of neurologically "normal" individuals will fail these items. If performance falls 1 to 2 standard deviations below average scores for age- and education-matched controls, one can conclude that an abnormality exists, especially if there is evidence that the relevant function was previously normal. The examination of gifted persons with mild but subjectively distressing impairment in the area of their talents is especially challenging. "Average" (or better) test scores may, nevertheless, represent deterioration when compared with past performance.

The organization and interpretation of the mental state examination can be simplified by dividing domains of mental functions into two categories based on their neuroanatomical affiliations (Chapter 1). The first group, the "state" functions, are influenced by the frontal network and the broadly projecting neuronal pathways of the ascending reticular activating system (ARAS). These anatomical systems mediate rapid modulations of the overall information-processing "tone" (Chapters 1 and 3) and their integrity is reflected in the maintenance of arousal and some aspects of attention, mood, and motivation. Metabolic disorders, medication effects, multifocal lesions, and frontal lobe damage (because of impaired top–down regulation) disrupt state-dependent mental functions. Primary deficits in state-dependent functions lead to impairments of relatively little localizing value. For example, the occasional misnaming of objects in a drowsy or inattentive patient has little localizing value whereas it would strongly suggest dysfunction within the left cerebral language network in an alert, attentive subject. Primary deficits in state functions affect performance of all other neuropsychological tasks and, therefore, influence the global interpretation of the mental state examination.

The second group, the "channel" functions, in contrast, rely on more discrete anatomical pathways with monosynaptic corticocortical connections organized into several overlapping large-scale distributed networks. Language, complex perceptual skills, and explicit memory are domains that are mediated by this type of arrangement.[117] Thus, primary deficits in the channel-dependent domains are more informative than those in the state-dependent functions for interpreting the putative anatomical substrate for an observed deficit. However, such interpretation should be further guided by the awareness that similar behavioral deficits can occur with lesions in any one of several anatomically distinct components of a distributed neurocognitive network. Hemispatial neglect, for example, can arise after lesions in frontal, parietal, or cingulate cortex (Chapter 3). In such instances, a cluster of "neighborhood signs" (e.g., hemianopia, hemiplegia) can guide more precise anatomic localization.

In general, the performance of each task in the examination is associated with an input route, an intermediate processing stage, and an output route. Reaching conclusions about the intermediate processing stage in patients who have an impairment of the input or output routes can be misleading. It may be impossible, for example, to know if a mute patient has aphasic speech, if an aphasic patient has abnormal thought processes, or if an extremely inattentive patient has retentive memory.

Inferences about brain–behavior correlations should follow the proper rules of induction. Consider the evidence that patients with left temporal lobe lesions are more likely to develop a material-specific verbal amnesia than those with right-sided temporal lesions. This evidence cannot be used to infer the presence of a left temporal lobe lesion in a patient who happens to have a verbal amnesia. It has only shown that an amnesia confined to verbal material could be used to predict the laterality of the lesion in patients with *documented* unilateral lesions confined to the temporal lobe.

Inferences about localization should also be confined to the legitimate population. For example, much of the information about the relationship between cognitive deficits and lesion site comes from the study of patients who develop such deficits as a consequence of single lesions acquired in adulthood. These relationships may not apply to chronic neurological disease or to diseases acquired early in life. For example, the intracarotid sodium amytal procedure (or Wada test) has demonstrated that the traditional pattern of left hemisphere dominance for language is much less frequent in right-handed patients with chronic epilepsy.[141] Similarly, patterns of deficits disclosed by neuropsychological tests are, by themselves, of questionable validity for identifying the putative anatomic distribution of cerebral dysfunction in such conditions as schizophrenia, depression, or usual aging.

II. GENERAL STRATEGY FOR THE MENTAL-STATE EXAMINATION AND REVIEW OF PRIMARY NEUROCOGNITIVE DOMAINS

The presenting symptoms and behavioral observations during the history-taking help to generate hypotheses about the nature of the primary disturbance and to plan a strategy for the examination. Identifying tasks that a patient can accomplish with approximately 75% accuracy avoids floor and ceiling effects and makes it possible to detect changes in performance over time. The examination should begin with an appraisal of the *level of arousal, mood, motivation, attention,* and *executive functions,* since primary deficits in these state-dependent functions will influence test selection and also interpretation. Next, *language and visual and auditory perceptual functions* should be reviewed since deficits in these functions are of localizing value and even mild deficits in these domains may affect performance on other tests that rely on language or sensory processing. *Explicit memory* and *reasoning* are tested next, with emphasis on verbal and nonverbal materials. *Judgment, insight,* and other aspects of *comportment* can be assessed based on direct observation and collateral information about the patient's daily living activities.

After the examination is completed, a "profile" can be constructed, contrasting domains of primary impairment with those in which test failure is secondary to another factor and with those in which performance is essentially normal. Performance in each domain can be rated: "mildly impaired" if objective test scores fall between 1 and 2 standard deviations below the mean for one's age and education, "moderately impaired" if between 2 and 3, and "severely impaired" if beyond 3.[174] Interpretation of performance requires comparison to the patient's premorbid level of ability. An estimated premorbid IQ can be derived from reading tests (e.g., *Wide Range Achievement Test–3 [WRAT-3]*[208] and the *American National Adult Reading Test [AMNART]*[68]) or from demographic variables.[6] In the absence of formal test scores, a profile can be based on clinical impressions.

Methods for informal bedside examination and for more formal objective testing are described in the sections that follow. Table 2–1 lists the tests and procedures discussed in this chapter and Table 2–2 is a quick reference to tasks at different levels of difficulty. Detailed descriptions, administration procedures, available norms, and summaries of research based on many of these measures are presented in Lezak[102] and in Spreen and Strauss.[174]

State-Dependent Domains

WAKEFULNESS/AROUSAL, SPAN, WORKING MEMORY AND THE ATTENTIONAL MATRIX

Wakefulness/arousal. The level of wakefulness ranges from deep coma to anxious hyperalertness and is characterized by the intensity of stimulation needed to elicit a meaningful response. In coma or stupor, for example, noxious stimulation is required to provoke a stereotyped response. This contrasts with the normal state of wakefulness in which the patient is responsive even to the subtlest of cues. "Comatose," "stuporous," "drowsy," "alert," and "hyperalert" are terms that can be used to describe the level of arousal. Interpretation of performance on mental state tests is substantially limited if the state of arousal is abnormal.

Attention/working memory/short-term memory. In Chapter 3, functions associated with the allocation of attention are divided into two broad categories. One category, generally associated with the function of the ARAS and of the frontal lobe, serves to maintain an overall attentional tone or "matrix." Terms such as "vigilance," "concentration," "short-term memory," and "working memory" refer to the positive aspects of the attentional matrix. "Working memory" refers to processes for the brief on-line holding and manipulation of information.[5] Only the former com-

TABLE 2–1. Mental State Tests According to Primary Domain

WAKEFULNESS, AROUSAL, AND THE ATTENTIONAL MATRIX

A. Concentration: Span/Vigilance/Working Memory
  -Continuous Performance Tests
  -Digit Span*[a], Visual Span[a]
  -**Paced Auditory Serial Attention Test**
  -Letter-Number Sequencing (WMS-III)[a]
  -**Sternberg Procedure**
B. Perseverance
  -Serial Recitation Tests (WMS-III)[a]
  -Word List Generation[a]
C. Resistance to Interference and Response Inhibition
  -Trail-Making Test[a]
  -Stroop Test
  -Alternating Sequences Test*
  -Go–No-Go Procedure*

MOOD

A. Self-Administered
  -MMPI-II
  -Beck Depression Inventory
  -Geriatric Depression Scale[a]
B. Examiner Administered
  -Hamilton Depression Rating Scale

MEMORY

  -Retrograde Memory Tests
  -Wechsler Memory Scale III[a]
  -**Rey Auditory Verbal Learning Test**[a]
  -**California Verbal Learning Test**[a]
  -RBANS Word List[a]
  -Hopkins Verbal Learning Test–Revised[a]
  -**Rey-Osterreith Complex Figure**[a]
  -**Selective Reminding Procedure**[a]
  -Warrington RMT[a]
  -Drilled Word Span Procedure*
  -Three Words–Three Shapes Procedure*

LINGUISTIC ASPECTS OF LANGUAGE

  -Boston Diagnostic Aphasia Examination (BDAE)
  -Western Aphasia Battery (WAB)
  -Peabody Picture Vocabulary Test
  -Token Test
  -Boston Naming Test[a]
  -Nelson Denny Reading Test
  -Wide Range Achievement Test–3 (WRAT-3)
  -Reading, Spelling subtests[a]

CALCULATION ABILITIES

  -BDAE—Supplementary Part[a]
  -WRAT-3, Arithmetic Subtest[a]
  -WAIS-III, Arithmetic Subtest[a]

(continued)

TABLE 2–1. Mental State Tests According to Primary Domain—
Continued

PERCEPTUAL TASKS

-Hooper Visual Organization Test
-Judgment of Line Orientation[a]
-Facial Recognition[a]
-Gollin Incomplete Figures
-Seashore Tests of Musical Talent
-Sound Recognition Test
-Visual Object and Space Perception Battery
-Woodcock Johnson Tests of Cognitive Ability[a]

CONSTRUCTIONAL TASKS

-WAIS-III—Block Design Subtest[a]
-Rey-Osterreith Complex Figure Test[a]
-3-D Cube Construction
-Copying a cube, drawing a Clock[a]

SPATIAL DISTRIBUTION OF ATTENTION

-Bilateral Simultaneous Stimulation (Visual, Auditory, Tactile)
-Verbal and Nonverbal Target Cancellation
-Blindfolded manual exploration

PARALINGUISTIC ASPECTS OF COMMUNICATION

-Discrimination, repetition, and production of affective and
 nonaffective prosody
-Profile of Nonverbal Sensitivity (PONS)
-Identification of Facial Affect

REASONING AND ABSTRACTIONS

-WAIS-III—Comprehension, Similarities, Matrices Subtests[a]
-Object and Form Sorting Tasks
-Visual-Verbal Test
-Wisconsin Card Sorting Test
-Raven Standard[a], *Colored**, **Advanced** Matrices

PLANNING AND SEQUENCING

-Alternating Sequences Test
-Drawing of a Clock
-Porteus Maze Test
-Tower of London

TESTING THE ELDERLY AND THE DIAGNOSIS OF DEMENTIA

-Short Mental State Tests
   1. Mini Mental State Examination*
   2. Blessed Dementia Scale*
-Brief Dementia Batteries
   1. Mattis Dementia Rating Scale
   2. Alzheimer's Disease Assessment Scale
   3. CERAD Battery
   4. Repeatable Battery for the Assessment of
      Neuropsychological Status

(continued)

TABLE 2–1.—Continued

-Assessment of Daily Living Activities
    1. Instrumental Activities of Daily Living
    2. Record of Independent Living
-Behavioral symptoms of dementia
    1. Neuropsychiatric Inventory
    2. BEHAVE-AD
-Clinical Severity Ratings/Stages
    1. Clinical Dementia Rating
    2. Global Deterioration Scale
    3. Functional Assessment Staging
-Assessment of the Patient with Superior Premorbid Intellectual
 Capacity or Special Talents
    1. Microcog
-Estimate of Premorbid IQ
    1. American National Adult Reading Test
    2. Demographic Formulae

---

    *= easy; Test names in Bold = hard.
    [a]= norms for older adults are available.

ponent is most clearly an attentional function whereas the latter is attributed to the "executive" functions of the brain. Disturbances of the attentional matrix are reflected in symptoms of impersistence, perseveration, distractibility, increased vulnerability to interference, and an inability to inhibit immediate but inappropriate response tendencies.

Vigilance, or sustained attention, is closely linked to arousal and can be measured with *continuous performance tests (CPTs)*. In the paradigmatic task, a target is repeatedly presented among a series of randomly occurring stimuli over an interval of several minutes. In a study where letters were visually presented at the rate of 1 per second, normal adults identified close to 90% of simple targets (e.g., the letter "X") and 80% of complex targets (e.g., the letter "X" preceded by an "A") while "brain-damaged" subjects identified an average of 80% and 60% of simple and complex targets, respectively. [157] Performance on this paradigm has been shown to be impaired in children with the attention deficit–hyperactivity disorder (ADHD).[66, 181, 187] Performance on *simple* vigilance tests is not likely to be influenced by IQ.[39] At the bedside, auditory or visual stimuli can be delivered via tape recorder, be read aloud, or be presented on a laptop computer.

There are several standardized variations of the basic CPT paradigm. The *Brief Test of Attention*[164,165] is presented on audio cassette, requires 8 minutes for administration, and has normative data for individuals up to age 81. The *Gordon Diagnostic Tests* are a series of automated visual continuous performance tests, some of which are sensitive to distractibility and the inability to inhibit inappropriate responses.[61,62] On the *Conners' CPT* the patient must respond to every letter, *except* the target and there are norms for adults with ADHD.[31] The *d2 Test* is a 10-minute, paper-and-pencil test of sustained visual attention in which a target letter "d" surrounded in any manner by two diacritical marks must be crossed out. [25] Foils include the let-

TABLE 2–2 Tasks by Level of Difficulty in Each Primary Domain*

Domain	Easy	Moderate	Hard
Attention	Counting 1–20, 20–1 Serial 2s	Months forward/ backward Serial 3s Category list generation	Serial 7s FAS list generation
Naming	Common objects + parts BNT, Items 1–20	BNT, items 21–40	BNT, items 41–60
Calculations	Simple addition, subtraction	Operations using >3-digit numbers	Word problems (e.g., What is 15% of 150?) WRAT-3 arithmetic
Comprehension	Do dogs fly?	Where is the source of illumination in this room?	Do you prefer a vehicle or a dwelling for transportation?
Repetition	The table	The book is on the table	No ifs, ands, or buts
Constructions	Copy a clock, simple geometric forms	Draw a clock, copy a cube	Copy Rey figure, Block Design (WAIS-III)
Visuoperception	Judge if pairs of faces, objects, angles are same or different	Facial Recognition (1–6) RBANS Line Orientation	Facial Recognition (7–13) Judgment of Line Orientation
Memory	Drilled Word Span procedure Three Words–Three Shapes	CERAD Word List Warrington RMT	Logical Memory (WMS-III) RAVLT, CVLT
Reasoning	Sort geometric forms or objects	Visual-Verbal Test	Raven's Matrices

*See text for explanation of abbreviations and references to published tests.

ters "p" and "b" and different numbers of diacritical marks around each letter. Age-related norms are available.[174] In addition to sustained attention, the above-named tests are also sensitive to perseveration and disinhibition. For example, some patients fail to catch the targets (errors of omission) whereas others keep responding to the foils (errors of commission).

The face validity of CPT tasks for assessing vigilance is illustrated with a clinical example: A 67-year-old man, in an acute confusional state secondary to a pulmonary empyema, identified only 15 of the 30 targets occurring among 300 stimuli in a 5-minute auditory letter detection task. One month after drainage of the empyema and antibiotic treatment, his score improved to 25, paralleling improvement on other tests of attention and resumption of his customary activities.

An alternate measure of attention/short term memory/working memory capacity is the *Digit Span* test.[111,194,195] Adults can normally repeat seven digits (plus or minus two) in forward sequence, a number that represents the average limit of human information processing capacity.[119] Backward span can also be measured and should not differ from forward span by more than two digits.[102] Digit span is influenced by education and age.[111,192] In adults over age 65, five digits forward and four backward is within "average" limits. Although often called a test of "short-term" memory or working "memory," digit span does not test explicit memory and amnestic patients usually have normal digit spans (Chapter 4). In aphasic patients, the nonverbal visual spatial attention span can be tested instead with the *Visual Span* subtest of the *Wechsler Memory Scale–III (WMS-III)*.[195] On this test, the examiner's pointing sequence on an irregular array of wooden blocks must be reproduced in the same order (forward span) or in reverse order (backward span). The nonverbal attention span assessed in this fashion is usually one or two items lower than the digit span.

The manipulative (or executive) aspects of working memory are emphasized in the *Letter-Number Sequencing* subtest of the *WMS-III*.[195] A string of letters intermixed with numbers (e.g., jw6h3a2) is presented aloud. The patient must repeat the stimuli in ascending order, with numbers first (viz., 236ahjw). The *Paced Auditory Serial Addition Test (PASAT)* is a much more demanding working memory task. Single digits are presented, one per 3 seconds, on an audiotape.[69] The patient must add each new number to the immediately preceding number, state the sum, and then add the next new number to the immediately preceding number in the string. For example, if the stimuli were "2, 6, 5, 3. . . ." the corresponding responses would be "8, 11, 8." Thus, the patient must hold one set of information on-line while simultaneously performing a mental calculation and discarding the answer before the next number in the sequence is delivered. The level of task difficulty can be further increased by increasing the rate of stimulus presentation.

The *Sternberg paradigm* provides a computerized chronometric method to measure working memory.[176] A stimulus set, containing from one to five digits, is first presented followed by a series of probe digits. The subject presses one response key if the probe is contained in the stimulus set and another if it is not. Decision time increases as a function of the size of the stimulus set. The slope of this function becomes steeper in patients with working memory deficits. Variables such as mood, motivation, aphasia, and motoric reaction time interfere with performance at all set sizes but do not influence the slope.

Perseverance and response inhibition. Tasks of self-initiated sustained behavioral output (e.g., *serial subtraction, word list generation*) can be used to detect impersistence. One popular measure, the *serial subtraction of 7 from 100*, can elicit errors in highly educated normal individuals.[171] Therefore, minor errors on serial 7s are not necessarily of significance. Other series generation tasks include, in ascending order of difficulty, reciting months of the year in reverse order, serial 3s, and reciting the alphabet in reverse order. On average, recitation of the months in forward sequence should require no more than 5–8 seconds in normal adults and no more than double the time for the reverse sequence. Forward serial 3s may require from 12 to 45 seconds depending on age.[193]

The generation of lists of words that either begin with a specified letter (lexical) or that are categorically related (semantic) can be used to assess perseverance, fluency, and mental retrieval. Spreen and Benton measured lexical generation of words beginning with the letters F, A, and S, each for a 60-second interval.[173] The *Controlled Oral Word Association Test (COWAT)* uses the letters C, F, and L.[14] On these tests, normal adults with a high-school education produce a total average of 36–40 words over the 3 minutes.[102,174] On tests of semantic list generation (animals) older adults can typically produce an average of about 18 ($\pm$ 5, depending upon age and education) in 60 seconds.[127] Successful performance on these tests implies normal perseverance and scanning of internal data stores. In the absence of aphasia, anomia, or amnesia, a reduction in the number of retrieved items, repetition of the same word, and listing of disqualified words (e.g., proper nouns in the lexical fluency task) are signs of difficulty with sustained output, concentration, and retrieval. Patients who cannot sustain behavioral output may also show generalized mental slowing and delayed response times. These are important features of the abulic state that is occasionally observed following frontal lobe lesions.

Susceptibility to interference and the inability to inhibit inappropriate automatic responses are assessed more specifically by tasks that provoke competing responses, such the *Stroop* procedure.[26,30,180] On this test, the time to read aloud a random sequence of color words (red, blue, green) in black and white print is measured. Next, the time to name the colors of an equal number of small rectangles (red, blue, green) is recorded. In the third—an "interference condition"—the words are printed in a nonmatching color and the task is to name the color of the text, inhibiting the equally strong, more automatic tendency to read the word. Response time is normally fastest in the word reading condition, slightly slower in the color-naming condition, and slowest in the interference condition (the "Stroop effect"). Errors of commission (i.e., reading the word) are evidence of the inability to inhibit the more automatic response tendency in the interference condition. On one early form of this test, the average time for adults to name 100 color dots, is 57 seconds, to read 100 color words is 42 seconds, and to name 100 colors in the interference condition, 109 seconds.[30] Several other standardized versions are available.[174]

The *Trail-Making Tests* also measure perseverance, response inhibition, and vulnerability to interference.[148] On Part A, on a sheet containing an irregular array of 25 numbered circles, the patient must draw a line connecting them in sequence (1-2-3, and so on). On Part B, numbers are intermixed with letters and must be connected in *alternating* sequence (1-a-2-b- and so on). Errors of perseveration may lead the patient to connect only numbers or only letters on part B. Performance on the *Trail-Making Tests* is influenced by IQ and age.[38,149] On average, high-school-educated 20-year-olds complete Part A in approximately 27 seconds and Part B in 59 seconds while similarly educated 60-year-olds require approximately 36 seconds and 81 seconds, respectively.[74,174]

A simple bedside test of the ability to inhibit inappropriate responses is the *Luria Alternating Sequences* task.[109] The patient must copy a short segment of connected alternating "m"s and "n"s (or alternating open triangles and squares) and then extend the pattern until the end of the page is reached, without lifting the pencil. Patients with attentional impairments may repeat the elements (perseveration) rather than alternate between them (Chapter 3, Fig. 3–2). A similar task is the quick repetitive alternation of a sequence of three hand postures–striking a table top with a clenched fist, an open palm, and the edge of the hand.[108] In the absence of an elementary motor disturbance this task assesses the capacity for sequencing and response inhibition.

A purer test of response inhibition is based on the "go–no-go" paradigm.[45] The patient is asked to quickly raise and immediately lower the index finger (hand palm-down on a flat surface) in response to a single tap of a pencil (the "go" signal) and to emit no response if the examiner taps twice in rapid succession (the "no-go" signal). We administered a series of 50 trials (30 "go" signals and 20 "no go" signals) to 20 cognitively normal subjects between 65 and 80 years of age who made, on average, three errors of commission (raising the finger following two taps) and no errors of omission with each hand. In this test, even a muscle flicker on the upper arm or hand should be considered an error.[79] In neurologically normal individuals, errors typically occur only in the initial trials. Patients with certain types of attentional problems cannot inhibit raising the finger in response to the "no-go" signal. In the case of a 60-year-old woman with a frontal meningioma, significant errors of commission on this task were reduced after surgical treatment.[101]

Perhaps the most important step in the mental state examination is to derive a measure of attention. Attention is required for the performance of all cognitive tasks and deficits can have repercussions throughout the mental state examination. A patient with a digit span of four may fail to repeat a ten-word sentence despite the absence of aphasia. Impulsive response tendencies could interfere with accurate responses to multiple choices. In patients with a primary impairment of attention, hour-to-hour and day-to-day fluctuations in performance are quite common. In general, inferences about localization based on abnormalities in the neuropsychological examination are far less dependable in the inattentive patient than in the patient who is fully alert and attentive. If attention is severely impaired, it may even be advisable to curtail the examination since the validity of findings would be questionable.

MOTIVATION AND MOOD

Cooperation with the examiner, the ability to sustain effort, and the spontaneous demonstration of initiative are among the observable aspects of motivation. Disturbances in motivation are described as "amotivational state," "apathy," and, in the more extreme cases, as "abulia." The abulic or apathetic patient may frequently reply "I don't know," offer terse responses, or take an inordinate amount of time to initiate a response. Unless the examiner allows sufficient time for a response, the number of primary impairments may be overestimated in these patients.

Mood and affect may be assessed during the course of the examination by traditional clinical methods of observation and questioning or with the help of standard questionnaires. Self-administered questionnaires such as the *Minnesota Multiphasic Personality Inventory–2*[67] and the *Beck Depression Inventory*[9,10] rely on the ability of the patient to read and understand the test items. These demands may exceed the limitations of many brain-damaged patients. The *Hamilton Depression Rating Scale*[70] is based on examiner ratings in an interview with the patient. Visual analogue scales are less dependent on verbal mediation and can be quite sensitive to temporal variations of mood.[51,122] On these tests, the patient is asked to indicate a point between the extremes of a line, each end representing polar aspects of mood (e.g., happy versus sad). These tests are not adequately standardized on brain-damaged populations but provide useful qualitative information.

In patients who appear to have a disturbance of motivation, mood, or affect, apathy must be distinguished from depression, and the ability to experience emotion must be distinguished from its display through speech prosody, facial expression, and body posture. In patients with pseudobulbar palsy or certain types of right hemisphere lesions, for example, the experience and expression of feeling may be dissociated (Chapter 6). Furthermore, some types of frontal lobe lesions and metabolic encephalopathies may lead to abulia, which can be mistaken for depression. Abnormalities of mood and motivation, like those in other state-dependent functions, are of limited localizing value but influence performance of mental state tests in other domains.

Channel-Dependent Domains

Linguistic aspects of language and related functions (praxis, calculations, right–left orientation, finger naming)

Linguistic processes in the brain can be broadly divided into (1) those that link thought (or meaning) to word forms ("lexical-semantic") and (2) those that sequence words and word endings to convey relationships among words ("syntactic"). "Aphasia" refers to a disturbance of either one of these components, reflected in abnormalities of oral or written communication (Chapter 5). The classical aphasia syndromes are based on patterns of deficits in *spontaneous speech, comprehension of oral and written language, repetition, naming, and writing*. The aim of the language examination is to identify whether lexical-semantic or syntactic processes are primarily affected and also to categorize the aphasia according to the classical syndromes.

Speech, repetition, and naming. Speech is "fluent" if the phrase length and melody are appropriate and "nonfluent" if phrase length is less than four words and the speech is halting or dysarthric. Nonfluent, agrammatical speech is usually associated with lesions anterior to the central sulcus (as in Broca's and transcortical motor aphasias), whereas fluent and paraphasic speech tends to be associated with more posterior lesions (as in Wernicke's, conduction, and transcortical sensory aphasias). Patients with the labored and agrammatical speech of a nonfluent aphasia may nevertheless convey meaning quite effectively in a "pithy" way whereas patients with fluent aphasia may produce almost incomprehensible speech which might be well articulated and fluent but quite devoid of informative nouns and verbs.

Errors in word production are referred to as "paraphasias." Sound substitutions within words (e.g., "ramp" instead of "lamp") are referred to as "phonemic" or "literal" paraphasias while substitutions of categorically similar words (e.g., "table" for "bench") are "semantic" paraphasias. Nonsensical words (e.g., "perset") are called "neologisms." Strings of such words or of improperly combined real words are referred to as "jargon aphasia." "Circumlocution" is the substitution of description for single words (e.g., "The thing you use to brush your teeth" instead of "toothbrush"). Lesions in the more posterior sectors of the language network result in more semantic paraphasias while anterior lesions are more often associated with phonemic paraphasias.

The ability to repeat spoken language is an important criterion for grouping the classical aphasia syndromes (Chapter 5). Aphasic repetition disorders are best elicited by asking the patient to repeat statements that vary in grammatical complexity. A progression from simple to more complex is: "The book," "The book is on the table," and "No ifs, ands or buts" (Table 2–2). Aphasic patients have the most difficulty repeating small grammatical words (e.g., "if," "or," "from"). In testing repetition, sentence length should not exceed the patient's immediate span of attention, otherwise, aphasic repetition disorders could not be distinguished from verbal working memory deficits. Repetition of "tongue twisters" such as "instrumental provincial artillery unit" or "hippopotamus" is not helpful with aphasic patients but rather can be used to evoke dysarthria and palilalia.

The ability to name objects is impaired in virtually all forms of aphasia and may also be an early symptom associated with dementia of the Alzheimer's type. Common objects (e.g., coat, skirt, eyeglasses) are convenient for bedside testing and component parts (e.g., lapel, hem, lens, frame) help to detect more subtle impairments. A quantitative measure of naming is provided by the *Boston Naming Test (BNT)*, which consists of 60 drawings of objects, graded in their level of difficulty.[88] Several sources of normative data are available.[80,174,182] Normal adults up to age 65 with a high school education can name an average of 55 words ($\pm$ 5); over age 75, 50 ($\pm$ 5) may be considered average. Those with less education may score five points lower.

Errors on the BNT could take the form of perceptual misidentifications, circumlocutions, semantic paraphasias, or phonemic paraphasias. Two types of cues are provided in the standard administration of this test. If the patient makes a visual identification error, a so-called "stimulus cue" is given that provides information about the object's identity. If the patient recognizes the object but cannot think of the name, a "phonemic cue" provides information about the initial sounds of the correct name. In a study designed to specifically evaluate the influence of perceptual difficulty on naming ability, Kirshner and colleagues presented pictured objects under four conditions ranging from a clear photograph of the object to a line drawing obscured by superimposed lines.[95] Patients with right cerebral lesions and those with dementia had more difficulty as perceptual distortion increased, and their spontaneous naming errors were predominantly based on perceptual misidentifications. Phonemic errors occurred only in the aphasic patients.

Occasionally, naming disorders can be selective (Chapter 5). For example, lesions in the lateral anterior temporal regions can give rise to specific inability to name tools or to name animals.[184] An isolated impairment of color naming is present in patients with the syndrome of alexia without agraphia. A naming deficit can be "one-way" (the patient cannot name but recognizes the name from choices) or "two-way" (the patient also cannot recognize the correct name when it is spoken). A patient with an aphasic two-way naming deficit can describe or demonstrate the use of the object whereas the patient with an object agnosia cannot (Chapters 1, 5, and 7).

Comprehension. The commonly used aphasia batteries, the *Boston Diagnostic Aphasia Examination (BDAE)*[60] and the *Western Aphasia Battery (WAB)*[91], test auditory language comprehension but do not differentiate between semantic and syntactic deficits. This is an important distinction since patients with nonfluent aphasias who score normally on comprehension subtests of the BDAE and the WAB may nevertheless have a specific inability to understand grammatically complex sentences containing the passive voice or embedded clauses. At bedside, semantic comprehension can be tested with questions that require a "Yes" or "No" response (e.g., "Do dogs fly?" or "Does it snow in summer?") and that depend on normal access to the meaning of nouns and verbs. Grammatical comprehension can be tested with questions that emphasize relational terms and morphological endings (e.g., "Do you put on your shoes *before* your socks" and "The girl was eat last night—is this correct?", respectively).

The *Token Test* assesses comprehension of conjoined sentences, adjectives, and prepositions.[40] It requires the manipulation of plastic pieces differing in color, geometric shape, and size in response to instructions of increasing complexity (e.g., "Put the yellow circle *behind* the red square, *before* you touch the black square") and is therefore sensitive to deficits in attention span. Short forms are also available.[80,174] The *Token Test* can detect subtle deficits of grammatical comprehension and has been particularly useful in the early stages of the primary progressive aphasia syndrome.[204] Patients with Broca's and transcortical motor aphasias show selective comprehension deficits for grammatical features of statements while those with Wernicke's and transcortical sensory aphasias lose the ability to understand the meanings of all types of words, whether grammatical or not. The "expressive-receptive" classification that is used in some clinical settings does not acknowledge these qualitative dissociations.

Reading and writing. Reading deficits may encompass all types of words as in the syndromes of "pure" and "central" alexia (Chapters 1 and 5). Wernicke's aphasia is usually accompanied by an alexia which is as severe as the comprehension deficit for spoken language whereas Broca's aphasia may be accompanied by a selective deficit for reading only grammatical words. Qualitative analysis of the reading errors of alexic patients has led to the definition of subtypes of alexia.[34] In "deep" alexia, the patient misreads but produces substitutes that are semantically similar to the target word (e.g., reading "buzz" as "bee"). In "phonological" alexia, there is a grapheme-to-phoneme conversion deficit, so the patient can read real words but not nonsense words (e.g., "forty" but not "flort"). In "surface" alexia the patient can read orthographically regular words but not irregular words (e.g., "blister" but not "colonel"). Reading aloud may be dissociated from silent reading comprehension and should be tested separately.

At the bedside, the patient can be asked "yes/no" questions about a brief newspaper passage that he/she has read silently. Many of the standard reading tests, such as the reading subtest of the *Wide Range Achievement Test–3 (WRAT-3)*,[208] reading sections of the *Woodcock-Johnson Tests of Achievement*,[212] and the *Nelson-Denny Reading Test* [27] were developed to assess reading achievement level. Aphasics' comprehension of printed words, sentences, and paragraphs is tested with the *BDAE*[60] and the *WAB*.[91] However, none of the standard reading tests distinguishes among the qualitative varieties of alexic errors outlined above. Experimental word lists can be used to study these distinctions.[153]

Aphasic writing deficits, or agraphia, may accompany alexia or may occur separately. "Phonological agraphia," a phoneme-to-grapheme transformation deficit, is characterized by the inability to spell nonsense words with preserved ability to spell real and regular words.[154,168] In "lexical agraphia" the patient can write nonsense words but not irregular words,[153] indicating a deficit at the level of the "whole word" approach, with preserved phonological access.

Agraphic errors can be linguistic or may reflect mechanical problems related to letter formation. Spontaneous writing, writing to dictation, and copying should be compared. Patients may spontaneously write a simple sentence without difficulty but be unable to write more complex material in response to dictation. Alternatively, some agraphic patients who cannot write spontaneously or to dictation may be able to slavishly copy printed text. The contribution of a defect in the mechanics of writing can be eliminated with the use of anagram letters or a typewriter. A disturbance of writing in the absence of aphasia, may be observed in patients in acute confusional states.[29] In most of these cases, symptoms consist mainly of perseverative repetition of letters and carelessness in the mechanical aspects of penmanship. Patients with callosal lesions may be agraphic only with the left hand. Patients with hemispatial neglect may fail to write in the neglected hemispace but this should not be considered a true agraphia.

Praxis. Liepmann defined three forms of apraxia.[103] "Melokinetic (or limb kinetic) apraxia" refers to a disturbance of fine movements, leading to awkward and inaccurate movement. This deficit can be observed not only when the patient is asked to carry out a pantomimed action but also in spontaneous limb usage. "Ideational apraxia" designates the inability to carry out a complex activity requiring a sequence of movements with real objects despite being able to correctly execute the individual components. This type of apraxia often occurs in acute confusional states and in dementia and probably represents a primary disturbance of attention and executive functions that interferes with the coherence of sequenced motor output. It can be tested by asking the patient to fold a letter, insert it in an envelope, and seal and stamp the envelope. An example of an error might be sealing the envelope prior to inserting the letter. "Ideomotor apraxia" refers to the inability to pantomime movements in response to verbal command despite the normal execution of the same movement in the naturalistic setting. Many apraxic patients can imitate the required movement when it is performed by the examiner, proving that the ideomotor apraxia is not based on a purely motor inability to execute the movement.

Testing for ideomotor apraxia should include commands aimed at buccofacial, limb, and whole body movements since there can be clear-cut dissociations.[4] Ideomotor apraxia usually encompasses only the first two types of movement. Buccofacial apraxia is common in patients with nonfluent aphasias. In response to commands such as "Cough," or "Show me how you would blow out a match," the patient may demonstrate an inappropriate movement or simply repeat the command (i.e., utter "Cough, cough").

Tests for ideomotor limb apraxia should emphasize movements that depend on fine distal actions of the foot and hand. These are more vulnerable to apraxia, perhaps because they are more dependent on the integrity of the pyramidal tract. To test for ideomotor limb apraxia, the patient can be asked to pantomime the use of common implements such as a toothbrush, comb, and scissors (e.g., "Show me how you would hold a comb and comb your hair"). In addition to a total inability to perform the movement, apraxic errors also include groping movements while trying to correctly position the hand, executing a movement in the wrong plane (e.g., sawing motion in a vertical orientation), and the substitution of a body part for the object (e.g., extending the index and middle fingers to represent the blades of a scissors) rather than positioning the hand in a way that is compatible with holding the imaginary implement. This last error type is a developmentally normal response for young children but its occurrence in adult patients may imply defective access to motor programs.[59]

Ideomotor apraxia can be seen bilaterally or, in the case of a right hemiplegia, in the nonhemiplegic left arm (also referred to as "sympathetic dyspraxia"). A prerequisite for diagnosing an apraxia is to confirm that the command was understood by having the patient choose the correct movement from among several performed by the examiner. In the patient with a generalized disturbance of comprehension, it is impossible to diagnose ideomotor apraxia. Whole body commands such as "Take the stance of a boxer" and axial commands directed at eye opening, sitting, and standing may be performed normally by severely aphasic and otherwise apraxic patients, suggesting that these movements may be mediated by different pathways. The comprehension and execution of axial commands are preserved in Wernicke's aphasia and these, therefore, should not be used to assess language comprehension. The ability to execute symbolic and conventional gestures may be dissociated from other types of movements and can be tested with such commands as "Salute" and "Wave good-bye."

Calculations, right–left orientation, finger identification. Lesions of the left inferior parietal lobule can interfere with calculation, right–left orientation, and finger identification. These functions can be impaired independently but when all are affected and are accompanied by dysgraphia, this symptom constellation is known as the Gerstmann syndrome (Chapter 1).

Knowledge of table values, execution of basic operations (i.e., adding, subtracting, "borrowing" or "carrying"), and numerical facts are some of the component processes for calculation, each of which can be selectively disrupted by brain damage.[190] Impairment of one or more of these components constitutes acalculia (or anarithmetria). Paper-and-pencil arithmetic examples can be used at bedside to test the fundamental operations of addition, subtraction, multiplication, and division. The supplementary section of the *BDAE* contains a more formal test with limited norms.[60] The *Arithmetic subtest* of the WRAT-3 has more challenging problems suitable for a range of mathematical abilities and provides norms for ages 5 to 75 years.[208] The *Arithmetic subtest* of the *Wechsler Adult Intelligence Scale–III (WAIS-III)* contains mathematical word problems presented orally for mental calculation with time constraints on oral responses.[194] None of these tests, however, distinguishes among types of calculation deficits which must be accomplished instead with experimental batteries.[43]

Performance on calculation tests can be impeded by several factors. Poor concentration interferes with mental calculation and can also result in careless errors in written calculation (e.g., failure to notice the sign). Aphasia and alexia may interfere with number reading and writing.[13] Hemispatial neglect interferes with perception of digits in the leftmost position or the proper alignment of numbers while calculating. Frontal lesions that interfere with the sequencing of activity may also disrupt calculation skill. Primary acalculia (anarithmetria) should not be diagnosed if calculation failure is secondary to any of these factors.

Consistent inability to differentiate "right" from "left" can represent an aphasic disturbance (i.e., incorrect labeling or understanding of the words "right" and "left") or a true disturbance of egocentric spatial orientation. Formal tests are available for assessing verbally mediated right–left discrimination.[16,60] The patient is asked to indicate and label right and left on his or her own body and on the examiner's. Complexity is increased with commands such as "Put your left hand on your right eye" or "Point with your left hand to my right ear." Even though these tests are used to assess "right–left disorientation," they really demonstrate that the patient has a specific *verbal labeling* disorder for right and left. To demonstrate deficits that represent spatial disorientation, the test of Culver can be used, in which the patient must decide the laterality of drawings of right and left limbs in various postures.[36] In normal young individuals, an average of 17 of the 20 items are correctly identified and for older groups the average score is about 15.[174] At the bedside, the patient can be asked to touch locations on his own limbs corresponding to those indicated on the examiner's body, without the use of words. Patients with the right–left naming disturbances of the Gerstmann syndrome are not impaired in their route-finding ability, suggesting that this is a lexical deficit rather than a manifestation of spatial disorientation. Right–left "disorientation" of the type seen in the Gerstmann syndrome is diagnosed only if it occurs either in the absence of aphasia or if its severity is out of proportion to the aphasia.

The testing of finger identification is important because of its association with the Gerstmann syndrome. The supplementary section of the *BDAE* includes several tests of finger naming, finger name comprehension, and visual finger matching.[60]

At the bedside, the examiner can ask the patient to match his own fingers to those demonstrated on an outline of a hand drawn on a piece of paper. As in the case of right–left orientation, a specific finger-identification disturbance is diagnosed only if it occurs in the absence of aphasia or when it is out of proportion to it.

PARALINGUISTIC ASPECTS OF COMMUNICATION

The formal linguistic components of communication outlined above are enhanced and modified by facial expressions, gestures, body posture, speech prosody, and other "paralinguistic" signals. The bedside examination of affective and attitudinal prosody, facial expressions, and gestures is described in detail in Chapter 6. Prosody can be tested informally by asking the patient to utter a simple declarative sentence (e.g., "Steve drives a *car*") with a particular affect (e.g., as though feeling anger or sadness) or emphasis (e.g., "Steve drives a *car*"). The examiner could also test comprehension of affect by asking the patient to identify the emotional tone of a sentence spoken with angry or happy intonation. The perception of facial affect can be tested by asking the patient to identify demonstrated expressions of affect or, in more objective detail, to match them with the Ekman and Friesen[46] photographs of actors depicting different emotions or attitudes. Patients with right-sided cerebral lesions may have specific deficits in the comprehension and production of both affective and emphatic prosody and with the nonverbal identification of facial affect.[76,186,202]

Right-sided cerebral lesions may also interfere with the ability to adjust interpersonal behavior to the social context. The *Profile of Nonverbal Sensitivity (PONS) Test* measures the ability to infer, from brief audio and video vignettes, the social setting for which certain tones of voice or body postures might be appropriate (e.g., returning an item to a store versus attending a wedding).[156] Benowitz and colleagues[12] demonstrated that patients with right cerebral lesions are deficient in this skill.

Impairments of turn-taking, switching speech styles to fit the audience, and maintaining appropriate interpersonal distance can also reflect a breakdown in the social uses of language. These features are apparent in the patient's interactions. In one case example, following a right temporal stroke, a 55-year-old man spoke in a pressured manner, using "legalese" instead of colloquial speech. When story recall was tested, he talked for 20 minutes, embellishing on the original story and punctuating his comments with terms such as "presumably" and "to whit." He also demonstrated problems with the discrimination of affective and nonaffective prosody. This patient was known to the examiner prior to his stroke and this speech style represented a dramatic change from his former interpersonal style and manner of speaking.

Although deficits in the paralinguistic features of communication are often subtle, they may have a profound impact on psychosocial adaptation, to the point that a patient who recovers from illness without motor, speech or memory deficits may be unable to return to work or sustain personal relationships.

Complex perceptual and spatial processes: visual and auditory
perception, constructions, dressing, spatial distribution of attention

Visual and auditory perception. Much of the cortical surface is devoted to the
transformation of sensory signals into complex percepts. The ability to discriminate
angles is one aspect of visual spatial perception that can be tested with *Judgment of
Line Orientation (JLO).*[16,20] In this test, the patient must select from a radial array of
lines those that match the angular orientation of two stimulus lines (Fig. 2–1, left).
Scores on this test are especially poor in patients with damage to right posterior
cerebral areas.[16] Performance of this task leads to activation within the right
temporoparieto-occipital region in control subjects.[71] Average *JLO* performance (25
of 30 items correct) is preserved until the age of 70 in well-educated individuals.
Over that age, 11% of subjects obtain lower scores.[18] This test is relatively free of
verbal mediation but is influenced by the level of education, and women may score,
on average, a few points lower than men.[16] If impulsiveness interferes with the
reliability of the patient's responses, the examiner can instead draw two oblique
lines side by side and ask if their slope is the same or different. A similar test with
even greater specificity for right hemisphere damage can be given in the somatosensory modality by having the blindfolded patient adjust two hinged rods to duplicate the angle of test rods examined by palpation.[115]

The mental synthesis of fragmented perceptual input can be measured with the
30 items on the *Hooper Visual Organization Test* (Fig. 2–1, right).[78] Young adults
obtain an average score of 25. In individuals over the age of 65 a score of 22 ($\pm$ 4)
may be considered normal.[124] Education may influence performance on this test.[174]
Sources of error on this test that *do not* imply primary deficits of perceptual synthesis include aphasia (failure to name the objects despite preserved recognition),
impulsivity (reaching premature conclusions based on a single fragment—see Fig.
2–1), and elementary visual deficits that interfere with information input.

Another test of complex visual perceptual processing is based on Warrington's[191]
observation that patients with right parietal lesions had difficulty identifying objects
photographed from an unusual perspective (see Fig. 2–2 for an example). Figure–
ground and contour discrimination were normal in these patients, suggesting that
the observed deficit represents a failure at the level of high-order perceptual analysis. The *Visual Object and Space Perception Battery*[189] and the *Visual Closure subtest*
of the *Woodcock-Johnson Tests of Cognitive Ability*[213] provide objective measures of
visual perception based on incomplete or transformed visual information. The *Gollin Incomplete Figures* are series of line drawings of common objects in which the
first item in the series has had most of the lines eradicated.[58] Subsequent drawings
of the same object provide increasingly more visual information, ending in full
exposure of the object. Patients who cannot generate a mental template of the object
on the basis of partial information may not be able to identify the object until it is
fully exposed. This test has also been used to assess implicit memory processes, as
described in Chapter 4.

A very specific type of form perception can be tested with *Facial Recognition*,
which requires the ability to *match* (rather than recognize) photographs of unfa-

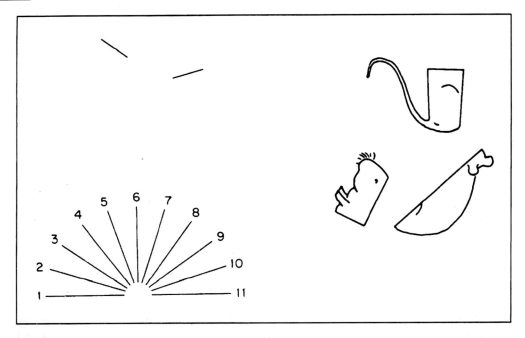

FIGURE 2–1. Left: Item from the *Judgment of Line Orientation Test*.[16, 20] The task is to choose from the 11 lines in the array (bottom) the two that match the orientation and direction of the stimulus lines at the top. (From *Contributions to Neuropsychological Assessment: Tests 5. Judgment of Line Orientation (Complete Test)* by Arthur L. Benton et al. Copyright. Used by permission of Oxford University Press, Inc.).

Right: Item from the *Hooper Visual Organization Test*. [78] The task is to identify the object, a mouse or rat, by mentally assembling the fragments. Responses such as "pipe" or "watering can" frequently occur when a premature conclusion is reached based on the top segment only. (Material from the *Hooper Visual Organization Test* copyright © 1957 by H. Elston Hooper. Reprinted by permission of the publisher, Western Psychological Services, 12031 Wilshire Boulevard, Los Angeles, California 90025, U.S.A. Not to be reprinted in whole or in part for any additional purpose without the expressed, written permission of the publisher. All rights reserved.)

miliar faces.[19] The first six items require an exact match. On subsequent items, a stimulus face must be matched to three nonidentical photographs of the same person taken from different angles and with different levels of shading (Fig. 2–3). The choices become more difficult as increasingly complex alterations of facial orientation and shading are introduced. The lesion for prosopagnosia, a defect of *face recognition*, is farther downstream from the anatomical areas necessary for perceptual discrimination of faces and so patients with prosopagnosia may perform normally on this test. As is true of other multiple choice tests, *Facial Recognition* may be failed by impulsive patients.

Nonverbal auditory perception is not routinely tested but can be impaired after damage to the auditory association areas. Such lesions may interfere with timbre and pitch discrimination and with memory for tonal patterns[120], functions that can

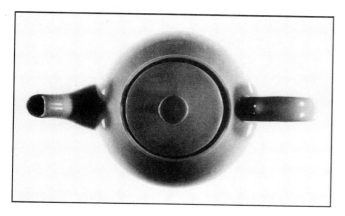

FIGURE 2–2. A teapot viewed from an unusual perspective. Correct identification probably requires mental rotation into a more familiar vantage point. Patients with right hemisphere dysfunction find this task difficult.

be measured with the *Seashore Tests* of musical talent.[150,166] Patients with left- or right-sided temporal lobe dysfunction may have difficulties with these tests.[23] The *Sound Patterns subtest* of the *Woodcock-Johnson Tests of Cognitive Ability* tests tonal pattern discrimination.[213] The ability to identify sounds characteristically associated with common objects can be impaired after right hemisphere damage and is referred to as "auditory agnosia."[172,173] At bedside the examiner can create sounds for the blindfolded patient by shaking a ring of keys, strumming the teeth of a comb, crumpling paper, or slamming a door. The patient can then be asked to open the eyes and point to the object that generated the sound from among a set of choices.

For the anatomic reasons listed in Chapter 1, unilateral lesions in auditory association cortex can escape clinical detection. The dichotic listening method may disclose such lesions. In one form of this task, two sets of three-digit numbers are simultaneously presented, one to each ear. Even normal subjects may fail to report all six digits: right-handed individuals are more accurate in digit perception in the right ear (approximately 3% to 10% higher scores than for the left ear).[92] This relative suppression of left-ear input probably reflects the dominance of the left hemisphere for speech perception. After left hemisphere lesions, dichotic listening shows a reduction in the right ear advantage while after right-sided lesions the left ear may be further suppressed.[93]

Constructional tasks. Constructional abilities entail complex perceptual, motor, and executive functions required by such tasks as drawing, assembling puzzles, and constructing designs from blocks or sticks. Because of the complexity of these tasks, damage to either hemisphere and to different regions within a hemisphere can produce constructional deficits. Paterson and Zangwill[133] noted *qualitative* differences in drawing deficits as a function of lesion side. Patients with right hemisphere lesions employed a disorganized and "piecemeal" approach which over-

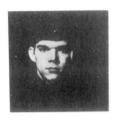

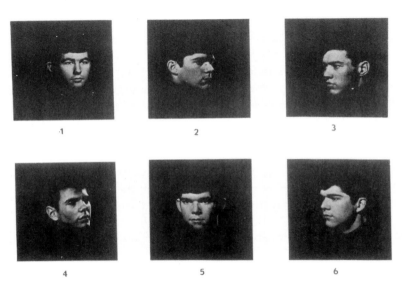

FIGURE 2–3. An item from the *Facial Recognition* test.[16,19] The task is to select from the six choices (bottom) three photographs of the individual depicted at the top. This task requires discrimination of the essential facial features and the ability to recognize them through various displacements of orientation and shading. (From *Contributions to Neuropsychological Assessment: Tests 4. Judgment of Line Orientation (Complete Test)* by Arthur L. Benton et al. Copyright. Used by permission of Oxford University Press, Inc.)

looked the "large picture" while those with left hemisphere lesions had more difficulty with internal details, omitting or misplacing them. On the *Block Design* subtest of the *WAIS*,[192] Kaplan and colleagues[89] noted similar qualitative differences in the performance of patients with right- or left-sided lesions. This study and studies of left- and right-hand performance of commissurotomized patients suggest that the right hemisphere contribution to this task lies in the maintenance of the overall configuration while that of the left lies in the processing of internal detail.[55]

These qualitative differences are not apparent from objective test scores alone, which may be similar after right or left cerebral damage. The *WAIS-R as a Neuro-psychological Instrument (WAIS-R NI)*[87] quantifies these qualitative distinctions and also contains controlled strategies for probing the nature of task failure, according to Kaplan's "Process Approach" to neuropsychological evaluation.[86] Severe deficits in three-dimensional block construction are much more common in patients with right hemisphere damage.[16]

The copy condition of the *Rey-Osterrieth Complex Figure* test[152] is a difficult test of constructions that is especially vulnerable to right hemisphere damage.[174] Patients with such lesions show a characteristic piecemeal copying strategy and tend to distort the overall contour of the figure (Fig. 2–4). Recently, stringent scoring criteria have been adapted for this test with normative data up to 89 years of age.[118]

At the bedside, constructional ability can be tested by asking the patient to copy simple figures (cube, daisy, house, clock). Problems with spatial planning can be demonstrated by having the patient fill in the numbers to create the face of a clock in a large circle provided by the examiner. In left-sided hemispatial neglect, all the numbers may be omitted from the left side of the clock (Fig. 3–3, Chapter 3). However, this performance can also represent a more general problem of poor planning, as evident in the example in Figure 2–5, taken from a patient with dementia and no neglect. Age and education both influence drawing ability. Goodglass and Kaplan[60] provide normative values for adults up to the age of 85 on tests of spontaneous drawing and copying of six simple objects, including a clock and a three-dimensional cube. Qualitative analysis of clock drawings has been carried out in a normative sample, 20 to 90 years of age, in patients with dementia and patients with focal cerebrovascular lesions.[52] Such factors as the placement of the hands, alignment of numbers, and the external contour were found to vary in patients as

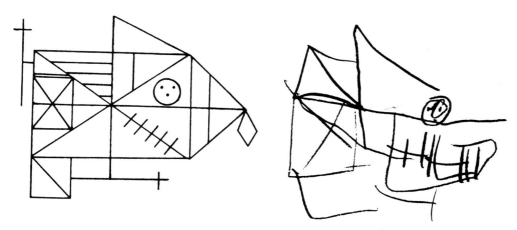

FIGURE 2–4. Left: The Rey-Osterrieth Complex figure.[151,152] Right: Copy of the figure by a 23-year-old man with a lifelong history of social emotional learning disability and a normal verbal IQ. Slowness and clumsiness of the left limbs during his performance of motor tasks suggested early damage to the right hemisphere of the brain.

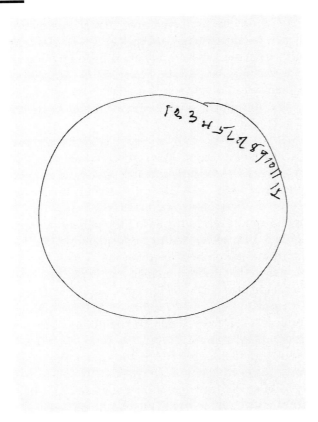

FIGURE 2–5. The clock drawing of an 85-year-old right-handed man with dementia and no evidence of spatial neglect on cancellation tests or on bilateral simultaneous stimulation. Poor planning, and not hemispatial neglect, is reflected in the irregular spacing of numbers within the circle. If the task had instead required a counterclockwise sequence, one might predict that the right side of the drawing would be empty.

a function of their diagnostic category and their age, illustrating the fact that numerous factors can interfere with clock drawing.

Dressing. Impairment of the ability to dress oneself, so-called "dressing apraxia," can occur with posterior parietal lesions, especially those involving the right hemisphere. A deficit exclusively for dressing the left side of the body could be a manifestation of hemispatial neglect. A more generalized dressing deficit has to do with the inability to align the axis of a garment with the body axis. At bedside, the patient can be handed a shirt or blouse that has been turned upside down, with one sleeve inside out. Errors attributable to dressing apraxia include inability to reorient the garment, to align it correctly to the body axis, and to properly introduce the arms into the sleeves (Chapter 7). A different type of dressing difficulty may emerge in patients who cannot execute a complex sequence of activities, as in confusional states. However, these patients can usually manage one piece of clothing at a time whereas patients with dressing apraxia cannot.

Spatial distribution of attention. In an earlier section of this chapter, the testing of the attentional *matrix* is described (Wakefulness/Arousal, Span, Working Memory, and the Attentional Matrix). This section deals with the testing of a *vector* aspect of attention, namely, its direction within the extrapersonal space. A dramatic impairment of this aspect of attention takes the form of left-sided hemispatial neglect and is seen after damage to any component of a neural network involving the dorsal visuofugal stream of processing in the right cerebral hemisphere (Chapter 3).

Contralesional extinction during bilateral simultaneous stimulation in the somatosensory, auditory, or visual modalities is considered evidence of sensory neglect, especially if it occurs in more than one sensory modality (reviewed in Chapter 3). Manifestations of neglect may also emerge as failure to read the left half of a sentence (hemialexia), creation of a wide margin on the left while writing, bisection of a horizontal line to the right of true center, and failure to copy the left side of figures or to place numbers on the left side of a clock face.

The extent and organization of manual exploration can be used to assess exploratory-motor aspects of neglect. The patient can be blindfolded, seated at a table and asked to "search" by palpation for a small object placed in different locations on the table surface. Patients with right hemisphere lesions and left-hemispatial neglect are less efficient and slower in locating the target on the left side using either hand whereas exploration is more systematic and rapid in the right side of space (Chapter 3).[200]

A variety of visual target cancellation tasks are available to objectively assess the exploratory-motor aspects of hemispatial neglect.[1,54,199,201,210] In one such task sensitive to hemispatial neglect, there are four forms consisting of structured and unstructured arrays of verbal and nonverbal stimuli, with target locations controlled in all forms (Fig. 2–6).[199] After being shown a sample of the target on a separate sheet of paper, patients must circle all the targets without moving the paper to the left or right. Exchanging the color of the pencil after every 10 targets circled allows the examiner to reconstruct the search path. Normal adults under the age of 65 can complete each of the four test conditions within 2 minutes without errors. Older patients can be allowed up to 3 minutes. On the random shape cancellation task, individuals over 65 may omit one or two in each field. Normal adults conduct a systematic search beginning on the left and proceeding to the right in horizontal or vertical rows even in the random arrays.[201]

Right-sided lesions result in a tendency to start on the right side of the page, to proceed in a disorganized manner, and to omit many targets from the left side of the page.[201] Overall, shape detection is less accurate than letter detection and more targets are omitted in the unstructured form (Chapter 3). Patients with left-sided lesions use the strategy employed by control subjects, may detect geometric shapes more quickly and accurately than letters, and do not omit more than a few targets from the right beyond the acute phase of stroke. Table 2–3 shows omission scores in various clinical groups.

In patients with subtle or resolving neglect, these cancellation tests can detect hemispatial inattention even when other similar tasks (such as the cancellation of lines) are performed well (Fig. 2–7). Abulic patients sometimes can fail to explore

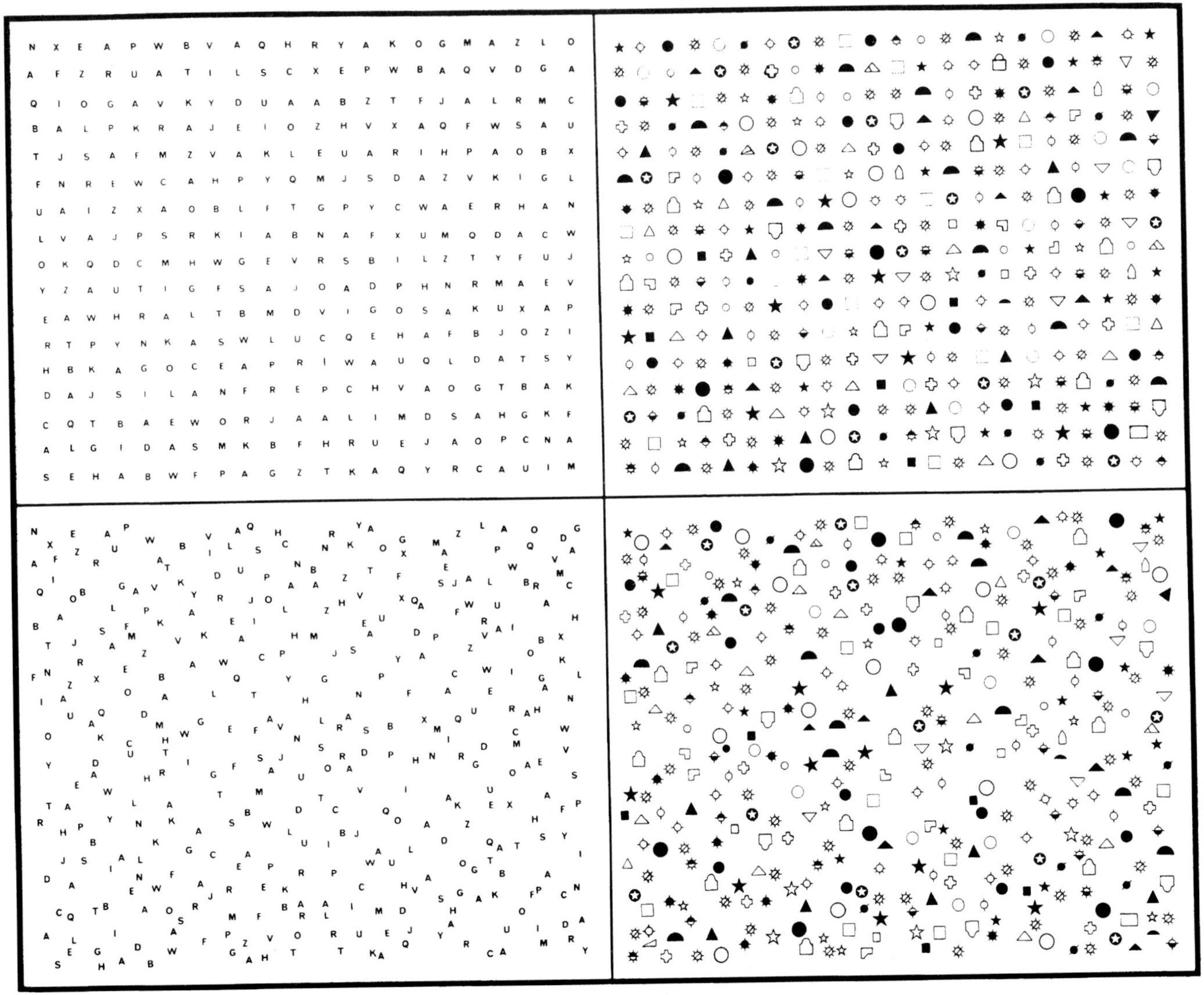

FIGURE 2–6. Four conditions of the target cancellation task[199]— two containing letters (target is "A") and two containing geometric forms (target is the circle with 8 external radii and an oblique diameter). In each condition, the targets are in identical locations and in mirror positions from left to right and top to bottom. The distractors are arranged in regular rows around the targets in the "structured" arrays and in irregular locations around the targets in the "unstructured" arrays. The patient is shown an example of the target on a separate piece of paper and asked to circle all the similar targets on the test forms. Pencils of different colors are exchanged after every ten targets circled to determine the origin (left versus right) and trajectory of the exploratory path (systematic versus unsystematic).

TABLE 2–3 Average Number of Target Omissions (with *Standard Deviations*) per Hemispace in Several Subject Groups on Visual Cancellation Tasks.†

	FORM							
	UNSTRUCTURED SHAPES		UNSTRUCTURED LETTERS		STRUCTURED SHAPES		STRUCTURED LETTERS	
	Left	*Right*	*Left*	*Right*	*Left*	*Right*	*Left*	*Right*
Right lesions	17.12	8.00	16.50	7.13	18.75	9.25	13.13	3.62
(N=8)	*9.98*	*6.53*	*13.66*	*7.38*	*11.99*	*8.94*	*12.78*	*3.93*
Left lesions	1.25	2.38	0.50	2.88	0.25	3.00	0.62	1.38
(N=8)	*1.75*	*2.72*	*0.54*	*5.40*	*0.45*	*5.11*	*1.41*	*2.32*
Controls <65	0.56	0.33	0.89	0.78	1.11	0.78	0.44	0.56
years	*0.68*	*0.68*	*1.10*	*0.79*	*0.99*	*0.91*	*0.51*	*0.68*
(N=9)								
Controls >65	0.29	0.33						
years	*0.72*	*0.80*						
(N=21)								
PRAD†	2.25	1.38						
(N = 29)	*3.13*	*1.75*						

†Patients with focal lesions were given as much time as they needed to complete these tasks. Control subjects under 65 years of age were given 2 minutes. Probable Alzheimer's disease (PRAD) patients and controls over the age of 65 (mean age=72) were allowed 3 minutes in which to complete the unstructured shape cancellation task.

a certain portion of the stimulus array, but this can be demonstrated to be a "pseudoneglect" since the "neglected" sector will shift from administration to administration.

EXPLICIT LEARNING AND RETROGRADE MEMORY

Memory loss is never global. Retrograde amnesia (loss of memory for remote events) can be dissociated from anterograde amnesia (deficit for learning new material); some amnesias may be modality- or material-specific; others may differentially affect registration or retrieval processes. Even in the most severe amnestic states, perceptual, habit, and skill learning, collectively referred to as "implicit" memory, may remain relatively intact (Chapter 4). The examination of explicit memory should survey orientation, awareness of current news, recall of past events, and the ability to learn and retain new verbal and nonverbal information in the auditory and visual modalities. In testing for amnesia, the challenge is to differentiate memory deficits that are primary (i.e., caused by limbic lesions) from those that are secondary to some other factor (i.e., inattentiveness, abulia, anomia).

Retrograde memory. Identification of famous personalities,[3] knowledge of public events,[167] recall of popular television programs,[175] and access to autobiographical information[98,99] have been used experimentally to test retrograde memory. The *Transient News Events Test* of O'Connor and colleagues is based on news items with

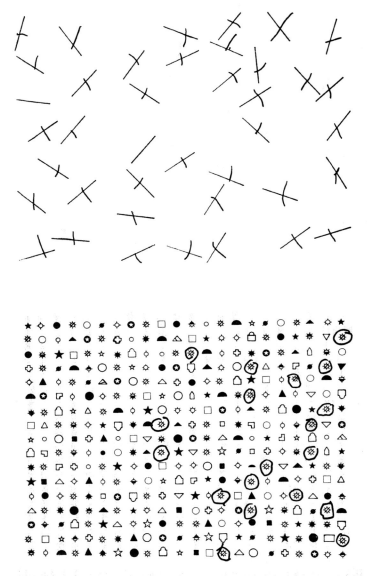

FIGURE 2–7. Top: The line-crossing test taken from a 66-year-old woman with a right frontal lesion. One line on the extreme left and another to the left of center are left uncrossed. Bottom: Performance of the same patient on the structured shape cancellation task, showing marked avoidance of the left side of the page. These examples illustrate that stimulus variables, such as target complexity and density, can influence the severity of the observed deficit.

time-limited exposure that have come to peak public attention during the past several decades, making it possible to estimate the approximate date at which these memories might have been stored.[130] All of these methods rely on the assumption that the information being tested was, in fact, acquired by the patient in the past and require corroboration from a reliable informant. The retrograde memory loss of the amnestic syndrome is characterized by a gradient whereby events that occurred closer in time to the onset of the amnesia are recalled least well (Ribot's Law), presumably due to their less extensive consolidation (Chapters 1 and 4).[3,167] In patients with dementia of the Alzheimer's type, recall of past events is disturbed without a time gradient in a more patchy fashion that worsens as the disease progresses.[2,211]

Anterograde memory. The acquisition (learning), retention, and recall (retrieval) of verbal and nonverbal material are key elements in the assessment of anterograde memory. The classic pattern of anterograde amnesia consists of normal immediate recall (due to preserved attention span, or working memory) and impaired delayed recall. Thus, the examiner should assure that a criterion level of immediate recall has been reached (e.g., 50%–75% of the information) before moving on to testing delayed recall.

A standardized battery, the *Wechsler Memory Scale–III (WMS-III)*, includes subtests that address attention, orientation, immediate verbal and nonverbal recall (including pictorial and spatial memory), learning efficiency, delayed recall, and recognition.[195] Individual subtest scores yield a profile of relative strengths and weaknesses and can be combined into composite indices that can also be compared with one another (e.g., immediate auditory memory index versus immediate visual memory index versus delayed general recall index, and so on). This test provides age-relevant norms.

Word lists are commonly used to assess memory functions. The words are presented over several learning trials and an increase in the number of words recalled on each successive trial is taken as a measure of learning. Amnestic patients with deficits at the point of learning, or encoding, show a "flat" learning curve whereby the number of words recalled does not increase from trial to trial. The *Rey Auditory Verbal Learning Test (RAVLT)*[152] and the *California Verbal Learning Test (CVLT)*[41] (presenting 15 unrelated or 16 categorically related words, respectively, over five trials) are among the most difficult of these tests and are most suitable for well-educated individuals with mild deficits. On both these tests, a second word list is introduced (single presentation only) after the fifth learning trial of list 1. Then recall for both lists is tested and the effects of proactive and retroactive interference are measured by the patient's contamination of one list by inclusion of items from the other. Normative data are available for both tests.[174] On the RAVLT, for example, young adults learn an average of 12 words on list 1 by the fifth trial while those over age 70 learn an average of eight or nine. After a delay of 20–30 minutes, younger individuals can recall an average of 11 words and those over 70, an average of six. Recognition of the words can be tested separately.

Shorter word lists (from ten to 12 items), better suited for patients with dementia or those with reduced attention spans, are provided on the battery from the *Consortium to Establish a Registry for Alzheimer's Disease (CERAD)*,[127] the *Repeatable Battery for the Assessment of Neuropsychological Status (RBANS)*,[138,139] the *Alzheimer's Disease Assessment Scale (ADAS)*,[155] and the *Hopkins Verbal Learning Test–Revised (HVLT-R)*.[11] The *Selective Reminding Procedure* [28,85] may present more of a challenge for patients with very mild deficits or high levels of premorbid ability. In one version of this test, a word list is presented over 12 trials or until it is correctly recalled on three consecutive trials. [72] The entire list is presented only on the first trial. On subsequent trials only those words not recalled on the immediately preceding trial are presented. Words recalled on two consecutive trials without "reminding" are presumed to be in long-term storage. Words recalled only after reminding are assumed to be retrieved via short-term, immediate recall. Recognition is also tested. Several variations of this test have been created.[174] Amnestic patients are impaired in the encoding of new information, as shown by their ability to recall only the words of which they are "reminded" during the immediately preceding trial.

Story recall, typically tested after only a single presentation, is another popular measure of learning and retention. The *Logical Memory subtest* of the *WMS-III*[195] presents two stories, each with 25 bits of information, for immediate and 30-minute-delayed recall. The second story is also presented a second time to assess the contribution of attentional deficits to recall. Although immediate recall may be reduced in the inattentive patient, there should be relatively little loss of information over time in the absence of a primary amnesia. The average percent retention on *Logical Memory* between the immediate and delayed recall conditions is approximately 80% for 30-year-olds, 75% for 65-year-olds, and 65% for 80-year-olds. The story from the *RBANS*[138] has only 12 elements and is appropriate for patients with limited education or those with moderate to severe mental-state compromise. This story is simple enough that individuals in their 70s can recall most of it even after a delay.

Nonverbal retrieval can be tested by the ability to reproduce geometric designs from memory. The *Visual Reproduction* subtest of the *WMS-III* contains relatively simple designs that are exposed briefly for immediate and delayed reproduction.[195] The recall component of the *Rey-Osterrieth Complex Figure* test[152] is more difficult and is vulnerable to deficits in planning and organization. One factor that reduces the impact of attentional deficits on performance is that the figure is first copied, rather than just examined. The test is scored on a 36-point scale and well-educated individuals over 70 obtain from 20 to 30 scorable elements for copying and 15–18 scorable elements on recall after a delay of up to 30 minutes.[102,174]

Pictorial memory can also be tested with a new subtest on the *WMS-III, Family Pictures*, in which a family is depicted in several scenes performing routine activities. Immediately after viewing each scene, the patient is asked to describe it and to point to the remembered locations of the characters on a blank page.[195] Recall is again tested 30 minutes later. Scoring provides separate measures of object and spatial memory.

Giving a patient three words and testing recall in 5–10 minutes is probably the single most common bedside test of memory used by the non-neuropsychologist. A more systematic variation of this test is the *Drilled Word Span* procedure, which uses a list of words equal to the patient's forward digit span minus one. This tailors the test to the patient's level of attention. The unrelated words are presented aloud by the examiner and the patient must immediately repeat them. This procedure is repeated until the patient repeats the list correctly three consecutive times (criterion). List size can be further decreased for the severely inattentive patient until criterion is reached. Sixty seconds after learning the list, during which the time the patient is instructed to remain silent, recall is tested. If the list is not recalled in its entirety at that point, this may signify that the patient is internally distracted or lacks initiative, and the list is presented again until criterion is reached. Recall is then tested after another interval of 60 seconds, during which the patient is distracted with a serial 3s task. Finally, it is tested after an interval of 3 minutes that is also filled with distracting activities. If the list is not recalled in its entirety after 60 seconds or 3 minutes, recognition from a list that includes test items and distracters can be tested.

The number of times the list needs to be presented to reach criterion (for immediate recall and also after the 60-second silent interval) is a measure of problems in attention. The effect of distraction is determined by comparing the number of words recalled following the silent and the distracted 60-second recall trials. Attentive amnestic patients can rehearse and thus retain information over a time interval if not distracted but lose the information once distracted, indicating an impairment of stable encoding. The rate of forgetting over time can be measured by comparing the number of words recalled after the two intervals with distraction, 60 seconds and 3 minutes. Table 2–4 contrasts the performance of a patient with a diagnosis of probable Alzheimer's disease, who reaches criterion in three trials but cannot retain information over time, with that of a patient in an acute confusional state, who can retain information despite initial registration problems.

Three Words–Three Shapes also provides a simple, flexible bedside technique for testing stages of learning and recall of verbal and nonverbal material.[199] The patient is first asked to copy the six stimuli. The paper is then removed and the patient is immediately asked to reproduce all six stimuli on a blank page. This step assesses incidental recall and working memory processes. If five or all six stimuli are reproduced correctly at that point, delayed recall is tested in 5, 15, and 30 minutes. If fewer than five items are recalled, the stimuli are reexposed for a 30-second study interval, following which immediate recall is again tested (study–recall trial). Study–recall trials are repeated until criterion is reached (at least five of the six items) or a maximum of five such trials have occurred, following which delayed recall is tested as above. Multiple choice recognition is tested after the 30-minute delay if spontaneous recall is faulty at that point.

This technique offers several advantages. First, verbal and nonverbal memory, usually tested in different modalities, are tested within the same modality. Secondly, incidental memory, the basis for recalling much of daily experience, is differentiated from volitional, rote memory. We recently demonstrated that incidental recall is impaired in patients with Alzheimer's disease but not in age-matched,

TABLE 2–4 Drilled Word Span Procedure*

A

STIMULUS LIST		MULTIPLE CHOICE FOILS	
Apple	Bench	Cheese	Garden
Shoe	Flower	Apron	Desk
Horse	Star	Tiger	Diamond
Truck	Paper	House	Park

B

	LEARNING TRIALS					DELAYED RECALL†			MULTIPLE CHOICE	
	1	2	3	4	5	60″S	60″D	3′D	Correct	False Positive
Patient 1										
Apple	+	+	+	+	+	+	+	+	+	None
Shoe	−	−	+	+	+	+	+	+	+	—
Horse	−	−	+	+	+	+	+	+	+	—
Truck	+	+	+	+	+	+	+	+	+	—
Patient 2										
Apple	+	+	+			+	+	+	+	Cheese
Shoe	+	+	+			+	−	+	+	Apron
Horse	+	+	+			+	+	−	−	—
Truck	+	+	+			+	+	−	+	—

*A. Stimulus List (select number of items equal to digit span minus one) and Multiple Choice Foils for Drilled Word Span Procedure (select number of items equal to word span and deliver intermixed with stimulus items). B. Performance in two patients with digit spans of five (word span=4). Patient 1, a 67-year-old man in an acute confusional state, required five initial learning trials to reach criterion but performance on all measures of delayed recall was intact. Patient 2, a 56-year-old woman with probable Alzheimer's disease, reached criterion in only three trials and retrieved all the words after the 60-seconds silent interval. Recall further diminished after 60 seconds (distracted) and 3 minutes and recognition was also impaired, including 2 false-positive identifications.

†S = Silent; D = Distracted; + = correct; − = incorrect.

nondemented subjects.[202a] Drilling to criterion helps to overcome attentional deficits and also to equalize the amount of encoded information for which recall is being tested across patients with different initial learning capacity. Several measures can be derived: incidental recall, number of study–recall trials to reach criterion (learning efficiency), delayed recall, and recognition. Normal young adults under 65 typically have full recall even in the incidental condition. Over the age of 65, one or two study exposures beyond initial copying may be required to reach criterion, and retention of four of the six items after 30 minutes is average. Patients with Alzheimer's dementia or Korsakoff's amnesia lose information even after 5 minutes and this is most marked for words. The test can be scored informally or formally by a method that allots points for accuracy.[202a] The test is easily adapted to different languages by pairing the shapes with words from the patient's native language. In addition, the difficulty level can be adjusted by increasing or decreasing the number of stimulus items used. Figures 2–8 and 2–9 illustrate examples of performance in two patients with different diagnoses.

Some tests of memory are based entirely on a recognition procedure. These are helpful in testing patients with language or constructional deficits. The *Recognition Memory Test* tests forced choice recognition of unfamiliar faces and of single words.[188] The 50 stimuli on each subtest are initially exposed without alerting the patient to the nature of the test; instead the patient is asked to rate each as "pleasant or unpleasant." The patient is then presented with pairs of items, one of which is the previously presented stimulus, and asked to choose the familiar one. A similar subtest with both short-term and delayed recognition is included in the *WMS-III*.[195] It is advisable to test both recall and recognition in order to differentiate among the varieties of memory disorders. For example, frontal lesions may disrupt recall but not recognition, whereas medial temporal lobe lesions may affect both.

The level of difficulty of a memory test is determined not only by the amount of information to be learned or its complexity but also by the way in which retention is tested. *Spontaneous* recall of information, especially of stories, is most difficult. *Cued* recall is less difficult. Thus, if a patient cannot spontaneously remember information, a cue (e.g., the category or first letter of the word) is provided to see if

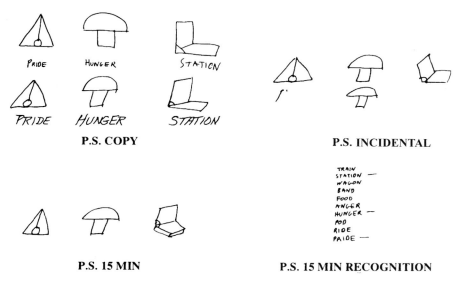

FIGURE 2–8. *Three Words–Three Shapes Test* in a 65-year-old man with a left frontal infarction. The patient copied the stimuli beneath the examiner's model (upper left). On incidental recall, the shapes were reproduced (with perseveration) but not the words (upper right). Despite repeated study-recall trials (not shown) the patient could not reproduce the words. The nonverbal stimuli were retained after a 15-minute delay (lower left). Despite a failure to spontaneously reproduce the words, he correctly recognized them by multiple choice from a list provided by the examiner (lower right). The conclusions from this performance would be that nonverbal memory is intact and that there is a retrieval deficit for verbal information.

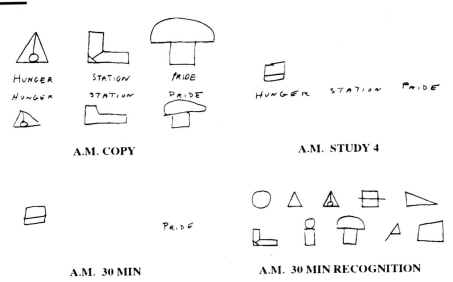

FIGURE 2–9. The *Three Words–Three Shapes Test* performance in a 72-year-old woman with dementia. The copy of the stimuli is adequate (upper left). She could reproduce none by incidental recall (not shown). She required four study–recall trials to reproduce the words and one design (upper right) but could learn none of the shapes even by the fifth study–recall trial (not shown). After a 30-minute delay, she recalled one word and her own design (lower left). Given a multiple choice, she recognized the words but none of the designs (lower right). This patient's performance illustrates a severe impairment of incidental memory, inability to store nonverbal information, and the temporal decay of verbal retrieval. Overall, nonverbal memory is worse than verbal memory since she was able to recognize the words but not the designs.

it can trigger recall. *Recognition* of the stimulus from among a set of choices is even easier. In the most severely impaired patient the examiner may have to resort to testing memory by hiding a few of the patient's personal belongings (e.g., wallet, watch, ring) around the examination room, making sure the patient can immediately locate them, and then asking for their retrieval after delays with and without distraction.

Nonexplicit memory. As described in Chapter 4, even the most severe amnestic state may still be compatible with relatively preserved ability to show priming and conditioning effects and to learn new motor skills. Motor (procedural) learning can be quantified with the use of the pursuit rotor. This electrical device consists of a rotating turntable with a metal contact on its surface. The task is to complete an electrical circuit between a hand-held stylus, and the revolving metal contact. The increase in the duration of time the contact is maintained from trial to trial is a measure of procedural learning. The amnestic patient HM was able to demonstrate learning on this task in the face of a severe explicit memory deficit.[32]

The *Gollin Incomplete Figures*, described earlier, can also be used to test priming effects in patients without primary visual perceptual deficits (see Fig. 4–3). Corkin[33] demonstrated that amnestic patients made fewer errors in stimulus identification upon a second presentation, implying that they had established perceptual learning despite the inability to consciously recall the task. Older nondemented individuals show a priming effect on this task, even 12 months after initial presentation, whereas those with the dementia of Alzheimer's disease show only short-term priming effects.[7]

REASONING/ABSTRACTION, COMPORTMENT, AND EXECUTIVE FUNCTIONS

Reasoning/abstraction. One of the most commonly used bedside tests of reasoning is *proverb interpretation*, which requires the formulation of a general principle from a concrete exemplar. Unfamiliar proverbs (e.g., "The good is the enemy of the best") are preferable, since the interpretation of common proverbs (e.g., "Strike while the iron is hot") may be overlearned. Another frequently used test is *Similarities*, which requires the abstraction of attributes common to superficially dissimilar objects and can be objectively measured on the *WAIS-III*.[194] When asked to compare two different objects (e.g., "How are a boat and a fish alike?"), elderly patients may tend to focus on physical attributes and state, "They are different." Restructuring the question (e.g., "What do a boat and a fish have in common?" or "Tell me one thing that is true about both a boat and a fish") may elicit more abstract responses. The disadvantages of both proverb interpretation and similarities tests is that they are influenced by education and cannot be used with aphasic patients.

The capacity for mental flexibility can be tested with object- and form-sorting tasks and matrix reasoning. A collection of objects or geometric forms can be subdivided into groups according to common function, color, shape, and constituent material.[42,57,197] Once an initial sort is made, the patient can be asked to regroup the stimuli in a different way. A more convenient test of mental flexibility at the bedside is represented in Figure 2–10, which illustrates an item similar to those on the *Visual-Verbal Test*.[48] The task is to divide the same set of items into two partially overlapping groups, wherein each group is defined by one common attribute. The ability to shift from one attribute to the second taps mental flexibility. Although aphasic patients may be unable to explain their groupings, they may display normal reasoning by being able to correctly point out the two groups. This test may therefore provide a probe for the dissociation of thought from language in aphasic patients.

The *Standard Progressive Matrices* is a standardized test of analogic reasoning

FIGURE 2–10. A method for testing reasoning similar to the items on the Visual-Verbal Test.[48] The patient is asked to select three of the four objects that share a single attribute (e.g., internal striped pattern). The patient is then asked to select a different group of three that share a different attribute, from among the same set of four objects (i.e., all forms with straight lines). Inability to shift to the second principle implies impaired mental flexibility.

that does not require verbal responses.[142] A children's version, the *Colored Matrices*, is appropriate for the more impaired or intellectually limited patient.[143] The test items consist of a 2×2 or 3×3 matrix with a missing element that must be selected from among six to eight choices. Early items are more dependent on visual pattern completion while later items emphasize numerical and spatial reasoning. This test is often considered a "test of nonverbal reasoning" but it undoubtedly engenders a great deal of internal verbal mediation. Figure 2–11 shows an example of a similar task.

The *Wisconsin Card Sorting Test (WCST)* requires abstraction, hypothesis testing, mental flexibility, and the ability to alter responses based on reinforcement.[65,75] Four stimulus cards, each with one of four geometric forms that differ in color and number, are aligned horizontally in front of the patient. Sixty-four test cards (or 128 in some versions) containing combinations of the three basic attributes (color, form, number) are presented one at a time. The task is to match each test card with one of the four stimulus cards (row 1, Fig. 2–12) on the basis of these attributes. The correct placement must be deduced from the examiner's feedback (i.e., "right" or

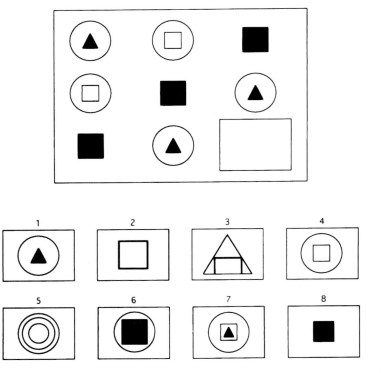

Figure 2–11. A matrix-type reasoning task. The patient must select, from the eight choices at the bottom, the design that best completes the logical matrix. In this instance, each row of the matrix contains the same elements but in a different sequence. The correct answer would be item 4. Patients with unilateral hemispatial neglect may fail to detect the choices on the left of the array. Patients who are impulsive may fail to examine all the possibilities prior to responding.

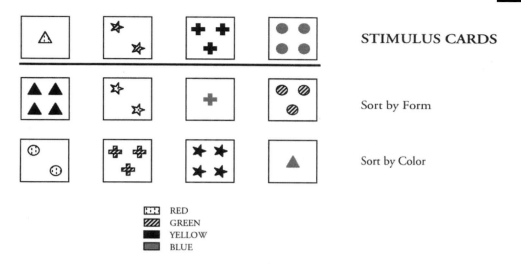

STIMULUS CARDS

Sort by Form

Sort by Color

RED
GREEN
YELLOW
BLUE

FIGURE 2–12. The four stimulus cards of the *Wisconsin Card Sorting Test* as seen from the patient's perspective (top row). The second row illustrates sorting by form and the third, by color. Illustrated with permission.

"wrong"). For example, if the reinforced category is form, the patient is expected to place cards that contain triangles (regardless of color or number) below the stimulus card with the triangle, cards that contain stars below the stimulus card with the stars, and so on (second row, Fig. 2–12). After a run of ten correct placements, the examiner switches the reinforced category without warning the patient. The patient must accordingly change the response strategy, again guided only by feedback. Patients with frontal lobe lesions achieve fewer categories and make more perseverative errors (i.e., continuing to sort by a category that is no longer being reinforced) than patients with lesions elsewhere in the brain.[121] In the 64-card version, adults should normally be able to switch categories at least four of the six possible times.[174] Conflicting results have been reported for the relative importance of the left and right frontal lobes in the performance of this task.[44,121] The *WCST* has been used extensively to study the deficits associated with schizophrenia and the functional specialization of the dorsolateral prefrontal cortex. Performance on the *WCST* is also sensitive to the attentional matrix of the patient and those who cannot inhibit immediate response tendencies do quite poorly.

Planning and sequencing. The ability to plan and sequence the individual components of complex, goal-directed activities is essential to normal mental functioning. Patients with frontal lobe damage and those in confusional states show deficits in this skill. One patient may fail to coordinate the individual steps of a recipe; another may have difficulty negotiating a busy intersection; still another patient may put on items of clothing in an inappropriate sequence. Patients with deficits in these areas may also have difficulty following instructions. The *Tower of London* is a puzzle that tests planning and sequencing skills.[169] The task is to move three

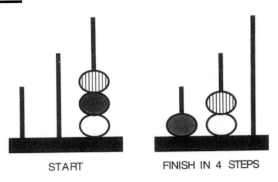

FIGURE 2–13. A schematic drawing similar to the *Tower of London* puzzle. The patient is given the apparatus as illustrated in the figure on the left and is shown a picture of the finished product on the right. The task is to move the beads (only one bead per step) among the pegs until they are in the same configuration depicted on the right, within four steps.

beads among three pegs to create the stimulus configuration in the least number of moves (see Fig. 2–13). Impulsive behavior may result in a trial-and-error approach and the failure to carry over strategies from the solution of one puzzle to the next. If this task is too difficult or lengthy, the examiner can also observe planning behavior while the patient performs the *Alternating Sequences Test* or draws a clock. *The Porteus Mazes* test the ability to plan a strategy for route-finding in a paper-and-pencil maze.[135] Taking the time to examine the maze prior to initiating a response (i.e., "Look before you leap") results in fewer errors and quicker response time. Liepmann's ideational apraxia may also be conceptualized as a deficit in the planning and sequencing of motor acts.

Comportment: judgment, insight, social appropriateness. The term "comportment" refers to complex mental processes that include insight, judgment, self-awareness, and social adaptation. There are no dependable objective measures of judgment. The patient's knowledge of solutions to everyday problems or emergencies (e.g., what to do if caught in a fire in a public building), measured by the *Comprehension subtest* of the WAIS-III,[194] does not necessarily predict the presence of good judgment in a real-life situation. Although an inadequate verbal response is likely to predict poor judgment, a correct response only reflects knowledge of the rules.[8] Dissociations between "knowing" and "behaving" are common in patients with frontal lobe pathology. Thus, it is advisable to question a relative for examples of poor judgment from the patient's daily life. Socially inappropriate behaviors, such as acting in an overly familiar manner with strangers or making off-color comments, are common manifestations of poor judgment. The ability to grasp the gist of a complex situation, to have empathy, and to catch the punch line of a joke or to decipher the humor in a cartoon sequence may also rely on mental faculties associated with judgment and social perception. Judgment and insight are closely related to one another. Denial or minimization of illness (anosognosia or anosodiaphoria) following right hemisphere lesions is a specific example of poor insight.

III. Testing the Elderly and the Diagnosis of Dementia

"Dementia" can be defined as a clinical condition in which there is the progressive decline of previously acquired cognitive and emotional capacities and comportment, interfering with the independent conduct of customary daily living activities. Its diagnosis usually requires abnormal neuropsychological test scores as well as evidence for an impairment of daily living activities (Chapter 10). The most common cause of this condition in individuals over 65 is Alzheimer's disease (AD) but there are other etiologies to be considered, especially under age 75, as described in Chapter 10.

There are some special considerations for testing mental state in older patients. First, "usual" aging is associated with some decline in mental functions, which must be taken into account when test performance is interpreted. Second, it is important to consider the possibility that a performance that is "normal for age" could still represent a decline from the patient's own prior level of ability (Chapter 10). Third, many standard tests are too difficult for elderly or moderately demented patients and there is a paucity of norms for older patients at different levels of education and from different racial and ethnic backgrounds. In order to meet this challenge, an increasing number of neuropsychological tests are being standardized on older community-dwelling individuals.[74,80–85,106,107,110,207] The goals of the neuropsychological investigation for dementia are to (1) differentiate between "benign" or age-linked change and more "malignant" symptoms indicative of disease and (2) identify a pattern of primary deficits in order to formulate a differential diagnosis.

On average, advancing age is associated with reduced scores on tests of reaction time, memory, cognitive flexibility, and some visuospatial skills.[21] The "classic" cognitive aging pattern on the WAIS is characterized by relative stability in the Verbal IQ (representing so-called "crystallized" mental abilities) across the life span.[111] In contrast, there is a linear decline in the Performance IQ (representing so-called "fluid" abilities)[24] that is not solely accounted for by the fact that it is based on timed tests.[177] Longitudinal and cross-sectional studies have shown that age-related change is not uniform, either across domains or across individuals, and that it does not threaten independence.[160–162] This lack of uniformity is reflected in an age-related increase in the magnitude of the standard deviation, a measure of within-group variability.[129,203] The increase in heterogeneity suggests that some individuals show a great deal of age-related change whereas others may show very little or none at all. For example, Benton and colleagues[18] observed that the magnitude of decline in scores in a group of nondemented 65–85-year-olds, compared to a younger index sample (16 to 65 years of age), was greatest on tests of memory (*Visual Retention*[17,170] and *Digit Sequence Tests*[16]) and least on tests of orientation, *Digit Span*[192], and *Judgment of Line Orientation*[16,20]. Furthermore, 33% of individuals in the oldest cohort (80 to 85 years) scored within the average range for the younger index sample on *all* of the tests.

There are two problems encountered in the diagnosis of dementia based on neuropsychological test scores. The first is that a patient may score in the "abnormal" range on testing, but this level of functioning may not represent a change from a prior level of performance. The second problem is that a patient's score may fall in the "normal" range but that patient may still be suffering from a dementia because the former level of functioning was much higher. There are two ways to assist the examiner in decision-making. First, an estimate of the patient's premorbid ability level can be derived, objectively, as outlined in section II, or subjectively, by considering the level of the patient's life accomplishments. A second strategy is to reexamine the patient after some time (6 months) has elapsed to obtain evidence of a decline over that interval of time which would be consistent with the impression of dementia.

A primary amnesia is the cardinal symptom of the dementia associated with the clinical syndrome of probable Alzheimer's disease (PRAD).[114] There may be a "preclinical" phase, during which individuals may not meet criteria for a diagnosis of dementia but may experience what has been variably referred to as "mild cognitive impairment"[134] or "age-associated memory impairment."[35] These patients may have abnormal memory test scores but may function relatively normally in daily life. In the longitudinal follow-up of this group of individuals, as many as 70% may go on to develop a frank dementia syndrome, so these abnormalities are important to detect for early diagnosis and intervention.[49,104]

Performance on delayed recall measures of explicit memory is the best discriminator between patients with a diagnosis of mild PRAD and nondemented control subjects.[128,178,179,205] Patients with early PRAD have normal immediate recall of the *Logical Memory* stories on the *WMS-R* but impaired delayed recall.[158] Because spontaneous recall is affected early in the course of the illness, it soon shows a floor effect and is not a good measure of disease progression. Recognition memory performance, usually preserved until later stages, can provide a better measure of disease progression.[105] Attentional deficits may sometimes occur early in PRAD, even prior to the onset of memory loss.[132,137] Forward digit span, however, tends to be preserved in the early stages.[104] Tasks requiring working memory, persistence, or divided attention are usually impaired in patients with mild to moderate dementia severity.[63,64]

Naming and verbal fluency deficits are also associated with dementia of the Alzheimer's type. Initially, patients may only perform poorly on the *BNT*, but many may go on to develop symptoms of fluent aphasias, including anomic, transcortical sensory, and Wernicke's types.[47,77,94,96,137] The score on the *BNT* is related to the rapidity of disease progression[97] and can be used to stage the disease.[105] Both lexical and semantic verbal fluency tasks are performed poorly by patients with PRAD.[123,185] The *Multilingual Aphasia Examination* can be used to screen for language deficits in adults up to 69 years of age.[15]

The examination for dementia begins with a careful history in which the nature of the onset (abrupt, subacute, insidious) and course (improving, static, fluctuating, progressive) of symptoms provide clues about the etiology. Descriptions of symptoms and their impact on daily living activities hint at the potential nature of the primary deficit (i.e., forgetfulness versus word-finding difficulty versus visual spatial disorientation). A quantitative score reflecting the overall severity of the dementia can be obtained with one of the very brief mental status screening tests available, the *Mini Mental State Examination (MMSE)*[50] or the *Blessed Dementia Scale (BDS)*.[22] The *Dementia Rating Scale (DRS)*[112,113] is more extensive and more sensitive to change over time[159] and has normative data for individuals over 89 years of age.[107,163] The mean score for high-school-educated individuals over 70 is 27/30 (27 out of a possible 30) on the MMSE, 34/37 on the BDS, and 137/144 on the DRS.[174] These scores need to be adjusted for education and age.[183] For example, in individuals over 80 without a high school education, the *MMSE* cutoff may be as low as 23. On the *MDRS*, a score of 130–133 is considered "average" for an 89-year-old.[107] In patients with PRAD, there is a characteristic annual rate of decline on these tests: an average of 3.24 points for the *Information-Memory-Concentration subtest* of the BDS, 2.81 points on the *MMSE*, and 11.38 points on the *DRS*.[159] The *Alzheimer's Disease Assessment Scale (ADAS)*[155] has been used extensively to measure medication effects on the symptoms of Alzheimer's dementia.

The *CERAD* test battery was designed to focus on the salient symptoms of dementia of the Alzheimer's type.[53,126,127,205,206] It includes a ten-word list presented visually for three learning trials, following which delayed recall is tested. Adults in their 70s recall a total average of 21/30 words over the three learning trials and at least six items after a delay of approximately 10 minutes. List generation (animals), constructions, and 15 items from the *BNT* are also included.

The *Instrumental Activities of Daily Living (IADL)*[100] and the *Record of Independent Living (RIL)*[196] are two scales that measure the impact of dementia on daily living activities in mildly demented, noninstitutionalized individuals. The *RIL* requires informants to rate the extent to which assistance is needed by the patient in carrying out routine activities. Verbal communication skills and changes in customary behaviors are also rated. The *Activities* and *Communication subtest* scores correlate with the *DRS* score but the *Behavior* score does not, suggesting that the first two are sensitive to the impact of the cognitive deficits of dementia while the third measures a different dimension. An adaptation of this test has been used to track progression of dementia in patients with PRAD.[105] There are also qualitative rating scales for the severity of dementia based on markers of functional capacity. The *Clinical Dementia Rating*[125] is most appropriate for earlier stages of dementia whereas the *Global Deterioration Scale (GDS)*[146,147] and the *Functional Assessment Staging (FAST)*[144] are more appropriate for moderate to late stages of illness when incontinence, immobility, and unresponsiveness emerge.

Patients with Alzheimer's disease may demonstrate poor performance on formal testing of visuospatial and language functions in the office even before significant change is observed in routine home or work activities. In contrast, many patients with frontal lobe dementia may score quite well on cognitive tests even when daily activities may be severely disrupted.[198] Discrepancies between office test performance and daily living activities can be reconciled by conducting a structured "home visit."[90]

"Noncognitive" behavioral symptoms, including apathy, disengagement from the environment, depression, agitation, and hallucinations can constitute the earliest symptoms of a dementia, as in the case of cortical Lewy body disease or frontal lobe dementia. The *Neuropsychiatric Inventory*, completed in an interview with a caregiver, provides a thorough review of these noncognitive symptoms.[37] The *Behavioral Pathology in Alzheimer's Disease Rating Scale (BEHAVEAD)* also provides a brief review of symptoms such as paranoia, depression, agitation, and hostility and the extent to which they cause distress to the caregiver.[73,116,145] The *Geriatric Depression Scale*[214] may not be as valid in patients with moderate to severe levels of dementia as it is in earlier stages.[56]

In cases of very early dementia, it is necessary to obtain objective testing to detect the mild deficits. However, patients with superior premorbid intellectual capacity or special talents pose a challenge for the detection of early dementia. Standard tests may yield a ceiling effect in these highly accomplished individuals. A detailed interview with family members or even with colleagues may establish further evidence for a change in functional capacity. Automated tests that include a measure of decision and reaction time, such as Microcog,[136] might be helpful in these instances. However, even the most diligent evaluation may yield no objective finding. These patients should be monitored at regular intervals and scores should be tracked over time for evidence of decline.

IV. TESTING LOBES AND HEMISPHERES

Sometimes it is desirable to organize the examination according to anatomical landmarks such as the major lobes of the brain.

Testing the Functions of the Temporal Lobe

The temporal lobes contain auditory cortex, visual association cortex, heteromodal association cortex, and the medially situated limbic and paralimbic structures. The left temporal lobe also contains Wernicke's area. Tests of naming and language comprehension can be used to assess the integrity of the left temporal lobe and its connections. Homologous parts of the right temporal lobe can be tested with nonverbal auditory tasks (e.g., identification of environmental sounds) and tasks of prosody. Exaggerated or unexpected ear asymmetries on dichotic listening can be used to detect unilateral lesions in auditory cortex. The integrity of limbic and paralimbic regions can be tested with verbal and nonverbal memory tests. Left-sided lesions tend to disrupt mostly verbal memory and right-sided lesions may disrupt nonverbal memory. Bilateral lesions that affect the visual association areas of the temporal lobe or their connections with other parts of the brain result in visual amnesia, visual anomia, prosopagnosia, achromatopsia, object agnosia, and alexia without agraphia. The anatomic correlates of these syndromes and methods of assessing them are reviewed in Chapters 1, 4, 5, and 7. The presence of an upper quadrantanopia is a helpful neighborhood sign indicating the presence of temporal lobe damage.

Occipital Lobe

The entire occipital lobe is occupied by the primary visual and visual association areas and the manifestations of damage to this part of the brain are confined to tasks in the visual modality. Depending on the selectivity of the lesion, occipital lobe damage is associated with visual field cuts, color perception deficits, and movement perception deficits (Chapters 1 and 7).

Parietal Lobe

The parietal lobe contains the somatosensory areas and the heteromodal association cortex of the posterior parietal region. Tests sensitive to left parietal lobe damage include naming, reading, writing, calculations, finger identification, and left–right naming. Equivalent lesions in the right hemisphere give rise to dressing difficulties, constructional difficulties, hemispatial neglect, and neglect of the body surface (Chapters 1, 3 and 7). Additional manifestations of parietal lobe damage, especially when bilateral, include Balint's syndrome as well as spatial and topographic disorientation (Chapter 7). An inferior quadrantanopia may be observed in patients with parietal lobe damage.

Frontal Lobe

Patients with selective frontal lobe damage usually display deficits in judgment, insight, mental flexibility, reasoning, abstraction, planning, sequencing, comportment, and the attentional matrix. Lesions that include the orbital (basal) part of the frontal lobes may also lead to declarative memory disturbances.

Left and Right Hemispheres

The two hemispheres of the human brain have distinctly different behavioral specializations. In most right-handed individuals, tests of linguistic function, ideomotor praxis, left–right identification, finger identification, calculation, and verbal memory are most sensitive to left hemisphere damage. Tests of dressing, constructions, complex nonverbal perceptual skills, the spatial allocation of attention, paralinguistic competence, and nonverbal memory are most sensitive to right hemisphere injury.

Assessment of Handedness

Some individuals perform all skilled manual functions (writing, combing, throwing a ball, using a scissors) with the right hand. Others may write with the right hand but use the left hand for certain skilled movements such as throwing a ball or combing. There is a tendency to classify such individuals as right-handed, since questions about activities other than writing are rarely asked during routine mental-state assessments. However, these individuals with mixed handedness may have a considerably different pattern of hemispheric specialization when compared with those who are fully right-handed. Specialized questionnaires are available for computing a quantitative index of handedness when such information becomes desirable.[131,140,209]

V. OVERVIEW AND CONCLUSIONS

The neuropsychological examination of mental state is a dynamic exploration of cognitive, behavioral, and emotional abnormalities resulting from neurological dysfunction. The examination methods and interpretation are firmly rooted in a model of behavioral neuroanatomy that links domains of complex mental activity to the large-scale neuroanatomical networks that subserve them. Flexibility is indispensible to effective neuropsychological assessment. Rigid attachment to test batteries that leave no room for improvisation should be avoided. Formulations based on the entire *pattern* of findings and guided by established principles of psychological and anatomical organization are favored over a catalogue of numerous putative lesion sites, each affixed to a single test finding. An assessment based on these considerations should provide a summary of the *primary* deficits, their *secondary* effects on test performance, their relevance to the structural integrity of the nervous system, their impact on daily living, and their implications for diagnosis and management.

REFERENCES

1. Albert, M: A simple test of visual neglect. Neurology 23:658–664, 1973.
2. Albert, M S, Butters, N and Brandt, J: Patterns of remote memory in amnesic and demented patients. Arch Neurol 38:495–500, 1981.
3. Albert, M S, Butters, N and Levin, J: Temporal gradients in the retrograde amnesia of patients with alcoholic Korsakoff's disease. Arch Neurol 36:211–216, 1979.
4. Alexander, M P, Baker, E, Naeser, M A, Kaplan, E and Palumbo, C: Neuropsychological and neuroanatomical dimensions of ideomotor apraxia. Brain 115 Pt 1:87–107, 1992.
5. Baddeley, A: Working Memory. Oxford University Press, Oxford, 1986.
6. Barona, A, Reynolds, C R and Chastain, R: A demographically based index of premorbid intelligence for the WAIS-R. J Consult Clin Psychol 52:885–887, 1984.
7. Beatty, W W, English, S and Winn, P: Long-lived picture priming in normal elderly persons and demented patients. J Int Neuropsychol Soc 4:336–341, 1998.
8. Bechara, A, Damasio, H, Tranel, D and Damasio, A R: Deciding advantageously before knowing the advantageous strategy. Science 275:1293–1295, 1997.
9. Beck, A, Ward, C, Mendelsohn, M, Mock, J and Erbaugh, J: An inventory for measuring depression. Arch Gen Psychiatry 4:561–571, 1961.
10. Beck, A T and Steer, R A: Beck Depression Inventory. Manual. Psychological Corporation, San Antonio, Texas, 1993.
11. Benedict, R H B, Schretlen, D, Groninger, L and Brandt, J: Hopkins Verbal Learning Test–Revised: Normative data and analysis of inter-form and test-retest reliability. Clin Neuropsychol 12:43–55, 1998.

12. Benowitz, L, Bear, D, Rosenthal, R, Mesulam, M-M, Zaidel, E and Sperry, R: Hemispheric specialization in nonverbal communication. Cortex 19:5–11, 1983.
13. Benson, D and Denckla, M: Verbal paraphasia as a source of calculation disturbance. Arch Neurol 21:96–102, 1969.
14. Benton, A L and Hamsher, K de S: Multilingual Aphasia Examination. University of Iowa, Iowa City, 1989.
15. Benton, A L, Hamsher, K de S and Sivan, AB: Multilingual Aphasia Examination, 3rd Ed. AJA, Iowa City, IA, 1994.
16. Benton, A L, Hamsher, K de S, Varney, N and Spreen, O: Contributions to Neuropsychological Assessment, 2nd Ed. Oxford University Press, New York, 1998.
17. Benton, A L: Revised Visual Retention Test, 4th Ed. Psychological Corporation, New York, 1974.
18. Benton, A L, Eslinger, P J and Damasio, A: Normative observations on neuropsychological test performances in old age. J Clin Neuropsychol 3:33–42, 1981.
19. Benton, A L and Van Allen, M W: Impairment in facial recognition in patients with cerebral disease. Cortex 4:344–358, 1968.
20. Benton, A L, Varney, N R and Hamsher, K de S: Visuospatial judgment: a clinical test. Arch Neurol 35:364–367, 1978.
21. Birren, J and Schaie, K (eds.): Handbook of the Psychology of Aging. Van Nostrand Reinhold, New York, 1977.
22. Blessed, G, Tomlinson, B E and Roth, M: The association between quantitative measures of dementia and of senile change in the cerebral grey matter of elderly subjects. Br J Psychiatry 114:797–811, 1968.
23. Boone, K B and Rausch, R: Seashore Rhythm Test performance in patients with unilateral temporal lobe damage. J Clin Psychol 45:614–618, 1989.
24. Botwinick, J: Intellectual abilities. In Birren, J E and Schaie, K W (Eds.): Handbook of the Psychology of Aging. Van Nostrand Reinhold, New York, 1977, pp. 580–605.
25. Brickenkamp, R: Test d2:/Aufmerksamkeits-Belastungs-Test (Handanweisung, 7th Ed.). Verlag fur Psychologie, C. J. Hogrefe, Gottingen, 1981.
26. Broverman, D: Dimensions of cognitive style. J Pers 28:167–185, 1960.
27. Brown, J I, Bennett, J M and Hanna, G: The Nelson-Denny Reading Test. Riverside, Chicago, 1981.
28. Buschke, H and Fuld, P A: Evaluating storage, retention, and retrieval in disordered memory and learning. Neurology 24:1019–1025, 1974.
29. Chedru, F and Geschwind, N: Writing disturbances in acute confusional states. Neuropsychologia 10:343–353, 1972.
30. Comalli, P J, Wapner, S and Werner, H: Interference effects of Stroop color-word test in childhood, adulthood, and aging. J Genet Psychol 100:47–53, 1962.
31. Conners, C K: Conners' Continuous Performance Test. Multi-Health Systems, Toronto, 1995.
32. Corkin, S: Acquisition of motor skill after bilateral medial temporal lobe excision. Neuropsychologia 6:225–266, 1968.
33. Corkin, S: Some relationships between global amnesias and memory impairments in Alzheimer's disease. In Corkin, S, Davis, K, Growdon, J, Usdin, E and Wurtman, R (Eds.): Alzheimer's Disease: A Report of Progress in Research. Raven Press, New York, 1982, pp. 149–164.
34. Coslett, H B: Acquired dyslexia. In Feinberg, T E and Farah, M J (Eds.): Behavioral Neurology and Neuropsychology. McGraw-Hill, New York, 1997, pp. 197–208.
35. Crook, T, Bahar, H and Sudilovsky, A: Age-associated memory impairment: diagnostic criteria and treatment strategies. Int Neurol 22:73–82, 1987.
36. Culver, C M: Test of right-left discrimination. Percept Mot Skills 29:863–867, 1969.
37. Cummings, J L, Mega, M, Gray, K, Rosenberg-Thompson, S, Carusi, D A and Gornbein,

J: The Neuropsychiatric Inventory: comprehensive assessment of psychopathology in dementia. Neurology 44:2308–2314, 1994.

38. Davies, A D: The influence of age on trail making test performance. J Clin Psychol 24: 96–98, 1968.

39. De Renzi, E and Faglioni, P: The comparative efficiency of intelligence and vigilance in detecting hemisphere damage. Cortex 1:410–433, 1965.

40. De Renzi, E and Vignolo, L: The Token Test: a sensitive test to detect disturbances in aphasics. Brain 85:665–678, 1962.

41. Delis, D, Kramer, J, Kaplan, E and Ober, B: The California Verbal Learning Test. The Psychological Corporation, San Antonio, Texas, 1987.

42. Delis, D C, Squire, L R, Bihrle, A and Massman, P: Componential analysis of problem-solving ability: performance of patients with frontal lobe damage and amnesic patients on a new sorting test. Neuropsychologia 30:683–697, 1992.

43. Deloche, G, Seron, X, Larroque, C, Magnien, C, Metz-Lutz, M N, Noel, M N, Riva, I, Schils, J P, Dordain, M, Ferrand, I Baeta, A, Basso, A, Cipolotti, L, Claros-Salinas, D, Howard, D, Gaillard, F, Goldenberg, G, Mazzucchi, A, Stachowiak, F, Tzavaras, A, Vendrell, J Bergego, C and Pradat-Diehl, P: Calculation and number processing: assessment battery; role of demographic factors. J Clin Exp Neuropsychol 16:195–208, 1994.

44. Drewe, E: The effect of type and area of brain lesion on Wisconsin Card Sorting Test performance. Cortex 10:159–170, 1974.

45. Drewe, E A: Go No-go learning after frontal lobe lesions in humans. Cortex 11:8–16, 1975.

46. Ekman, P and Friesen, W: Pictures of Facial Affect. Consulting Psychologists Press, Palo Alto, California, 1975.

47. Faber-Langendoen, K, Morris, J C, Knesevich, J W, LaBarge, E, Miller, J P and Berg, L: Aphasia in senile dementia of the Alzheimer type. Ann Neurol 23:365–370, 1988.

48. Feldman, M J and Drasgow, J: The Visual-Verbal Test. Western Psychological Services, Los Angeles, 1959.

49. Flicker, C, Ferris, S H and Reisberg, B: Mild cognitive impairment in the elderly: predictors of dementia. Neurology 41:1006–1009, 1991.

50. Folstein, M, Folstein, S and McHugh, P: "Mini-mental state." A practical method for grading the cognitive state of patients for the clinician. J Psychiatr Res 12:189–198, 1975.

51. Folstein, M F and Luria, R: Reliability, validity, and clinical application of the Visual Analogue Mood Scale. Psychol Med 3:479–486, 1973.

52. Freedman, M, Leach, L, Kaplan, E, Winocur, G, Shulman, K and Delis, D: Clock Drawing: A Neuropsychological Analysis. Oxford University Press, New York, 1994.

53. Galasko, D, Edland, S D, Morris, J C, Clark, C, Mohs, R and Koss, E: The Consortium to Establish a Registry for Alzheimer's Disease (CERAD). Part XI. Clinical milestones in patients with Alzheimer's disease followed over 3 years. Neurology 45:1451–1455, 1995.

54. Gauthier, L, DeHaut, F and Joanette, Y: The Bells Test: a quantitative and qualitative test for visual neglect. Int J Clin Neuropsychol 11:49–50, 1989.

55. Geschwind, N: Specializations of the human brain. Sci Am 241:180–199, 1979.

56. Gilley, D W and Wilson, R S: Criterion-related validity of the Geriatric Depression Scale in Alzheimer's disease. J Clin Exp Neuropsychol 19:489–499, 1997.

57. Goldstein, K and Scheerer, M: Abstract and concrete behavior: an experimental study with special tests. Psychol Monogr 53:No 239:1941.

58. Gollin, E: Developmental studies of visual recognition of incomplete objects. Percept Mot Skills 11:289–198, 1960.

59. Goodglass, H and Kaplan, E: Disturbance of gesture and pantomime in aphasics. Brain 86:703–720, 1963.

60. Goodglass, H and Kaplan, E: The Assessment of Aphasia and Related Disorders, 2nd Ed. Lea & Febiger, Philadelphia, 1983.

61. Gordon, M: The Gordon Diagnostic System. Gordon Systems, DeWitt, New York, 1983.

62. Gordon, M, McClure, F D and Post, E M: Interpretive guide to the Gordon Diagnostic System. Gordon Systems, Syracuse, 1986.

63. Grady, C L, Grimes, A M, Patronas, N, Sunderland, T, Foster, NL and Rapoport, SI: Divided attention, as measured by dichotic speech peformance, in dementia of the Alzheimer type. Arch Neurol 46:317–320, 1989.

64. Grady, C L, Haxby, J V, Horwitz, B, Sundaram, M, Berg, G, Schapiro, M, Friedland, R P and Rapoport, S I: Longitudinal study of the early neuropsychological and cerebral metabolic changes in dementia of the Alzheimer type. J Clin Exp Neuropsychol 10:576–596, 1988.

65. Grant, D A and Berg, E: The Wisconsin Card Sort Test Random Layout: Directions for administration and scoring. Wells Printing, Madison, Wisconsin, 1980.

66. Grant, M L, Ilai, D, Nussbaum, NL and Bigler, ED: The relationship between continuous performance tasks and neuropsychological tests in children with attention-deficit hyperactivity disorder. Percept Mot Skills 70:435–445, 1990.

67. Greene, R L: The MMPI-2/MMPI: An Interpretive Manual. Psychological Assessment Resources, Odessa, FL, 1992.

68. Grober, E and Sliwinski, M: Development and validation of a model for estimating premorbid verbal intelligence in the elderly. J Clin Exp Neuropsychol 13:933–949, 1991.

69. Gronwall, D and Sampson, H: The Psychological Effects of Concussion. Auckland University Press, Auckland, New Zealand, 1974.

70. Hamilton, M: Development of a rating scale for primary depressive illness. Br J Soc Clin Psychol 6:278–296, 1967.

71. Hannay, H J, Falgout, J C, Leli, D A, Katholi, C R, Halsey, J H Jr and Wills, E L: Focal right temporo-occipital blood flow changes associated with judgment of line orientation. Neuropsychologia 25:755–763, 1987.

72. Hannay, H J and Levin, H S: Selective reminding test: an examination of the equivalence of four forms. J Clin Exp Neuropsychol 7:251–263, 1985.

73. Harwood, D G, Ownby, R L, Barker, W W and Duara, R: The behavioral pathology in Alzheimer's Disease Scale (BEHAVE-AD): factor structure among community-dwelling Alzheimer's disease patients. Int J Geriatr Psychiatry 13:793–800, 1998.

74. Heaton, R, Grant, I and Matthews, C: Comprehensive norms for an expanded Halstead-Reitan Battery: Demographic corrections, research findings and clinical applications. Psychological Assessment Resources, Odessa, Florida, 1992.

75. Heaton, R K, Chelune, G J, Talley, J L, Kay, G G and Curtis, C: Wisconsin Card Sorting Test (WCST) Manual Revised and Expanded. Psychological Assessment Resources, Odessa, Florida, 1993.

76. Heilman, K M, Bowers, D, Speedie, L and Coslett, H B: Comprehension of affective and nonaffective prosody. Neurology 34:917–921, 1984.

77. Hier, D B, Hagenlocker, K and Shindler, A G: Language disintegration in dementia: effects of etiology and severity. Brain Lang 25:117–133, 1985.

78. Hooper, H: The Hooper Visual Organization Test Manual. Western Psychological Services, Los Angeles, 1958.

79. Hoshiyama, M, Koyama, S, Kitamura, Y, Shimojo, M, Watanabe, S and Kakigi, R: Effects of judgement process on motor evoked potentials in Go/No-go hand movement task. Neurosci Res 24:427–430, 1996.

80. Ivnik, R J, Malec, J F, Smith, G E, Tangalos, E G and Petersen, R C: Neuropsychological tests' norms above age 55: COWAT, BNT, MAE Token, WRAT-R Reading, AMNART, Stroop, TMT, and JLO. Clin Neuropsychol 10:262–278, 1996.

81. Ivnik, R J, Malec, J F, Smith, G E, Tangalos, E G, Petersen, R C, Kokmen, E and Kurland, L T: Mayo's older Americans normative studies: WAIS-R norms for ages 56 through 97. Clin Neuropsychol 6(Suppl):1–30, 1992.

82. Ivnik, R J, Malec, J F, Smith, G E, Tangalos, E G, Petersen, R C, Kokmen, E and Kurland,

L T: Mayo's older Americans normative studies: WMS-R norms for ages 56 through 94. Clin Neuropsychol 6 (Suppl):49–82, 1992.

83. Ivnik, R J, Malec, J F, Tangalos, E G, Petersen, R C, Kokmen, S and Kurland, L T: The Auditory Verbal Learning Test (AVLT): norms for ages 55 and older. Psychological Assessment 2:304–312, 1990.

84. Ivnik, R J, Malec, J F, Tangalos, E G, Petersen, R C, Kokmen, S and Kurland, L T: Mayo's older Americans normative studies: updated AVLT norms for ages 56–97. Clin Neuropsychol 6(Suppl):83–104, 1992.

85. Ivnik, R J, Smith, G E, Lucas, J A, Tangalos, E G, Petersen, R C and Kokmen, E: Free and Cued Selective Reminding Test: MOANS norms. J Clin Exp Neuropsychol 19:676–691, 1997.

86. Kaplan, E: A process approach to neuropsychological assessment. In Boll, T and Bryant, B K (Eds.): Clinical Neuropsychology and Brain Function: Research, Measurement and Practice. American Psychological Association, Washington, DC, 1988.

87. Kaplan, E, Fein, D, Morris, R and Delis, D C: WAIS-R NI Manual. The Psychological Corporation, San Antonio, Tx, 1991.

88. Kaplan, E, Goodglass, H and Weintraub, S: The Boston Naming Test. Lea and Febiger, Philadelphia, 1983.

89. Kaplan, E, Palmer, E, Weinstein, C, Baker, E and Weintraub, S: Block design: a brain–behavior based analysis. Paper presented at the International Neuropsychological Society Annual European Meeting, Bergen, 1981.

90. Kapust, L R and Weintraub, S: The home visit: field assessment of mental status impairment in the elderly. Gerontologist 28:112–115, 1988.

91. Kertesz, A: Aphasia and Associated Disorders. Grune & Stratton, New York, 1979.

92. Kimura, D: Cerebral dominance and the perception of verbal stimuli. Can J Psychol 15: 166–171, 1961.

93. Kimura, D: Some effects of temporal lobe damage on auditory perception. Can J Psychol 15:156–165, 1961.

94. Kirshner, H S and Bakar, M: Syndromes of language dissolution in aging and dementia. Compr Ther 21:519–523, 1995.

95. Kirshner, H S, Casey, P F, Kelly, M P and Webb, W G: Anomia in cerebral diseases. Neuropsychologia 25:701–705, 1987.

96. Kirshner, H S, Webb, W G and Kelly, M P: The naming disorder of dementia. Neuropsychologia 22:23–30, 1984.

97. Knesevich, J W, LaBarge, E and Edwards, D: Predictive value of the Boston Naming Test in mild senile dementia of the Alzheimer type. Psychiatry Res 19:155–161, 1986.

98. Kopelman, M, Wilson, B and Baddeley, A: Autobiographical Memory Interview. Psychological Assessment Resources, Odessa, Florida, 1996.

99. Kopelman, M D: Remote and autobiographical memory, temporal context memory and frontal atrophy in Korsakoff and Alzheimer patients. Neuropsychologia 27:437–460, 1989.

100. Lawton, M P and Brody, E M: Assessment of older people: self-maintaining and instrumental activities of daily living. Gerontologist 9:179–186, 1969.

101. Leimkuhler, M E and Mesulam, M M: Reversible go–no go deficits in a case of frontal lobe tumor. Ann Neurol 18:617–619, 1985.

102. Lezak, M: Neuropsychological Assessment, 3rd Ed. Oxford University Press, New York, 1995.

103. Liepmann, H: Das Krankheitsbild der Apraxie ("motorischen Asymbolie") auf Grund eines Falles von einseitiger Apraxie. Monatsschrift fur Psychlgie und Neurologie 8:15–44, 102–132, 188–197, 1900.

104. Linn, R T, Wolf, P A, Bachman, D L, Knoefel, J E, Cobb, J L, Belanger, A J, Kaplan, E F and D'Agostino, R B: The 'preclinical phase' of probable Alzheimer's disease. A 13-year prospective study of the Framingham cohort. Arch Neurol 52:485–490, 1995.

105. Locascio, J J, Growdon, J H and Corkin, S: Cognitive test performance in detecting, staging, and tracking Alzheimer's disease. Arch Neurol 52:1087–1099, 1995.
106. Lucas, J A, Ivnik, R J, Smith, G E, Bohac, D L, Tangalos, E G, Graff-Radford, N R and Petersen, R C: Mayo's older Americans normative studies: category fluency norms. J Clin Exp Neuropsychol 20:194–200, 1998.
107. Lucas, J A, Ivnik, R J, Smith, G E, Bohac, D L, Tangalos, E G, Kokmen, E, Graff-Radford, N R and Petersen, R C: Normative data for the Mattis Dementia Rating Scale. J Clin Exp Neuropsychol 20:536–547, 1998.
108. Luria, A: Higher Cortical Functions in Man. Basic Books, New York, 1966.
109. Luria, A: Human Brain and Psychological Processes. Harper & Row, New York, 1966.
110. Manly, J J, Jacobs, D M, Sano, M, Bell, K, Merchant, C A, Small, S A and Stern, Y: Cognitive test performance among nondemented elderly African Americans and whites. Neurology 50:1238–1245, 1998.
111. Matarazzo, J: Wechsler's Measurement and Appraisal of Adult Intelligence, 5th Ed. Williams & Wilkins, Baltimore, 1972.
112. Mattis, S: Mental state examination for organic mental syndromes in the elderly patient. In Bellak, L and Karasu, T E (Eds.): Geriatric Psychiatry. Grune & Stratton, New York, 1976, pp. 77–121.
113. Mattis, S: Dementia Rating Scale: Professional Manual. Psychological Assessment Resources, Odessa, Florida, 1988.
114. McKhann, G, Drachman, D, Folstein, M, Katzman, R, Price, D and Stadlan, E: Clinical diagnosis of Alzheimer's disease: Report of the NINCDS-ADRDA Work Group* under the auspices of Department of Health and Human Services Task Force on Alzheimer's Disease. Neurology 34:939–944, 1984.
115. Meerwaldt, J D and van Harskamp, F: Spatial disorientation in right hemisphere infarction. J Neurol Neurosurg Psychiatry 45:586–590, 1982.
116. Mendez, M F, Perryman, K M, Miller, B L and Cummings, J L: Behavioral differences between frontotemporal dementia and Alzheimer's disease: a comparison on the BEHAVE-AD rating scale. Int Psychogeriatr 10:155–162, 1998.
117. Mesulam, M-M: Large-scale neurocognitive networks and distributed processing for attention, language, and memory. Ann Neurol 28:597–613, 1990.
118. Meyers, J and Meyers, K: Rey Complex Figure Test and Recognition Trial. The Psychological Corporation, San Antonio, Tx, 1995.
119. Miller, G A: The magical number seven, plus or minus two: some limits on our capacity for processing information. Psychol Rev 63:81–97, 1956.
120. Milner, B: Laterality effects in audition. In Mountcastle, V (Eds.): Interhemispheric Relations and Cerebral Dominance. Johns Hopkins Press, 1962, pp. 177–195.
121. Milner, B: Effects of different brain lesions on card-sorting. Arch Neurol 9:90–100, 1963.
122. Monk, T H: A Visual Analogue Scale technique to measure global vigor and affect. Psychiatry Res 27:89–99, 1989.
123. Monsch, A U, Bondi, M W, Butters, N, Salmon, D P, Katzman, R and Thal, L J: Comparisons of verbal fluency tasks in the detection of dementia of the Alzheimer type. Arch Neurol 49:1253–1258, 1992.
124. Montgomery, K and Costa, L: Neuropsychological test performance of a normal elderly sample. Paper presented at the International Neuropsychological Society Meeting Mexico City, Mexico, 1983.
125. Morris, J C: The Clinical Dementia Rating (CDR): current version and scoring rules. Neurology 43:2412–2414, 1993.
126. Morris, J C, Edland, S, Clark, C, Galasko, D, Koss, W, Mohs, R, van Belle, G, Fillenbaum, G and Heyman, A: The Consortium to Establish a Registry for Alzheimer's Disease (CERAD). Part IV. Rates of cognitive change in the longitudinal assessment of probable Alzheimer's disease. Neurology 43:2457–2465, 1993.

127. Morris, J C, Heyman, A, Mohs, R C, Hughes, J P, van Belle, G, Fillenbaum, G, Mellits, E D and Clark, C: The Consortium to Establish a Registry for Alzheimer's Disease (CERAD). Part I. Clinical and neuropsychological assessment of Alzheimer's disease. Neurology 39:1159–1165, 1989.

128. Morris, J C, McKeel, D W, Jr., Storandt, M, Rubin, E H, Price, J L, Grant, E A, Ball, M J and Berg, L: Very mild Alzheimer's disease: informant-based clinical, psychometric, and pathologic distinction from normal aging. Neurology 41:469–478, 1991.

129. Nelson, E A and Dannefer, D: Aged heterogeneity: fact or fiction? The fate of diversity in gerontological research. Gerontologist 32:17–23, 1992.

130. O'Connor, M G, Cermak, L S Sieggreen, M A, Bachna, K, Kaplan, B, and Ransil, B J: The effects of age and gender on the long-term retention of Transient News Events. J Int Neuropsychol Soc, 5:117, 1998.

131. Oldfield, R C: The assessment and analysis of handedness: the Edinburgh inventory. Neuropsychologia 9:97–113, 1971.

132. Parasuraman, R, Greenwood, P M, Haby, J V and Grady, C L: Visuospatial attention in dementia of the Alzheimer's type. Brain 115:711–733, 1992.

133. Paterson, A and Zangwill, O L: Disorders of visual space perception associated with lesions of the right cerebral hemisphere. Brain 67:331, 1944.

134. Petersen, R C, Smith, G E, Waring, S C, Ivnik, R J, Kokmen, E and Tangelos, E G: Aging, memory, and mild cognitive impairment. Int Psychogeriatr 9 (Suppl) 1:65–69, 1997.

135. Porteus, S D: Porteus Mazes Tests: Fifty Years Applications. The Psychological Corporation, San Antonio, TX, 1965.

136. Powell, D H, Kaplan, E F, Whitla, D, Weintraub, S, Catlin, R and Funkenstein, H H: Manual for MicroCog: Assessment of Cognitive Functioning. The Psychological Corporation, San Antonio, TX, 1993.

137. Price, B H, Gurvit, H, Weintraub, S, Geula, C, Leimkuhler, E and Mesulam, M: Neuropsychological patterns and language deficits in 20 consecutive cases of autopsy-confirmed Alzheimer's disease. Arch Neurol 50:931–937, 1993.

138. Randolph, C: Repeatable Battery for the Assessment of Neuropsychological Status (RBANS). The Psychological Corporation, San Antonio, TX, 1998.

139. Randolph, C, Tierney, M C, Mohr, E and Chase, T: The Repeatable Battery for the Assessment of Neuropsychological Status (RBANS): preliminary clinical validity. J Clin Exp Neuropsychol 20:310–319, 1998.

140. Ransil, B J and Schachter, S C: Test-retest reliability of the Edinburgh Handedness Inventory and Global Handedness preference measurements, and their correlation. Percept Mot Skills 79:1355–1372, 1994.

141. Rasmussen, T and Milner, B: Clinical and surgical studies of the cerebral speech areas in man. In Zulch, K, Creutzfeld, O and Gallagher, G (Eds.): Cerebral Localization. Springer Verlag, New York, 1975, pp. 238–257.

142. Raven, J: Guide to the Standard Progressive Matrices. The Psychological Corporation, New York, 1956.

143. Raven, J: Guide to using the Coloured Progressive Matrices. The Psychological Corporation, New York, 1956.

144. Reisberg, B: Functional assessment staging (FAST). Psychopharmacol Bull 24:653–659, 1988.

145. Reisberg, B, Auer, S R and Monteiro, I M: Behavioral pathology in Alzheimer's disease (BEHAVE-AD) rating scale. Int Psychogeriatr 8:301–308; discussion 351–354, 1996.

146. Reisberg, B, Ferris, S H, de Leon, M J and Crook, T: The Global Deterioration Scale for assessment of primary degenerative dementia. Am J Psychiatry 139:1136–1139, 1982.

147. Reisberg, B, Ferris, S H, de Leon, M J and Crook, T: Global Deterioration Scale (GDS). Psychopharmacol Bull 24:661–663, 1988.

148. Reitan, R M: Validity of the Trail-Making Test as an indication of organic brain damage. Percept Mot Skills 8:271–276, 1958.

149. Reitan, R M: Correlations between the Trail-Making Test and the Wechsler-Bellevue Scale. Percept Motor Skills 9:127–130, 1959.

150. Reitan, R M and Wolfson, D: The Seashore Rhythm Test and brain functions. Clin Neuropsychol 3:70–78, 1989.

151. Rey, A: L'examen psychologique dan les cas d'encephalopathie traumatique. Arch Psychol 28 (112): 1941.

152. Rey, A: L'examen clinique en psychologie. Presses Universitaires de France, Paris, 1970.

153. Roeltgen, D P and Heilman, K M: Lexical agraphia. Further support for the two-system hypothesis of linguistic agraphia. Brain 107:811–827, 1984.

154. Roeltgen, D P, Sevush, S and Heilman, K M: Phonological agraphia: writing by the lexical-semantic route. Neurology 33:755–765, 1983.

155. Rosen, W G, Mohs, R C and Davis, K L: A new rating scale for Alzheimer's disease. Am J Psychiatry 141:1356–1364, 1984.

156. Rosenthal, R, Hall, J, Archer, D, DiMatteo, M and Rogers, P: The PONS Test Manual. Irvington Publishers, New York, 1979.

157. Rosvold, H, Mirsky, A, Sarason, I, Bransome, E Jr and Beck, L: A continuous performance test of brain damage. J Clin Consulting Psychol 20:343–350, 1956.

158. Rubin, E H, Storandt, M, Miller, J P, Kinscherf, D A, Grant, E A, Morris, J C and Berg, L: A prospective study of cognitive function and onset of dementia in cognitively healthy elders. Arch Neurol 55:395–401, 1998.

159. Salmon, D P, Thal, L J, Butters, N and Heindel, W C: Longitudinal evaluation of dementia of the Alzheimer type: a comparison of 3 standardized mental status examinations. Neurology 40:1225–1230, 1990.

160. Schaie, K E: Longitudinal Studies of Adult Psychological Development. The Guilford Press, New York, 1983.

161. Schaie, K W: The Seattle Longitudinal Study: a thirty-five-year inquiry of adult intellectual development. Z Gerontol 26:129–137, 1993.

162. Schaie, K W: The course of adult intellectual development. Am Psychol 49:304–313, 1994.

163. Schmidt, R, Freidl, W, Fazekas, F, Reinhart, B, Grieshofer, P, Koch, M, Eber, B, Schumacher, M, Polmin, K and Lechner, H: The Mattis Dementia Rating Scale: normative data from 1,001 healthy volunteers. Neurology 44:964–966, 1994.

164. Schretlen, D, Bobholz, J H and Brandt, J: Development and psychometric properties of the Brief Test of Attention. Clin Neuropsychol 10:80–89, 1996.

165. Schretlen, D, Brandt, J and Bobholz, J H: Validation of the Brief Test of Attention in patients with Huntington's Disease and amnesia. Clin Neuropsychol 10:90–95, 1996.

166. Seashore, C E, Lewis, D and Saetveit, D L: Seashore Measures of Musical Talent (rev. ed.). The Psychological Corporation, New York, 1960.

167. Seltzer, B and Benson, D F: The temporal pattern of retrograde amnesia in Korsakoff's disease. Neurology 24:527–530, 1974.

168. Shallice, T: Phonological agraphia and the lexical route in writing. Brain 104:413–429, 1981.

169. Shallice, T: Specific impairments of planning. Philos Trans R Soc Lond Biol 298:199–209, 1982.

170. Sivan, A B: Benton Visual Retention Test, 5th Ed. The Psychological Corporation, San Antonio, TX, 1992.

171. Smith, A: The serial sevens substraction test. Arch Neurol 17:78–80, 1967.

172. Spinnler, H and Vignolo, L: Impaired recognition of meaningful sounds in aphasia. Cortex 2:337–348, 1966.

173. Spreen, O and Benton, A: Neurosensory Center Comprehensive Examination for Aphasia. Neuropsychological Laboratory, Department of Psychology, University of Victoria, Victoria, BC, 1969.

174. Spreen, O and Strauss, E: A Compendium of Neuropsychological Tests. Oxford University Press, New York, 1998.

175. Squire, L, Chace, P and Slater, P: Retrograde amnesia following electroconvulsive therapy. Nature 260:775–777, 1976.
176. Sternberg, D: High-speed scanning in human memory. Science 153:652–654, 1966.
177. Storandt, M: Age, ability level and methods of administering and scoring the WAIS. J Gerontology 32:175, 1977.
178. Storandt, M: Neuropsychological assessment in Alzheimer's disease. Exp Aging Res 17:100–101, 1991.
179. Storandt, M and Hill, R D: Very mild senile dementia of the Alzheimer type. II. Psychometric test performance. Arch Neurol 46:383–386, 1989.
180. Stroop, J: Studies of interference in serial verbal reactions. J Exp Psychol 18:643, 1935.
181. Sykes, D, Douglas, V, Weiss, G and Munde, K: Attention in hyperactive children and the effect of methylphenidate (Ritalin). J Child Psychol Psychiatry 12:129–139, 1971.
182. Tombaugh, T N and Hubley, A M: The 60-item Boston Naming Test: norms for cognitively intact adults aged 25 to 88 years. J Clin Exp Neuropsychol 19:922–932, 1997.
183. Tombaugh, T N and McIntyre, N J: The mini-mental state examination: a comprehensive review (see comments). J Am Geriatr Soc 40:922–935, 1992.
184. Tranel, D, Damasio, H and Damasio, A R: A neural basis for the retrieval of conceptual knowledge. Neuropsychologia 35:1319–1327, 1997.
185. Troster, A I, Salmon, D P, McCullough, D and Butters, N: A comparison of the category fluency deficits associated with Alzheimer's and Huntington's disease. Brain Lang 37:500–513, 1989.
186. Tucker, D M, Watson, R T and Heilman, K M: Discrimination and evocation of affectively intoned speech in patients with right parietal disease. Neurology 27:947–950, 1977.
187. van Leeuwen, T H, Steinhausen, H C, Overtoom, C C, Pascual-Marqui, R D, van't Klooster, B, Rothenberger, A, Sergeant, J A and Brandeis, D: The continuous performance test revisited with neuroelectric mapping: impaired orienting in children with attention deficits. Behav Brain Res 94:97–110, 1998.
188. Warrington, E: Recognition Memory Test Manual. NFER-Nelson, Windsor, England, 1984.
189. Warrington, E and James, M: Visual Object and Space Perception Battery. Thames Valley Test Company, Bury St. Edmunds, Suffolk, England, 1991.
190. Warrington, E K: The fractionation of arithmetical skills: a single case study. Q J Exp Psychol [A] 34:31–51, 1982.
191. Warrington, E K: Neuropsychological studies of object recognition. Philos Trans R Soc Lond Biol 298:15–33, 1982.
192. Wechsler, D: Manual for the Wechsler Adult Intelligence Scale. The Psychological Corporation, New York, 1955.
193. Wechsler, D: Wechsler Memory Scale–Revised Manual. The Psychological Corporation, San Antonio, Texas, 1987.
194. Wechsler, D: Wechsler Adult Intelligence Scale—Third Edition. The Psychological Corporation, San Antonio, Texas, 1997.
195. Wechsler, D: Wechsler Memory Scale–III. The Psychological Corporation, San Antonio, Texas, 1998.
196. Weintraub, S: The Record of Independent Living: an informant-completed measure of activities of daily living and behavior in elderly patients with cognitive impairment. Am J Alzheimer Care 1:35–39, 1986.
197. Weintraub, S: Mental state testing. In Samuels, M A and Feske, S (Eds.): Office Practice of Neurology. Churchill Livingstone, New York, 1995, pp. 698–705.
198. Weintraub, S and Kapust, L R: Non-amnestic dementias: special considerations for clinicians and caregivers. Am J Alzheimer Care 4:6–11, 1989.
199. Weintraub, S and Mesulam, M-M: Mental state assessment of young and elderly adults in behavioral neurology. In Mesulam, M-M (Eds.): Principles of Behavioral Neurology. FA Davis, Philadelphia, 1985, pp. 71–123.

200. Weintraub, S and Mesulam, M-M: Right cerebral dominance in spatial attention. Further evidence based on ipsilateral neglect. Arch Neurol 44:621–625, 1987.
201. Weintraub, S and Mesulam, M-M: Visual hemispatial inattention: stimulus parameters and exploratory strategies. J Neurol Neurosurg Psychiatry 51:1481–1488, 1988.
202. Weintraub, S, Mesulam, M-M and Kramer, L: Disturbances in prosody. A right hemisphere contribution to language. Arch Neurol 38:742–744, 1981.
202a. Weintraub, S, Peavy, G M, O'Connor, M, Johnson N A, Acar D, Guinessey, J and Janssen, I: Three words-Three shapes: A clinical test of memory. J Clin Exp Neuropsychol, in press.
203. Weintraub, S, Powell, D. and Whitla, D: Successful cognitive aging: individual differences among physicians on a computerized test of mental state. J Geriatr Psychiatry 28: 15–34, 1994.
204. Weintraub, S, Rubin, N P and Mesulam, M-M: Primary progressive aphasia. Longitudinal course, neuropsychological profile, and language features. Arch Neurol 47:1329–1335, 1990.
205. Welsh, K A, Butters, N, Hughes, J P, Mohs, R C and Heyman, A: Detection and staging of dementia in Alzheimer's disease. Use of the neuropsychological measures developed for the Consortium to Establish a Registry for Alzheimer's Disease. Arch Neurol 49:448–452, 1992.
206. Welsh, K A, Butters, N, Mohs, R C, Beekly, D, Edland, S, Fillenbaum, G and Heyman, A: The Consortium to Establish a Registry for Alzheimer's Disease (CERAD). Part V. A normative study of the neuropsychological battery. Neurology 44:609–614, 1994.
207. Welsh, K A, Fillenbaum, G, Wilkinson, W, Heyman, A, Mohs, R C, Stern, Y, Harrell, L, Edland, S D and Beekly, D: Neuropsychological test performance in African-American and white patients with Alzheimer's disease. Neurology 45:2207–2211, 1995.
208. Wilkinson, G S: The Wide Range Achievement Test–3. Administration Manual. The Psychological Corporation, San Antonio, Texas, 1993.
209. Williams, S M: Handedness inventories: Edinburgh versus Annett. Neuropsychology 5: 43–48, 1991.
210. Wilson, B A, Cockburn, J and Halligan, P: The Behavioral Inattention Test. Thames Valley Test, Reading, England, 1987.
211. Wilson, R S, Kazniak, A W and Fox, J H: Remote memory in senile dementia. Cortex 17:41–48, 1981.
212. Woodcock, R W and Johnson, M B: Woodcock-Johnson Tests of Achievement. Riverside, Chicago, 1989.
213. Woodcock, R W and Johnson, M B: Woodcock-Johnson Tests of Cognitive Ability. Riverside, Chicago, 1989.
214. Yesavage, J A, Brink, T L, Rose, T L, Lum, O, Huang, V, Adey, M and Leirer, V O: Development and validation of a geriatric depression screening scale: a preliminary report. J Psychiatric Res 17:37–49, 1983.

3

Attentional Networks, Confusional States and Neglect Syndromes

M.-Marsel Mesulam

I. Introduction

In a now lost manuscript written in the fifth-century B.C.E., Empedocles is quoted as having stated that "the nature of God is like a circle of which the center is everywhere and the circumference nowhere." The omnipresence that Empedocles envisaged would have engendered an all-encompassing awareness: Nothing would be ignored, nothing could be brought into sharper focus, all events would be registered in parallel, everything would have full access to instantaneous action, and the global would be identical to the focal. Anything short of such omnipresence creates the need to choose which of many suitable mental or external events will have preferential access to the narrow portals of consciousness and action. "Attention" is a generic term that can be used to designate the entire family of processes that mediate this choice. The presence of attentional modulation is inferred when identical events elicit differential responses according to momentary and reversible shifts in their significance. At the psychological level, attention implies a preferential allocation of processing resources and response channels to events that have become behaviorally relevant. At the neural level, attention refers to alterations in the selectivity, intensity and duration of neuronal responses to such events.

The span of human attention is subject to numerous biological constraints. Sensory organs have narrow beams of optimal acuity which need to be reoriented to focalize events of relevance. Processing capacity is limited and does not permit us to heed more than a tiny fraction of external and internal events at any given time. Access to response channels imposes another bottleneck: We have only two hands and it is usually impossible to simultaneously engage them in two independent tasks. These constraints create a state of constant competition for the scarce processing resources of the central nervous system (CNS). Small brains cope with this type of challenge by shifting the burden of selection to peripheral organs. In the frog, for example, the inner ear is selectively tuned to spectral and temporal properties of species-specific mating calls,[46] and the retinotectal projection contains "bug perceiver" fibers that respond best when a dark object, smaller than a receptive field, enters that field, stops, and moves about intermittently.[199] Although this sort of automatic pattern detection maximizes the limited processing capacity of the CNS, it also restricts the range of events that can be identified and the flexibility with which they become interpreted. The situation is vastly different in more advanced species, especially primates, where the filtering shifts from the periphery to the CNS. The increased complexity of the synaptic pathways involved in this process creates a situation where the same stimulus can elicit intense attentiveness or complete indifference according to context and past experience.

During wakefulness, the individual is bombarded by a great many sensory signals emanating from outside and from within. The inexhaustible supply of memory traces and thought sequences generated by the brain itself provides additional sources of potential stimuli. The part of the stimulus space that is most relevant for achieving goals of immediate importance (and these goals could range from food scavenging to resolving deep ethical dilemmas) keeps shifting from moment to moment in a manner that reflects the inner needs of the individual, the state of the environment, and the experience gained in the past. Attentional modulations select the part of the stimulus space that is to capture the center of awareness while holding the other stimuli, which have now become potential sources of distractibility, at bay—at least temporarily. Aspects of attention-related processes include arousal (the general level of responsivity), orientation (the realignment of sensory organs), selective attention (the preference for some stimuli over others), sustained attention (vigilance), and divided attention (the simultaneous heeding of several events). Attention can be distributed globally or focally, it can act upon stimuli in parallel or serially, and it can be attracted exogenously by external events or directed endogenously by mental phenomena related to motivation and volition.

The work of attention is part of everyday experience. The focusing on one out of many simultaneous conversations in a cocktail party setting or the detection of infrequent blips on a radar screen are paradigmatic activities showing attention at work. Keeping an evolving line of thought in sharp focus, scanning mental content in search of a specific memory or word, resisting distraction, shifting awareness from one sensory modality to another, from one part of the body to another, from one part of the extrapersonal space to another, and from one moment of time to another are among the innumerable manifestations of attention. Orientation, exploration, concentration, and vigilance are positive aspects of attention, whereas distractibility, impersistence, confusion, and neglect reflect attentional deficits. It is not difficult to see why Ferrier,[105] William James,[172] and Sherrington,[322] among others, could have singled out attention not only as the climax of mental integration but also as the most important prerequisite for the manifestation of intellectual and reflective powers.

From the vantage point of psychological processes, the boundaries of attention intersect those of consciousness, arousal, affect, motivation, memory, and perception. The contents of consciousness are determined by the targets of selective attention. The influences of arousal, mood, and motivation on attention are intuitively obvious. Although some might consider arousal and attention virtually synonymous, this can be debated, since attentional deficits can occur in perfectly awake individuals and since extreme levels of arousal—as in pain or terror—may impair the flexibility of attention. Attention may also influence perceptual operations. It is common knowledge among neurologists that sensory examinations are virtually impossible to perform on inattentive subjects. Furthermore, alterations in critical sensory fusion thresholds can arise not only from disturbances along sensory pathways but also from variations in the level of vigilance. Intact attention is also an important requisite for many cognitive processes, especially memory. The relevance of these interactions to the testing of mental state is discussed in Chapter 2.

Attentional modulations can be divided into those that are domain-specific and domain-independent. Visual neurons mediate domain-specific attentional responses to visual stimuli, face neurons to faces, posterior parietal neurons to spatial targets, language areas to words, and so on. Domain-independent modulations are exerted predominantly through the bottom-up influence of the ascending reticular activating system (ARAS) and the top-down influence of the cerebral cortex, especially the frontal lobes (Fig. 3–1). Through these two channels, domain-specific modula-

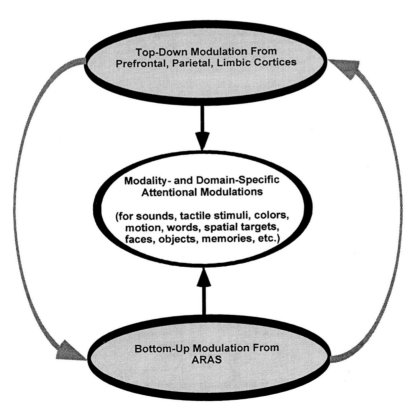

FIGURE 3–1. A schematic representation of the three compartments that regulate the attentional matrix.

tions become responsive to arousal levels, motivational valence, cognitive state, and volition. The overall "attentional matrix" (as reflected by phenomena such as detection efficiency, focusing power, concentration span, vigilance level, novelty-seeking tendencies, resistance to interference, on-line processing capacity, and signal-to-noise ratio) is the collective manifestation of all domain-specific and domain-independent attentional modulations. The clinical syndrome of "acute confusional state" reflects a global impairment of the attentional matrix whereas the syndrome of "spatial neglect" reflects the impairment of a domain-specific system that distributes attention within the extrapersonal space. This chapter reviews these two syndromes and their neurobiological bases.

II. CONFUSIONAL STATES AS DISORDERS OF THE ATTENTIONAL MATRIX

Generalized disturbances of the attentional matrix are part of everyday experience. The behavior that follows a sudden awakening from sleep by an unexpected telephone call is a fairly common example. Although the individual may give the external appearance of being awake, it may be difficult to focus on the telephone conversation, to avoid distractibility, or to organize thought and speech coherently. It may even be difficult to recruit all the information necessary for proper orientation in time and space. What should have been a simple action, such as using a pen to write down a message, suddenly requires undue effort and may result in a great deal of fumbling and perhaps even in a few attempts at writing with the wrong end of the pen. Finding the correct word or controlling immediate but inappropriate response tendencies may prove impossible. If such an individual were administered tests that place a premium on attentional functions, the performance could be quite unflattering. Such an individual can be said to be in an acute confusional state. Naturally, no medical intervention is necessary, since either voluntary mental effort or a few more hours of sleep will effectively reverse all of these difficulties.

Acute confusional states may also arise as pathologic alterations of mental state, especially in patients with a wide variety of toxic and metabolic encephalopathies. This is probably the single most common neurologically based mental-state disturbance that most physicians will see. An acute confusional state is also known as delirium, organic psychosis, or acute organic brain syndrome. It can be defined simply as a change of mental state in which the most salient deficits involve the overall attentional tone. This does not mean that attentional deficits necessarily emerge in isolation. Indeed, patients in acute confusional states commonly have additional cognitive and behavioral disturbances such as memory loss, agitation, and hallucinations. Some of these are secondary to the attentional difficulties, whereas some others may arise independently. It is also important to realize that not all patients with attentional disturbances can automatically be described as being in a confusional state. For example, patients with the typical form of Alzheimer's disease commonly also have attentional difficulties. However, they cannot be said to exhibit a confusional state since the salient feature is amnesia rather than inattention. Many patients in confusional states are also disoriented. However, this is not a necessary feature of the condition, and it is possible to see patients in confusional states who maintain orientation. It is the salience of a global attentional deficit rather than the presence of disorientation that is the sine qua non for the diagnosis of a confusional state. The central role of the attentional disorder in confusional states has been emphasized in many clinical descriptions of this condition.[1,50,98,237] Although most acute confusional states occur in the context of a toxic–metabolic encephalopathy, the two conditions are not synonymous since this syndrome has many other causes.

Clinical Picture

The clinical picture of a patient in an acute confusional state is familiar to most physicians. There are usually no focal neurologic signs of a motor or sensory nature, with the possible exception of a coarse tremor, myoclonus, or asterixis. Attentional deficits arise at several levels of behavior. Vigilance is defective. Attention either wanders aimlessly or is suddenly focused with inappropriate intensity, even if for only a fleeting moment, on an irrelevant stimulus that becomes the source of distractibility. Thought and skilled movement also become vulnerable to interference, impersistence, and perseveration. The patient may volunteer that "concentration" and "thinking straight" require great effort. The stream of thought loses its coherence because of the frequent intrusions by competing thoughts and sensations. Sequences associated with skilled movement, even those as automatic as dialing the telephone or using eating utensils, lose their coherence and show signs of disintegration, perseveration, and impersistence. Tests which assess the various components of sustained attention, divided attention, selective attention, the on-line holding of information (working-memory), inhibition of inappropriate responses, and resistance to distractibility reveal considerable impairment. Thus performance in attentional tasks such as the *Digit Span Test*, the *Stroop Interference Test*, and the *Alternating Sequences Task* (Chapter 2) is impaired. When asked to recite the months of the year in reverse order, the patient may say, "December, November, October, September . . . October, November, December, January," showing the inability to withhold the more customary response tendencies in this test of working memory. This clinical description highlights the three cardinal features of confusional states: (1) disturbance of vigilance, heightened distractibility, and impaired working-memory, (2) inability to maintain a coherent stream of thought, and (3) inability to carry out a sequence of goal-directed movements.

Difficulties in additional aspects of mental function are also common in confusional states. Perceptual distortions may lead to illusions. Hallucinations, ideas of reference, misidentifications of place and people, delusions, and agitation may arise. The patient is often, but not always, disoriented and shows evidence of faulty memory. Mild anomia, dysgraphia, dyscalculia, and constructional deficits are common. Judgment may be faulty, insight appears blunted, and affect is quite labile with a curious tendency for facetious witticism.[50,237] Some of these deficits are probably secondary to attentional difficulties. For example, if the patient is allowed sufficient drilling during the acquisition stage of a learning task, memory improves. Calculations that appear devastated when tested mentally may prove to be quite accurate when the patient is allowed the use of a pencil and paper. Other deficits of mental state, however (e.g., poor judgment and hallucinations), may be affected independently by the underlying pathogen. It is important to realize, however, that in confusional states these additional deficits are usually of lesser importance than the attentional difficulties.

Some confusional states are characterized by apathy; others, especially when related to alcohol, barbiturate, or opiate withdrawal, lead to extreme agitation. In their more severe forms, confusional states may lead to stupor and coma. This gives rise to the widely held opinion that confusional states are disorders of wakefulness and arousal. However, in the early stages of most confusional states attention is impaired out of proportion to the drowsiness, suggesting that the mechanisms of attention are impaired independently. Two other characteristics of confusional states are the rapid fluctuation of mental state that may occur from one hour to the next and the rather typical nocturnal exacerbation (sundowning).

It is important to differentiate confusional states from other conditions such as Wernicke's aphasia, depression, schizophrenia, and dementia. Vigilance may be impossible to assess in patients with Wernicke's aphasia, and the speech output could give the impression of an incoherent stream of thought (Chapter 5). However, the salience of paraphasias in spontaneous speech and the attentiveness with which the patient performs commands aimed at axial musculature (roll over, sit up, close your eyes) differentiate Wernicke's aphasia from confusional states. Depressed patients also have attentional disturbances, but the changes in mood dominate the clinical picture. In contrast, the patient in a confusional state may also be transiently sad and tearful, but this is not sustained over time and the affect lacks associative depth. The hallucinations of the acute confusional state are usually visual whereas those of schizophrenia are usually auditory. The onset late in life and the lack of previous psychiatric history are characteristics of the acute confusional state but not of schizophrenia. Dementia is a descriptive term that refers to a heterogeneous group of patients who have in common a progressive deterioration of cognitive and behavioral faculties (Chapter 10). Some patients with dementia have attentional impairment as the most salient deficit of mental state and can therefore be considered to be in a chronic confusional state. It is also possible to consider a toxic-metabolic confusional state, especially when it lasts for weeks to months, a reversible dementia.

Prevalence, Causes and Pathophysiology

An acute confusional state can occur at any age but its prevalence is higher above the age of 65. Up to 20%–25% of patients above the age of 65 admitted to a general hospital may develop an acute confusional state during the hospital stay.[5] The causes of confusional states can be divided into at least six major groups: *(1)* toxic-metabolic encephalopathies, *(2)* environmental stressors in vulnerable individuals, (3) multifocal brain lesions, (4) epileptic seizures, (5) space-occupying lesions, and (6) focal brain lesions. These pathological factors lead to confusional states through the mediations of at least three different mechanisms: (1) interference with the bottom-up influence of the ARAS on the attentional matrix; (2) interference with the top-down influences of frontal, parietal, and limbic cortices on the attentional matrix; (3) and multifocal partial damage distributed throughout the cerebral cortex in a way that influences all domain-specific attentional modulations.

Confusional states are most commonly caused by *toxic–metabolic encephalopathies*. The adequate function of the central nervous system depends on the metabolic integrity of its constituent neurons and glia. Any condition that interferes with the nutritional requirements, acid–base balance, or electrolyte environment of these cells could interfere with nervous function. It is therefore not surprising that metabolic disturbances ranging from renal insufficiency to hepatic failure, anemia, endocrinopathies, hyperglycemia, anoxia, acidosis, and alkalosis, may each cause an encephalopathy. Withdrawal from alcohol, barbiturates, or opiates as well as the intake of various psychoactive drugs including analgesics, hypnotics, sedatives, tranquilizers, neuroleptics, antidepressants, and antihypertensives can also cause a toxic encephalopathy. Among antihypertensives, the β-blockers are frequently implicated although the objective data establishing such a relationship are not always consistent.[86] In cardiac intensive care units, lidocaine can lead to acute and psychotic confusional states, probably because of its selective activation of the limbic system.[230]

In some of the toxic and metabolic encephalopathies the common denominator appears to be an interference with neurotransmitter action.[101] Toxins and drugs that interfere with cholinergic transmission are particularly apt to produce confusional states. In the surgical service of a general hospital, Tune and associates[349] found that seven of eight patients who developed a postoperative confusional state had serum anticholinesterase activity higher than 1.5 pM atropine equivalents, whereas only four of the 17 patients who were not in a confusional state had levels in that range. Marked anticholinergic activity is a property of numerous traditional neuroleptics, antidepressants, and antihistamines but not of the selective serotonin reuptake inhibitors and newer antipsychotics. Many drugs, alcohol, and several anesthetic agents have their greatest depressant effect on the reticular formation and on high-order association cortex,[165,279] suggesting that these two critical modulators of the attentional matrix may have a selective vulnerability to factors that induce toxic–metabolic encephalopathies.

Environmental stressors such as sensory deprivation (as in cataract surgery), immobilization (as in the treatment of multiple trauma), and interference with circadian rhythms (as in intensive care units) can lead to acute confusional states, especially in the elderly and in those with preexisting neurological diseases. The intensive care and postsurgical settings, especially after cardiotomy, are particularly prone to trigger acute confusional states.[237,327] *Multifocal brain diseases* such as those seen in meningitis, encephalitis, anoxia, vasculitis, disseminated intravascular coagulation, fat embolism, and closed head injury can result in confusional states—especially in the acute period.[56,87] These conditions are characterized by a myriad of small tissue lesions spread throughout the brain. Although none of these lesions is large enough to cause specific impairments such as aphasia, neglect, agnosia, or amnesia, they can collectively cause attentional deficits in multiple domains and lead to the clinical picture of a confusional state.

Patients with *epilepsy* may develop confusional states either postictally or in the course of nonconvulsive complex partial seizures, some of which may be very difficult to record by scalp electrodes.[212] Patients with *space-occupying lesions*, especially subdural hematoma, may come to medical attention in a confusional state. Epilepsy and space-occupying lesions trigger confusional states at least in part because they disrupt the electrical or structural integrity of the ARAS. *Focal brain lesions* in the parahippocampal-fusiform-lingual gyri (on either side of the brain) or in the posterior parietal and inferior prefrontal regions of the right hemisphere can also cause confusional states, probably because they interfere with the top-down modulation of the attentional matrix.[78,160,225,239]

Work-up, Vulnerability, and Clinical Course

An acute confusional state may sometimes be the presenting clinical sign of an underlying disease outside of the CNS. We have seen patients in whom the clinical diagnosis of a confusional state prompted a thorough medical investigation that uncovered occult pulmonary empyema, heart failure, cholecystitis, or even spinal epidural abscess. Patients in a confusional state may not give a coherent history and may show an insensitivity to pain which could interfere with such clinical signs as rebound tenderness or neck stiffness. When the underlying cause is unclear, an extensive search should be undertaken with appropriate blood tests, radiological procedures, and especially lumbar puncture even if the patient is afebrile. Otherwise, reversible disease processes can be missed. When a pronounced confusional state is present and a toxic–metabolic encephalopathy is suspected, an electroencephalogram (EEG) may be helpful. If the EEG is normal, a toxic–metabolic cause can virtually be ruled out and another etiology should be considered.

There are great individual variations in the susceptibility to confusional states induced by toxic–metabolic encephalopathy. In general, the elderly and those with preexisting brain disease—especially dementia—seem more vulnerable to developing acute confusional states in response to even mild metabolic stresses.[200,237] In young patients, only severe toxic–metabolic insults can induce a confusional state, and the removal of the underlying cause results in rapid and dramatic improvement. The elderly, however, are much more vulnerable to milder forms of toxic–metabolic perturbations. In some, improvement may not start for days after the correction of the underlying condition and may last for months (Fig. 3–2). Furthermore, some of these patients may never regain a fully normal mental state despite prolonged improvement. It is not clear why recovery can take so long after the presumptive offending agent has been removed or why it is sometimes incomplete. Perhaps this reflects the state of diminished neural reserve characteristic of the aging brain and also the fact that some toxic–metabolic encephalopathies lead to at least some irreversible neural damage. It is also con-

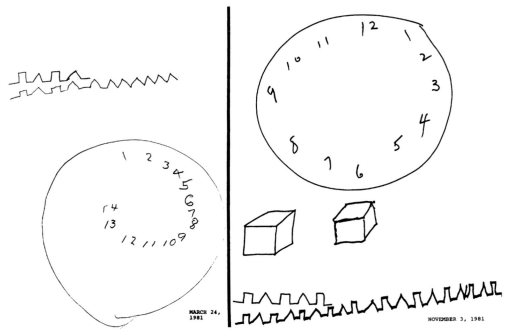

FIGURE 3–2. An 83-year-old man with congestive heart failure developed a confusional state which interfered with all daily living activities. Left: His clock drawing on the day of presentation (March 24, 1981) shows poor planning and marked perseveration. The tracings above the clock show his performance in the alternating sequences task. The very top tracing is the examiner's model. The patient is asked to copy it and then to continue with the same pattern until he reaches the end of the page. The patient performs reasonably well during the copying phase. However, he subsequently cannot resist the immediate response tendency to repeat the segment just drawn. This results in a series of perseverative triangles instead of the alternating square-triangle pattern. Right: The congestive heart failure responded to treatment and disappeared in a matter of a few days. However, the improvement of the confusional state was gradual and took approximately 6 months to reach a plateau. By that time, he was driving and successfully performing customary daily living activities. His performance 7 months later (November 3, 1981) in the alternating sequences and in drawing a clock is much improved. He can even copy a cube reasonably well, a task he had found impossible during the acute episode.

ceivable that individuals who show this pattern of extreme vulnerability and indolent recovery may have a preexisting degenerative brain disease which had not yet reached its full clinical manifestations. In fact, the most florid confusional states take the form of a "beclouded dementia" in patients already afflicted with dementing CNS diseases. Even an occult urinary tract infection may be sufficient to induce a severe exacerbation of mental-state impairment in this group of patients. Although the presence of a preexisting dementia precludes a return to complete normalcy, the treatment of the toxic–metabolic encephalopathy can be very beneficial because it leads to an improvement of the superimposed confusional state.

III. Biology of the Attentional Matrix

More than a hundred years ago, Ferrier[105] and then Bianchi[25] observed that bilateral frontal lobe lesions in macaque monkeys severely impaired attentiveness. These reports generated considerable interest in the relationship of the cerebral cortex to the process of attention. However, the report of Dempsey and Morison[72] in 1942 on the recruiting response obtained by thalamic stimulation, and that of Moruzzi and Magoun[253] in 1949 on EEG desynchronization and the ARAS, rapidly shifted emphasis to the brainstem. Although these workers did not directly conclude that the brainstem was the seat of attention or of consciousness, such an implication subsequently dominated the literature for many years. For example, the landmark experiments of Broadbent[38] and Hernandez-Peón[155] suggested that selective attention was exerted by a peripheral filter that, under the control of the brainstem reticular activating system, inhibited unattended messages at the level of the sensory receptor. Such early selection models of attention have since attracted sharp criticism. For example, it has been shown that complex semantic and affective components of a verbal message strongly influence the effectiveness of selective attention in dichotic listening experiments.[246,347] Since peripheral receptors could not possibly identify such complex aspects of the message, the filter appeared to be located at considerably more downstream components of the neuraxis, perhaps at cortical levels. Today, although vestiges of a predominantly subcortical theory of attention can still be detected, there is an emerging sense that neocortex, thalamus, and brainstem are collectively involved in the modulation of selective attention and that the more complex aspects of this function are executed by neocortical mechanism.

One of the most coherent frameworks for understanding the relationship between cortex and the ARAS in the regulation of attention was proposed by Sokolov.[330] Based on an original observation by Pavlov, Sokolov described an "orienting reflex," which includes an increase in the level of arousal (as denoted by EEG desynchronization and galvanic skin responses), an alignment of sensory receptors toward the source of stimulation, and a facilitation of neural responses to sensory stimuli. Sokolov postulated that this reflex required an interaction between neocortical and brainstem reticular components, the relative contribution of each component varying according to the nature of the stimulus. In the case of painful stimuli, for example, arousal can be elicited directly through the stimulation of the reticular core by collaterals of ascending pathways without much need for cortical participation. The orienting response to a novel stimulus or to a significant word, however, requires initial identification of novelty and significance at neocortical levels. Descending impulses from the cortex are subsequently sent to the reticular formation, which then becomes mobilized to generate the appropriate attentional and arousal tone by influencing thalamic and cortical activity. As repeated exposure to an event decreases its novelty value, an inhibitory signal originates in cortex and dampens the level of reticular core activation, thus leading to habituation. Sokolov's arguments were strengthened by a massive body of evidence showing that cortical lesions markedly interfered with the habituation of the orienting response, especially when the stimulus was particularly complex.[208, 320, 330]

Figure 3–1 outlines an organization which is also based on pivotal interactions between the cerebral cortex and the ARAS. According to this model, virtually all parts of the cerebral cortex participate in attentional modulation although no neuron is necessarily dedicated to this function. Attentional functions are thus distributed, just as memory storage is distributed. Every cortical area appears to support attentional modulation in its own domain of specialization in a way that maintains the fidelity of the initial encoding. These domain-specific modulations are then subjected to two regulatory influences—the bottom-up influence of the ARAS and top-down influence of heteromodal and limbic cortices.

Domain-specific Attentional Modulation in the Cerebral Cortex

Domain-specific attentional modulations can be detected at all levels of the cerebral cortex. Neural responses in primary auditory and visual cortex of the cat, for example, increase when the animal attends to the source of stimulation or when it is aroused by a pinch of the tail.[163,202] In the primary somatosensory cortex of monkeys, the behavioral relevance of a vibratory stimulus influences neuronal responsivity.[167] When human subjects are asked to make a difficult discrimination in one of three simultaneously presented modalities, the primary area in the attended modality shows the most activation, indicating the presence of attentional enhancement even at the first cortical synapse of sensory pathways.[304]

The attentional modulations in primary sensory cortex are relatively modest when compared to those seen at the more downstream synaptic relays of sensory pathways.[166,167,190,320] Neurons in movement-sensitive visual association areas MT (V5) and MST, for example, give distinctly enhanced responses to dots moving in their preferred direction if the animal is engaged in a task that requires attentiveness to the moving stimuli.[348] Furthermore, visual association neurons in V4 and inferotemporal cortex display larger and more selective responses to attended visual stimuli, and such response enhancements are associated with improved performance in the behavioral task.[113,335]

Modality-specific modulations have also been observed in tasks of selective attention where optimal performance necessitates the suppression of the unattended input channels. In a mental arithmetic task performed on a background of auditory distractors, the filtering of the irrelevant auditory input was associated with decreased activity in auditory association cortices.[117] Furthermore, selective attention to visual stimuli led to decreased activity in auditory and somatosensory association cortices.[323] In the monkey, neurons in V4 and inferotemporal visual association cortex (but not in primary visual area V1) show a dramatic reduction of responses to unattended visual stimuli within their receptive fields, indicating that this part of visual association cortex may play a role in filtering out irrelevant information.[245] In fact, monkeys with inferotemporal lesions show learning deficits caused by an inability to ignore irrelevant visual information, and a similar condition may exist in the human as illustrated by a patient who displayed excessive visual distractibility following an infarct of the visual association areas in the right temporal lobe.[229,332]

When subjects who were exposed to concurrent visual, auditory, and somato-sensory stimulation were asked to ignore two of the modalities while making a difficult discrimination in the third, the unimodal association area in the attended modality displayed the most activation.[304] However, the association cortices in the two deliberately ignored modalities continued to display some activation as well, showing that attentional filtering is unlikely to follow a strict "early selection" pattern and that it occurs on a representation that has already been subjected to considerable cortical processing. Such "late selection" would tend to increase the flexibility of attentional modulation when compared to an arrangement where the unattended channel is prevented from accessing the cerebral cortex.

Domain-specific attentional effects can also be identified in cortical areas specialized for more complex functions such as face and object recognition, spatial attention, and language. When compared to a passive viewing condition, for example, the attentive examination of faces (but not of houses) increased the activation of the fusiform face area.[370] In the inferior parietal lobule, neurons give enhanced responses to behaviorally relevant extrapersonal targets that are likely to attract visual and manual grasp but not to neutral stimuli at identical spatial locations.[40,227] Furthermore, words at an attended location elicit greater P300 responses in the posterior parts of the left hemisphere, suggesting that language cortex gives enhanced neural responses to attended words.[218]

Modality- and domain-specific attentional modulations are also seen in conjunction with working memory and novelty-seeking behaviors. Working memory is a special type of attentional process which enables the on-line holding of information. In a typical task of working memory, also known as delayed matching to sample, a monkey is first briefly shown a sample cue (a color, pattern, or location), exposed to a variable delay, and rewarded for responding to a subsequent test stimulus only if it matches the sample. The crucial component of working memory is the delay period of up to 20 seconds, during which the animal has to maintain an on-line mental representation of a cue which is no longer visible. Each part of unimodal association cortex seems to participate in the maintenance of working memory in its own area of specialization. For example, neurons with increased activity during delay periods are seen in inferotemporal cortex in experiments where the stimuli are colors or visual patterns and in posterior parietal cortex when the stimuli are spatial locations.[58, 111] Furthermore, working-memory performance in visual and auditory tasks is severely impaired after damage to visual and auditory unimodal association cortices, even when the lesions leave sensory abilities in the relevant modality relatively intact.[57,159]

Preferential attention to novel events is one of the most characteristic features of the primate brain. In humans, sensory deprivation and monotony induce restlessness and even vivid hallucinations.[156] Monkeys will work hard in a setting where the only reward is a peek through a window, and human subjects who are given a choice between familiar and simple versus novel and complex patterns will consistently spend more time viewing the latter.[22,41] Nearly all cortical areas respond preferentially to novel stimuli in their specific domains of specialization. In the monkey, inferotemporal neurons give greater responses to the sight of unfamiliar objects and show decremental responses to repeated presentations of the same geometric shape.[39,99] Furthermore, face-responsive inferotemporal cells alter their firing to a face as it becomes more familiar.[306] In the human brain, enhanced responses to novel visual events are quite conspicuous in V4 and the fusiform gyrus.[346]

Despite the presence of these anatomically segregated domain-specific attentional modulations, however, domain-specific attentional deficits are relatively rare in clinical practice. The reason for this apparent discrepancy is probably based on the fact that focal lesions, such as those caused by occlusive cerebrovascular lesions, lead to syndromes of aphasia, amnesia, or prosopagnosia, thus precluding the assessment of attentional functions in the pertinent domains. Unilateral neglect presents an exception to this pattern because it is the outcome of damage to a network which targets extrapersonal events for spatial representation and action. As shown later, unilateral focal damage to components of this network gives rise to a domain-specific impairment of spatial attention.

In contrast to cerebrovascular lesions which tend to cause a relatively complete but focal destruction of the afflicted area, toxic–metabolic encephalopathies induce a state of partial dysfunction in many parts of the cerebral cortex. Partial lesions are expected to trigger neural processing inefficiencies that can interfere with attentional modulations in the relevant domains. The multifocal but partial lesions induced by toxic–metabolic encephalopathy can thus collectively lead to multiple domain-specific attentional impairments and to the emergence of confusional states.

Domain-specific attentional impairments in memory and language could potentially arise in conjunction with partial lesions such as those associated with degenerative diseases. At the early stages of Alzheimer's disease, for example, neurofibrillary degeneration is confined to the limbic system, where it involves only some of the neurons (Chapter 10). At these initial stages, the patient tends to experience fluctuating inefficiencies of memory retrieval. This retrieval deficit could be conceptualized as a domain-specific disorder in the attentive scanning and activation of internal data stores related to declarative memory. Similarly, the initial stages of primary progressive aphasia are associated with partial lesions within the language network. At these stages of the disease, the patient cannot name an object but can point to it when the correct name is provided by the examiner. This one-way anomia could represent an attentional disorder confined to the internal activation of lexical linkages. This interpretation is supported by the observation that an object which cannot be named at one moment may be named successfully a few minutes later, indicating that the failure stems from an inability to selectively activate existing lexical associations.

This brief survey shows that each cortical area can display attentional modulations in the modalities and domains for which it is specialized. Attention to a given event is not encoded by a special group of dedicated neurons but by modulations in the activity of neurons normally involved in the processing of the relevant category or modality. Such modulations are much more prominent in downstream and transmodal parts of association cortex, where they help to construct a personally edited representation of the world based on significance rather than appearance. The magnitude and timing of these domain-specific attentional modulations are influenced by domain-independent regulatory neurons located in the ARAS and high-order association cortices.

The Ascending Reticular Activating System (ARAS)—Bottom-up Modulation of Attentional Tone

The ARAS contains two major axes:

1. A reticulothalamocortical pathway, the activation of which promotes cortical arousal by facilitating the transthalamic passage of sensory information towards the cerebral cortex. Acetylcholine is the major transmitter along the reticulothalamic component of this pathway and excitatory amino acids are the transmitters along the thalamocortical component. The intralaminar and reticular nuclei are the thalamic components most closely associated with this axis of the ARAS.

2. Transmitter-specific extrathalamic pathways which originate in the brainstem and basal forebrain and which send direct projections to the cerebral cortex. The brainstem components include dopaminergic projections from the substantia nigra–ventral tegmental area, serotonergic projections from the raphe nuclei, and noradrenergic projections from the nucleus locus coeruleus. The basal forebrain components include cholinergic and GABAergic pathways which originate in the nucleus basalis. Collectively these pathways exert a major influence on all aspects of arousal and attentional modulation (Chapter 1).

The ARAS exerts a domain-independent global influence upon attentional modulation without displaying any selectivity for sensory modality or cognitive domain. Its relevance to human attention was shown in a functional imaging experiment where the transition from relaxed wakefulness to intense attentiveness was associated with the activation of the midbrain reticular formation and the intralaminar thalamic nuclei.[187] The ARAS was one of the first neural systems to be investigated systematically from the vantage point of behavioral physiology. Soon after the introduction of EEG recording, spontaneous electrical rhythms were found to be very sensitive to levels of consciousness and attentional states. High-voltage slow waves, for example, were associated with drowsiness and certain sleep states, whereas desynchronized fast activity was associated with arousal, excitement, attentiveness, and rapid eye movement (REM) sleep. The pacemakers for these EEG rhythms were found to be located in components of the ARAS such as the brainstem reticular formation, the thalamus, and the nucleus basalis.[232]

Neurons in the midbrain reticular core and in the intralaminar thalamic nuclei tend to have higher firing rates during states of EEG desynchronization (waking and REM sleep) than during slow-wave sleep.[122,339–341] The firing rates decrease just before the appearance of the first EEG spindles during the transition from waking to sleep and increases just before EEG desynchronization and behavioral waking. Increased activity in these midbrain reticular neurons is correlated with a facilitation of the transthalamic transmission of sensory information toward the cerebral cortex and with an increased depolarization of cortical output neurons. The activity of these brainstem pacemakers and the concurrent desynchronization of the EEG thus correspond to a state where sensory events can have a greater impact upon cortical circuitry and also where the cortex has an enhanced readiness for efferent responses. Damage to these brainstem neurons leads to permanent states of stupor and coma.[286] Neuronal activity in the midbrain reticular core is high not only during wakefulness but also during REM sleep. Some have argued that REM sleep is characterized by intense attentiveness to internal rather than external stimuli, but this is a difficult hypothesis to test. A more cautious interpretation suggests that the activation of the midbrain reticular core is necessary but not sufficient for wakefulness and attentiveness.

In a task where monkeys had to emit a rapid bar press to a visual cue in order to obtain reward, the shortest reaction times occurred within a restricted range of multiunit activity in the mesencephalic reticular formation.[125] This range was above the level of activity seen during slow-wave sleep but below the level seen in states of extreme arousal such as startle. However, not all reaction times that occurred within this range of midbrain activity were short. These experiments suggested that there may be an inverted-U relationship between reticular activity and reaction times and that reticular formation activity within the optimal range is necessary but not sufficient for rapid responses indicative of attentiveness. The activity of neurons in the reticular formation of monkeys engaged in a fixed foreperiod go–no-go task showed systematic changes in activity 543 ± 246 ms prior to the presentation of the cue and returned to control levels after the cue.[293] The suggestion was made that these neurons could encode an anticipatory set for the temporal and spatial shifting of selective attention. Taken together, these studies suggest that the neurons of the brainstem reticular core may influence not only the maintenance of wakefulness but also the fine tuning of attentional tone during wakefulness.

The brainstem reticular core receives collaterals from a large number of ascending and descending pathways in a way that would enable it to integrate a wide spectrum of neural information related to the extrapersonal world and the internal milieu.[313] The ARAS influences the cerebral cortex both directly and also through thalamic relays. The projection from the brainstem to the thalamus is mostly cholinergic and originates from the pedunculopontine and laterodorsal tegmental nuclei of the brainstem reticular formation.[234] The activation of this cholinergic projection tends to promote the transfer of information from the thalamus to the cerebral cortex. The cholinergic innervation from the reticular formation reaches all thalamic nuclei but is particularly intense within the intralaminar, reticular, and limbic nuclei.[144,291] The pathways emanating from the intralaminar nuclei are widely distributed within the cerebral cortex (as opposed to the much more focal projections of sensory relay nuclei), tend to favor layer I, can have a widespread and bilateral influence on cortical activity, and may modulate signal-to-noise ratios during attentional focusing and sensory discrimination.[291]

The reticular nucleus of the thalamus receives projections from the brainstem and cerebral cortex but does not project back to the cerebral cortex.[177] It gives rise to GABAergic projections which inhibit the activity of the other thalamic nuclei.[132] Cholinergic innervation has an excitatory influence upon all thalamic nuclei except for the reticular nucleus, where it exerts an inhibitory effect. Stimulation of the cholinergic projection from the brainstem to the thalamus thus releases the specific thalamic nuclei from the inhibition of the reticular nucleus at the same time that it activates them directly. The descending projections from the cerebral cortex to the reticular nucleus are excitatory and therefore suppress thalamocortical transmission. These characteristics suggest that the reticular nucleus may act as an attentional valve for regulating thalamocortical transmission according to the integrated influence of the cortex and the brainstem reticular core.

It should be pointed out that the brainstem core and the nucleus reticularis thalami share the designation "reticular" by accident rather than by design. According to Meyer,[240] the thalamic reticular nucleus had already been designated the "stratum reticulatum" by Arnold in 1838, whereas the brainstem core received the designation "formatio reticularis" by Deiters in 1865 and by Forel in 1877—without any implication of common function. Although the traditional view tends to associate the connectivity of the intralaminar and reticular nuclei with the designations of "diffuse" and "nonspecific," modern neuroanatomical methods have shown that their projections obey a topographical organization. Perhaps the word "widespread" would provide a better characterization of these projections.

The ARAS contains transmitter-specific pathways which innervate the cerebral cortex without a thalamic relay. As reviewed in Chapter 1, these pathways include noradrenergic projections from the nucleus locus coeruleus, serotonergic projections from the raphe nuclei, dopaminergic connections from the substantia nigra–ventral tegmental area, cholinergic and GABAergic projections from the nucleus basalis of Meynert, and probably also histaminergic projections from the hypothalamus. Each of these pathways has a specific influence upon the surface EEG and attentional behaviors.

The cholinergic projection from the nucleus basalis, for example, is necessary to maintain arousal-related low voltage fast activity in the surface EEG.[353] Inhibiting cholinergic neurotransmission interferes with numerous attention-related processes such as spatial working memory, the generation of novelty-related P300 potentials, covert shifts of spatial attention, and performance in sustained attention tasks.[82,138,337,354] Changes in the activity of neurons in the nucleus locus coeruleus and the brainstem raphe are also closely correlated with changes in EEG activity, usually preceding them by several seconds.[202,353] The neurons of the nucleus locus coeruleus fire slowly during drowsiness and slow-wave sleep and in rapid bursts during wakefulness and REM sleep.[51] Noradrenaline increases the postsynaptic evoked response relative to spontaneous activity, thus enhancing the signal-to-noise ratio in neural transmission.[251] Agents that increase central noradrenergic activity, such as dextroamphetamine enhances attentiveness whereas noradrenergic depletion alters the focusing of attention and novelty-seeking behaviors.[37,292,318]

The electrical stimulation of the serotonergic brainstem raphe neurons can induce an arousal-related pattern of low-voltage fast activity in the cerebral cortex.[90] Serotonergic agonists reduce distractibility in a two-choice runway task, suggesting that serotonin may modulate the sensory gating of behaviorally relevant cues in the environment.[33] Dopaminergic projections to the prefrontal cortex promote working memory, and the dopaminergic cells of the substantia nigra–ventral tegmental area are selectively responsive to motivationally relevant stimuli and to cues that signal their existence.[110,124,316] Histaminergic projections from the hypothalamus to the cerebral cortex have been implicated in the regulation of cortical arousal.[356] These extrathalamic components of the ARAS provide a set of parallel channels which collectively influence almost all aspects of attentional modulation in all parts of the cerebral cortex. Pathological conditions which interfere with the functions of the ARAS, but which are not severe enough to cause stupor or coma, can thus disrupt attentional functions throughout the cerebral cortex and may give rise to generalized (domain-independent) attentional deficits with clinical characteristics of confusional states.

Frontal Lobes and the Top-Down Modulation of Attention

Parietal, limbic, and especially prefrontal cortices mediate the top-down modulation of attentional responses in ways that are sensitive to context, motivation, acquired significance, and conscious volition. The metabolic activation of prefrontal and posterior parietal cortex is a common correlate of almost all attentional tasks, regardless of modality or domain. In one experiment, for example, a task of sustained attention (vigilance) led to the activation of the superior parietal lobule and of prefrontal cortex in Brodmann areas (BA) 8, 9, 44, and 46 regardless of the sensory modality that was used for stimulation.[270] In another experiment, sustained attention led to inferior parietal lobule (BA40) activation whereas divided attention was associated with prefrontal (BA46) activation.[175] In a selective attention task where one of three modalities had to be attended and the other two ignored, prefrontal activation occurred regardless of the modalities that were ignored or attended.[304] These observations suggest that prefrontal and posterior parietal cortices exert a top-down influence upon all types of domain-specific attentional modulations in a manner that may mediate the volitional regulation of the attentional focus.

As noted above, many cortical areas display modulations related to working memory in their specific domain of specialization. Prefrontal and posterior parietal cortices, however, influence working memory in all domains (Chapter 1). Thus, in delayed-matching-to-sample tasks, prefrontal neurons display delay firing for faces, inanimate objects, and spatial locations. An individual prefrontal neuron responsive to the presentation of a cue is usually also the one that displays the delay activity, as if it were prolonging the attentional focusing on the cue even when it is no longer part of ambient reality. One of the most remarkable properties of these prefrontal neurons is a resistance to interference. For example, in an A•B•C•D•A paradigm (where the cue and its match are separated by distractors), a prefrontal neuron which is known to emit a selective delay activity following the presentation of A continues to show high delay activity after B, C, and D and maintains it until the reappearance of A.[75] Prefrontal neurons may therefore play a critical role in protecting the contents of working memory from distraction. Lesions of prefrontal cortex in the monkey impair performance in all types of working memory tasks and also decrease the selectivity of delay activity in other parts of the cerebral cortex, suggesting that domain-specific working memory activities are subject to top-down modulations emanating from prefrontal cortex.[75,112]

The importance of the human prefrontal cortex to working memory had been inferred from cases of brain damage and was confirmed more than 25 years ago by a functional imaging experiment which found that reverse digit span tasks resulted in hemodynamic activations that were maximal over the frontal lobes.[295] Since then, numerous studies have reconfirmed the presence of domain-independent frontal lobe activation during working-memory tasks based on verbal, perceptual, and spatial stimuli.[106,219] Working memory is usually divided into two groups of processes: the on-line maintenance of information and its active manipulation. The latter aspect is attributed to the function of a "central executive" agency. In human subjects, tasks which emphasize the executive aspects of working memory elicit the preferential activation of prefrontal dorsolateral cortex whereas tasks based on the on-line maintenance of information elicit the activation of both prefrontal cortex and posterior parietal cortex.[53,65,194]

As noted above, many areas of the brain give enhanced responses to novel or unexpected events within their specific domain of specialization. The frontal lobe plays a particularly critical role in this realm of function and influences novelty-related activity in all realms of processing. Damage to frontal cortex, for example, induces a placid disinterest in the environment. Furthermore, the P300 response elicited by novel or deviant stimuli is critically dependent on the integrity of prefrontal cortex; an N2–P3 response which is maximal over prefrontal cortex appears to determine the attentional resources that will be allocated to novel events; and the region of the frontal eye fields belongs to a distributed network specialized for exploring the extrapersonal space and seeking motivationally relevant targets.[67,191,227]

Mood and motivation strongly influence the allocation of attentional resources. The degree of hunger, for example, enhances the response of the orbitofrontal taste area to food items.[305] Many of these mood- and motivation-related modulations are mediated through top-down projections emanating from limbic structures (Chapter 1). For example, amygdaloid activity modulates the response of extrastriate visual cortex to faces displaying certain types of emotional expression.[249] Limbic structures can thus induce widespread attentional modulations which modify the impact of sensory events according to their emotional and motivational relevance. Other limbic structures such as the cingulate gyrus may also exert a generalized influence on attentional modulation.[280a] Thus, selective and divided attention elicit anterior cingulate activation regardless of the stimulus modality, and cingulate activation is associated with improved performance in tasks of vigilance and spatial atten-tion.[60,63,186,259]

In addition to limbic areas, prefrontal and parietal cortices also participate in mediating the effect of motivation upon neural responses. Identical sensory stimuli, for example, can elicit dramatically different responses from lateral prefrontal neurons when their relationships to reward are altered.[310] Furthermore, an arbitrary sensory cue elicits greater responses from dorsolateral prefrontal neurons when it signals the impending delivery of a preferred food item such as a piece of apple or cabbage than when it signals a less favorite food such as a raisin.[358] In posterior parietal cortex, neurons increase firing as the animal looks at food when hungry and liquid when thirsty.[206]

Limbic, parietal, and prefrontal cortices can thus collectively modulate the neural impact (and, hence, attentional valence) of sensory events. These regions are in a position to exert a global top-down influence on attentional modulations in all modalities and domains. Damage to these parts of the brain may thus provide another setting for the emergence of multiple attentional deficits and may explain why focal lesions in prefrontal cortex, posterior parietal cortex, and medial temporal cortex cause acute confusional states.[160,225,239]

The reticular nucleus of the thalamus receives projections from all cortical areas, including the prefrontal and posterior parietal cortex. Furthermore, the nuclei which give rise to the transmitter-specific extrathalamic corticopetal pathways of the ARAS receive cortical projections from components of the limbic system. The sources of top-down attentional modulation shown in Figure 3–1 can therefore also influence the sources of bottom-up modulation emanating from the ARAS. In turn, the components of the ARAS also innervate the prefrontal, parietal, and limbic cortices, and can thus exert a reciprocal influence upon the top-down modulation of the attentional matrix.

The top-down control of the attentional matrix by prefrontal and parietal cortices displays a pattern of right hemisphere specialization. Thus, sustained and divided attention tasks in any sensory modality elicit greater activation in the right posterior parietal and prefrontal cortices.[175,270] Furthermore, the posterior parietal or prefrontal lesions that give rise to confusional states are almost always located in the right hemisphere.[103,131,239,278] Support for the specialization of the right hemisphere in the regulation of the attentional matrix has been gathered from several additional sources. First, simple reaction times to ipsilateral visual stimuli are faster with the left hand.[10] Second, patients with right hemisphere lesions are more likely to have bilateral deficits in reaction times.[162] Third, in split-brain patients, vigilance is more effective when the task is being mediated by the right hemisphere.[85] Fourth, patients with right hemisphere damage show less physiological arousal (as measured by galvanic skin responses) to sensory stimulation than patients with equivalent damage to the left hemisphere.[147,252] As will be shown, a similar pattern of right hemispheric specialization can also be identified in the domain of spatial attention.

IV. NEGLECT SYNDROMES AS DISORDERS OF SPATIAL ATTENTION

A most important aspect of selective attention is the ability to shift the focus of awareness from one extrapersonal event to another. The neural systems associated with this function would be expected to face sensory–motor as well as cognitive challenges. The sensory–motor challenge is based on the innumerable ways in which the position of the target can shift with respect to the limbs, trunk, and sensory organs. If the eyes move, for example, there is a shift in the retinal representation of the target although its relationship to the body and limbs remains the same. If the trunk rotates in the absence of head and eye movements, the target will maintain its retinal representation but will need to elicit a different trajectory to be grasped by the hand. The neural structures that control visuospatial attention must therefore translate retinocentric information into body-centered and spatial frames of reference so that the pertinent events can become targeted for effective focusing, exploration, and action.

The distribution of spatial attention also entails complex cognitive processes for detecting motivational relevance, compiling mental representations, planning search strategies, and volitionally shifting the attentional focus from one target to another. Although shifts of spatial attention imply overt redirections of the attentional focus within the extrapersonal space, such shifts can also occur covertly as in the process of attending to the periphery without moving the eyes or of mentally planning a route for reaching a familiar destination. A flexible zooming of the attentional span from a global to a local perspective is another essential component of spatial attention. In everyday experience, for example, a global sort of awareness encompasses much of the ambient extrapersonal space and allows the rapid (automatic) detection of deviance from uniformity, as in the case of a windswept piece of paper entering the peripheral field of view while driving, or the emergence of a rustling sound behind the head while immersed in a book. The subsequent narrowing (focalization) of the attentional focus and its redirection to the relevant event for more detailed exploration can occur covertly without any head or eye deviation or overtly through a reorientation of the sense organs and limbs. In addition to such reflexive shifts triggered by exogenous events, the movement of the attentional focus can also be initiated endogenously, as in the anticipation of impending events or in the course of searching for missing objects.

Each of these sensory–motor and cognitive aspects of spatial attention becomes severely impaired in patients with the syndrome of contralesional unilateral neglect. Severe contralesional neglect occurs almost exclusively after right hemisphere lesions, so the clinical examples below will be confined to patients with left neglect. Under normal circumstances, the probability of attracting attention tends to be determined by the novelty or significance of an event, irrespective of its location. In the neglect syndrome, the probability of attracting attention, entering awareness, influencing mental representations, or becoming a target for action decreases in proportion to the relative leftness of an event or response. Events that appear to be neglected, however, may nevertheless exert an implicit influence on numerous aspects of cognitive function. Neglect is said to exist when the impact of sensory events upon explicit behaviors displays a spatially addressed bias that cannot be explained by elementary sensory–motor deficits.

Many models of neglect have been proposed, ranging from the phenomenological to the computational. Few, if any, have been able to account for the entire spectrum of clinical manifestations, leading some authors to question the existence of an identifiable neglect syndrome. Contrary to some of the models that have been proposed in the past, it is becoming increasingly clear that neglect cannot be attributed to a unitary deficit of arousal, orientation, representation, or intention. Instead it reflects the collective and interactive outcome of multiple impairments encompassing all of these processes. As in the case of aphasia and amnesia, neglect is a "network syndrome." It represents damage to one or more components of a distributed network where each component has a different pattern of physiological and anatomical specialization. The following account reviews the clinical, neuropsychological, and physiological bases of the neglect syndrome from the vantage point of a distributed neurocognitive network located along the dorsal sensory–fugal streams of processing reviewed in Chapter 1 and revolving around cortical epicenters in the posterior parietal cortex, frontal eye fields, and cingulate gyrus.

The Neuropsychology of Neglect

The left neglect syndrome is characterized by a reduction of neural resources that can be mobilized by sensory events located on the left and by motor plans directed to the left. When the neglect is severe, the patient may behave as if one-half of the universe had abruptly ceased to exist in any meaningful form. One patient may shave, groom, and dress only the right side of the body; another may fail to eat food placed on the left side of the tray; another may omit to read the left side of words printed anywhere on the page; still another may fail to copy detail on the left side of a drawing and may show a curious tendency to leave an uncommonly wide margin on the left when asked to write (Fig. 3–3). When the examiner approaches the bed from the neglected left side and initiates a conversation, the patient may briskly orient to the right side and initiate a fruitless but determined search for the source of the voice. Even without specific stimulation, some patients display a tonic rotation toward the right side of the bed, as if in response to the irresistible magnetism exerted by events located on the right.

In other patients, the unilateral neglect is much more subtle and might not be detected by observation of spontaneous behavior. In those cases, it may be necessary to use specialized bedside maneuvers such as bilateral simultaneous stimulation or target cancellation tasks in order to reveal the presence of neglect. Although the most dramatic and observable aspects of neglect occur in the visual sphere, the phenomenon can be multimodal, so the patient may also display a rightward bias during the detection of auditory, somatosensory, and even olfactory targets. Many patients with unilateral neglect may also have hemianopia, hemihypesthesia, or hemiparesis. However, the possibility that neglect is caused by a combination of elementary sensory-motor deficits can be dismissed on the basis of several obser-

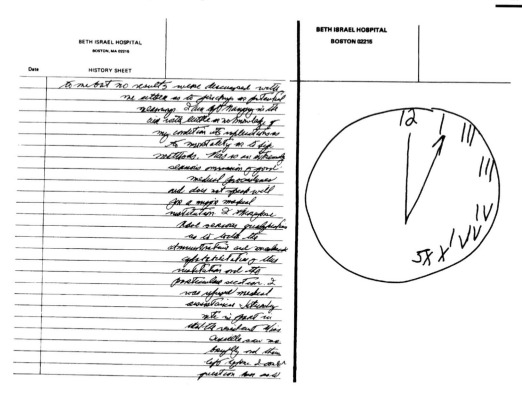

FIGURE 3–3. This figure shows two characteristic manifestations of unilateral neglect. Left: A spontaneous writing sample from a 55-year-old right-handed man who developed left unilateral neglect following a right temporoparietal infarct. The margin on the left side of the sheet is uncommonly wide and indicates the presence of neglect. Right: This clock was drawn by a 47-year-old right-handed airline pilot who developed left unilateral neglect following a subarachnoid hemorrhage. In addition to a tendency for perseveration, the clock drawing shows marked neglect of the left side.

vations. The extent of sensory loss, for example, does not correlate with the severity of neglect.[47,114,148,369] In fact, while some patients with a homonymous hemianopia neglect the blind field, others show no neglect or even a compensatory over-exploration of the blind side.[16] Hemianopia is thus neither necessary nor sufficient for the emergence of neglect (Fig. 3–4). Furthermore, left-sided neglect sometimes encompasses olfactory stimuli although primary olfactory pathways are uncrossed and the olfactory inattention should have occurred on the right rather than the left side if primary sensory loss, however subtle, had been responsible for the deficit.[21,227] Hemiparesis is another factor which is not essential since patients show neglect for the left side even when they are asked to use the intact right limb during tasks of manual exploration. Unilateral neglect may also occur in the absence of any perceptible limitation of eye movements, so gaze paresis is not a necessary component either. Neglect is therefore not a disorder of seeing, hearing, or moving but one of looking, detecting, listening, and exploring. Neuropsychological tests

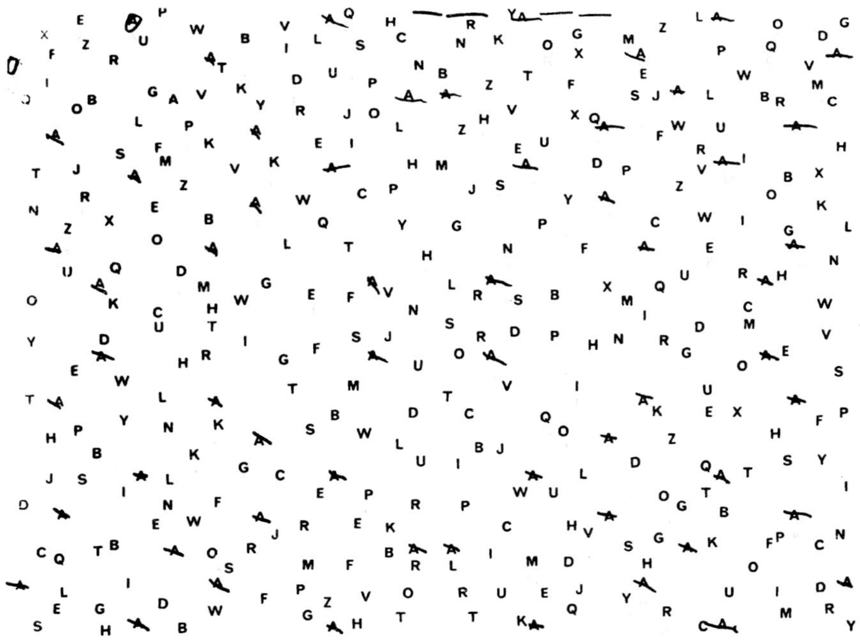

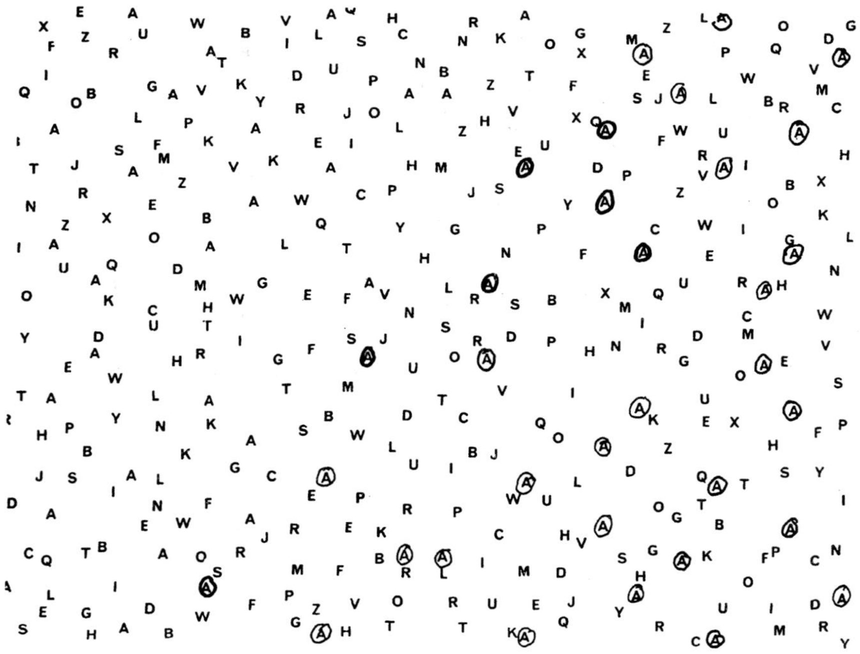

help to classify neglect behaviors into sensory–representational, motor–exploratory, and limbic–motivational components.[228] No test is absolutely specific for assessing a single component of neglect. However, each of the tests described below emphasizes one of these three behavioral components more than the other two.

REPRESENTATIONAL (PERCEPTUAL) COMPONENT OF NEGLECT—EXTINCTION,
LINE BISECTION, MENTAL VISUALIZATION AND COVERT SHIFTS OF ATTENTION

Patients with unilateral neglect behave as if sensory events within the left extrapersonal hemispace had lost their impact on awareness, especially when competing events are present on the right side. This aspect of neglect can be probed with tests of extinction, line bisection, and covert attentional shifts. Extinction is said to exist when patients who respond accurately to unilateral stimulation from either side consistently ignore the stimulation on the left under conditions of bilateral simultaneous stimulation. If extinction occurs in only one modality, it can conceivably reflect a subtle disruption of relevant sensory pathways or even a callosal disconnection syndrome.[97,333] However, multimodal extinction almost always reflects the representational aspect of neglect.

Extinction can be quantified by measuring the critical difference in size, brightness, loudness, or duration which overcomes the neglect. In the bedside setting, for example, extinction based on the traditional bilateral presentation of moving fingers can be overcome in some cases if the magnitude of the left sided stimulus is intensified by moving the whole hand or the whole arm. In some patients, the tendency for extinction may be so powerful that the mere presence of ambient visual input on the right may elicit left neglect. In such cases, even unilateral stimuli on the left may appear to be ignored, raising the possibility of a hemianopia. It may be useful to test these patients in a darkened room where brief flashes of light can be presented as stimuli, allowing the examiner to make a more definitive distinction between neglect and hemianopia. Extinction can occur in any sensory modality but intermodality dissociations constitute the rule rather than the exception. Extinction can also be cross-modal. For example, contralesional tactile extinction in the hand may be elicited by ipsilesional visual stimulation, especially if the visual stimulation is presented close to the hand.[81]

The line bisection test offers one of the most versatile methods for assessing

FIGURE 3–4. This figure shows the performance of two different patients on the random-letter cancellation task. An 8 × 10 sheet of paper containing 15 A's in each quadrant is placed directly in front of the patient, who is then asked to check or encircle all the A's without moving the sheet of paper. Top: A 59-year-old right-handed woman suffered a left-sided stroke that left her with a dense right homonymous hemianopia. Despite the blind right hemifield, she does not miss any targets on the right. Bottom: A right-handed woman in her 70s had an infarct in the right frontal region. She developed a hemiparesis. Visual field testing did not reveal any hemianopia. However, she has marked neglect for targets on the left. These two patients demonstrate that there is no obligatory relationship between hemianopia and unilateral neglect.

unilateral neglect. In the traditional version, patients are asked to mark the mid-point of a horizontal line drawn on a sheet of paper. Neurologically intact subjects tend to place the bisection mark slightly left of the true center. Patients with left hemineglect tend to place their mark rightward of center (Fig. 3–5 left). The magnitude of the rightward deviation is monotonically related to the length of the line although the proportionality constant varies from patient to patient.[244,258] This relationship to total length implies that the sensory information from the entire line is being apprehended and that the neglect is a postsensory phenomenon directed to an internal representation. In fact, patients with left hemianopia but no hemineglect tend to bisect the line leftward of center (probably as a compensatory strategy), showing that the rightward deviation in the bisection does not arise from a lack of sensory input from the left side.[16]

The rightward bisection error suggests that the left side of the line is being underestimated (neglected) by the patient. It is as if the representational salience of the left side becomes diminished and that it takes a greater length of line on the left to balance the salience of a shorter segment on the right. Confirmation for this interpretation comes from two variants of the line bisection task. In the "landmark" test where the task is to point to the shorter side of a correctly prebisected line, patients with left hemineglect choose the left side as the shorter, indicating its lesser salience.[140] In another task, where patients are required to set the end points of an imaginary horizontal line on the basis of a dot that is to be considered as its midpoint, patients with left neglect place the end points so as to make the left segment longer, as if more distance is needed on the left to match the salience of a shorter distance on the right.[30]

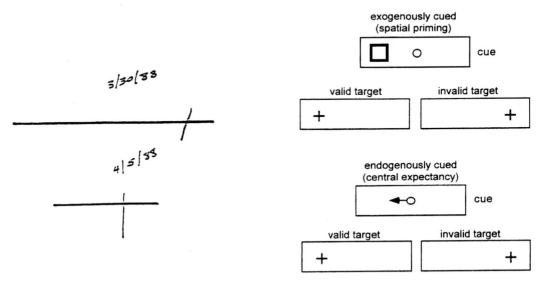

FIGURE 3–5. Left: Line bisection at two points in time by a patient with right hemisphere damage and left neglect. From Robertson and Eglin.[298] Right: Standard paradigms for exogenous and endogenous shifts of covert attention as developed by Posner and colleagues.[287]

The field of left neglect was thrown into considerable turmoil when it was reported that lines shorter than 5 cm were bisected leftward of the true midpoint.[214] According to one explanation of the line bisection task, the orientation of patients with left neglect is automatically directed to the rightmost point of the line from whence it is volitionally pulled back and moved as far to the left as the excessive attentional pull of the right permits. The patient then places the bisection mark at the subjective midpoint of the segment between the right end of the line and the "attentional horizon" reached on the left.[133,170] If the line is long enough, its left end remains beyond the attentional horizon and the bisection mark is placed rightward of true center. If the line is shorter, the attentional horizon extends beyond the left endpoint of the line, inducing a confabulatory completion of the missing segment (between the true left end point and the attentional horizon), and a subsequent bisection of the resulting distance (between the true right end point and the left end point of the confabulated segment), often leading the patient to place the midpoint leftward of true center. Such confabulatory completion on the left has been noted in the context of neglect dyslexia, especially for very short words.[48] According to a different and less elaborate interpretation, bisection errors diminish with decreasing line length, so the inconsistent and small crossover effect for short lines could represent the resurfacing of the normal tendency for making bisection errors slightly leftward of center.[258] Mathematical and computational models of line bisection have been described, some of which also account for the crossover effect elicited by short lines.[9,48,244,258]

Under normal circumstances, it is reasonable to assume that each segment of the extrapersonal space has equal claim to mental representation and that there are synaptic mechanisms which flexibly enhance the representational salience of spatial locations containing significant events. For example, the representation of the space behind the body is relatively muted in the course of most daily activities. While driving a car, however, this part of the extrapersonal space acquires as much behavioral relevance as any other segment of the environment and becomes continuously updated by information obtained through the rearview mirror. In patients with left unilateral neglect, it appears that the inner representation becomes permanently skewed toward the right hemispace. Extinction and line bisection errors are two manifestations of this phenomenon. Another manifestation is elicited when patients with left neglect are asked to close their eyes and point toward the body midline. In this task, the patients usually point right of midline, illustrating a relative shrinkage of the mental representation of the left hemispace.[146] This mental devaluation of the left side has numerous additional manifestations: When patients with hemineglect develop delirium, their hallucinations remain confined to the right side of space; when they dream, their rapid eye movements are directed to the right; and when they are exposed to a small stationary spot of light in the dark, the illusory movement they report is almost always directed to the right.[17,88,227]

The rightward skewing of spatial representations was demonstrated directly in a study where patients were asked to mentally retrieve prominent features along the Piazza del Duomo in Milan as they imagined themselves looking toward the cathedral. Patients with left neglect were much more accurate in listing the details which would have been situated on the right side of the square when viewed from that vantage point. Upon being asked to imagine looking at the square while facing away from the cathedral, the patients again showed better recall of the items that would have appeared to be on the right, although these were the less readily recalled details during the assumption of the former vantage point. Thus, the impaired evocation of left sided details in the first part of the experiment was not caused by an obliteration of the information but by an inability to activate the part of the representation which fell to the left of the imaginary perspective.[28] It is as if the internally directed attentional spotlight fails to illuminate left-sided features which, moments later, become noticeable when a mental remapping places them on the right side of the mind's eye.

In addition to this difficulty in *activating* the left side of existing representations, patients with left neglect also display a relative deficit in *constructing* a representation of the left side. In one experiment, for example, patients with right hemineglect were asked to judge if two members of a pair of geometric shapes were identical or not. The stimuli were presented through a centrally placed slit under which the objects were passed at a constant rate, one at a time. The subject had to reconstruct the entire object mentally and store its representation for comparison to the subsequent member of the pair. The results showed that patients were less accurate in detecting differences in the left side of objects, regardless of whether the objects had moved leftward or rightward under the slit during the presentation.[29] Since sensory input was centrally situated, the outcome cannot be attributed to the neglect of actual events in extrapersonal space. Rather, it resulted from a faulty construction (or reactivation) of the left side of the object as represented mentally, even though the constituent information had originated centrally. In most cases, patients with representational neglect also have neglect for events on the left side of the environment. In one instance, however, a patient who no longer neglected external events on the left continued to neglect the left side of internal representations, showing that the distribution of attention to external events and to their internal representations may be based on different mechanisms.[23]

A task developed by Posner and colleagues for the covert shifting of spatial attention has played a very influential role in this field.[287] No eye movements are allowed, so attentional shifts remain covert and move within a mental representation of the ambient visual scene (Fig. 3–5, right). In one form of this task, the cue takes the form of a brief change in the luminance of one of two peripheral locations and generates an *exogenous* shift of the attentional focus through the process of priming. Targets that appear at the primed location (valid trials) are detected more rapidly than targets that appear in the opposite side (invalid trials). In a second version, a centrally placed directional arrow generates an *endogenous* shift of spatial expectancy so that subsequently presented targets in that direction (valid trials) are normally detected more rapidly than targets in the opposite direction (invalid trials).

The invalid conditions in both forms of the task induce an extinction-like phenomenon since they generate a rivalry between the cued location and the target. Normal subjects display no major rightward or leftward difference in the magnitude of the "invalidity effect," defined as the prolongation of the reaction time when attention is cued to one side but must be moved to a target that appears on the opposite side. As expected, patients with left hemineglect show much longer reaction times when responding to targets on the left. The "invalidity effect" in trials where attention becomes cued to the right but must be shifted to a target on the left is also disproportionately prolonged, showing that patients with left unilateral neglect have an excessive difficulty disengaging attention from the right hemispace when the task requires a subsequent leftward shift.[289]

MOTOR-EXPLORATORY ASPECTS OF UNILATERAL NEGLECT—VISUAL AND
TACTILE SEARCH AND NEGLECT DYSLEXIA

Many of the tasks listed above involve the shifting of the attentional focus in a covert fashion, without overt head and eye movements. In everyday life, however, the effective distribution of attention almost always requires active orienting, scanning, and searching. These motor-exploratory aspects of attention are also impaired in unilateral neglect. Patients with left neglect display a pervasive reluctance to scan and explore the left hemispace even in the absence of obvious gaze or limb paresis. This aspect of neglect reflects not only a lack of interest in the left side but also a rightward bias in the tuning of motor systems involved in exploration. Even in total darkness, for example, patients with left neglect confine oculomotor scanning to the right side.[161]

The impairment of search behavior is readily elicited by tasks which require the patient to circle or check targets on a sheet of paper.[2,3,366] Neurologically normal subjects (at least those whose native language is written from left to right) tend to start target cancellation from the upper left corner and proceed systematically from left to right (as in reading), in vertical sweeps, or "as the ox plows" (back and forth—left to right, right to left, and so on). Patients with left hemineglect omit many more targets on the left, need more time to find targets on the left, use a disorganized scanning strategy, tend to start the task from the right side of the page, make fewer and lower-amplitude eye movements to the left, and have longer visual fixation times on right-sided targets.[20,366] In some types of tasks, detection performance follows the power function (targets canceled = K[targets presented]^B) where the constant and exponent are derived empirically.[49] This relationship implies that the patient has some covert awareness of the total number of targets and that the neglect is a postsensory phenomenon.

Target detection tasks have received a great deal of emphasis in the definition of left neglect. Patients without left sided target detection failures are usually described as having no neglect, even if they have extinction. This chapter takes a different approach and assumes that extinction is one of many components of the neglect syndrome and that it may or may not be accompanied by other manifestations of neglect. Target cancellation tasks vary in design. As expected, more difficult tasks are more sensitive for eliciting neglect. Thus, contralesional detection failures in patients with left neglect are more extensive when the patient needs to detect letters rather than lines, complex shapes rather than letters, and when the targets are embedded among foils or scattered without clear arrangement into rows or columns. A patient who may show considerable left hemineglect in detecting complex shapes, for example, may perform almost normally when the targets are simple lines.[367]

The observation that targets oriented randomly on the page are less efficiently detected than targets organized into rows and columns implies that an inability to endogenously impose an orderly scanning strategy contributes to the severity of the neglect (Fig. 3–6). Neglect of left sided targets is also more severe if the target identification requires "attentive" serial search (as in the case of the search for an individual letter embedded among other letters) than if it can be based on "preattentive" pop-out features (as in the case of a slanted line embedded among straight lines), suggesting that global attention may be less impaired than focal search.[2] In general, patients with left hemineglect miss most of the targets on the left side of the page, and also some on the right side, at least in part because these targets enter the left visual field as the head and eyes turn rightward during the search task (Fig. 3–6).

Left-sided target detection failures reflect two interactive factors, a decreased tendency to explore the left side and also an excessive attraction exerted by stimuli on the right. If patients are given two versions of a cancellation task, one where they have to mark the detected targets and another where they have to erase them, performance is considerably better in the second version, probably because it gradually eliminates the hypersalience of the right sided targets which are also the first to be detected and erased.[211] When paper-and-pencil tasks are used, neglect may reflect not only a reluctance to visually scan the left side but also a reluctance to move the arm leftward to make the cancellation mark. The use of a 90° mirror, which reverses the direction of a manual movement needed to mark a target from the direction of the visual attentional shift that leads to its detection, shows that target cancellation impairments reflect a failure to look left in some patients and a failure to reach to the left in others.[345]

As noted earlier, patients asked to point straight ahead without visual feedback tend to point slightly to the right of the body midline.[145] This phenomenon has been attributed to an alteration in the representational midpoint of extrapersonal space, a mechanism that has also been invoked to explain the rightward error in line bisection. However, patients who were required to estimate the body midline by looking at a laterally moving spot and indicating when it should be stopped made rightward errors when the spot was traveling leftward but no errors when it was traveling rightward, suggesting that the resistance to leftward movement (with the arm in the pointing task or the eyes in this version of the task) may be more important than a representational shift in causing the rightward deviation of the estimated body midline.[102]

Left neglect may also entail a failure to read words on the left side of the page. At least some of this neglect dyslexia may reflect the impairment of visual search on the left. Some patients also neglect the left part of words written on the right side of the page, and they sometimes produce confabulatory completions of the neglected segment.[189] In some patients the fragmentation of the word into the neglected and perceived parts respects morphemic boundaries and lexical structure; in others nonwords are more prone to neglect than real words.[257] These aspects of

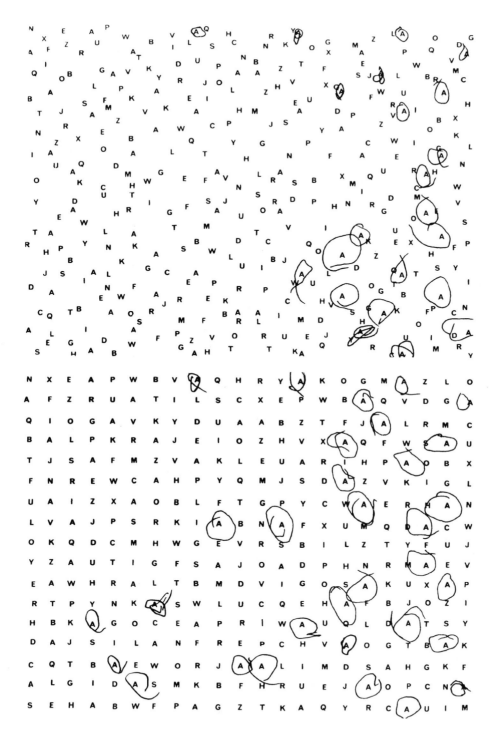

FIGURE 3–6. This shows the random-letter cancellation task performance of a 40-year-old man who sustained a severe head injury that damaged widespread frontoparieto-occipital regions of the right hemisphere. The accident occurred 7 years prior to this testing. Top: Performance in the random letter cancellation task shows severe left neglect. Bottom: When the same letters are arranged in an orderly fashion, performance improves.

neglect dyslexia indicate that the entire word is first encoded, in some implicit lexical form, and that the neglect is superimposed upon this representation. Thus neglect dyslexia is influenced by two interactive factors: the spatial location of the word (the low-level or bottom-up factor) and its morphemic and lexical structure (the high-level or top-down factor).[257]

Patients with left unilateral neglect can also experience difficulties in manual exploration and tactile target detection. Blindfolded search for small objects by manual palpation is intact on the right side of the table not only with the right hand but also with the left hand, whereas it becomes ineffective on the left side of the table even when the intact right hand is being used.[365] These observations show that left neglect is associated with impaired tactile exploration within the left hemispace regardless of the limb that is being used. Thus motor programs involved in exploration appear to be organized according to the hemispace within which the movement is to be discharged rather than the muscle groups that are being activated.[10,357]

Patients with hemineglect display a reluctance to direct movements into the left side, whether or not such movements have any exploratory purpose. This has been designated hypokinesia and contributes to the emergence of "intentional" neglect.[153] In some paradigms and in some patient groups, hypokinesia makes a major contribution to the emergence of target detection failures whereas in others it seems to play a minor role. For example, in a reaction time experiment, response times to left sided targets improved considerably when the hand had to move rightward to reach the response button.[92] In another group of patients, however, where the stimulus sheet had to be moved by the subject under a fixed central slit (so that targets on the right were exposed under the slit by moving the sheet to the left) more targets were detected on the right side, indicating that hypokinesia toward the left was not an important factor.[241] In the context of left neglect, "hypokinesia" and "intentional neglect" tend to be used to designate general impairments of leftward movements whereas "exploratory deficit" refers to more complex breakdowns of systematic search strategies within the extrapersonal space.

MOTIVATIONAL ASPECTS OF UNILATERAL NEGLECT

A major role of any attentional system is to shift the attentional searchlight toward emotionally and motivationally significant events. While expecting a phone call or knock on the door, for example, the relevant segment of space becomes hypersalient so that otherwise insignificant stimuli in the vicinity of the phone or door assume an enhanced ability to attract attention. Patients with unilateral neglect devalue the left side of the world and behave not only as if nothing is actually happening in the left but also as if nothing of importance could be expected to emanate from that side. The influence of this factor can be probed by varying motivational valence. For example, a patient showed marked improvement in detecting targets on the left when he was promised one penny for each accurate detection (Fig. 3–7). Although several alternative explanations may come to mind, one possibility is to attribute this improvement to a reward-induced motivational enhancement of targets on the left. Another patient with severe left hemineglect failed to reach for

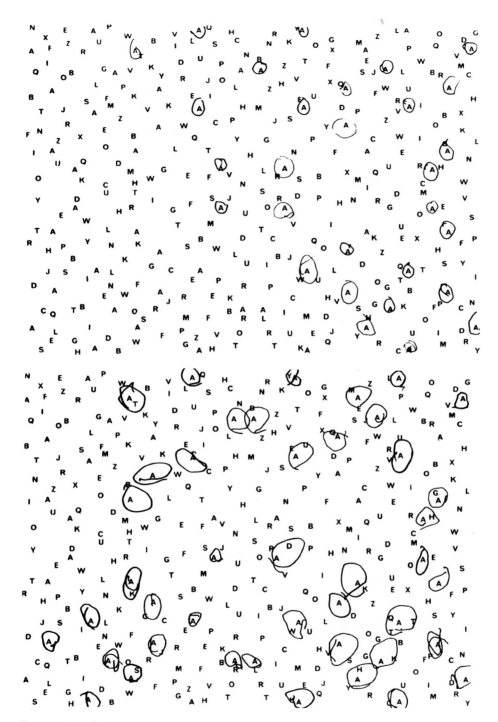

FIGURE 3–7. Same patient as in Figure 3–6, but during a different testing session, approximately a year later. Top: The performance in the random-letter cancellation task shows the diagonal effect. Bottom: Following the performance shown on the top, the patient was promised one penny for each correct detection. The bottom figure shows how this incentive diminishes the neglect. Performance a few minutes later was back to baseline, so practice effects are unlikely to account for this difference.

food on the left side of the tray and would bitterly complain that his tea had been left out. On a day when the nurse was instructed to withhold breakfast, the patient became unusually hungry by noontime but did not show any change in the severe neglect of left-sided targets in a letter cancellation task. When his lunch tray was brought, however, he had no reluctance to reach for his tea on the left side of the tray. These anecdotal observations suggest that a devaluation of sensory events on the left may contribute to the emergence of neglect and that the relationship between neglect and motivation may be material-specific so that hunger decreases the spatial distribution of neglect for edible items but not for letters.

THE GATING IN NEGLECT IS CENTRAL, NOT PERIPHERAL—EVIDENCE BASED ON IMPLICIT PROCESSING

In some patients with extinction, reaction times are longer to unilateral right sided stimuli than to bilateral stimuli although both are reported as unilateral right-sided stimulation by the patient, indicating that the extinguished stimulus gains access to the CNS and exerts a covert influence on behavior.[80] In other patients neglected sensory stimuli can elicit cortical evoked potentials.[352] Furthermore, the observations that the rightward error in line bisection is proportional to total line length, that the number of neglected targets is a power function of the total number of targets, and that neglect dyslexia respects morphemic and lexical boundaries strongly indicate that many manifestations of neglect represent top-down spatial biases imposed upon percepts that are already encoded in the CNS.

Additional support for this interpretation comes from experiments showing that events which appear to be neglected in traditional detection tasks can continue to influence cognitive processes. In one experiment, left-sided objects which were easily identified when presented alone became ignored through the process of extinction when paired with meaningless patterns on the right. Nonetheless, the patients were much faster in detecting centrally presented words which were semantically related to the extinguished object, showing that the stimulus had been able to trigger covert semantic priming.[222] Furthermore, a patient with left hemineglect who was shown line drawings of two houses, one of which had flames coming out of the left side, judged the two drawings to be visually identical but chose the one without flames when asked to select the house she would prefer to live in;[213] and another patient who was shown two banknotes, one of which was torn on the left, could not tell that the two were different but preferred the intact one without being able to explain the reasons for the choice.[45] These observations provide further evidence that conscious, declarative awareness is not an obligatory outcome of perceptual encoding and that behavior may be influenced implicitly by stimuli that are not accessible to explicit consciousness. The covert impact of neglected stimuli upon behavior is analogous to phenomena such as blindsight in hemianopia, implicit memory in the amnestic syndrome, and the autonomic responsivity to familiar faces in prosopagnosia (Chapters 1, 4, and 7).

Determinants of Neglect: The Burden of Being on the Left

At the age of 73, the legendary filmmaker Federico Fellini suffered a stroke that left him with severe left hemineglect.[45] Because of his fame and talent as a cartoonist, he became a favorite target of his physicians, who extracted innumerable drawings, providing one of the most artistic documentation of the hemispatial neglect syndrome. Fellini drew clocks with human limbs for hands but without numbers on the left, lines (depicted as seesaws) bisected by fulcrums displaced to the right, and thinly clad exemplars of the opposite gender with details missing on the left. In one such drawing, probably produced spontaneously, he sketched himself speeding toward his own right, asking himself, *"Dov'é la sinistra?"* (Where is the left?) With this question, Fellini displayed as great an insight into the neuropsychology of neglect as he had for filmmaking (Fig. 3–8).

In the preceding account, the word "left" has deliberately been used without further qualification as if it constituted a fixed attribute such as color or texture. This is clearly not the case since there can be no left or right without a specific frame of reference. At least four interrelated frames of reference can define the leftness of an extrapersonal event : "egocentric" (defined with respect to the observer), "allocentric" (defined with respect to another extrapersonal event), "world-centered" (defined with respect to a fixed landmark), and "object-centered" (defined with respect to a principal axis in the canonical representation on an object). Furthermore, since the eyes, head, and trunk can rotate and tilt with respect to each other, the egocentric frame of reference contains "retinocentric," "cephalocentric," "somatocentric," and "gravitational" coordinates so that an event which is in the left according to one egocentric coordinate could be on the right according to another. Perceptual and conceptual factors also influence the segmentation of the stimulus field into individual clusters with their own left and right sides. In general it can be said for patients with left neglect that a location in one of the egocentric lefts, in the allocentric left, in the world-centered left, in the object-centered left, and in the segmentational left diminishes perceptual salience and the probability

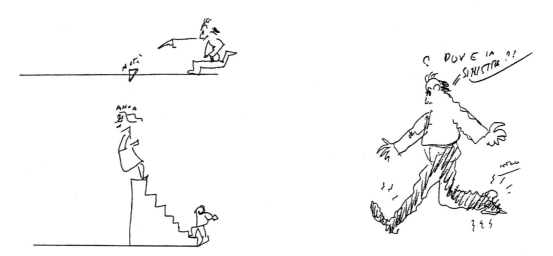

FIGURE 3–8. Left: Fellini's line bisection performance. The bisection point is rightward of true center. The whimsical embellishments are on the right side of both lines. The left sides of the lines remain unadorned. Right: Fellini looking for the lost left side of the world as he asks himself, *"Dov'é la sinistra?"* (Where is the left?) From Cantagallo and Della Sala.[45]

that it will trigger action. A location on the right side of any of these frames of reference has the opposite effect of promoting salience and access to action.

EGOCENTRIC COORDINATES

Because of the mobility of the eyes with respect to the head, the head with respect to the body, and the body with respect to the earth, it is necessary to subdivide egocentric coordinates into retinocentric, cephalocentric, somatocentric, and gravitational components. The retina is the obligatory entry zone for all visual information. Almost all visual neglect therefore displays some retinotopic mapping which then interacts with other egocentric frames of reference. Turning the eyes to the right, for example, brings more of the right hemispace into the left visual field and can interfere with the detection of targets within the right somatocentric hemispace. Conversely, turning the head and eyes into the left or providing vestibular or proprioceptive stimulations which promote such rotations can reduce the number of target detection failures on the left side of a test sheet placed in front of the patient.[180,308] These effects are also seen in accessing mental representations. Thus, neglect of the left side of an imagined scene improved when head and eyes were deviated to the left, apparently because this maneuver triggered an analogous movement of the mind's eye.[223] A similar phenomenon was observed in another left hemineglect patient who displayed a dramatic improvement in naming cities on the western coast of an *imagined* map of France upon left vestibular stimulation with cold water, a procedure that would have induced leftward deviations of the head and eyes (Fig. 3–9, top left).[277]

The distribution of neglect is also influenced by the somatocentric and cephalocentric frames of reference. Thus, detection of stimuli presented to the left visual field improves when the eyes and targets are moved 30° to the right so that the stimuli (still directed to the same part of the retina) become located in the right side of the somatocentric coordinates.[192] Rightward errors in line bisection and left-sided detection failures during blindfolded tactile exploration improve when the line or tactile maze is placed on the right side of the body, and saccadic reaction times to targets in the left visual field improve if the trunk is rotated to the left so that all visual stimuli (even those directed to the left visual field) fall on the right of the body midline.[24,150,181] The rightward line bisection error indicative of neglect is less prominent when the patients are tested in the supine position.[285] This observation suggests that the boundaries between left and right may be sharper in the erect posture and illustrates the influence of the gravitational frame of reference in determining the extent of neglect.

ALLOCENTRIC FACTORS AND RELATIVE LEFTNESS

Extinction is traditionally assessed by simultaneously presenting one stimulus to the left visual field and another to the right, each with identical horizontal eccentricity. However, double simultaneous stimulation can also be confined to a single visual field. In such experiments, the leftmost of two stimuli presented in either the left or right field becomes extinguished in patients with left neglect.[80,116] This creates a setting where the same right-field stimulus that is detected when paired with a

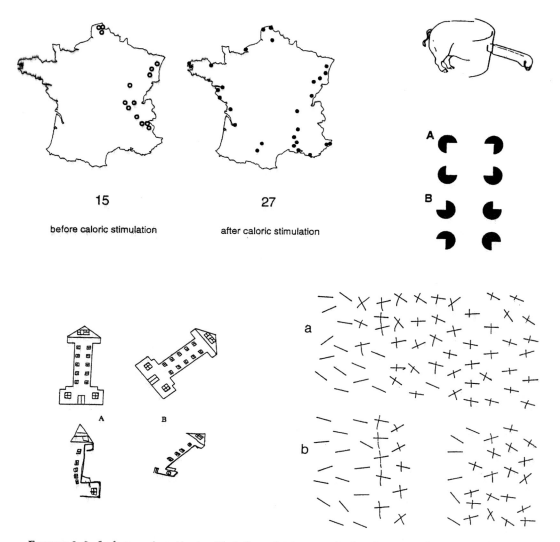

15
before caloric stimulation

27
after caloric stimulation

A

B

a

b

FIGURE 3–9. Left top: A patient with left neglect was asked to imagine the map of France and name as many towns as possible within 2 minutes. Before caloric stimulation, only towns on the east side of France are named. After cold-water stimulation to the left ear, towns in the west are also named. From Perenin.[277] Left bottom: A patient with left neglect neglects detail on the left when asked to copy an upright tower (A). When the tower is tilted, the patient omits detail on the left on the principal axis although some of the information is now in the right side (B). From Halligan and Marshall.[137] Right top: A patient with left neglect traced with her finger the contour of this chimeric figure accurately but identified it as a pan. When questioned about the left side, she suggested that it "must be vegetables in the pan; parsnips or maybe potatoes." From Young, and associates.[373] Right middle: A patient with left extinction was asked to indicate verbally the number of incomplete circles. He reported four targets in A where they formed a Kanisza rectangle, but only two (presumably those on the right) in B where no Kanisza figure was formed. From Mattingley and colleagues.[216] Right bottom: A patient with left hemiplegia and left neglect was asked to place a mark on all the lines in the display. When the display contains a uniform distribution of lines (a), only lines on the left of the workspace are neglected. When the display is broken into two focal workspaces (b), lines on the left of the right-sided cluster are neglected although they were detected in the former arrangement. From Driver and Halligan.[91]

stimulus on its left becomes ignored when paired with a stimulus to its right, even under identical conditions of head, eye, and trunk positioning. An analogous phenomenon has been reported in the somatosensory modality. Thus, when patients with left neglect were administered simultaneous taps at the same two horizontally aligned spots on the wrist, the left sided tap was consistently extinguished but shifted from one of the spots to the other depending on whether the arm was prone or supine. This experiment shows that tactile information emanating from the same spot of skin, located on the right arm and within the right egocentric hemispace, becomes heeded or ignored depending on whether it is located on the left or right of another simultaneously administered stimulus.[254] It appears, therefore, that being on the left of another event increases the probability of neglect, even when both events are in the right hemispace.

Allocentric effects are also seen in target detection tasks. This was shown in an experiment where patients with left extinction were asked to attend to horizontally aligned peripheral target sites with different eccentricities. All target sites were visible throughout the experiment but only one contained the stimulus that needed to be detected in any given trial and all trials were initiated during central fixation. In contrast to normals who are faster in detecting more centrally located targets, patients with left extinction displayed faster reaction times to the right sided targets with the greater eccentricity, presumably because they were located in the allocentric right of the other targets.[196]

The influence of relative leftness provides another reason why the left sides of words and chimeric faces become neglected even when the experimental paradigm is designed to insure that the entire stimulus falls within the right visual field.[19,373] Another example of a similar phenomenon is provided by a patient with left hemineglect who was given a chimeric drawing made up of a pig's bottom (distinguished by the characteristic tail) on the left and a saucepan (distinguished by its handle) on the right. The patient traced the contours on both sides accurately with the fingers of the right hand but identified the entire picture as a saucepan (Fig. 3–9, right top). When pressed to account for the details of the left contour she suggested that the left part might depict "vegetables in the pan, parsnips or maybe potatoes."[373] Although the information from the entire chimeric contour is likely to have entered the CNS through the intact left hemisphere during the process of tracing, its allocentric left side became subject to neglect.

Allocentric coordinates influence not only the impact of sensory input but also the effectiveness of motor responses. In one experiment, subjects saw a "1" or a "2" in the center of the visual field and had to press a key with the right index finger for one of the numbers and the right middle finger for the other. In the conventional position of the hand, the index finger was on the left of the middle finger. In a second condition, the keyboard was rotated 180° so that the relative position of the two fingers with respect to each other was reversed. In each condition, responses were slower with the finger on the relative left position. Thus, the effectiveness of performance was based on the relative leftness of the responding digit rather than on any change in the location of the sensory input.[197] In these experiments, the linkage of the fingers to motor cortex had obviously remained unaltered, suggesting that the changes in response speed are imposed at an advanced level of the neuraxis where motor output is mapped according to the spatial location where the movement is discharged rather than the anatomical location of the muscles that contract. It should be noted, however, that none of the experiments cited in this section have totally dissociated allocentric from egocentric factors since events located to the left of other events in these tasks were also located further to the left within egocentric coordinates.

EFFECT OF EYE MOVEMENTS UPON NEGLECT—THE GLOBAL AND FOCAL WORKSPACES

In testing patients with neglect, the eyes are usually allowed to move, creating complex interactions between retinotopic and other egocentric coordinates. At the beginning of a target cancellation task, for example, targets on the right of central fixation are detected accurately and the eyes move in that direction. However, the rightward bias for internal representations, the fact that more and more of the test sheet enters the left visual field as the eyes move rightward, and the reluctance to scan leftward collectively result in a failure to return fixation all the way back to the starting point. The second fixation point is therefore slightly rightward of the first. This rightward drift of the starting point gives rise to the characteristic diagonal line of demarcation between the area of neglect and that of accurate detection (Fig. 3–7 top). This phenomenon explains why placing the entire test sheet on the right side of the patient does not eliminate the neglect of targets on the left side of the sheet. Although this maneuver may initially improve performance, the diagonal effect becomes gradually established as parts of the test sheet enter the left hemifield in the course of rightward oculomotor scanning. Asking the patient to look to the left is also of limited benefit, since a similar diagonal will soon be established as the endogenously prompted leftward excursion of the head and eyes becomes gradually more limited.

A test sheet placed in front of the patient defines the "global workspace." As the eyes move, the point of regard defines a "focal workspace" with its own allocentric left and right. Depending on the task, the focal workspace may include each face, word, or other target placed within the global workspace. Left neglect operates within both the global and focal workspaces. Thus, as the patient looks at a face or word on the right side of the test sheet, the face or word constitutes the focal workspace and its left side becomes vulnerable to neglect. Furthermore, the point of the pen or pencil defines the center of the focal workspace in drawing and copying tasks. In such tasks, the patient tends to omit detail on the left of each drawing even when all the activity is confined to the right side of the test sheet and even when the right side of items further to the left are drawn quite accurately. One patient with left neglect who was asked to draw a map of the British Isles from memory, for example, omitted the west coast of England and Scotland while including Ireland in his map.[135]

WORLD- AND OBJECT-BASED COORDINATES

In a target detection experiment done in patients with left neglect, the position of the targets remained the same but the subjects were asked to perform the task when sitting and when reclining to the left. As expected, target detection in the sitting position was least effective in the two quadrants located in the somatocentric left. While reclining, however, subjects continued to neglect targets in the same two quadrants although one of these (the former upper left quadrant) was now in the right visual field and within the right somatocentric hemispace of the subjects.[42] These results may reflect the tendency to represent the environment with respect to the canonical gravitational vantage point of the erect posture or with respect to a fixed environmental landmark. Stimuli on the left side of this representation are then neglected even when they are no longer on the left side with respect to egocentric coordinates.

An analogous phenomenon can be seen at the level of individual objects (Fig. 3–9, lower left). Thus a patient did not draw the detail on the left side of the canonical vertical axis of a tower, even when the model was inclined 45° to the right so that part of the detail on the left of the canonical axis fell in the right side of the patient.[137] In another experiment, the ability to determine if two random tower-like shapes were same or different deteriorated when the critical detail was on the left side of the canonical axis even when the object was inclined to the right and the canonical left entered the egocentric right.[91] These observations indicate that the definition of left and right in the neglect syndrome is influenced by the subjective canonical representations of objects and further support the conclusion that neglect operates at the level of internalized perceptual representations. Although object-centered effects have been reported in several settings, they may become influential in determining the distribution of neglect only in the case of stimuli with very prominent canonical axes or lateral asymmetries.[18,100]

SEGMENTATION AND CONCEPTUALIZATION EFFECTS
The distribution of neglect is also influenced by the perceptual (gestalt) and conceptual (top-down) segmentations of the stimulus field (Fig. 3–9, right middle). Thus, four black circles with a missing quadrant resisted extinction when they collectively formed an illusory Kanizsa rectangle, presumably because they were being processed as a single entity rather than four distinct stimuli.[216] Furthermore, asking a patient to copy a pot containing two daisies emanating out of a common stem led to the omission of the entire left flower whereas erasing the convergence into a common stem and the pot below it (so that the patient saw two separate unattached daisies) led to a drawing where both daisies were drawn but each with details missing on its left half.[136] In another setting, when a target cancellation task was administered in conventional form and also after erasing the central targets so as to give the impression of two distinct clusters of targets, the patient omitted targets on the left of the right-sided cluster although the same targets were detected when they were part of a single array.[91] This experiment further emphasizes the influence of the focal workspace in determining the distribution of neglect within the larger global workspace (Fig. 3–9, lower right).

Top-down conceptual processing of the sensory input also influences the distribution of neglect. Thus, neglect of the left side of a letter string is less likely if the letters form a word than a nonword,[325] and the ability to use information from the left side of a chimeric face increases if the information on the right side is degraded.[373] In these cases, the knowledge that the stimuli are words and faces, and that their identity cannot be resolved without access to further left-sided information is likely to have triggered a top-down push of the attentional horizon further to the left. This is consistent with the notion that neglect represents an impairment in the "automatic" allocation of attention to the left and that this bias can be overcome, at least partially and transiently, under specific "cognitive" states. For example, left extinction can be diminished when the subject is instructed to ignore the right-sided stimulus and line bisection improves when the subject is made to read a number on the left end of the line.[80,171]

FAR-SPACE VERSUS NEAR-SPACE

Unilateral neglect represents a distortion in the lateral distribution of attention along the x axis. Some component of vertical neglect along the y axis can also be identified, suggesting that patients with neglect have greater difficulty with the detection of targets in the lower quadrants.[283] However, vertical neglect is much less pronounced than lateral neglect and its clinical and anatomical determinants remain to be clarified. Several observations indicate that the distribution of neglect may also show variations along the z-axis and that there may be dissociable states of neglect for peripersonal, near-, and far-spaces. Thus some patients have left neglect only for the near-space within an arm's reach, whereas others neglect only left-sided events in far-space, beyond an arm's reach.[134,355]

Many patients with unilateral neglect also display a "peripersonal" neglect of the body. Sometimes this leads to dressing apraxia, to a denial of left-sided hemiparesis, and, on occasion, even to the delusion that the paralyzed limb belongs to somebody else. The latter two features are known as anosognosia.[13] Another related phenomenon is motor neglect (negligence motrice), which is used to describe a reluctance to use the contralateral limbs even in the absence of discernible weakness. Specific commands to use that limb usually overcome this resistance. Motor neglect is confined to the limb contralateral to the lesion, regardless of the hemispace or direction of the movement. Thus, motor neglect and directional hypokinesia are not identical phenomena.

V. RIGHT HEMISPHERE DOMINANCE FOR SPATIAL ATTENTION

Clinical evidence based on thousands of patients shows that contralesional neglect is more frequent, severe, and lasting after right hemisphere lesions than after equivalent lesions in the left hemisphere.[47,70,73,114,266,365] Furthermore, reversible cerebral inactivation by intracarotid injections of sodium amytal caused visual neglect and tactile extinction only after the inhibition of the right hemisphere.[224,334] A simple neural model based on a right hemisphere specialization for the spatial distribution of attention may help to account for this asymmetry (Fig. 3–10). This model is based on three sets of postulates:

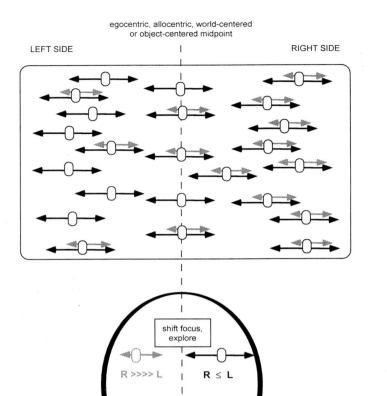

egocentric, allocentric, world-centered
or object-centered midpoint

LEFT SIDE

RIGHT SIDE

shift focus,
explore

R >>>> L

R ≤ L

set salience,
map targets

R >>>> L

R ≤ L

LEFT HEMISPHERE
(ATTEND TO RIGHT SIDE)

RIGHT HEMISPHERE
(ATTEND TO BOTH SIDES)

FIGURE 3–10. A right hemisphere specialization model for shifting spatial attention and representing salience. The large rectangle corresponds to the global workspace and the small rectangles with the curved corners represent multiple focal workspaces (such as individual faces, words, or stimulus clusters) distributed within the global workspace. The arrows depict the directional probability of attentional shifts and representational salience, gray for the left hemisphere, black for the right hemisphere. Within a given workspace, global or focal, the left hemisphere attentional mechanisms are more likely to endow the right side of events with salience, and tend to coordinate the distribution of attention almost exclusively within the right hemispace, especially in a contraversive direction. In contrast, right hemisphere attentional mechanisms are more likely to distribute salience and attentional shifts more equally within both hemispaces and in both directions, although there is a slight leftward predominance. In the normal brain all points in the extrapersonal space have an equal probability of claiming salience and attentional shifts although there may be a slight leftward bias because of the greater right hemisphere involvement in attentional tasks. When the left hemisphere is damaged, a mild leftward bias emerges but does not cause neglect because attention and salience can still be distributed in all directions. When the right hemisphere is damaged, a strong rightward bias emerges and keeps pushing the attentional focus rightward. The setting of salience and the mapping of extrapersonal targets for intended foveation, attentional grasp, and exploration are more closely allied with the function of neurons in posterior parietal cortex, whereas the selection, sequencing, and execution of attentional shifts and exploratory behaviors are more closely allied with the functions of neurons in the frontal lobe.

1. The left hemisphere attributes salience predominantly to the right side of events, coordinates the distribution of attention mainly within the right hemispace, and shifts attention mostly in a contraversive rightward direction.

2. The right hemisphere attributes salience to both sides of events, coordinates the distribution of attention within both hemispaces, and shifts attention in both the contraversive and ipsiversive directions with only a slight contralateral and contraversive bias.

3. The right hemisphere devotes more neuronal resources to spatial attention, and attentional tasks are more likely to engage right hemisphere mechanisms.

According to this model, each hemisphere has a greater tendency to shift attention in a contraversive direction and within the contralateral hemispace, but the asymmetry is more pronounced in the left hemisphere. In the intact state, the attentional spotlight can be shifted to any motivationally relevant location but there may also be a slight bias favoring the left because the right hemisphere is more likely to be engaged by attentional tasks. Left hemisphere lesions are not expected to give rise to much contralesional neglect since the ipsiversive attentional shifting ability of the right hemisphere and its capacity to coordinate the distribution of attention within both hemispaces are likely to compensate for the loss. Right hemisphere lesions, however, are likely to yield severe contralesional neglect because the left hemisphere has relatively little ability to endow left-sided events with salience, to trigger leftward attentional shifts, or to coordinate the distribution of spatial attention within the left side. Following right hemisphere lesions, left-sided events would thus lose representational salience and the focus of attention would keep being pushed rightward, toward the rightmost boundary of the global workspace, under the unopposed influence of the left hemisphere. The constitutive role of the right hemisphere in the ipsilateral distribution of attention and the paucity of left hemisphere mechanisms for shifting attention ipsiversively, even within the right hemispace, explains why right hemisphere damage also gives rise to mild but detectable attentional impairments within the ipsilesional right hemispace (Fig. 3–11).

The model in Figure 3–10 predicts that the right hemisphere should participate in encoding and activating the representation of sensory events throughout the extrapersonal space, whereas the left hemisphere should confine its influence to contralateral right-sided events. In support of this prediction, the left hemisphere displays event-related potentials, EEG desynchronizations, and metabolic activation only after stimulation of the right side whereas the right hemisphere shows such changes after stimulation of either side.[76,151,270,294] Retrieval of spatial information also leads to greater right hemisphere activation, regardless of the extrapersonal location of the information that is being retrieved, and right hemisphere lesions can give rise to states of global topographical disorientation encompassing the entire extrapersonal space, suggesting that the right hemisphere plays a critical role in activating the mental representation of both sides of space.[209,255,343] This organization is consistent with a proposed dichotomy according to which the field of view and perceptual style of the right hemisphere is "global" whereas that of the left

INTRACAROTID AMYTAL TEST (IAT)

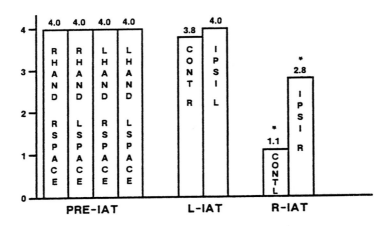

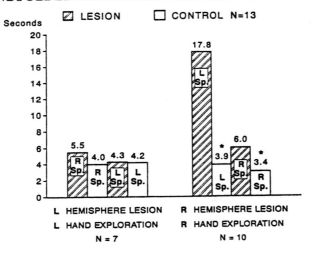

FIGURE 3–11. Top: Target detection during the intracarotid amytal test (IAT) in 32 right-handed patients with left hemisphere dominance for language. Patients used the ipsi-injectional hand for detection. A score of 4 indicates perfect performance. Inactivation of the left hemisphere (L-IAT) caused no significant target detection failure in either the contrainjectional right hemispace (CONT R) or the ipsi-injectional left hemispace (IPSI L). Inactivation of the right hemisphere (R-IAT) in the same subjects caused a severe contrainjectional (CONT L) left-sided target detection failure and a lesser but significant (*) target detection failure in the ipsi-injectional (IPSI R) right side.[334] Bottom: Tactile exploration in controls and patients with unilateral lesions in the left hemisphere (L HEMISPHERE LESION) and in the right hemisphere (R HEMISPHERE LESION). Exploration was directed to targets in the right (R Sp.) and left (L Sp.) hemispaces. The y-axis shows the time for detection. The longer the time, the worse the performance. Lesions in the left hemisphere do not interfere with tactile exploration in either hemispace although the patients had to use the nonpreferred left hand. Lesions in the right hemisphere cause a significant (*) slowing of tactile exploration in the left as well as right hemispaces.[365]

216

hemisphere is more "focal."[299] Furthermore, the line bisection errors in patients with left hemineglect can be described by a mathematical model where the right hemisphere encodes salience in both hemispaces whereas the left hemispace encodes salience in only the contralateral left hemispace.[9]

The model summarized above leads to two predictions concerning cerebral activations during attentional shifts: (1) The right hemisphere should show relatively greater activation when attention is shifted symmetrically to the right and to the left. (2) The left hemisphere should be activated mostly when attention shifts within the contralateral right side, especially in a contraversive rightward direction, whereas the right hemisphere should be activated when attention shifts within either hemispace and in either direction. Both predictions are supported by the available evidence: Functional imaging experiments where neurologically intact subjects were asked to shift attention equally to the left and to the right, showed greater activation in the right hemisphere;[260] increased cortical activation in the left hemisphere was noted only after covert attentional shifts within the contralateral right side whereas activations in the right hemisphere were seen after shifts within either hemispace;[61] and a blindfolded manual exploration task showed right hemisphere activation even when the exploration occurred on the ipsilateral right side.[119] Furthermore, damage or transcranial magnetic stimulation of the right hemisphere diminished the speed and accuracy of saccades to actual and remembered targets in both directions whereas left hemisphere damage had a much more modest effect and was confined to saccades made in the contralesional rightward direction.[267,282] In keeping with these observations, left hemisphere dysfunction caused by stroke or barbiturization did not impair target detection even in the right hemispace, whereas right hemisphere dysfunction caused severe target detection failures in the left hemispace and lesser but statistically significant target detection failures in the right hemispace (Fig. 3–11).

The model depicted in Figure 3–10 suggests that the attentional functions of the two hemispheres can be classified not only on the basis of a "place code" which signals the location of the attentional focus but also on the basis of a "vector code" which signals the direction of attentional shifts from any point of origin. Experimental support for the vectorial part of this organization is somewhat mixed. A functional imaging study found that the laterality of cerebral activation depended on the hemispace within which attention was being shifted rather than on the direction of the shifts within the hemispace.[61] However, other experiments showed that unilateral brain damage interferes with contraversive shifts of covert attention irrespective of the hemispace or field within which the shift occurred, although the effect is more pronounced in the contralesional field.[11,288]

At least two distinct explanations have been proposed to account for the hemispheric asymmetry in neglect-causing lesions. According to Kinsbourne, each hemisphere promotes contralateral orientation and imbalance is normally prevented through interhemispheric reciprocal inhibition. However, the rightward orientation promoted by the left hemisphere is normally more potent, so its disinhibition by right hemisphere lesions causes a greater rightward bias than the leftward bias caused by equivalent left hemisphere lesions. This is why the left neglect caused by right hemisphere lesions is more profound than the right neglect caused by equivalent left hemisphere lesions.[188] According to another explanation, the left hemisphere attends only to the contralateral right hemispace whereas the right hemisphere attends to the entire extrapersonal space. Consequently, damage to the right hemisphere causes contralesional neglect whereas damage to the left hemisphere does not.[152,227] The model depicted in Figure 3–10 does not depend on interhemispheric reciprocal inhibition and adds a vectorial component to the control of attentional shifts. The lack of reciprocal interhemispheric interactions is consistent with the observation that callosal resection does not yield prominent neglect syndromes.[115]

The physiological basis for the right hemisphere specialization in directed attention is poorly understood. Parts of the human posterior parietal cortex may be larger on the right side of the brain and may provide a structural substrate for this specialization.[173] Functional asymmetry is probably also based on dynamic factors which influence the timing of neural engagement and the proportion of neurons with contraversive versus ipsiversive sensory and motor fields. As noted in the section on confusional states (section II), the right hemisphere may also have a specialized role in modulating the domain-independent aspects of the overall attentional matrix.

There is relatively little information on the hemispheric specialization of directed attention in left-handers. In the case of language, approximately 60% of left-handers maintain the typical pattern of left hemisphere dominance for language-related functions. An analogous persistence of the typical asymmetry pattern occurs in attentional functions, so most left-handers display a right hemisphere specialization for directed attention.[334] Even when there is right hemisphere dominance for language, neglect arises after right hemisphere inactivation, suggesting that right hemisphere specialization for directed attention may be more tightly conserved than left hemisphere specialization for language.[334] Rarely, marked right-sided neglect may occur after a unilateral left hemisphere lesion in a dextral patient. This is designated "crossed neglect."[109] The most striking instances of right unilateral hemineglect, however, have been described in patients with bilateral injury to the brain.[364] Severe neglect for the right hemispace should therefore raise the suspicion of bihemispheric lesions.

VI. FUNCTIONAL ANATOMY OF UNILATERAL NEGLECT

Influential papers on left neglect by Brain,[35] Patterson and Zangwill[273] and McFie and colleagues.[220] designated the parietal lobe as a principal site of damage although many of the patients had either multilobar infarcts or major head trauma or large neoplasms. Hécaen and associates[143] subsequently described the emergence of unilateral neglect in patients who underwent excision of the right inferior parietal lobule for the control of focal epilepsy. This localization acquired even greater certitude when unilateral neglect was described following infarctions in the region of the inferior parietal lobule in individuals without a history of prior neurologic im-

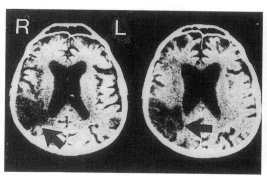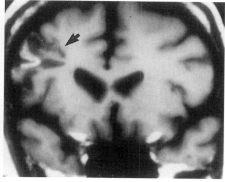

FIGURE 3–12. Left: The right-sided inferior parietal lobule infarct which caused Fellini's left neglect. From Cantagallo and Della Sala.[45] Right: A right-sided frontal lesion in the region of the FEF caused severe left neglect.[66]

pairment.[64,74,148] Based on this evidence, textbooks of neurology have traditionally referred to left neglect as a "parietal sign" and encouraged the diagnosis of parietal lobe pathology in patients with this syndrome. Subsequent clinical reports, however, described left neglect in patients with lesions in the frontal lobes, cingulate gyrus, striatum, and thalamus (Fig. 3–12). This multiplicity of lesion sites raised the concern that neglect-causing lesions may have no anatomical specificity. However, the availability of a macaque monkey model for contralesional neglect helped to show that each of these areas had a special contribution to make to the function of directed attention and that they collectively formed an interconnected network organized according to the principles of selectively distributed processing.[227] It is therefore no longer accurate to designate left neglect as a "parietal syndrome." The more accurate designation would be to characterize it as an "attentional network syndrome," realizing that the responsible lesion can be anywhere within the network shown in Figure 3–13.

The Parietal Component of the Attentional Network

The phylogenetic expansion of the human parietal lobe rivals that of the frontal lobe. Posterior parietal cortex is situated at the confluence of visual, auditory, somatosensory, and vestibular unimodal areas. It also contains heteromodal cortices which support multi-modal integration. The posterior parietal lobe can be divided into four major topographic components. (1) *The superior parietal lobule* (spl in Figure 1–7 of Chapter 1) contains somatosensory association cortex in BA5 and anterior BA7, and heteromodal cortex in posterior BA7. (2) *The inferior parietal lobule* (ipl in Figure 1–7 of Chapter 1) contains the supramarginal (sg) and angular (ag) gyri, corresponding to BA39 and 40, respectively. Most of the inferior parietal lobule would appear to have properties of heteromodal cortex although an anterior rim of the supramarginal gyrus can probably be characterized as somatosensory association cortex. (3) *The intraparietal sulcus* is one of the most important landmarks of

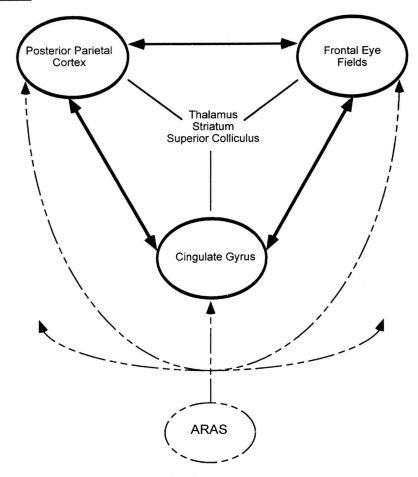

FIGURE 3–13. A large-scale distributed network for spatial attention.

the posterior parietal cortex. It separates the inferior from the superior parietal lobules and has many secondary branches which extend into both lobules. The intraparietal sulcus is very deep and contains a large amount of cortex along its banks. Its functional affiliations are likely to be sensory–motor anteriorly and visuospatial posteriorly. (4) *The medial parietal cortex* (mpo in Fig. 1–7 of Chapter 1) contains somatosensory association cortex (BA5 and 7) anteriorly and heteromodal cortex (BA7 and 31) posteriorly. In addition to its rich sensory associations, posterior parietal cortex is interconnected with premotor cortex, the frontal eye fields (FEFs), the superior colliculus, the parahippocampal gyrus, and several paralimbic areas including the cingulate gyrus, insula, and orbitofrontal cortex.[235,238,248,269] The cingulate connection is the strongest of these paralimbic connections. This pattern of connectivity, inferred from neuroanatomical experiments in macaque monkeys, shows that posterior parietal cortex is well positioned to mediate the type of sensory–motor and cognitive integration that would be needed for spatial attention.

Small lesions confined to parietal cortex rarely cause conspicuous neglect. Persistent and severe neglect in the context of parietal lobe damage almost always indicates a large lesion with considerable subcortical extension. Such lesions can give rise to each of the manifestations of neglect described earlier, although the specific cluster of deficits varies greatly from patient to patient. The large lesion size in most patients has made it difficult to identify the region of the parietal lobe that is most critical for the emergence of contralesional neglect. Functional imaging studies in neurologically intact subjects show that tasks of covert visuospatial attention,[61,262] tactile exploration,[119] oculomotor search,[120] and auditory target detection[226] elicit cortical activation in the superior and inferior parietal lobules, the banks of the intraparietal sulcus, and, less frequently, medial parietal cortex.

The one component of the posterior parietal cortex that is most consistently activated in all of these tasks lies within the banks of the intraparietal sulcus and in its immediate vicinity.[118] This activation occurs in tasks of covert attention (whether attention is shifted endogenously through voluntary modulations of expectation or exogenously through sensory priming) and also in tasks of overt tactile and oculomotor search.[118–120,185,260] The banks of the intraparietal sulcus may thus constitute the parietal core of the attentional network in the human brain although the adjacent parts of the inferior, superior, and medial parietal lobules are also likely to participate in the relevant neural activities. These regions of posterior parietal cortex have also been activated during the execution of tasks closely related to spatial attention, such as the initiation of visually guided saccades, the mental reactivation of spatial maps, visually guided reaching, and the detection of sound movement.[27,52,129,169,204,209,254]

In the monkey, damage to the inferior parietal lobule causes contralesional extinction and reaching deficits whereas damage that involves the banks of the immediately adjacent superior temporal sulcus causes neglect of contralesional stimuli.[207,363] Lesions involving the inferior parietal lobule also interfere with the ability to solve a tactile visuomotor maze and impair the ability to determine allocentric spatial relations among objects.[281,350] Although precise functional homologies between human and monkey brains are difficult to establish, these lesion experiments show that there are considerable interspecies similarities in the behavioral affiliations of posterior parietal cortex and therefore suggest that the physiological properties of neurons in this portion of the monkey brain may help to reveal the neural bases of directed attention and neglect in the human.

As in the human brain, the posterior parietal cortex of the macaque includes the *superior parietal lobule* (involved mostly in somatosensory function), the *inferior parietal lobule* (involved mostly in heteromodal integration, but with a visual bias posteriorly and a somatosensory bias anteriorly), the *intraparietal sulcus* (involved in visuomotor integration and limb reaching), and *medial parietal cortex*. The extensive cortex along the intraparietal sulcus of the macaque brain has been subdivided into a mosaic of functionally distinct regions known as LIP, MIP, VIP, and AIP (lateral, medial, ventral, and anterior intraparietal).[312] Among these areas, the posterior part of the inferior parietal lobule (BA 7a in the monkey) and area LIP show the closest relationship to visuospatial attention whereas the superior parietal lobule

(BA5), the anterior part of the inferior parietal lobule (BA7b), MIP, VIP, and AIP are more closely related to manual reaching and grasping (Fig. 3–14).

Ingenious experiments based on the recording of individual neurons in awake and behaving macaque monkeys show that these areas collectively display two properties that are of critical importance for shifting attention from one extrapersonal target to the other. (1) They form a representation of the external space based on motivational salience rather than on shape, color, or object identity. (2) They enable the mapping not of absolute spatial position but of "kinetic plans" for exploring, grasping, and foveating salient events. Neurons in the posterior inferior parietal lobule and adjacent intraparietal sulcus, for example, increase their firing rates when the animal detects, looks at, or reaches toward a motivationally relevant object such as food when hungry or liquid when thirsty.[40,166,206,256,302] These neurons are not as responsive if the visual event has no motivational significance or if equivalent eye and limb movements are performed passively or spontaneously.[126,206] Furthermore, some neurons are more active before a targeted saccadic eye movement whereas others are more active before a reaching movement toward the same stimulus, indicating that the encoding is contingent on the nature of the intended action rather than on spatial position alone.[328] Many of these neurons display both sensory and motor contingencies, explaining why so many manifestations of uni-

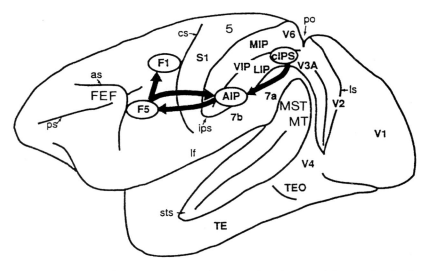

FIGURE 3–14. The location of cortical areas related to spatial attention in the macaque brain. Modified from Sakata et al.[311] Abbreviations: as=arcuate sulcus; cIPS=caudal intraparietal sulcus; cs=central sulcus; FEF=frontal eye field; F1=primary motor area; F5= hand region of ventral premotor cortex; ips=intraparietal sulcus; lf= lateral (sylvian) fissure; LIP = lateral intraparietal area; ls=lunate sulcus; MIP=medial intraparietal area; po=parieto-occipital sulcus; MT (V5), MST=motion-sensitive visual areas of the superior temporal sulcus; ps=principal sulcus; sts=superior temporal sulcus; S1=primary somatosensory area; TE and TEO=inferotemporal visual association areas; VIP=ventral intraparietal area; V1–4, V6=the primary, secondary, third, fourth, and sixth visual areas; 5, 7a, 7b=Brodmann areas.

lateral neglect resulting from parietal lesions reflect a breakdown of sensory–motor integration rather than an isolated disruption of perception or movement.

Area LIP, located in the lateral bank of the intraparietal sulcus, is known as the "posterior eye field" because of its critical role in coordinating eye movements. It is closely interconnected with the FEF and the superior colliculus, triggers saccadic eye movements in response to microstimulation, and gives directionally tuned responses prior to saccadic eye movements directed to visual targets or their remembered sites.[6] Neurons in LIP have sensory, motor, and memory fields. They respond when the monkey intends to make a saccade that will bring a behaviorally relevant stimulus (or its remembered site) into their receptive fields.[94] The activity during the delay period before a saccade indicates that these neurons encode covert shifts of the attentional focus, the intention to shift the attentional focus, or the activation of a motor plan to move the eyes toward the target.

In the monkey, area 7a of posterior parietal cortex is monosynaptically interconnected with LIP. This area seems to have a closer relationship to the encoding of attentional factors than to the control of saccadic eye movements. Thus, 7a neurons have fewer connections with FEF, give fewer presaccadic responses, and do not trigger saccadic eye movements upon stimulation.[329] These neurons have large receptive fields and relatively little sensitivity for color, shape, orientation, or object identity. They respond to behaviorally relevant events whether or not such events become targeted for reaching or foveation. This was demonstrated by training monkeys to maintain central fixation while a spot of light appeared in the peripheral field. In some trials, detection of subsequent dimming of the peripheral spot was rewarded while in other trials, identically placed spots had no such behavioral relevance. Even in the absence of any head and eye movements, the response of these neurons to the onset of the light spot was much more vigorous when reward was made contingent on the detection of subsequent dimming.[40] These neurons may therefore play a major role in encoding a map of salience which can be used by LIP to generate motor plans.

Neurons in posterior parietal cortex can be said to represent the extrapersonal world according to the motor output needed for grasping and exploring behaviorally salient events. The visual (or auditory) information emanating from these events is initially registered in retinocentric (or head-centered) coordinates. However, coordinate transformations become necessary because the relevant motor output needs to be planned in egocentric and spatial coordinates. Such remappings seem to take place at various sites within posterior parietal cortex, especially in areas 7a and LIP. Neurons in these two regions have visual receptive fields with strong gradients of excitability distributed according to foveal eccentricity. The gradient is retinotopic but the base level of excitability is gaze-dependent. Groups of these neurons can thus encode spatial position in a head-centered frame of reference by combining retinotopic information with information about eye position.[7]

Some of these neurons can also use proprioceptive information related to head position to create a body-centered representation and vestibular information in order to create a world-centered representation.[6] There are even some neurons which encode events in world-centered coordinates based on environmental landmarks

rather than proprioceptive or vestibular inputs.[8] Many LIP neurons with presaccadic activity for movements toward sources of sound display directional preferences that move with the eyes, indicating that they can bring auditory and visual
information into a common frame of reference in a way that promotes a holistic
sense of a single spatial dimension.[8] There may also be a segregation of neurons
sensitive to different frames of reference. For example, LIP is more closely involved
in constructing a body-centered representation based on proprioceptive input
whereas area 7a is more closely involved in constructing a world-centered representation based on vestibular input and environmental landmarks.[329] Posterior parietal cortex thus has the computational capability for the multimodal mapping of
salient events in multiple frames of reference. Damage to these neurons may account for the multimodal aspects of neglect and their manifestations according to
multiple coordinate frames.

Neurons in 7a and LIP participate not only in tasks that require an actual or
intended overt movement of the attentional focus but also in tasks that require
covert shifts of attention. Many of these neurons are excited by the appearance of
a cue which initiates a shift of covert attention. The subsequent appearance of a
target excites area 7a neurons only if it is at a location different from that of the
cue.[301,338] Thus neurons of area 7a and adjacent intraparietal sulcus provide signals
for redirecting the attentional focus even when the shift involves no head or eye
movements. The lack of response to targets located at the same site as the cue
indicates that these neurons are more closely involved in shifting the attentional
focus than in registering the presence or location of a significant event in the extrapersonal space.

Neurons in posterior and medial parietal cortex play an important role in additional aspects of spatial attention such as reaching, grasping, tactile search, and
manual exploration. For example, neurons in BA5 have somatosensory receptive
fields with directionally tuned responses coded in arm- or body-centered coordinates. These neurons give responses that are more closely related to the significance
of the stimulus and the motor planning it elicits than the actual execution of the
movement.[44] Thus in a go–no-go reaching task, neurons of BA5 were activated
during the delay period before an impending movement, regardless of whether the
animal was instructed to go or not, suggesting that "thinking" of the motor plan
was sufficient to induce the neural activity.[179] Neurons in area MIP, located in the
posterior portion of the medial bank of the intraparietal sulcus, fire optimally when
the animal reaches toward a visual target. This sector of the intraparietal sulcus
projects selectively to the arm region of premotor cortex where neurons encode
motor programs in arm-centered coordinates.[54] Area AIP, located in the anterior
part of the lateral bank of the intraparietal sulcus, is interconnected with ventral
premotor area F5 and coordinates the manual grasping of complex visual objects.
Furthermore, neurons in VIP have corresponding tactile and visual selectivities, so
a neuron with a foveal visual receptive field will have a somatosensory receptive
field around the mouth, suggesting that it may integrate the process of buccal grasp
under visual guidance.[54] Area 7b also contains neurons with corresponding tactile
and visual receptive fields: If the tactile field is on the hand the visual field is also

near the hand, even when the hand moves but the eyes do not.[127] Such neurons would be expected to play an important role in behaviors where tactile search is conducted under visual guidance.

The medial parietal cortex contains a parieto-occipital area, PO, also known as V6. Area V6 and adjacent regions of medial parietal cortex contain neurons which participate in the encoding of stimulus location in body-centered coordinates. These neurons project to dorsal premotor cortex, provide sites for visuosomatomotor integration, and contribute to target localization under conditions where visual scanning needs to be coordinated with manual reaching.[176] Neurons medial and posterior to LIP, in a region known as the parietal reach region, fire during visually guided arm movements and may play a role in manual grasping and tactile exploration in a manner that is analogous to the role of LIP in visual search and gaze.[328] Posterior parietal cortex thus contains many areas which coordinate manual reaching and tactile exploration. Damage to these areas may be responsible for the hypokinesia, intentional neglect, and tactile exploration deficits in patients with neglect.

These observations suggest that the brain does not have a unitary "spatial map." Instead, posterior parietal cortex contains several mappings of behaviorally relevant targets in terms of the motor strategies that would be needed to reach or foveate them. If there is a sensory "representation" in parietal cortex, it appears to be encoded in terms of strategies aimed at shifting the focus of attention to a behaviorally relevant target. Posterior parietal cortex plays a relatively minor role in identifying the perceptual or semantic nature of the stimulus that has been chosen as the target of attentional focusing. This latter function is carried out by more ventral association areas. The two streams of processing become integrated through multiple interconnections, including those that have been described between inferotemporal cortex and are 7a.[238]

The Temporo-Occipitoparietal Area, the Superior Temporal Sulcus, and the Encoding of Visual Motion

Because extrapersonal events and the observer can move with respect to each other, the neural mechanisms that direct attention to external targets must be sensitive to motion of the self and of the target. In the macaque, motion-sensitive neurons are located in the banks of the superior temporal sulcus, in areas known as MT (V5), MST and FST. On topographical grounds, these areas, especially MST and FST, can be considered as part of the inferior parietal lobule. Neurons in MST and FST have larger receptive fields than those in MT. They also have response properties which suggest they use information about real or inferred motion to generate signals for smooth pursuit eye movements.[95,168] The neurons of MST have preferred movement directions, encode complex motion patterns, enhance their responses to behaviorally relevant stimuli, and show a reduction of directional selectivity if attention is attracted to a point outside their receptive fields.[348] Neurons in MST are also responsive to optic flow, so they can encode self-motion and the direction of heading.[198] These neurons may help to direct attention toward targets that are in motion, select a heading for approaching targets, and navigate the body among solid objects in the environment.

In the macaque brain area MST (and perhaps also FST) is interconnected with the inferior parietal lobule–intraparietal sulcus region, the frontal eye fields, and the cingulate gyrus.[14,34,238,268] Areas MST and FST are also interconnected with the adjacent heteromodal cortex of the superior temporal sulcus and inferotemporal visual association cortex.[34] The MST and FST thus provide neural bridges between the dorsal and ventral streams of visual processing. Neurons in the posterior part of the inferior parietal lobule and in area VIP also participate in optic flow analysis.[36,324] Neurons in VIP are more sensitive to motion in near-space, whereas MST neurons may be more sensitive to motion in far space.[36,54] This difference may provide one of the several potential neural substrates for the dissociation of neglect for near-space from neglect for far-space.

Some of these motion-sensitive areas are likely to have been damaged as part of the superior temporal sulcus ablations that cause contralesional neglect in the macaque.[363] In the cat, the reversible inactivation of an area equivalent to MT (V5) causes severe contralesional visual neglect.[275] The extent to which these areas are part of the attentional network in the human has not yet been fully settled. Tasks of covert attentional shifts have led to activations at the confluence of the temporal, parietal, and occipital lobes in the most posterior aspects of the middle temporal gyrus.[118,185] This activation falls within a region designated as MT+ which probably includes the human homologues of MT (V5), MST, and FST.[79] In one patient, damage confined to this region led to left-sided target cancellation deficits even 4 years after the cerebrovascular accident, and even in the absence of any visual field cut.[141] It appears, therefore, that this temporo-occipitoparietal area may play an important role in the attentional network, at least for certain types of spatial attention.

The Frontal Connection in Neglect

Numerous clinical reports have shown that lesions confined to the right frontal lobe can cause states of contralesional neglect which are just as severe as those caused by parietal lesions.[66,149,164,326] Although this type of neglect had initially been attributed to head and eye deviations caused by a weakness of neck and eye muscles, clinical observations showed that the head and eye deviation were secondary to the inattention rather than its cause.[15] The critical frontal area responsible for the emergence of the neglect syndrome has been difficult to infer. Some authors have implicated the region of the FEF, and others the inferior frontal gyrus.[66,164,227]

Many functional imaging experiments based on tasks of either overt of covert shifts of directed attention reported activation in the region of FEF, usually extending into adjacent premotor and prefrontal cortex.[61,119,185,262] As opposed to the FEF of the monkey which is located in the posterior part of BA8, the human FEF is located in BA6 at the junction of the precentral and superior frontal sulci.[14,69,274] Activation in the human FEF has been seen during covert attention shifts even when potentially confounding factors such as working memory, intense foveal fixation, inhibition of eye movements, and the conditional (go–no-go) aspects of the task have been controlled.[118] A definitive demonstration of FEF activation in covert attention shifting tasks has been hampered by the inability to monitor eye movements during the imaging. This has posed a potential dilemma since occasional eye movements, either reflexive or induced by blinks, do occur even when the subject is instructed to keep the eyes still and could conceivably account for the observed FEF activation. As an indirect test of this hypothesis, we compared the activation in the covert attentional task to activation in a task where the subject was instructed to make non-attentional saccadic eye movements to the left and right.[261] When the activation in the saccade task was subtracted from the activation in the covert attentional shifting task, residual FEF activation was still seen. Since the surreptitious and rare saccades in the covert task could not possibly have involved more eye movements than the deliberate saccades, the residual FEF activation in this experiment suggested that at least some of the FEF activation must have been related to the attentional shifts rather than the eye movements. It appears, therefore, that tasks of spatial attention, overt as well as covert, lead to FEF activation and that this region can be considered as the frontal core of the attentional network. In many reports, tasks of spatial attention elicit additional frontal activation in a medial premotor area known as the supplementary motor cortex and in lateral prefrontal cortex. These two areas may need to be included within the frontal component of the attentional network.

In the macaque monkey, lesions in the area of the FEF have been known to result in marked contralateral neglect.[25,182,362,368] Animals with such lesions do not orient toward the contralateral hemispace, fail to retrieve motivationally relevant objects from the contralesional side even with the intact arm, and show poor orientation and exploration within the contralesional hemispace even in the absence of competing stimuli from the intact side. As in humans, the lack of response to events in the neglected hemispace may be so profound that it may be difficult to distinguish hemianopia from neglect.[182]

The FEF of the monkey is interconnected with posterior parietal cortex, peristriate and inferotemporal cortex, the cingulate gyrus, other prefrontal areas, and the dorsomedial and medial pulvinar nuclei of the thalamus.[14] The reciprocal parietal connections of FEF are directed predominantly to LIP and, to a lesser extent, to area 7a. The FEF also sends efferent projections to premotor cortex as well as to the striatum, superior colliculus and subthalamic nucleus.[12,236] These projections provide direct access to pathways that control head, eye, and limb movements necessary for visual scanning and other exploratory activities. Up to 51% of all the afferent input into the caudal portion of the FEF originates in unimodal visual association areas in the peristriate and inferotemporal regions.[14] This pattern suggests that the FEF may be profoundly influenced by (and probably also profoundly influences) visual information at a relatively early stage of analysis. This may explain why a lesion so far removed from traditional visual pathways may appear to result in a major disturbance of visually guided behavior. Parts of the frontal eye fields also receive auditory input, and this connection may mediate orientation to auditory stimuli.[14] Furthermore, the frontal eye fields receive extensive limbic inputs from the cingulate cortex. This connection may be important in directing exploratory movements toward motivationally relevant segments of the extrapersonal space. It is interesting that posterior parietal cortex and the FEF receive inputs from overlapping groups of cingulate neurons.[247] This arrangement would ensure that the frontal and parietal regions that are important for attention receive similar information about the distribution of motivational relevance.

The FEF and the superior colliculus contain units that could be considered command neurons for eye movements, and combined lesions in both of these areas yield a severe depression of contralaterally directed saccades.[123,314,371] It has been suggested that the superior colliculus may mediate the foveation of peripheral stimuli, whereas the frontal eye fields may mediate the internal planning and spatial organization of exploration with the head and eyes and perhaps also with the limbs.[55,227] In the monkey, FEF neurons give a burst of activity just before a saccade to a behaviorally relevant target or to its remembered site. Spontaneous saccades not directed toward a relevant object do not elicit such bursts. These neurons have relatively large and mostly contralateral visual fields. The direction of a saccade that will occur upon microstimulation of a particular neuron is independent of orbital eye position and can be predicted by mapping its visual field.[123] As in the case of LIP, with which it is tightly interconnected, the FEF can thus play a crucial role in foveating and visually exploring behaviorally relevant visual targets. In addition to generating contraversive saccades, the FEF neurons also play major roles in maintaining fixation and suppressing inappropriate saccades.[83,331] Neurons in the FEF also participate in the on-line retention of spatial information in tasks that require saccadic eye movements toward the remembered sites of relevant targets. These neurons may thus encode the type of sensory–motor working memory which is essential for the systematic exploration of a visual scene under the guidance of mental representations.

Unilateral inactivation of the FEF leads to a selective impairment of contraversive saccades. After such inactivation, the same spot in head-centered contralateral space is more successfully targeted by ipsiversive saccades originating from an eccentric contralateral fixation point than by contraversive saccades originating from central fixation points.[331] The deficit is not necessarily for making saccades within the contralateral head-centered space but for making them in a contraversive direction anywhere in the extrapersonal space, showing that the FEF uses a "vector" code signaling the direction of saccades rather than a strictly "place" code signaling their destination.[331] These properties are consistent with the vectorial properties of the model illustrated in Figure 3–10.

The supplementary eye field (SEF) is an oculomotor area on the dorsomedial surface of the frontal lobe. As in the case of the FEF, the human SEF becomes activated by real as well as imagined saccadic eye movements.[32] Its relationship to eye movements is slightly more complex than that of the FEF, since SEF stimulation induces eye movements with a dependence on the position of the eyes in the orbit. Neurons in SEF discharge before saccadic eye movements and are active during the learning of associations between visual cues and the direction of eye movements.[263] In a task where macaque monkeys were required to make eye movements to the right or left of a horizontal bar, SEF neurons fired differentially as a function of the end to which the eye movement was made regardless of the direction of the movement.[263] Thus, neurons in the SEF appear to have motor action fields defined relative to an object-centered frame of reference. Such neurons may participate in encoding external events in object-centered coordinates and may contribute to the emergence of the object-centered aspects of neglect.

In addition to their role in reaching and grasping, neurons of the ventral premotor cortex respond preferentially to visual stimuli in the space near the arms and face whereas FEF neurons respond to more distant stimuli, thus providing another potential neural substrate for the distinction between near and far neglect. Neurons in ventral premotor cortex also encode the egocentric location of objects, even after the light is turned off, in a way that may underlie the ability to reach toward or avoid objects in the dark.[128]

A review of LIP and FEF neurons may occasionally give the impression that the two have nearly identical properties. Both areas have neurons with visual as well as saccade-related discharges, saccades are obtained by microstimulation in both areas, both project to the intermediate layers of the superior colliculus and both display predictive remapping of receptive fields prior to an impending eye movement. However, neurons with exclusively sensory responses to stimuli are more common in LIP whereas neurons that display exclusively presaccadic discharges are more common in FEF. Furthermore, the FEF projection to the superior colliculus arises predominantly from saccade-related neurons, whereas the LIP projection comes predominantly from neurons with visual activity.[272] It appears, therefore, that the FEF signal conveys a more advanced sensory-to-motor transformation and may therefore exert a greater influence upon the collicular encoding of eye movement commands.[272,317] Although this information appears to imply that LIP is more "sensory" and FEF more "motor," both areas support sensory–motor integration, explaining why frontal as well as parietal lesions can lead to neglect syndromes with sensory as well as motor manifestations.

The Limbic Connection in Neglect

Patients who develop neglect on the basis of lesions confined to the cingulate gyrus are rare.[154] However, functional imaging studies in neurologically normal subjects engaged in tasks of covert shifts of attention, overt oculomotor exploration, and manual search have consistently shown an anterior cingulate focus of activation.[118,185,262] Subjects who are most effective in shifting spatial attention also show significant activation in the posterior cingulate gyrus.[186] The cingulate component of the attentional network may thus have two parts: an anterior part which may reflect a global attentional engagement, and a posterior part which may participate in more differentiated lateralized shifts of motivational relevance and focalized attention.

In cats, stimulation of the cingulate region suppresses searching head and eye movements toward the contralateral side.[174] In monkeys, unilateral lesions of the cingulum bundle and adjacent cingulate cortex result in contralateral somatosensory extinction.[360] Monosynaptic connections link the cingulate gyrus to the FEF,

BA7a, and perhaps also the superior colliculus.[14,193,238] The cingulate projection may enable FEF and BA7a neurons to encode the behavioral relevance of extrapersonal events.

The cingulate gyrus displays a complex organization of architecture, connectivity, and function. Its multiple behavioral affiliations are predominantly limbic in the ventral cingulate, visuospatial in the posterodorsal cingulate, and somatomotor in the anterodorsal cingulate. Neurons in the dorsal part of the anterior cingulate fire in response to behaviorally relevant cues and during the planning and execution of reaching movements.[264] Neurons of the posterior cingulate gyrus fire tonically during steady gaze at a rate determined by the direction of preceding eye movement and the current angle of the eye in the orbit.[264] Their activity increases immediately following saccadic eye movements. Saccadic eye movements to the same target can elicit different firing intensities if they are based on contraversive versus ipsiversive saccades.[264] These neurons are therefore encoding the direction of displacement rather than the location of the target. Since their activity is postsaccadic, they are likely to be monitoring rather than controlling overt shifts in the direction of visual attention. The predominance of postsaccadic activity is reminiscent of neuronal activity in BA7a whereas the vectorial encoding is reminiscent of neuronal activity in FEF.

Subcortical Neglect and Phylogenetic Corticalization of Attention

Unilateral neglect in the human has been reported after lesions of the thalamus.[43,290,315,359] The deficit has been attributed to an impairment in *engaging* the contralesional target and has been contrasted to the *disengagement* deficit associated with parietal lesions.[290] In some patients the medial dorsal and medial pulvinar nuclei were at the focus of the neglect-causing thalamic lesion. Functional imaging during tasks of attentional shifts has shown activations in the ventral lateral nucleus and in a region that is at the junction of the medial pulvinar and the mediodorsal nucleus.[118] Pulvinar activation is also seen in tasks of selective attention to objects and seems to encode the behavioral salience or relevance of stimuli.[195,250] In the monkey, the receptive fields of neurons in the medial pulvinar nucleus are quite large. They show attentional modulation when the stimulus is made behaviorally relevant and may help to generate visual salience by increasing the signal-to-noise ratio.[280,300] In concert with BA7a, with which it is interconnected, the pulvinar nucleus may thus participate in establishing a representational map of salience. The medial pulvinar is the major thalamic nucleus for BA7a whereas the mediodorsal nucleus provides the major thalamic input to the FEF. However, both thalamic nuclei project to FEF, 7a, and the cingulate gyrus.[14,238]

Unilateral striatal damage has also been associated with contralateral neglect.[68,142,205] Functional imaging has shown caudate and putaminal activation during overt and covert shifts of spatial attention.[118,119] Striatal dysfunction induced by interrupting the dopaminergic nigrostriatal pathway yields contralateral neglect in cats, rats, and monkeys.[104,203,215,243] Unilateral Parkinson's disease, especially when it affects the right nigrostriatal system, leads to manifestations of contralesional neglect.[96] Some neurons in the caudate and putamen of the macaque monkey are preferentially active in relationship to cues which direct spatial attention, whereas others are selectively active following cues which instruct a motor act.[183] These neurons are sensitive to the behavioral relevance of the cue but not to its color and participate in the construction of spatial plans for the sequential distribution of attention-related oculomotor and limb movements.[184,243]

The intermediate layers of the superior colliculus play a critical role in initiating eye movements, foveating visual targets, and releasing ocular fixation when a new target must be foveated.[89] The superior colliculus receives input directly from the retina, from primary visual cortex, from LIP, from the FEF, and perhaps also from the cingulate gyrus.[193] Its intermediate (oculomotor) layers receive partially overlapping input from the FEF and LIP.[319] Lesions of the superior colliculus can lead to contralesional neglect in the cat.[336] There are no analogous human cases. Functional imaging shows more superior colliculus activation in tasks of overt oculomotor exploration than in those of covert attentional shifts.[120]

Several functional imaging studies had detected cerebellar activation even in tasks of covert attentional shifts, suggesting that the cerebellum may play an important role in spatial attention. However, an experiment which employed stringent controls for all motor activities involved in the task failed to show cerebellar activation associated with covert shifts of attention.[118] This is consistent with studies which show that cerebellar lesions do not cause deficits in covert shifts of attention.[372] Conceivably, the cerebellum may play a more important role in tasks that involve overt exploration.

Components of the ARAS such as the intralaminar thalamic nuclei, the brainstem raphe nuclei, the nucleus locus coeruleus, the ventral tegmental area–substantia nigra, and the nucleus basalis project to each cortical component of the attentional network. These projections modulate the activation state of the attentional network. In keeping with this relationship, unilateral lesions in the intralaminar nuclei and even in the mesencephalic reticular formation trigger contralateral neglect in the cat and in the monkey.[265,361,362]

Prefrontal lesions cause neglect in monkeys and humans but not in cats, and the parietal neglect in the monkey is mild compared to the neglect that is seen after analogous lesions in the human brain. It appears, therefore, that cerebral cortex assumes an increasingly more critical role in spatial attention in the course of phylogenetic evolution. In humans, even those neglect syndromes that arise in conjunction with subcortical lesions could conceivably reflect an associated state of cortical dysfunction caused by the interruption of corticocortical connection pathways running in the white matter or diaschisis-induced remote cortical hypometabolism. In fact, neglect-causing subcortical lesions have been reported to induce distal hypometabolism in frontal and parietal cortex.[107]

VII. DISSOCIATIONS AND SUBTYPES—IS THERE PARIETAL VERSUS FRONTAL NEGLECT?

The symptoms and signs of neglect are so numerous that no individual patient is likely to manifest them all. Dissociations among the behavioral components are the rule rather than the exception. Some patients display extinction but no other symptom of neglect while others display most of the other manifestations of neglect except for extinction.[66,201,365] Patients who only display extinction can direct focal attention anywhere in the extrapersonal space, but only when there is one target at a given time. These patients seem to have a relatively selective impairment of global attention. Thus, when the extrapersonal space contains multiple events which need to be detected in parallel, events on the left side lose their salience and become ignored.

Other patients display no extinction upon bilateral simultaneous stimulation but fail to detect targets on the left. Such patients presumably have a relatively preserved global awareness of the extrapersonal space but cannot direct focal attention to the left. In addition to the dissociation of extinction from the other manifestations of neglect, other dissociations have also been reported, including those of clock drawing from target cancellation,[366] visual from tactile or auditory extinction,[71,342] directional hypokinesia from perceptual representation,[31,241] and perceptual representation from target cancellation.[23,62,210]

These dissociations could conceivably represent clinical "subtypes" of neglect, each with a different anatomical substrate within the attentional network. Some evidence suggests that reaching deficits, extinction, and extinction-like phenomena (such as attentional disengagement in tasks of covert attentional shifts) may be associated with superior parietal lobule lesions whereas the distortions of spatial representation and perhaps other manifestations of neglect may be associated with inferior parietal lobule lesions.[242,289,351] However, functional imaging experiments have not yet supported this correlation and clinical reports indicate that directional reaching may be impaired after inferior parietal lesions as well.[118,119,217]

Despite the overwhelming evidence which now links both posterior parietal cortex and the FEF to sensory–motor integration, traditional neurology still tends to associate the parietal lobe with "sensory" and the frontal lobe with "motor" function. A relatively attractive hypothesis has therefore evolved around the possibility that "parietal neglect" might be predominantly perceptual whereas "frontal neglect" might be predominantly motor. In support of this possibility, several studies have shown that "perceptual" tasks such as extinction and line bisection are more likely to be associated with parietal lesions whereas "motor" tasks such as target cancellation are more likely to be associated with frontal lesions.[26,66,201] Since the traditional line bisection task requires a manual response for placing the bisection point and since target cancellation tasks need to unfold within a perceptual template of the stimulus display, ingenious experiments with pulleys and mirrors have been devised to dissociate the representational from the motor aspects of these tasks. Some of these experiments have shown that errors in these tasks can be attributed to representational biases in patients with parietal lesions and to directional hypokinesia in patients with frontal lesions.[31,345] Other studies, however, have not been able to confirm the presence of a relationship between directional hypokinesia and frontal lesions,[217] or have identified behavioral subtypes without being able to fit them into anatomical subtypes.[221] A definitive study based on tasks that isolate the representational from the exploratory aspects of spatial attention remains to be done in patients with small lesions confined to the frontal or parietal lobes.

Even if such a study were done, however, it is unrealistic to expect a strict dichotomy between parietal and frontal lesions, with the former displaying a pure sensory subtype of the neglect syndrome and the latter a pure motor subtype. The frontal and parietal components of the attentional network subserve a level of sensory–motor integration where the boundaries between action and perception become blurred. At a behavioral level, sensory representations are necessary for guiding exploration, and exploration is necessary for updating representations.[93,227] At a physiological level, parietal and FEF neurons have motor as well as sensory fields. Thus both parietal and frontal lesions would be expected to yield neglect syndromes with sensory–representational as well as motor–exploratory components. Furthermore, the strong interconnectivity between the frontal and parietal components of the attentional network raises the possibility that damage to one may induce distal dysfunction in the other through the process of diaschisis. This would further reduce the possibility of seeing anatomically segregated subtypes of neglect. A narrow sensory versus motor dichotomy in relationship to parietal versus frontal lesions is therefore unlikely and has not been supported by either animal or human studies on neglect. The most that could be expected is to find a relative (and probably quite subtle) predominance of representational features in the manifestations of the neglect caused by parietal lesions and a relative predominance of exploratory (not just intentional) features in the manifestations of the neglect caused by frontal lesions.

VIII. A NEURAL NETWORK FOR THE DISTRIBUTION OF SPATIAL ATTENTION

The evidence reviewed earlier has led to the hypothesis that directed attention to the extrapersonal space is organized at the level of a distributed large-scale network revolving around three cortical epicenters (or local networks). Each of these epicenters supports a slightly different but interactive and complementary type of neural encoding. The collective activity of these three epicenters allows behaviorally salient targets in the environment to be represented mentally and to become the targets of further action and exploration.[227] Lesions within any component of the network in Figure 3–13 or to its interconnections can result in contralesional neglect. Depending on the exact site of the lesion, the resulting neglect syndrome can be multimodal or modality-specific and can lead to clinical patterns that differ from patient to patient even if there is no fixed and universal relationship between lesion site and clinical subtype. In general, lesions that encroach upon network epicenters are likely to cause multimodal deficits whereas those that disconnect the network from specific afferents could cause modality-specific attentional disorders.

The attentional network depicted in Figure 3–13 is organization according to the computational principles outlined in Chapter 1. This was determined in the macaque brain by injecting two different retrogradely transported fluorescent tracers, one in the FEF and the other in the region of the intraparietal sulcus and BA7a.[247] The results showed that these two epicenters of the attentional network were interconnected not only with each other and the cingulate gyrus but also with an identical set of 12 additional areas in the premotor, lateral prefrontal, orbitofrontal, lateral and inferior temporal, parahippocampal, and insular cortex. All of these areas appear to participate in the coordination of spatial attention. However, the FEF, posterior parietal cortex, and cingulate gyrus play a more critical role than the others since they are the only sites where damage consistently leads to contralesional neglect. The fact that FEF and posterior parietal cortex have common connections with exactly the same set of additional areas creates an arrangement which supports parallel processing and through which the entire network can execute a very rapid survey of a vast informational landscape related to motivational salience, spatial representations, and motor strategies. Attention can thus be shifted adaptively from one site to another according to behavioral relevance.

In these anatomical experiments, double labeling with both retrograde tracers (indicating that the same neuron projects to both injection sites through axonal collaterals) was very rare and confined to only a few neurons in the FEF, posterior parietal cortex, and cingulate gyrus.[247] Thus the information directed to the two epicenters of the attentional network from a common cortical source needs to be integrated by local circuit neurons, providing greater computational flexibility than if this integration were mediated by collateral axons of the same neurons. Anatomical experiments in the monkey also found that the medial pulvinar and parts of the mediodorsal nucleus project to both the FEF and posterior parietal cortex and that both of these cortical areas send interdigitating projections to the striatum, suggesting that these subcortical structures may play an important role in integrating the activity of network components.[231]

Assigning an identifiable "task" to each component of this network raises the specter of anthropomorphism but serves a heuristic purpose. Thus, the posterior parietal component (centered around the intraparietal sulcus but including adjacent cortex of the inferior and superior parietal lobules) may encode salient events in egocentric, allocentric, environment-centered and perhaps object-centered coordinates. The resulting mental representation would allow behaviorally relevant environmental events to be mapped with respect to each other and with respect to the observer so that they can be targeted for covert shifts of the attentional focus, overt foveation, oculomotor scanning, tactile exploration, reaching, and manual grasp. The dual functional role of the parietal component is to create a dynamic representation of salience and to compute provisional strategies (or plans) for shifting attention from one salient target to the other.

The parietal component of the attentional network contains the heteromodal region designated "P" in Figure 1–11b of Chapter 1. This region acts as a critical gateway for spatial attention in ways that are analogous to the critical role of Wernicke's area in language comprehension and of the hippocampo–entorhinal complex in declarative memory. Wernicke's area (indicated by "W" in Figure 1–11b of Chapter 1), for example, assumes a critical role in language comprehension, not as the convergent site of a mental lexicon, but as a transmodal gateway for linking word forms in multiple sensory modalities to the distributed associations that encode their meaning.[233] The hippocampo–entorhinal complex (indicated by "L" in Figure 1–11b of Chapter 1) assumes its critical role in memory not as the site of memory storage but as a gateway for binding distributed fragments of events and experiences into coherent entities that can support declarative recall. In a similar fashion, posterior parietal cortex would seem to play its key role in spatial attention not as the repository of a multimodal spatial map but as a critical gateway for linking distributed channels of spatially relevant information with each other and with multiple channels of motor output related to orienting, reaching, grasping, scanning, and exploration. When the parietal component of the attentional network is destroyed, the individual input and output channels may remain quite intact but they cannot be integrated into a coherent template that can sustain flexible shifts of spatial attention.

The frontal component of the attentional network (centered around the FEF but including adjacent premotor and perhaps prefrontal cortex) may play its critical role in the attentional network by converting plans and intentions into specific sequences of motor acts that shift the focus of attention. There is no single set of spatial codes upon which all kinetic strategies for exploration, foveation, and grasping converge. Instead, there are multiple circuits, such as LIP–FEF and AIP–F5, each specialized for specific input–output relationships related to looking, grasping, searching, and so on. The parietal and frontal components of the attentional network provide gateways for accessing and coordinating these circuits. They also constitute "bottlenecks" where lesions have the most severe impact on the integrity of directed attention. It might be said that the posterior parietal cortex sculpts a salience- and trajectory-based template of the extrapersonal space, whereas the FEF selects and sequences the individual acts needed to navigate and explore the resultant landscape. The role of the cingulate component is the least well understood. As a limbic component of the attentional network, the cingulate gyrus may play a critical role in identifying the motivational relevance of extrapersonal events and in sustaining the level of effort during the execution of attentional tasks.

The frontal and parietal components of this network have a collective mechanism for specifying whether (and how) an event in ambient or imagined space will become the target of enhanced neuronal impact, visual grasp, manipulation, or exploration. Each of the three cortical components in Figure 3–13 serves a dual purpose: It provides a local network for regional neural computations and also a nodal point for the linkage of distributed information. Functional imaging experiments suggest that all three core components are probably engaged simultaneously and interactively by attentional tasks (Fig. 3–15). It is therefore unlikely that there is a temporal or processing-level hierarchy among components of the attentional network. The phenomenon of spatial attention is not the sequentially additive product of perception, motivation, and exploration but an emergent (i.e., relational) quality of the network as a whole.

IX. OVERLAP WITH OTHER NETWORKS: EYE MOVEMENTS, WORKING MEMORY, AND TEMPORAL EXPECTATION

Advanced primates interact with the environment predominantly through visually guided behaviors. In fact, the direction of gaze is almost always aligned with the direction of attention, except perhaps when there is a conscious intent to deceive an observer. Even auditory, tactile, and olfactory stimuli attract automatic visual orientation. It is therefore reasonable to expect a close relationship between the network for spatial attention and the network which controls eye movements. All components of the attentional network shown in Figure 3–13, the FEF, posterior parietal cortex, cingulate gyrus, superior colliculus, striatum, pulvinar, and mediodorsal nucleus, have been implicated in either the control or monitoring of eye movements.[4,8,89,303,317] When a covert spatial attention task was compared to a task of nonattentional repetitive saccadic eye movements, the components of the attentional network were found to be activated by both tasks although most activations were greater for the attentional than the saccadic task.[59,261] It appears, therefore, that the network for spatial attention is at least partially embedded within the sensory–motor network for oculomotor control, irrespective of whether the attentional task involves any eye movements. In keeping with this formulation, the covert lateral shifting of attention causes a contralateral deviation of vertical saccades, suggesting that shifts of spatial attention may automatically engage oculomotor mechanisms even when the attentional shifts do not involve eye movements.[321]

A second type of overlap occurs with the networks subserving working memory and temporal expectancy. A conjunction analysis of two tasks, one based on covert shifts of spatial attention and the other on working memory for letters, showed that the frontal and parietal epicenters of the attentional network displayed a nearly complete overlap with the areas activated by the working-memory task, although the working-memory task led to additional prefrontal activation, and the attentional task to additional parietal and temporal activation.[194] Furthermore, a task that manipulated temporal expectancy by directing attention to different temporal intervals led to the activation of all three cortical epicenters of the attentional network.[260] In further support of this overlap, it is interesting to note that estimates of time duration are particularly vulnerable to the same lesions that are most effective in causing neglect, namely premotor and posterior parietal lesion in the right hemisphere.[139]

One common denominator of the functions subserved by these overlapping networks located along the dorsal visuofugal streams of processing is that they *move* attention: from one location to another, from one point in time to another, and from

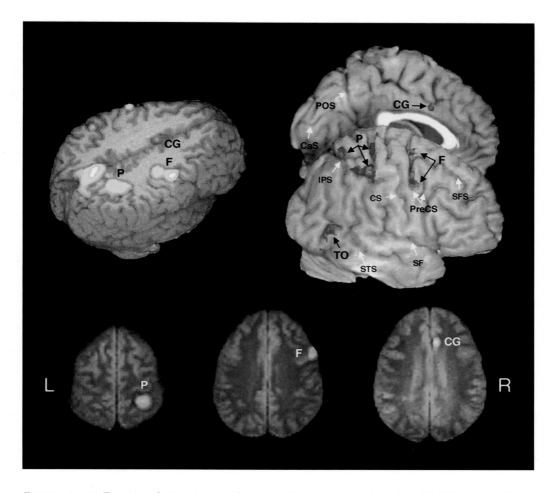

FIGURE 3–15. Functional imaging with magnetic resonance imaging (fMRI). Top left: Functional MRI of a subject engaged in a task of covert shifts of spatial attention. All three cortical components of the attentional network (parietal [P], FEF [F] and cingulate [CG]) are activated, and there is more activation in the right hemisphere although the task required symmetrical attentional shifts to the left and right.[121] Top right: Another subject performing the same task. The parietal component (P) is centered around the banks of the intraparietal sulcus (IPS). There is activation in a temporo-occipito-parietal (TO) area functionally corresponding to MT+.[121] Bottom: Functional PET study in a subject engaged in a task of manual exploration of the right hemispace with the right hand. As in the case of tasks based on covert shifts of visuospatial attention, this task of overt manual exploration leads to the activation of the same cortical epicenters of the attentional network: parietal (P), FEF (F), and cingulate (CG). The activations are almost exclusively right-sided although the task was being performed in the right hemispace with the right hand, a result which is consistent with the model depicted in Figure 3–10.[119] Additional abbreviations: CaS = calcarine fissure; CS = central sulcus; POS = parietoccipitol PreCS = precentral sulcus; SF = sylvian fissure; SFS = superior frontal sulcus; STS = superior temporal sulcus.

an external source of input to its internal on-line representation. It appears, therefore, that the network shown in Figure 3–13 subserves a general function of shifting the attentional focus in space, in time, and in mental domains. In comparison, the attentional function of the ventral streams of sensory processing is based on locking onto a specific object and filtering out irrelevant input.[245]

The network for spatial attention also displays partial overlap with cortical areas which coordinate additional aspects of attention. For example, tasks of selective attention (as assessed by the *Stroop* test), and divided attention cause cingulate and prefrontal activation.[60,63,271,344] Furthermore, nonspatial sustained attention tasks are impaired in patients with frontal or posterior parietal lesions and there is a strong correlation between the impairment of sustained attention and the severity of contralesional neglect, suggesting that the two aspects of attention may have intersecting anatomical substrates.[297,309] However, the overlap between the two sets of cortical areas is not complete. Thus, tasks of sustained attention display frontal activation predominantly in BA8–9–46 (rather than in FEF) and parietal activation predominantly in BA40 (rather than in the intraparietal sulcus).[175,270] These results are consistent with clinical observations indicating that damage to the inferior parietal lobule and to the inferior prefrontal cortex may lead to confusional states in patients who have no manifestations of unilateral neglect.[239]

X. Causes, Course, and Treatment of Unilateral Neglect and Relationship to Other Components of the Right Hemisphere Syndrome

Left unilateral neglect commonly occurs in conjunction with additional behavioral manifestations attributed to right hemisphere injury. These include denial of illness (anosognosia), constructional deficits, and dressing difficulty (apraxia). The correlation coefficients are 0.64 between extinction and apraxia, 0.46 between extinction and anosognosia, and 0.4 between extinction and defective block designs.[157] Unilateral neglect can arise not only as a consequence of focal structural lesions of the brain but also as a manifestation of seizures.[146] Toxic–metabolic encephalopathy, subdural hematoma, or head injury almost never give rise to unilateral neglect. Most patients recover from unilateral neglect caused by cerebrovascular accidents. Life-table analyses indicated that the median time required for 50% of the patients to recover from neglect behavior varied from 9 to 43 weeks.[158] The most persistent cases of neglect occur after large lesions which also extend to subcortical structures.

In macaque monkeys, the period of contralesional neglect following FEF lesions corresponds to the period of diaschisis-induced metabolic depression in subcortical areas synaptically related to the area of destruction. The recovery of neglect is linked to the normalization of metabolism in these distant regions.[77] In keeping with these experimental results, clinical recovery in some patients with neglect has been associated with the resolution of distal hypometabolism, especially in cortical areas that belong to the attentional network.[284] In other patients, clinical recovery has been associated with a resolution of distal hypometabolism in the contralateral left hemisphere.[276]

The nature of the behavioral deficits may give the impression that unilateral neglect would be amenable to behavioral modification. In individual cases, behavioral strategies such as sensory cueing and verbal instructions may indeed improve performance.[84,296] However, these gains are rarely lasting. Fresnel prisms, cold caloric stimulation to the contralesional ear, and vibratory stimulation to the contralesional neck muscles lead to temporary improvement of neglect because they realign the relationship between egocentric frames of reference and targets in the extrapersonal space.[178,180,307] Transient improvement has also been obtained by patching the ipsilesional eye, based on the assumption that this can cause a relatively greater deafferentation of the contralesional superior colliculus whose uninhibited activity has been blamed for the hyperattentiveness to the ipsilesional right hemispace.[296]

Since unilateral dopaminergic denervation can cause contralesional neglect, therapeutic trials with dopamine agonists have been initiated. One study reported improvement in two patients.[108] However, a larger study showed an opposite result, namely a worsening of contralesional visual search following the administration of bromocriptine.[130] The suggestion was made that systemically administered dopaminergic agents might help neglect syndromes caused by damage to the presynaptic component of ascending dopaminergic pathways but that they might have adverse effects in neglect syndromes caused by damage to the postsynaptic striatal and cortical components.[130]

XI. OVERVIEW AND CONCLUSIONS

Attention permeates all aspects of behavior. A flexible interplay between concentration and distractibility is one of the most essential prerequisites for advanced mental activity. Excess in either direction can lead to cognitive impairment. The judicious deployment of attentional resources is a difficult skill to master, and the directive to "pay attention" is ubiquitous in the education of children. In fact, attentional deficits probably constitute the single most common type of developmental learning disability of childhood.

Although no neuron is exclusively devoted to attention, all areas of the cerebral cortex display attentional modulations. These modulations are more prominent in downstream components of sensory pathways and within limbic and heteromodal association areas. Through such attentional modulations, the mental representation of experience transcends surface appearances and becomes sensitive to behavioral relevance. Domain-specific attentional responses are under the bottom-up influence of the ARAS and the top-down influence of frontoparietal and limbic cortices. Focal lesions which interfere with the bottom-up or top-down regulation of attention or multifocal partial lesions which disrupt multiple domain-specific attentional modulations give rise to the clinical syndrome of acute confusional states.

Contralesional neglect represents a domain-specific impairment of spatial attention. A large-scale distributed network with cortical epicenters in the posterior parietal cortex, FEF, and the cingulate gyrus mediates the transformation of extrapersonal events into internal representations which can then be targeted for attentional shifts. Damage to any cortical or subcortical component of this network leads to contralesional neglect. In the human brain, this network displays a distinctly asymmetrical organization. The left hemisphere directs attention mostly within the contaraletal hemispace and in a predominantly contraversive direction whereas the right hemisphere directs attention more evenly within both sides of space and in both direction. As a consequence of this organization, prominent contralesional neglect is seen almost exclusively after right hemisphere lesions. The neural network for spatial attention displays a partial overlap with other networks involved in moving the attentional focus from one point in time to another and from one mental domain to another.

The organization of the attentional network is similar to that of networks associated with language and memory. The advent of functional imaging, the ability to use identical attentional tasks in animals and humans, and the existence of an animal model for the attentional network have made this area of research particularly fruitful for exploring the organizing principles of large-scale neurocognitive networks in the human brain. A better understanding of these principles could potentially lead to more rational and effective therapeutic interventions for patients with spatial neglect and other cognitive deficits.

This work was supported in part by NS 30863 and NS 20285 from National Institutes for Neurological Disease and Stroke and AG 13854 from National Institute on Aging.

REFERENCES

1. Adams, R D and Victor, M: Delirium and other confusional states. In Wintrobe, M M, Thorn, G W, Adams, R D, Braunwald, E, Isselbacher, K J and Petersdorf, R G (Eds.): Principles of Internal Medicine. McGraw-Hill, New York, 1974, pp. 149–156.

2. Aglioti, S, Smania, N, Barbieri, C and Corbetta, M: Influence of stimulus salience and attentional demands on visual search patterns in hemispatial neglect. Brain Cogn 34:388–403, 1997.

3. Albert, M L: A simple test of visual neglect. Neurology 23:658–664, 1973.

4. Alexander, G E, Crutcher, M D and DeLong, M R: Basal ganglia-thalamocortical circuits: parallel substrates for motor, oculomotor, "prefrontal" and "limbic" functions. Prog Brain Res 85:119–146, 1990.

5. American Psychiatric Association: Diagnostic and Statistical Manual of Mental Disorders, DSM-IV. American Psychiatric Association, Washington, DC, 1994.

6. Andersen, R A: Encoding of intention and spatial location in the posterior parietal cortex. Cereb Cortex 5:457–469, 1995.

7. Andersen, R A, Essick, G K and Siegel, R M: Encoding of spatial location by posterior parietal neurons. Science 230:456–458, 1985.

8. Andersen, R A, Snyder, L H, Bradley, D C and Xing, J: Multimodal representation of

space in the posterior parietal cortex and its use in planning movements. Ann Rev Neurosci 20:303–330, 1997.

9. Anderson, B: A mathematical model of line bisection behaviour in neglect. Brain 119: 841–850, 1996.

10. Anzola, G P, Bertoloni, G, Buchtel, H A and Rizzolatti, G: Spatial compatibility and anatomical factors in simple and choice reaction times. Neuropsychologia 15:295–302, 1977.

11. Arguin, M and Bub, D: Modulation of the directional attention deficit in visual neglect by hemispatial factors. Brain Cogn 22:148–160, 1993.

12. Arikuni, T, Sakai, M, Hamada, I and Kubota, K: Topographical projections from the prefrontal cortex to the post-arcuate area in the rhesus monkey, studied by retrograde axonal transport of horseradish peroxidase. Neurosci Lett 19:155–160, 1980.

13. Babinski, J: Contribution a l'étude des troubles mentaux dans l'hémisplégie organique cerebrale (anosognosie). Rev Neurol (Paris) 27:845–848, 1914.

14. Barbas, H and Mesulam, M-M: Organization of afferent input to subdivisions of area 8 in the rhesus monkey. J Comp Neurol 200:407–431, 1981.

15. Bard, L: De l'origine sensorielle de la déviation conjuguée des yeux avec rotation de la tête chez les hémiplégiques. Semin Med 24:9–13, 1904.

16. Barton, J J S and Black, S E: Line bisection in hemianopia. J Neurol Neurosurg Psychiatry 64:660–662, 1998.

17. Battersby, W S, Khan, R L, Pollock, M and Bender, M B: Effects of visual, vestibular, and somatosensory-motor deficit on autokinetic perception. J Exp Psychol 52:398–410, 1956.

18. Behrmann, M and Moscovitch, M: Object-centered neglect in patients with unilateral neglect: effects of left-right coordinates of objects. J Cog Neurosci 6:1–16, 1994.

19. Behrmann, M, Moscovitch, M, Black, S E and Mozer, M: Perceptual and conceptual mechanisms in neglect dyslexia. Brain 113:1163–1183, 1990.

20. Behrmann, M, Watt, S, Black, S E and Barton, J J S: Impaired visual search in patients with unilateral neglect: an oculographic analysis. Neuropsychologia 35:1445–1458, 1997.

21. Bellas, D N, Novelly, R A, Eskenazi, B and Wasserstein, J: The nature of unilateral neglect in the olfactory sensory system. Neuropsychologia 26:45–52, 1988.

22. Berlyne, D: Conflict, Arousal and Curiosity. McGraw-Hill, New York, 1960.

23. Beschin, N, Cocchini, G, Sala, S D and Logie, R H: What the eyes perceive, the brain ignores: a case of pure unilateral representational neglect. Cortex 33:3–26, 1997.

24. Beschin, N, Cubelli, R, Sala, S D and Spinazzola, L: Left of what? The role of egocentric coordinates in neglect. J Neurol Neurosurg Psychiatry 63:483–489, 1997.

25. Bianchi, L: The functions of the frontal lobes. Brain 18:497–522, 1895.

26. Binder, J, Marshall, R, Lazar, R, Benjamin, J and Mohr, J P: Distinct syndromes of hemineglect. Arch Neurol 49:1187–1194, 1992.

27. Binkofski, F, Dohle, C, Posse, S, Stephan, K M, Hefter, H, Seitz, R J and Freund, H-J: Human anterior intraparietal area subserves prehension. Neurology 50:1253–1259, 1998.

28. Bisiach, E, Capitani, E, Luzzatti, C and Perani, D: Brain and conscious representation of outside reality. Neuropsychologia 19:543–551, 1981.

29. Bisiach, E, Luzzatti, C and Perani, D: Unilateral neglect, representational schema and consciousness. Brain 102:609–618, 1979.

30. Bisiach, E, Rusconi, M L, Peritti, A and Vallar, G: Challenging current accounts of unilateral neglect. Neuropsychologia 32:1431–1434, 1994.

31. Bisiach, G, Geminiani, G, Berti, A and Rusconi, M: Perceptual and premotor factors of unilateral neglect. Neurology 40:1278–1281, 1990.

32. Bodis-Wollner, I, Bucher, S F, Seelos, K C, Paulus, W, Reiser, M and Oertel, W H: Functional MRI mapping of occipital and frontal cortical activity during voluntary and imagined saccades. Neurology 49:416–420, 1997.

33. Boulenguez, P, Foreman, N, Chauveau, J, Segu, L and Buhot, M-C: Distractability and locomotor activity in rat following intracollicular injection of a serotonin 1B-1D agonist. Behav Brain Res 67:229–239, 1995.

34. Boussaoud, D, Ungerleider, L G and Desimone, R: Pathways for motion analysis: cortical connections of the medial superior temporal sulcus and fundus of the superior temporal visual areas in the macaque. J Comp Neurol 296:462–495, 1990.

35. Brain, W R: Visual disorientation with special reference to lesions of the right cerebral hemisphere. Brain 64:244–272, 1941.

36. Bremmer, F, Duhamel, J-R, Hamed, S B and Graf, W: The representation of movement in near extra-personal space in the macaque ventral intraparietal area (VIP). In Thier, P and Karnath, H-O (Eds.): Parietal Lobe Contributions to Orientation in 3D Space. Springer, Berlin, 1997, pp. 619–630.

37. Britton, D R, Ksir, C, Britton, K T, Young, D and Koob, G F: Brain norepinephrine depleting lesions selectively enhance behavioral responsiveness to novelty. Physiol Behav 33:473–478, 1984.

38. Broadbent, D E: Perception and Communication. Pergamon Press, New York, 1958.

39. Brown, M W, Wilson, F A and Riches, I P: Neuronal evidence that inferotemporal cortex is more important than hippocampus in certain processes underlying recognition memory. Brain Res 409:158–162, 1987.

40. Bushnell, M C, Goldberg, M E and Robinson, D L: Behavioral enhancement of visual responses in monkey cerebral cortex: 1. Modulation in posterior parietal cortex related to selective visual attention. J Neurophysiol 46:755–771, 1981.

41. Butler, R A: Discrimination learning by rhesus monkeys to visual-exploration motivation. J Comp Physiol Psychol 46:95–98, 1953.

42. Calvanio, R, Petrone, P N and Levine, D N: Left visual spatial neglect is both environment-centered and body-centered. Neurology 37:1179–1183, 1987.

43. Cambier, J, Elghozi, D and Strube, E: Lésion du thalamus droit avec syndrome de l'hémisphère mineur. Discussion du concept de négligence thalamique. Rev Neurol (Paris) 136:105–116, 1980.

44. Caminiti, R, Ferraina, S and Johnson, P B: The sources of visual information to the primate frontal lobe: a novel role for the superior parietal lobule. Cortex 319–328, 1996.

45. Cantagallo, A and Della Sala, S: Preserved insight in an artist with extrapersonal spatial neglect. Cortex 34:163–189, 1998.

46. Capranica, R R: Auditory processing in anurans. Fed Proc 37:2324–2328, 1978.

47. Chain, F, Leblanc, M, Chedru, F and Lhermitte, F: Négligence visuelle dans les lésions posterieures de l'hémisphère gauche. Rev Neurol (Paris) 135:105–126, 1979.

48. Chatterjee, A: Cross-over, completion and confabulation in unilateral spatial neglect. Brain 118:455–465, 1995.

49. Chatterjee, A, Mennemeier, M and Heilman, K M: A stimulus-response relationship in unilateral neglect: the power function. Neuropsychologia 30:1101–1108, 1992.

50. Chedru, F and Geschwind, N: Disorders of higher cortical functions in acute confusional states. Cortex 8:395–411, 1972.

51. Chu, N and Bloom, F E: Norepinephrine-containing neurons: changes in spontaneous discharge patterns during sleeping and waking. Science 179:907–910, 1973.

52. Clower, D M, Hoffman, J M, Votaw, J R, Faber, T L, Woods, R P and Alexander, G E: Role of posterior parietal cortex in the recalibration of visually guided reaching. Nature 383:618–621, 1996.

53. Cohen, J D, Peristein, W M, Braver, T S, Nystrom, L E, Noll, D C, Jonides, J and Smith, E E: Temporal dynamics of brain activation during a working memory task. Nature 386: 604–606, 1997.

54. Colby, C L and Duhamel, J-R: Spatial representations for action in parietal cortex. Cog Brain Res 5:105–115, 1996.

55. Collin, N G, Cowey, A, Latto, R and Marzi, C: The role of frontal eye-fields and superior colliculi in visual search and non-visual search in rhesus monkeys. Behav Brain Res 4: 177–193, 1982.

56. Collins, R C, Al-Monddhiry, H, Chernik, N L and Posner, J B: Neurological manifestations of intravascular coagulation in patients with cancer. Neurology 25:795–806, 1975.

57. Colombo, M, Rodman, H R and Gross, C G: The effects of superior temporal cortex lesions on the processing and retention of auditory information in monkeys (*Cebus apella*). J Neurosci 16:4501–4517, 1996.

58. Constantinides, C and Steinmetz, M A: Neuronal activity in posterior parietal area 7a during the delay periods of a spatial memory task. J Neurophysiol 76:1352–1355, 1996.

59. Corbetta, M, Akbudak, E, Conturo, T E, Snyder, A Z, Ollinger, J M, Drury, H A, Linenweber, M R, Petersen, S E, Raichle, M E, Van Essen, D C and Shulman, G L: A common network of functional areas for attention and eye movements. Neuron 21:761–773, 1998.

60. Corbetta, M, Miezin, F M, Dobmeyer, S, Shulman, G L and Petersen, S: Selective and divided attention during visual discriminations of shape, color, and speed: functional anatomy by positron emission tomography. J Neurosci 11:2383–2402, 1991.

61. Corbetta, M, Miezin, F M, Shulman, G L and Petersen, S E: A PET study of visuospatial attention. J Neurosci 13:1202–1226, 1993.

62. Coslett, H B: Neglect in vision and visual imagery: a double dissociation. Brain 120: 1163–1171, 1997.

63. Coull, J T: Neural correlates of attention and arousal: insights from electrophysiology, functional neuroimaging and psychopharmacology. Prog Neurobiol 55:343–361, 1998.

64. Critchley, M: The Parietal Lobes. Edward Arnold, London, 1953.

65. D'Esposito, M, Detre, J A, Alsop, D C, Shin, R K, Atlas, S and Grossman, M: The neural basis of the central executive system of working memory. Nature 378:279–281, 1995.

66. Daffner, K R, Ahern, G L, Weintraub, S and Mesulam, M M: Dissociated neglect behavior following sequential strokes in the right hemisphere. Ann Neurol 28:97–101, 1990.

67. Daffner, K R, Mesulam, M-M, Scinto, L F M, Cohen, L G, Kennedy, B F, West, W C and Holcomb, P J: Regulation of attention to novel stimuli by frontal lobes: an event-related potential study. Neuroreport 9:787–791, 1998.

68. Damasio, A R, Damasio, H and Chui, H C: Neglect following damage to frontal lobe or basal ganglia. Neuropsychologia 18:123–132, 1980.

69. Darby, D G, Nobre, A C, Thangaraj, V, Edelman, R R, Mesulam, M-M and Warach, S: Cortical activation in the human brain during lateral saccades using EPISTAR functional magnetic resonance imaging. Neuroimage 3:53–62, 1996.

70. De Renzi, E, Falioni, P and Scotti, G: Hemispheric contribution to exploration of space through the visual and tactile modality. Cortex 6:191–203, 1970.

71. De Renzi, E, Gentilini, M and Pattacini, F: Auditory extinction following hemisphere damage. Neuropsychologia 22:613–617, 1984.

72. Dempsey, E W and Morrison, R S: The production of rhythmically recurrent cortical potentials after localized thalamic stimulation. Am J Physiol 135:293–300, 1942.

73. Denes, G, Semenza, C, Stoppa, E and Lis, A: Unilateral spatial neglect and recovery from hemiplegia. Brain 105:543–552, 1982.

74. Denny-Brown, D and Chambers, R A: The parietal lobe and behavior. Proceedings of the Association for Research in Nervous and Mental Disease 36:35–117, 1958.

75. Desimone, R: Neural mechanisms for visual memory and their role in attention. Proc Natl Acad Sci USA 93:13494–13499, 1996.

76. Desmedt, J E: Active touch exploration of extrapersonal space elicits specific electrogenesis in the right cerebral hemisphere of intact right handed man. Proc Natl Acad Sci USA 74:4037–4040, 1977.

77. Deuel, R and Collins, R: Recovery from unilateral neglect. Exp Neurol 81:733–748, 1983.

78. Devinsky, O, Bear, D and Volpe, B: Confusional states following posterior cerebral artery infarction. Arch Neurol 45:160–163, 1988.

79. DeYoe, E, Carman, G J, Bandettini, P, Glickman, S, Wieser, J, Cox, R, Miller, D and Neitz, J: Mapping striate and extrastriate visual areas in human cerebral cortex. Proc Natl Acad Sci USA 93:2382–2386, 1996.

80. Di Pellegrino, G and De Renzi, E: An experimental investigation of the nature of extinction. Neuropsychologia 33:153–170, 1995.

81. Di Pellegrino, G, Làdavas, E and Farné, A: Seeing where your hands are. Nature 388: 730, 1997.

82. Dias, E C, Compaan, D M, Mesulam, M-M and Segraves, M A: Selective disruption of memory-guided saccades with injecton of a cholinergic antagonist in the frontal eye field of monkey. Soc Neurosci Abstr 22:418, 1996.

83. Dias, E C, Kiesau, M and Segraves, M A: Acute activation and inactivation of macaque frontal eye field with GABA-related drugs. J Neurophysiol 74:2744–2748, 1995.

84. Diller, L and Weinberg, J: Hemi-inattention in rehabilitation: the evolution of a rational remediation program. Adv Neurol 18:63–80, 1977.

85. Dimond, S J: Depletion of attentional capacity after total commissurotomy in man. Brain 99:347–356, 1976.

86. Dimsdale, J E, Newton, R P and Joist, T: Neuropsychological side effects of β-blockers. Arch Intern Med 149:514–525, 1989.

87. Dines, D E, Louis, W, Burgher and Okazaki, H: The clinical and pathological correlation of fat embolism syndrome. Mayo Clin Proc 50:407–411, 1975.

88. Doricchi, F, Guariglia, C, Paolucci, S and Pizzamiglio, L: Disappearance of leftward rapid eye movements during sleep in left visual hemi-attention. Neuroreport 2:285–288, 1991.

89. Dorris, M C, Paré, M and Munoz, D P: Neuronal activity in monkey superior colliculus related to the initiation of saccadic eye movements. J Neurosci 17:8566–8579, 1997.

90. Dringenberg, H C and Vanderwolf, C H: Neocortical activation: modulation by multiple pathways acting on central cholinergic and serotonergic systems. Exp Brain Res 116:160–174, 1997.

91. Driver, J and Halligan, P W: Can visual neglect operate in object-centered coordinates? An affirmative single case study. Cog Neuropsychol 8:475–496, 1991.

92. Driver, J and Mattingley, J B: Parietal neglect and visual awareness. Nature Neurosci 1: 17–22, 1998.

93. Droogleever-Fortuyn, J: On the neurology of perception. Clin Neurol Neurosurg 81:97–107, 1979.

94. Duhamel, J-R, Colby, C L and Goldberg, M E: The updating of the representation of visual space in parietal cortex by intended eye movements. Science 255:90–92, 1992.

95. Dürsteler, M R and Wurtz, R H: Pursuit and optokinetic deficits following chemical lesions of cortical areas MT and MST. J Neurophysiol 60:940–965, 1988.

96. Ebersbach, G, Trottenberg, T, Hattig, H, Schelosky, L, Schrag, A and Poewe, W: Directional bias of initial visual exploration. A symptom of neglect in Parkinson's disease. Brain 119:79–87, 1996.

97. Eidelberg, E and Schwartz, A S: Experimental analysis of the extinction phenomenon in monkeys. Brain 94:91–108, 1971.

98. Engel, G L and Romano, J: Delirium. A syndrome of cerebral insufficiency. J Chron Dis 9:260–277, 1959.

99. Fahy, F L, Riches, I P and Brown, M W: Neuronal activity related to visual recognition memory: long-term memory and the encoding of recency and familiarity information in the primate anterior and medial inferior temporal and rhinal cortex. Exp Brain Res 96: 457–472, 1993.

100. Farah, M J, Brunn, J L, Wong, A B, Wallace, M A and Carpenter, P A: Frames of reference for allocating attention to space: evidence from the neglect syndrome. Neuropsychologia 28:335–347, 1990.

101. Faraj, B A, Bowen, P A, Isaacs, J W and Rudman, D: Hypertyraminemia in cirrhotic patients. N Engl J Med 294:1360–1364, 1976.

102. Farnè, A, Ponti, F and Làdavas, E: In search of biased egocentric reference frames in neglect. Neuropsychologia 36:611–623, 1998.

103. Fealey, M P, O'Harre, J, Veale, D and Calloghan, M: Episodes of acute confusion or psychosis in familial hemiplegic migraine. Acta Neurol Scand 65:369–375, 1982.

104. Feeney, D M and Wier, C S: Sensory neglect after lesions of substantia nigra or lateral hypothalamus: differential severity and recovery of function. Brain Res 178:329–346, 1979.

105. Ferrier, D: Functions of the Brain. G. P. Putnam's Sons, New York, 1876.

106. Fiez, J A, Raife, E A, Balota, D A, Schwarz, J P and Raichle, M E: A positron emission tomography study of the short-term maintenance of verbal information. J Neurosci 16: 808–822, 1996.

107. Fiorelli, M, Blin, J, Bakchine, S, Laplane, D and Baron, J C: PET studies of cortical diaschisis in patients with motor hemi-neglect. J Neurol Sci 104:135–142, 1991.

108. Fleet, W S, Valenstein, E, Watson, R T and Heilman, K M: Dopamine agonist therapy for neglect in humans. Neurology 37:1765–1770, 1987.

109. Fujimori, M, Wakisaka, K, Yamadori, A, Imamura, T, Uehara, T, Yamashita, K and Tabuchi, M: Crossed non-dominant hemisphere syndrome in a right-hander. Behav Neurol 7:123–126, 1994.

110. Furey, M L, Pietrini, P, Haxby, J V, Alexander, G E, Lee, H C, VanMeter, J, Grady, C L, Shetty, U, Rapoport, S I, Schapiro, M B and Freo, U: Cholinergic stimulation alters performance and task-specific regional cerebral blood flow during working memory. Prod Natl Acad Sci USA 94:6512–6516, 1997.

111. Fuster, J M: Inferotemporal units in selective visual attention and short-term memory. J Neurophysiol 64:681–697, 1990.

112. Fuster, J M, Bauer, R H and Jervey, J P: Functional interactions between inferotemporal and prefrontal cortex in a cognitive task. Brain Res 330:299–307, 1985.

113. Fuster, J M and Jervey, J P: Inferotemporal neurons distinguish and retain behaviorally relevant features of visual stimuli. Science 212:952–955, 1981.

114. Gainotti, G, Messerli, P and Tissot, R: Qualitative analysis of unilateral spatial neglect in relation to laterality of cerebral lesions. J Neurol Neurosurg Psychiatry 35:545–550, 1972.

115. Gazzaniga, M S: Perceptual and attentional processes following callosal section in humans. Neuropsychologia 25:119–133, 1987.

116. Gazzaniga, M S and Ladavas, E: Disturbances in spatial attention following lesion or disconnection of the right parietal lobe. In Jeannerod, M (Eds.): Neurophysiological and Neuropsychological Aspects of Spatial Neglect. Elsevier, Amsterdam, 1987, pp. 203–213.

117. Ghatan, P H, Hsieh, J C, Petersson, K M, Stone-Elander, S and Ingvar, M: Coexistence of attention-based facilitation and inhibition in the human cortex. Neuroimage 7:23–29, 1997.

118. Gitelman, D R, Nobre, A N, Parrish, T B, LaBar, K S, Kim, Y-H, Meyer, J R and Mesulam, M-M: A large-scale distributed network for spatial attention: an fMRI study with stringent behavioral controls. Brain 122:1093–1106, 1999.

119. Gitelman, D R, Alpert, N M, Kosslyn, S M, Daffner, K, Scinto, L, Thompson, W and Mesulam, M-M: Functional imaging of human right hemispheric activation for exploratory movements. Ann Neurol 39:174–179, 1996.

120. Gitelman, D R, Kim, Y-H, Parrish, T B, Nobre, A C, Meyer, J R, Hallam, D, Callahan, C, Russell, E J and Mesulam, M-M: Superior colliculus activation by overt but not covert spatial attention tasks, visualization by functional magnetic resonance imaging. Neuroimage 5:S61, 1997.

121. Gitelman, D R, Nobre, A C, Meyer, J R, Parrish, T B, Callahan, C, Russell, E J and Mesulam, M-M: Functional magnetic resonance imaging of covert spatial attention. Hum Brain Map 3:S180, 1996.

122. Glenn, L L and Steriade, M: Discharge rate and excitability of cortically projecting in-

tralaminar thalamic neurons during waking and sleep states. J Neurosci 2:1387–1404, 1982.

123. Goldberg, M E and Bushnell, M C: Behavioral enhancement of visual responses in monkey cerebral cortex: II. Modulation in frontal eye fields specifically related to saccades. J Neurophysiol 46:773–787, 1981.

124. Goldman-Rakic, P S and Friedman, H S: The circuitry of working memory revealed by anatomy and metabolic imaging. In Levin, H S, Eisenberg, H M and Benton, A L (Eds.): Frontal Lobe Function and Dysfunction. Oxford University Press, New York, 1991, pp. 72–91.

125. Goodman, S J: Visuo-motor reaction times and brain stem multiple-unit activity. Exp Neurol 22:367–378, 1968.

126. Gottlieb, J P, Kusunoki, M and Goldberg, M E: The representation of visual salience in monkey parietal cortex. Nature 391:481–484, 1998.

127. Graziano, M S A and Gross, C G: Spatial maps for the control of movement. Curr Opin Neurobiol 8:195–201, 1998.

128. Graziano, M S A, Hu, X T and Gross, C G: Coding the locations of objects in the dark. Science 277:239–241, 1997.

129. Griffiths, T D, Rees, G, Rees, A, Green, G G R, Witton, C, Rowe, D, Büchel, C, Turner, R and Frackowiak, R S J: Right parietal cortex is involved in the perception of sound movement in humans. Nat Neuroscience 1:74–79, 1998.

130. Grujic, Z, Mapstone, M, Gitelman, D R, Johnson, N, Weintraub, S, Hays, A, Kwasnica, C, Harvey, R and Mesulam, M-M: Dopaminergic agonists reorient visual exploration away from the neglected hemispace. Neurology 51:1395–1398, 1998.

131. Guard, O, Delpy, C, Richard, D and Dumas, R: Une cause mal connue de confusion mentale: le ramollissemant temporal droit. Rev Med 40:2115–2121, 1979.

132. Guillery, R W, Feig, S L and Lozsádi, D A: Paying attention to the thalamic reticular nucleus. Trends Neurosci 21:28–32, 1998.

133. Halligan, P W and Marshall, J C: How long is a piece of string? A study of line bisection in a case of visual neglect. Cortex 24:321–328, 1988.

134. Halligan, P W and Marshall, J C: Left neglect for near but not far space in man. Nature 350:498–500, 1991.

135. Halligan, P W and Marshall, J C: Left visuo-spatial neglect: a meaningless entity? Cortex 28:525–535, 1992.

136. Halligan, P W and Marshall, J C: When two is one: a case study of spatial parsing in visual neglect. Perception 22:309–312, 1993.

137. Halligan, P W and Marshall, J C: Toward a principled explanation of unilateral neglect. Cog Neuropsychol 11:167–206, 1994.

138. Hammond, E J, Meador, K J, Aunq-Din, R and Wilder, B J: Cholinergic modulation of human P3 event-related potentials. Neurology 37:346–350, 1987.

139. Harrington, D L, Haaland, K Y and Knight, R T: Cortical networks underlying mechanisms of time perception. J Neurosci 18:1085–1095, 1998.

140. Harvey, M, Milner, A D and Roberts, R C: An investigation of hemispatial neglect using the landmark task. Brain Cogn 27:59–78, 1995.

141. Hasselbach, M and Butter, C M: Ipsilesional displacement of egocentric midline in neglect patients with, but not in those without, extensive right parietal damage. In Thier, P and Karnath, H-O (Eds.): Parietal Lobe Contributions to Orientation in 3D Space. Springer, Berlin, 1997, pp. 579–595.

142. Healton, E B, Navarro, C, Bressman, S and Brust, J: Subcortical neglect. Neurology 32: 776–778, 1982.

143. Hécaen, H, Penfield, W, Bertrand, C and Malmo, R: The syndrome of apractognosia due to lesions of the minor cerebral hemisphere. Arch Neurol Psychiatry 75:400–434, 1956.

144. Heckers, S, Geula, C and Mesulam, M-M: Cholinergic innervation of the human thalamus: dual origin and differential nuclear distribution. J Comp Neurol 325:68–82, 1992.

145. Heilman, K M, Bowers, D and Watson, R T: Performance on hemispatial pointing task by patients with neglect syndrome. Neurology 33:661–664, 1983.
146. Heilman, K M and Howell, G J: Seizure-induced neglect. J Neurol Neurosurg Psychiatry 43:1035–1040, 1980.
147. Heilman, K M, Schwartz, H D and Watson, R T: Hypoarousal in patients with the neglect syndrome and emotional indifference. Neurology 28:229–232, 1978.
148. Heilman, K M and Valenstein, E: Auditory neglect in man. Arch Neurol 26:32–35, 1972.
149. Heilman, K M and Valenstein, E: Frontal lobe neglect in man. Neurology 22:660–664, 1972.
150. Heilman, K M and Valenstein, E: Mechanisms underlying hemispatial neglect. Ann Neurol 5:166–170, 1979.
151. Heilman, K M and Van Den Abell, T: Right hemispheric dominance for mediating cerebral activation. Neuropsychologia 17:315–321, 1979.
152. Heilman, K M and Van Den Abell, T: Right hemisphere dominance for attention: the mechanism underlying hemispheric asymmetries of inattention (neglect). Neurology 30:327–330, 1980.
153. Heilman, K M, Watson, R T and Valenstein, E: Neglect and related disorders. In Heilman, K M and Valenstein, E (Eds.): Clinical Neuropsychology. Oxford University Press, New York, 1985, pp. 279–336.
154. Heilman, K M, Watson, R T, Valenstein, E and Damasio, A R: Localization of lesions in neglect. In Kertesz, A (Ed.): Localization in Neuropsychology. Academic Press, New York, 1983, pp. 455–470.
155. Hernandez-Peón, R, Scherrer, H and Jouvet, M: Modification of electric activity in cochlear nucleus during "attention" in unanesthetized cats. Science 123:331–332, 1956.
156. Heron, W: The pathology of boredom. Sci Am 196:52–56, 1957.
157. Hier, D B, Mondlock, J and Caplan, L R: Behavioral abnormalities after right hemisphere stroke. Neurology 33:337–344, 1983.
158. Hier, D B, Mondlock, J and Caplan, L R: Recovery of behavioral abnormalities after right hemisphere stroke. Neurology 33:345–350, 1983.
159. Horel, J A: Cold lesions in inferotemporal cortex produce reversible deficits in learning and retention of visual discriminations. Physiol Psychol 12:259–270, 1984.
160. Horenstein, S, Chamberlin, W and Conomy, J: Infarction of the fusiform and calcarine regions: agitated delirium and hemianopia. Trans Am Neurol Assoc 92:85–89, 1967.
161. Hornak, J: Ocular exploration in the dark by patients with visual neglect. Neuropsychologia 30:547–552, 1992.
162. Howes, D and Boller, F: Simple reaction time: evidence for focal impairment from lesions of the right hemisphere. Brain 98:317–332, 1975.
163. Hubel, D H, Henson, C O, Rupert, A and Galambos, R: "Attention" units in the auditory cortex. Science 129:1279–1280, 1959.
164. Husain, M and Kennard, C: Visual neglect associated with frontal lobe infarction. J Neurol 243:652–657, 1996.
165. Hyvärinen, J, Laakso, M, Roine, R, Leinonen, L and Sippel, H: Effect of ethanol on neuronal activity in the parietal association cortex of alert monkeys. Brain 101:701–715, 1978.
166. Hyvärinen, J and Poranen, A: Function of the parietal associative area 7 as revealed from cellular discharges in alert monkeys. Brain 97:673–692, 1974.
167. Hyvärinen, J, Poranen, A and Jokinen, Y: Influence of attentive behavior on neuronal responses to vibration in primary somatosensory cortex of the monkey. J Neurophysiol 43:870–882, 1980.
168. Ilg, U A and Thier, P: MST neurons are activated by smooth pursuit of imagery targets. In Thier, P and Karnath, H-O (Eds.): Parietal Lobe Contributions to Orientation in 3D Space. Springer, Berlin 1997, pp. 173–184.
169. Inoue, K, Kawashima, R, Satoh, K, Kinomura, S, Goto, R, Koyama, M, Sugiura, M, Ito,

M and Fukuda, H: PET study of pointing with visual feedback of moving hands. J Neurophysiol 79:117–125, 1998.

170. Ishiai, S, Furukawa, T and Tsukagoshi, H: Visuospatial processes of line bisection and the mechanisms underlying unilateral spatial neglect. Brain 112:1485–1502, 1989.

171. Ishiai, S, Sugishita, M, Odajima, N, Yaginuma, M, Gono, S and Kamaya, T: Improvement of unilateral spatial neglect with numbering. Neurology 40:1395–1398, 1990.

172. James, W: The Principles of Psychology. Holt, New York, 1890.

173. Jäncke, L, Schlaug, G, Huang, Y and Steinmetz, H: Asymmetry of planum parietale. Neuroreport 5:1161–1163, 1994.

174. Jansen, J, Andersen, P and Kaada, B P: Subcortical mechanisms in the "searching" or "attention" response elicited by prefrontal cortical stimulation in unanesthetized cats. Yale J Biol Med 28:331–341, 1955.

175. Johannsen, P, Jakobsen, J, Bruhn, P, Hansen, SB, Gee, A, Stødkilde-Jørgensen, H and Gjedde, A: Cortical sites of sustained and divided attention in normal elderly humans. Neuroimage 6:145–155, 1997.

176. Johnson, P B, Ferraina, S, Garasto, M R, Battaglia-Mayer, A, Ercolani, L, Burnod, Y and Caminiti, R: From vision to movement: cortico-cortical connections and combinatorial properties of reaching-related neurons in parietal areas V6 and V6A. In Thier, P and Karnath, H-O (Eds.): Parietal Lobe Contributions to Orientation in 3D Space. Springer, Berlin 1997, pp. 221–236.

177. Jones, E G: Some aspects of the organization of the thalamic reticular complex. J Comp Neurol 162:285–308, 1975.

178. Kaada, B R, Pribram, K H and Epstein, J A: Respiratory and vascular responses in monkeys from temporal pole, insula, orbital surface and cingulate gyrus. J Neurophysiol 12:348–356, 1949.

179. Kalaska, J F and Crammond, D J: Deciding not to go: neuronal correlates of response selection in a GO/NOGO task in primate premotor and parietal cortex. Cereb Cortex 5:410–428, 1995.

180. Karnath, H-O: Neural encoding of space in egocentric coordinates? In Thier, P and Karnath, H-O (Eds.): Parietal Lobe Contributions to Orientation in 3D Space. Springer, Berlin 1997, pp. 497–520.

181. Karnath, H O, Schenkel, P and Fischer, B: Trunk orientation as the determining factor of the 'contralateral' deficit in the neglect syndrome and as the physical anchor of the internal representation of body orientation in space. Brain 114:1997–2014, 1991.

182. Kennard, M A: Alterations in response to visual stimuli following lesions of frontal lobe in monkeys. Arch Neurol Psychiatry 41:1153–1165, 1939.

183. Kermadi, I and Boussaoud, D: Role of the primate striatum in attention and sensorimotor processes: comparison with premotor cortex. Neuroreport 6:1177–1181, 1995.

184. Kermadi, I and Joseph, J P: Activity in the caudate nucleus of monkey during spatial sequencing. J Neurophysiol 74:1995.

185. Kim, Y-H, Gitelman, D R, Nobre, A C, Parrish, T B, LaBar, K S and Mesulam, M-M: The large scale neural network for spatial attention displays multi-functional overlap but differential asymmetry. Neuroimage 9:269–277, 1999.

186. Kim, Y-H, Gitelman, D R, Parrish, T B, Nobre, A C, LaBar, K S and Mesulam, M-M: Posterior cingulate activation varies according to the effectiveness of attentional engagement. Neuroimage 7:S67, 1998.

187. Kinomura, S, Larsson, J, Gulyás, B and Roland, P E: Activation by attention of the human reticular formation and thalamic intralaminar nuclei. Science 271:512–515, 1996.

188. Kinsbourne, M: Mechanisms of unilateral neglect. In Jeannerod, M (Eds.): Neurophysiological and Neuropsychological Aspects of Spatial Neglect. Elsevier, New York, 1987, pp. 69–86.

189. Kinsbourne, M and Warrington, E K: A variety of reading disability associated with right hemisphere lesion. J Neurol Neurosurg Psychiatry 25:339–344, 1962.

190. Knight, R: Electrophysiology in behavioral neurology. In Mesulam, M-M (Ed.): Principles of Behavioral Neurology. FA Davis, Philadelphia, 1985, pp. 327–346.

191. Knight, R T: Decreased response to novel stimuli after prefrontal lesions in man. Electroenceph alogr Clin Neurophysiol 59:9–20, 1984.

192. Kooistra, C A and Heilman, K M: Hemispatial visual inattention masquerading as hemianopia. Neurology 39:1125–1127, 1989.

193. Künzle, H: Regional and laminar distribution of cortical neurons projecting to either superior or inferior colliculus in the hedgehog tenrec. Cereb Cortex 5:338–352, 1995.

194. LaBar, K, Gitelman, D R, Parrish, T B, Kim, Y H and Mesulam, M-M: Overlap of frontoparietal activations during covert spatial attention and verbal working memory in the same set of subjects: an fMRI study. Soc Neurosci Abstr 24:1896, 1998.

195. LaBerge, D and Buchsbaum, M S: Positron emission tomographic measurements of pulvinar activity during an attention task. J Neurosci 10:613–619, 1990.

196. Làdavas, E: Selective spatial attention in patients with visual extinction. Brain 113:1527–1538, 1990.

197. Làdavas, E, Farné, A, Carletti, M and Zeloni, G: Neglect determined by the relative location of responses. Brain 117:705–714, 1994.

198. Lappe, M: Analysis of self-motion by parietal neurons. In Thier, P and Karnath, H-O (Eds.): Parietal Lobe Contributions to Orientation in 3D Space. Springer, Berlin, 1997, pp. 597–618.

199. Lettvin, J Y, Maturana, H R, McCulloch, W S and Pitts, W H: What the frog's eye tells the frog's brain. Proceedings of the Institute of Radio Engineers 47:1940–1951, 1959.

200. Lipowski, Z J: Delirium (acute confusional state). In Frederiks, J A M (Ed.): Handbook of Clinical Neurology. Elsevier, Amsterdam, 1985, 2, pp. 523–559.

201. Liu, G T, Bolton, A K, Price, B H and Weintraub, S: Dissociated perceptual-sensory and exploratory-motor neglect. J Neurol Neurosurg Psychiatry 55:701–706, 1992.

202. Livingstone, M S and Hubel, D H: Effects of sleep and arousal on the processing of visual information in the cat. Nature 291:554–561, 1981.

203. Ljungberg, T and Ungerstedt, U: Sensory inattention produced by 6-hydroxydopamine-induced degeneration of ascending dopamine neurons in the brain. Exp Neurol 53:585–600, 1976.

204. Luna, B, Thulborn, K R, Strojwas, M H, McCurtain, B J, Berman, R A, Genovese, C R and Sweeney, J A: Dorsal cortical regions subserving visually guided saccades in humans: an fMRI study. Cereb Cortex 8:40–47, 1998.

205. Luria, A R, Karpov, B A and Yarbuss, A L: Disturbances of active visual perception with lesions of the frontal lobes. Cortex 2:202–212, 1966.

206. Lynch, J C: The functional organization of posterior parietal association cortex. Behav Brain Sci 3:485–499, 1980.

207. Lynch, J C and McLaren, J W: Deficits of visual attention and saccadic eye movements after lesions of parietooccipital cortex in monkeys. J Neurophysiol 61:1989.

208. Lynn, R: Attention, Arousal and the Orientation Reaction. Pergamon Press, Oxford, 1966.

209. Maguire, E A, Burgess, N, Donnett, J G, Frackowiak, RSJ, Frith, C D and O'Keefe, J: Knowing where and getting there: a human navigation network. Science 280:921–924, 1998.

210. Manoach, D S, O'Connor, M and Weintraub, S: Absence of neglect for mental representations during the intracarotid amobarbital procedure. Arch Neurol 53:333–336, 1996.

211. Mark, V W, Kooistra, C A and Heilman, K M: Hemispatial neglect affected by non-neglected stimuli. Neurology 38:1207–1211, 1988.

212. Markand, O N, Wheeler, G L and Pollack, S L: Complex partial status epilepticus (psychomotor status). Neurology 28:189–196, 1978.

213. Marshall, J C and Halligan, P W: Blindsight and insight in visuo-spatial neglect. Nature 336:766–767, 1988.

214. Marshall, J C and Halligan, P W: When right goes left: An investigation of line bisection in a case of visual neglect. Cortex 25:503–515, 1989.

215. Marshall, J F: Somatosensory inattention after dopamine-depleting intracerebral 6-OHDA injections: spontaneous recovery and pharamacological control. Brain Res 177:311–324, 1979.

216. Mattingley, J B, Davis, G and Driver, J: Preattentive filling-in of visual surfaces in parietal extinction. Science 275:671–674, 1997.

217. Mattingley, J B, Husain, M, Rorden, C, Kennard, C and Driver, J: Motor role of human inferior parietal lobe revealed in unilateral neglect patients. Nature 392:179–182, 1998.

218. McCarthy, G and Nobre, A C: Modulation of semantic processing by spatial selective attention. Electroencephalogr Clin Neurophysiol 88:210–219, 1993.

219. McCarthy, G, Puce, A, Constable, R T, Krystal, J H, Gore, J C and Goldman-Rakic, P: Activation of human prefrontal cortex during spatial and nonspatial working memory tasks measured by functional MRI. Cereb Cortex 6:600–611, 1996.

220. McFie, J, Percy, M D and Zangwill, O L: Visual-spatial agnosia associated with lesions of the right cerebral hemisphere. Brain 73:167–190, 1950.

221. McGlinchey-Berroth, R, Bullis, D P, Milberg, W P, Verfaellie, M, Alexander, M and D'Esposito, M: Assessment of neglect reveals dissociable behavioral but not neuroanatomical subtypes. J Int Neuropsychol Soc 2:441–451, 1996.

222. McGlinchey-Berroth, R, Milberg, W P, Verfaellie, M, Alexander, M and Kilduff, P T: Semantic processing in the neglected visual field: evidence from a lexical decision task. Cog Neuropsychol 10:79–108, 1993.

223. Meador, K J, Loring, D W, Bowers, D and Heilman, K M: Remote memory and neglect syndrome. Neurology 37:522–526, 1987.

224. Meador, K J, W., L D, Lee, G P, Brooks, B S, Thompson, E E, Thompson, W O and Heilman, K M: Right cerebral specialization for tactile attention as evidenced by intracarotid sodium amytal. Neurology 38:1763–1766, 1988.

225. Medina, J L, Rubino, F A and Ross, A: Agitated delirium caused by infarction of the hippocampal formation and fusiform and lingual gyri: a case report. Neurology 24:1181–1183, 1974.

226. Medvedev, S V, Vorobiev, V A, Roudas, M S, Pakhomov, S V, Alho, K, Naatanen, R, Reinikainen, K and Tervaniemi, M: Human brain structures involved in sustaining lateralized auditory attention: two PET studies comparison. Neuroimage 5:S78, 1997.

227. Mesulam, M-M: A cortical network for directed attention and unilateral neglect. Ann Neurol 10:309–325, 1981.

228. Mesulam, M-M: Attention, confusional states and neglect. In Mesulam, M-M (Ed.): Principles of Behavioral Neurology. F A Davis, Philadelphia, 1985, pp. 125–168.

229. Mesulam, M-M: Patterns in behavioral neuroanatomy; association areas, the limbic system, and hemispheric specialization. In Mesulam, M-M (Ed.): Principles of Behavioral Neurology. F A Davis, Philadelphia, 1985, pp. 1–70.

230. Mesulam, M-M: Lidocaine toxicity and the limbic system [letter]. Am J Psychiaty 144:1623–1624, 1987.

231. Mesulam, M-M: Large-scale neurocognitive networks and distributed processing for attention, language, and memory. Ann Neurol 28:597–613, 1990.

232. Mesulam, M-M: Cholinergic pathways and the ascending reticular activating system of the human brain. Ann N Y Acad Sci 757:169–179, 1995.

233. Mesulam, M-M: From sensation to cognition. Brain 121:1013–1052, 1998.

234. Mesulam, M-M, Geula, C, Bothwell, M A and Hersh, L B: Human reticular formation: cholinergic neurons of the pedunculopontine and laterodorsal tegmental nuclei and some cytochemical comparisons to forebrain cholinergic neurons. J Comp Neurol 283:611–633, 1989.

235. Mesulam, M-M and Mufson, E J: The insula of Reil in man and monkey. In Peters, A and Jones, E G (Ed.): Cerebral Cortex. Plenum Press, New York, 1985, 4, pp. 179–226.

236. Mesulam, M-M: Tetramethyl benzidine for horseradish peroxidase neurohistochemistry: a non-carcinogenic blue reaction product with superior sensitivity for visualizing neural afferents and efferents. J Histochem Cytochem 26:106–117, 1978.

237. Mesulam, M-M and Geschwind, N: Disordered mental states in the postoperative period. Urol Clin North Am 3:199–215, 1976.

238. Mesulam, M-M, Van Hoesen, G W, Pandya, D N and Geschwind, N: Limbic and sensory connections of the inferior parietal lobule (area PG) in the rhesus monkey: a study with a new method for horseradish peroxidase histochemistry. Brain Res 136:393–414, 1977.

239. Mesulam, M-M, Waxman, S G, Geschwind, N and Sabin, T D: Acute confusional states with right middle cerebral artery infarctions. J Neurol Neurosurg Psychiatry 39:84–89, 1976.

240. Meyer, A: Historical Aspects of Cerebral Anatomy. Oxford University, London, 1971.

241. Mijovic, D: Mechanisms of visual spatial neglect. Brain 114:1575–1593, 1991.

242. Milner, A D: Neglect, extinction, and the cortical streams of visual processing. In Thier, P and Karnath, H-O (Ed.): Parietal Lobe Contributions to Orientation in 3D Space. Springer, Berlin, 1997, pp. 3–22.

243. Miyashita, N, Hikosaka, O and Kato, M: Visual hemineglect induced by unilateral striatal dopamine deficiency in monkeys. Neuroreport 6:1257–1260, 1995.

244. Monaghan, P and Shillcock, R: The cross-over effect in unilateral neglect. Modelling detailed data in the line bisection task. Brain 121:907–921, 1998.

245. Moran, J and Desimone, R: Selective attention gates visual processing in the extrastriate cortex. Science 229:782–784, 1985.

246. Moray, N: Attention in dichotic listening: affective cues and the influence of instructions. Q J Exp Psychol 11:56–60, 1959.

247. Morecraft, R J, Geula, C and Mesulam, M-M: Architecture of connectivity within a cingulo-fronto-parietal neurocognitive network for directed attention. Arch Neurol 50: 279–284, 1993.

248. Morecraft, R J, Geula, C and Mesulam, M-M: Cytoarchitecture and neural afferents of orbitofrontal cortex in the brain of the monkey. J Comp Neurol 323:341–358, 1992.

249. Morris, J S, Friston, K J, Buchel, C, Frith, C D, Young, A W, Calder, A J and Dolan, R J: A neuromodulatory role for the human amygdala in processing emotional facial expressions. Brain 121:47–57, 1998.

250. Morris, J S, Friston, K J and Dolan, R J: Neural responses to salient visual stimuli. Proc R Soc Lond [Biol] 264:769–775, 1997.

251. Morrison, J H and Magistretti, P J: Monoamines and peptides in cerebral cortex. Trends Neurosci 6:146–151, 1983.

252. Morrow, L, Vrtunski, P B, Kim, Y and Boller, F: Arousal responses to emotional stimuli and laterality of lesion. Neuropsychologia 19:65–71, 1981.

253. Moruzzi, G and Magoun, H W: Brain stem reticular formation and activation of the EEG. Electroencephalogr Clin Neurophysiol 1:459–473, 1949.

254. Moscovitch, M and Behrmann, M: Coding of spatial information in the somatosensory system: evidence from patients with neglect following parietal lobe damage. J Cog Neurosci 6:151–155, 1994.

255. Moscovitch, M, Kapur, S, Köhler, S and Houle, S: Distinct neural correlates of visual long-term memory for spatial location and object identity: a positron emission tomography study in humans. Proc Nat Acad Sci USA 92:3721–3725, 1995.

256. Mountcastle, V B, Lynch, J C, Georgopoulous, A, Sakata, H and Acuna, A: Posterior parietal association cortex of the monkey: command functions for operations within extrapersonal space. J Neurophysiol 38:871–908, 1975.

257. Mozer, M C and Behrmann, M: On the interaction of selective attention and lexical knowledge: a connectionistic account of neglect dyslexia. J Cog Neurosci 2:96–123, 1994.

258. Mozer, M C, Halligan, P W and Marshall, J C: The end of the line for a brain-damaged model of unilateral neglect. J Cog Neurosci 9:171–190, 1997.

259. Naito, E, Kinomura, S, Kawashima, R, Geyer, S, Zilles, K and Roland, PE: Correlation of the rCBF in anterior cingulate cortex with reaction time. Neuroimage 7:S948, 1998.

260. Nobre, A C, Coull, J T, Mesulam, M-M and Frith, C D: The neural system for directing spatial and temporal attention compared with PET. Soc Neurosci Abstr 23:300, 1997.

261. Nobre, A C, Dias, E C, Gitelman, D R and Mesulam, M-M: The overlap of brain regions that control saccades and covert visual attention revealed by fMRI. Neuroimage 7:S9, 1998.

262. Nobre, A C, Sebestyen, G N, Gitelman, D R, Mesulam, M-M, Frackowiak, R S J and Frith, C D: Functional localization of the system for visuospatial attention using positron emission tomography. Brain 120:515–533, 1997.

263. Olson, C R and Gettner, S N: Object-centered direction selectivity in the macaque supplementary eye field. Science 269:985–988, 1995.

264. Olson, C R, Musil, S Y and Goldberg, M E: Posterior cingulate cortex and visuospatial cognition: properties of single neurons in the behaving monkey. In Vogt, B A and Gabriel, M (Eds.): Neurobiology of Cingulate Cortex and Limbic Thalamus: A Comprehensive Handbook. Birkhäuser, Boston, 1993, pp. 366–380.

265. Orem, J, Schlag-Rey, M and Schlag, J: Unilateral visual neglect and thalamic intralaminar lesions in the cat. Exper Neurol 40:784–797, 1973.

266. Oxbury, J M, Campbell, D C and Oxbury, S M: Unilateral spatial neglect and impairments of spatial analysis and visual perception. Brain 97:551–564, 1974.

267. Oyachi, H and Ohtsuka, K: Transcranial magnetic stimulation of the posterior parietal cortex degrades accuracy of memory-guided saccades in humans. Invest Ophthalmol Vis Sci 36:1441–1449, 1995.

268. Pandya, D N, Van Hoesen, G W and Mesulam, M-M: Efferent connections of the cingulate gyrus in the rhesus monkey. Exp Brain Res 42:319–330, 1981.

269. Pandya, D N and Yeterian, E H: Architecture and connections of cortical association areas. In Peters, A and Jones, E G (Eds.): Cerebral Cortex. Plenum Press, New York, 1985, 4, pp. 3–61.

270. Pardo, J V, Fox, P T and Raichle, M E: Localization of a human system for sustained attention by positron emission tomography. Nature 349:61–64, 1991.

271. Pardo, J V, Pardo, P J, Janer, K W and Raichle, M E: The anterior cingulate cortex mediates processing selection in the Stroop attentional conflict paradigm. Proc Natl Acad Sci USA 87:256–259, 1990.

272. Paré, M and Wurtz, R H: Monkey posterior parietal cortex neurons antidromically activated from superior colliculus. J Neurophysiol 78:3493–3497, 1997.

273. Patterson, A and Zangwill, O L: Disorders of visual space perception associated with lesions of the right cerebral hemisphere. Brain 67:331–358, 1944.

274. Paus, T: Location and function of the human frontal eye-field: a selective review. Neuropsychologia 34:475–483, 1996.

275. Payne, B R, Lomber, S G, Geeraerts, S, van der Gucht, E and Vandenbussche, E: Reversible visual hemineglect. Proc Natl Acad Sci USA 93:290–294, 1996.

276. Perani, D, Vallar, G, Paulesu, E, Alberoni, M and Fazio, F: Left and right hemisphere contribution to recovery from neglect after right hemisphere damage—an [18F] FDG PET study of two cases. Neuropsychologia 31:115–125, 1993.

277. Perenin, M-T: Optic ataxia and unilateral neglect: clinical evidence for dissociable spatial functions in posterior parietal cortex. In Thier, P and Karnath, H-O (Eds.): Parietal Lobe Contributions to Orientation in 3D Space. Springer, Berlin, 1997, pp. 289–308.

278. Peroutka, S J, Sohmer, B H, Kumar, A J, Folstein, M and Robinson, R G: Hallucinations and delusions following a right temporoparieto-occipital infarction. Johns Hopkins Med J 151:181–185, 1982.

279. Perrin, R G, Hockman, C H, Kalant, H and Livingston, K E: Acute effects of ethanol on spontaneous and auditory evoked electrical activity in cat brain. Electroencephalogr Clin Neurophysiol 36:19–31, 1974.

280. Petersen, S E, Robinson, D L and Keys, W: Pulvinar nuclei of the behaving rhesus monkey: visual responses and their modulation. J Neurophysiol 54:867–886, 1985.

280a. Peterson, B S, Skudlarski, P Gatenby, J C, Zhang, H, Anderson, A W and Gore, J C: An fMRI study of stroop word-color interference: Evidence for cingulate subregions subserving multiple distributed attentional systems. Biol Psychiatry 45: 1237–1258, 1999.

281. Petrides, M and Iversen, S D: Restricted posterior parietal lesions in the rhesus monkey and performance on visuospatial tasks. Brain Res 161:63–77, 1979.

282. Pierrot-Deseilligny, C, Rivaud, S, Gaymard, B and Agid, Y: Cortical control of reflexive visually-guided saccades. Brain 114:1473–1485, 1991.

283. Pitzalis, S, Spinelli, D and Zoccolotti, P: Vertical neglect: behavioral and electrophysiological data. Cortex 33:679–688, 1997.

284. Pizzamiglio, L, Perani, D, Cappa, S F, Vallar, G, Paolucci, S, Grassi, F, Paulesu, E and Fazio, F: Recovery of neglect after right hemispheric damage. Arch Neurol 55:561–568, 1998.

285. Pizzamiglio, L, Vallar, G and Doricchi, F: Gravitational inputs modulate visuospatial neglect. Exp Brain Res 117:341–345, 1997.

286. Plum, F and Posner, J B: The Diagnosis of Stupor and Coma. F A Davis, Philadelphia, 1972.

287. Posner, M I: Orienting of attention. Q J Exp Psychol 32:3025, 1980.

288. Posner, M I, Walker, J A, Friedrich, F A and Rafal, R D: How do the parietal lobes direct covert attention? Neuropsychologia 25:135–145, 1987.

289. Posner, M I, Walker, J A, Friedrich, J F and Rafal, R D: Effects of parietal injury on covert orienting of attention. J Neurosci 4:1863–1874, 1984.

290. Rafal, R D and Posner, M I: Deficits in human visual spatial attention following thalamic lesions. Proc Natl Acad Sci USA 84:7349–7353, 1987.

291. Raos, V C, Dermon, C R and Savaki, H E: Functional anatomy of the thalamic centrolateral nucleus as revealed with the [14C]deoxyglucose method following electrical stimulation and electrolytic lesion. Neurosci 68:299–313, 1995.

292. Rapoport, J L, Buchsbaum, M S, Zahn, T P, Weingartner, H, Ludlow, C and Mikkelsen, E J: Dextroamphetamine: cognitive and behavioral effects in normal prepubertal boys. Science 199:560–563, 1978.

293. Ray, C L, Mirsky, A F and Pragay, E B: Functional analysis of attention-related unit activity in the reticular formation of the monkey. Exp Neurol 77:544–562, 1982.

294. Reivich, M, Gur, R C and Alavi, A: Positron emission tomographic studies of sensory stimulation, cognitive processes and anxiety. Hum Neurobiol 2:25–33, 1983.

295. Risberg, J and Ingvar, D H: Patterns of activation in the grey matter of the dominant hemisphere during memorizing and reasoning—a study of regional cerebral blood flow changes during psychological testing in a group of neurologically normal patients. Brain 96:737–756, 1973.

296. Robertson, I H, Halligan, P W and Marshall, J C: Prospects for the rehabilitation of unilateral neglect. In Robertson, I H and Marshall, J C (Eds.): Unilateral Neglect: Clinical and Experimental Studies. Lawrence Erlbaum, Hillside, New Jersey, 1993, pp. 279–292.

297. Robertson, I H, Manly, T, Beschin, N, Daini, R, Haeske-Dewick, H, Hömberg, V, Jehkonen, M, Pizzamiglio, G, Shiel, A and Weber, E: Auditory sustained attention is a marker of unilateral spatial neglect. Neuropsychologia 35:1527–1532, 1997.

298. Robertson, L C and Eglin, M: Attentional search in unilateral visual neglect. In Robertson, I H and Marshall, J C (Eds.): Unilateral Neglect: Clinical and Experimental Studies. Lawrence Erlbaum, Hillside, New Jersey, 1993, pp. 169–191.

299. Robertson, L C, Lamb, M R and Knight, R T: Effects of lesions of temporal-parietal junction on perceptual and attentional processing in humans. J Neurosci 8:3757–3769, 1988.

300. Robinson, D L: Functional contributions of the primate pulvinar. Prog Brain Res 95:371–380, 1993.

301. Robinson, D L, Bowman, E M and Kertzman, C: Covert orienting of attention in macaques. II. Contribution of parietal cortex. J Neurophysiol 74:698–712, 1995.

302. Robinson, D L, Goldbert, M E and Stanton, G B: Parietal association cortex in the primate: sensory mechanisms and behavioral modulations. J Neurophysiol 41:910–932, 1978.

303. Robinson, D L and McClurkin, J W: The visual superior colliculus and pulvinar. Rev Oculomot Res 3:337–360, 1989.

304. Roland, P E: Cortical regulation of selective attention in man. J Neurophysiol 48:1059–1078, 1982.

305. Rolls, E T: Information representation, processing, and storage in the brain: analysis at the single neuron level. In Changeux, J-P and Konishi, M (Eds.): The Neural and Molecular Bases of Learning. John Wiley New York, 1987, pp. 503–540.

306. Rolls, E T, Baylis, C G, Hasselmo, M E and Nalwa, V: The effect of learning on the face selective responses of neurons in the cortex in the superior temporal sulcus of the monkey. Exp Brain Res 76:153–164, 1989.

307. Rossi, PW, Kheyfets, S and Reding, M J: Fresnel prisms improve visual perception in stroke patients with homonymous hemianopia or unilateral visual neglect. Neurology 40:1597–1599, 1990.

308. Rubens, A B: Caloric stimulation and unilateral visual neglect. Neurology 35:1019–1024, 1985.

309. Rueckert, L and Grafman, J: Sustained attention deficits in patients with lesions of posterior cortex. Neuropsychologia 36:653–660, 1997.

310. Sagakami, M and Niki, H: Encoding of behavioral significance of visual stimuli by primate prefrontal neurons: relation to relevant task conditions. Exp Brain Res 97:423–436, 1994.

311. Sakata, H, Taira, M, Kusunoki, M, Murata, A and Tanaka, Y: The parietal association cortex in depth perception and visual control of hand action. Trends Neurosci 20:350–357, 1997.

312. Sakata, H, Taira, M, Murata, A, Gallese, V, Tanaka, Y, Shikata, E and Kusunoki, M: Parietal visual neurons coding three-dimensional characteristics of objects and their relation to hand action. In Thier, P and Karnath, H-O (Eds.): Parietal Lobe Contributions to Orientation in 3D Space. Springer-Verlag, Berlin, 1997, pp. 237–254.

313. Scheibel, M E and Scheibel, A B: Anatomical basis of attention mechanisms in vertebrate brains. In Quarton, G C, Melnechuk, T and Schmitt, F O (Eds.): The Neurosciences. Rockefeller University Press, New York, 1967, pp. 577–602.

314. Schiller, P H, True, S D and Conway, J L: Effects of frontal eye field and superior colliculus ablations on eye movements. Science 206:590–592, 1979.

315. Schott, B, Laurent, B, Mauguiere, F and Chazot, G: Négligence motrice par hematome thalamique droit. Rev Neurol (Paris) 137:1981.

316. Schultz, W: Dopamine neurons and their role in reward mechanisms. Curr Opin Neurobiol 7:191–197, 1997.

317. Segraves, M A and Goldberg, M E: Functional properties of corticotectal neurons in the monkey's frontal eye field. J Neurophysiol 58:1387–1419, 1987.

318. Selden, N R W, Robbins, T W and Everitt, B J: Enhanced behavioral conditioning to context and impaired behavioral and neuroendocrine responses to conditioned stimuli following ceruleocortical noradrenergic lesions: support for an attentional hypothesis of central noradrenergic function. J Neurosci 10:531–539, 1990.

319. Selemon, L D and Goldman-Rakic, P D: Common cortical and subcortical targets of the dorsolateral prefrontal and posterior parietal cortices in the rhesus monkey: evidence for a distributed neural network subserving spatially guided behavior. Neuroscience 8:4049–4068, 1988.

320. Sharpless, S and Jasper, H: Habituation of the arousal reaction. Brain 79:655–680, 1956.

321. Sheliga, B M, Riggio, L and Rizzolatti, G: Spatial attention and eye movements. Exp Brain Res 105:261–275, 1995.

322. Sherrington, C S: Man on His Nature. Cambridge University Press, Cambridge, England, 1951.
323. Shulman, G L, Corbetta, M, Buckner, R L, Raichle, M E, Fiez, J A, Miezin, F M and Petersen, S E: Top-down modulation of early sensory cortex. Cereb Cortex 7:193–206, 1997.
324. Siegel, R M and Read, H L: Analysis of optic flow in the monkey parietal area 7a. Cereb Cortex 7:327–346, 1997.
325. Sieroff, E, Pollatsek, A and Posner, M I: Recognition of visual letter strings following injury to the posterior visual spatial attention system. Cog Neuropsychol 5:427–449, 1988.
326. Silberpfenning, J: Contribution to the problem of eye movements. Confin Neurol 4:1–13, 1941.
327. Smith, L W and Dimsdale, J E: Postcardiotomy delirium: conclusions after 25 years? Am J Psychiat 146:452–458, 1989.
328. Snyder, L H, Batista, A P and Andersen, R A: Change in motor plan, without a change in the spatial locus of attention, modulates activity in posterior parietal cortex. J Neurophysiol 79:2814–2819, 1998.
329. Snyder, L H, Grieve, K L, Brotchie, P and Andersen, R A: Separate body- and world-referenced representations of visual space in parietal cortex. Nature 394:887–891, 1998.
330. Sokolov, E N: Neuronal models and the orienting reflex. In Brazier, M (Ed.): The Central Nervous System and Behavior. Madison Printing, Madison, NJ, 1960, pp. 187–276.
331. Sommer, M A and Tehovnik, E J: Reversible inactivation of macaque frontal eye field. Exp Brain Res 116:229–249, 1997.
332. Soper, H V, Diamond, I T and Wilson, M: Visual attention and inferotemporal cortex in rhesus monkeys. Neuropsychologia 13:409–419, 1975.
333. Sparks, R and Geschwind, N: Dichotic listening in man after section of neocortical commissures. Cortex 4:3–16, 1968.
334. Spiers, P A, Schomer, D L, Blume, H W, Kleefield, J, O'Reilly, G, Weintraub, S, Osborne-Shaefer, P and Mesulam, M-M: Visual neglect during intracarotid amobarbital testing. Neurology 40:1600–1606, 1990.
335. Spitzer, H, Desimone, R and Moran, J: Increased attention enhances both behavioral and neuronal performance. Science 240:338–340, 1988.
336. Sprague, J M and Meikle, T H, Jr.: The role of the superior colliculus in visually guided behavior. Exp Neurol 11:115–146, 1965.
337. Steckler, T, Inglis, W, Winn, P and Sahgal, A: The pedunculopontine tegmental nucleus: a role in cognitive processes? Brain Res Rev 19:298–318, 1994.
338. Steinmetz, M A: Contributions of posterior parietal cortex to cognitive functions in primates. Psychobiology 26:109–118, 1998.
339. Steriade, M: State-dependent changes in the activity of rostral reticular and thalamocortical elements. Neurosci Res Prog Bull 18:83–91, 1980.
340. Steriade, M: EEG desynchronization is associated with cellular events that are prerequisites for active behavioral states. Behav Brain Sci 4:489–492, 1981a.
341. Steriade, M: Mechanisms underlying cortical activation: neuronal organization and properties of the midbrain reticular core and intralaminar thalamic nuclei. In Pompeiano, O and Ajmone Marson, C (Eds.): Brain Mechanisms and Perceptual Awareness. Raven Press, New York, 1981, pp. 327–377.
342. Stone, S P, Halligan, P W, Marshall, J C and Greenwood, R J: Unilateral neglect: a common but heterogeneous syndrome. Neurology 50:1902–1905, 1998.
343. Takahashi, N, Kawamura, M, Shiota, J, Kasahata, N and Hirayama, K: Pure topographic disorientation due to right retrosplenial lesion. Neurology 49:464–469, 1997.
344. Taylor, S F, Huang, G, Tandon, R and Koeppe, R A: Letter naming among distractors activates anterior cingulate cortex in a selective attention task. Neuroimage 7:S94, 1998.
345. Tegnér, R and Levander, M: Through a looking glass. A new technique to demonstrate directional hypokinesia in unilateral neglect. Brain 114:1943–1951, 1991.

346. Tootell, R B H, Hadjikhani, N K, Mendola, J D, Marrett, S and Dale, A M: From retinotopy to recognition: fMRI in human visual cortex. TICS 2:174–182, 1998.

347. Treisman, A M: Verbal cues, language and meaning in selective attention. Am J Psychol 77:206–219, 1967.

348. Treue, S and Maunsell, J H R: Attentional modulation of visual signal processing in the parietal cortex. In Thier, P and Karnath, H-O (Eds.): Parietal Lobe Contributions to Orientation in 3D Space. Springer, Berlin, 1997, pp. 355–384.

349. Tune, L E, Damlouji, N F, Holland, A, Gardner, T J, Folstein, M F and Coyle, J T: Association of postoperative delirium with raised serum levels of anticholinergic drugs. Lancet 2:651–653, 1981.

350. Ungerleider, L G and Brody, B A: Extrapersonal spatial orientation: the role of posterior parietal, anterior frontal, and inferotemporal cortex. Exper Neurol 56:265–280, 1977.

351. Vallar, G: The anatomical basis of spatial hemineglect in humans. In Robertson, I H and Marshall, J C (Eds.): Unilateral Neglect: Clinical and Experimental Studies. Lawrence Erlbaum, Hillside, New Jersey, 1993, pp. 27–59.

352. Vallar, G, Sandroni, P, Rusconi, M L and Barbieri, S: Hemianopia, hemianesthesia, and spatial neglect: a study with evoked potentials. Neurology 41:1918–1922, 1991.

353. Vanderwolf, C H and Stewart, D J: Thalamic control of neocortical activation: a critical re-evaluation. Brain Res Bull 20:529–538, 1988.

354. Voytko, M L, Olton, D S, Richardson, R T, Gorman, L K, Tobin, J R and Price, D L: Basal forebrain lesions in monkeys disrupt attention but not learning and memory. J Neurosci 14:167–186, 1994.

355. Vuilleumier, P, Valenza, N, Mayer, E, Reverdin, A and Landis, T: Near and far visual space in unilateral neglect. Ann Neurol 43:406–410, 1998.

356. Wada, H, Inagaki, N, Yamatodani, A and Watanabe, T: Is the histaminergic neuron system a regulatory center for whole-brain activity? Trends Neurosci 14:415–418, 1991.

357. Wallace, R J: Spatial S-R compatibility effects involving kinesthetic cues. J Exp Psychol 93:163–168, 1972.

358. Watanabe, M: Reward expectancy in primate prefrontal neurons. Nature 382:629–632, 1996.

359. Watson, R T and Heilman, K M: Thalamic neglect. Neurology 29:690–694, 1979.

360. Watson, R T, Heilman, K M, Cauthen, J C and King, F A: Neglect after cingulectomy. Neurology 23:1003–1007, 1973.

361. Watson, R T, Heilman, K M, Miller, D and King, F A: Neglect after mesencephalic reticular formation lesions. Neurology 24:294–298, 1974.

362. Watson, R T, Miller, B D and Heilman, K M: Nonsensory neglect. Ann Neurol 3:505–508, 1978.

363. Watson, R T, Valenstein, E, Day, A and Heilman, K M: Posterior neocortical systems subserving awareness and neglect. Arch Neurol 51:1014–1021, 1994.

364. Weintraub, S, Daffner, K R, Ahern, G, Price, B H and Mesulam, M-M: Right sided hemispatial neglect and bilateral cerebral lesions. J Neurol Neurosurg Psychiatry 60:342–344, 1996.

365. Weintraub, S and Mesulam, M-M: Right cerebral dominance in spatial attention. Further evidence based on ipsilateral neglect. Arch Neurol 44:621–625, 1987.

366. Weintraub, S and Mesulam, M-M: Visual hemispatial inattention: stimulus parameters and exploratory strategies. J Neurol Neurosurg Psychiatry 51:1481–1488, 1988.

367. Weintraub, S and Mesulam, M-M: Neglect: hemispheric specialization, behavioral components and anatomical correlates. In Boller, F and Grafman, J (Eds.): Handbook of Neuropsychology. Elsevier, Amsterdam, 1989, 2, pp. 357–374.

368. Welch, K and Stuteville, P: Experimental production of unilateral neglect in monkeys. Brain 81:341–347, 1958.

369. Willanger, R, Danielsen, U T and Ankerhus, J: Denial and neglect of hemiparesis in right-sided apopleptic lesions. Acta Neurol Scand 64:310–326, 1981.

370. Wojciulik, E, Kanwisher, N and Driver, J: Covert visual attention modulates face-specific activity in human fusiform gyrus: an fMRI study. J Neurophysiol 79:1574–1578, 1998.
371. Wurtz, R H and Goldberg, M E: Activity of superior colliculus in behaving monkey. III. Cells discharging before eye movements. J Neurophysiol 35:575–585, 1972.
372. Yamaguchi, S, Tsuchiya, H and Kobayashi, S: Visuospatial attention shift and motor responses in cerebellar disorders. J Cog Neurosci 10:95–107, 1998.
373. Young, A W, Hellawell, D J and Welch, J: Neglect and visual recognition. Brain 115:51–71, 1992.

4

Memory and Amnesia

Hans J. Markowitsch

I. Introduction

Memory is the glue that holds together our thoughts, impressions, and experiences. Without it, past and future would lose their meaning and self-awareness would be lost as well. In the 1950s the case description of H. M. by Scoville and Milner[182] alerted scientists all over the world to the fact that certain circumscribed brain lesions within the limbic system may destroy the ability to form new memories, while leaving other intellectual functions untouched. The following two case reports are intended to display the symptoms of memory disturbance that may arise after bilateral damage to limbic structures.

II. The Classic Limbic Amnesic Syndrome

Medial Temporal Lobe Damage: Case H. M. (Scoville and Milner)

The description of H. M. (despite the existence of similar previous reports whose significance for the neurobiology of memory remained largely unappreciated) is a milestone in the history of neuropsychological research that aims to understand how the brain functions as it engages in long-term information storage.

In the early 1950s, the neurosurgeon William B. Scoville performed a series of operations on patients with pharmacologically intractable epilepsies. One of these patients was a 23-year old right-handed man of normal intelligence (IQ above 100) who received a bilateral resection of the anterior parts of his medial temporal lobes on September 1, 1953 (Fig. 4–1). This surgery reduced the frequency of his preoperatively severe epileptic attacks and enabled their control by drugs. However, H. M. thereafter lost his ability to form new stable memories. Consequently, while still displaying adequate social skills and expressing himself verbally better than most people, time appeared to have stopped for him. He could no longer keep up with what day or year it was, or with events happening in the world and in his own life. He was able to reflect on his condition by stating, for example, "Every

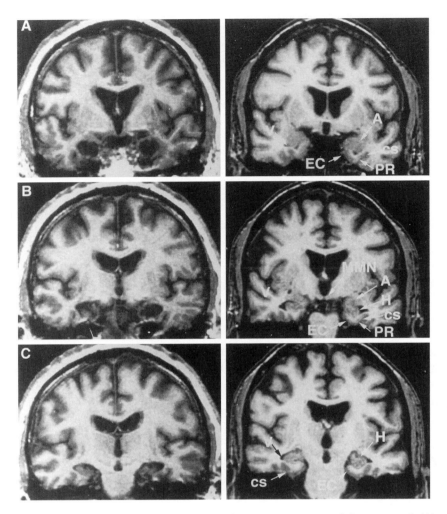

FIGURE 4–1. This series of T1-weighted images is arranged from rostral (A) to caudal (C) through the temporal lobe of H. M. (shown on left) and of a 66-year-old man (on the right) who has served as a control subject in neuropsychological studies. Sections from the control brain were selected to match as closely as possible the levels illustrated from H. M.'s brain. The control brain illustrates the structures that are likely to have been eliminated in H. M.'s brain. Level A: The amygdala (A) and entorhinal cortex (EC) are heavily damaged at this level. The collateral sulcus (cs) is barely visible; therefore, little of the perirhinal (transento-rhinal) cortex (PR) is likely to be intact at this level. Level B: This is the rostral level of the hippocampal formation (H), which is missing bilaterally in H. M. The entorhinal cortex is also missing at this level. Because the collateral sulcus is visible, some perirhinal (PR) cortex is likely to be intact at this level. The medial mammillary nucleus (MMN) is present at this level and appears to be slightly shrunken in H. M. Level C: This level shows the body of the hippocampal formation and the temporal horn of the ventricle (v). Most of the hippocampal formation, including the entorhinal cortex, is missing at this level in H. M. Note throughout that H. M.'s cerebral neocortex demonstrates relatively little sulcal widening and that sulcal widening is more pronounced in the cognitively normal control subject. (Reproduced with permission from Fig. 5 of Corkin et al.[31] from *The Journal of Neuroscience* 17:3671, 1997.)

day is alone, whatever enjoyment I've had, and whatever sorrow I've had" (p. 217).[136]

H. M.'s "intellect" (as defined by the IQ) remained intact after surgery, and there were no major emotional or behavioral changes. His working memory (also known as short-term or immediate memory or attention span) was intact; he retained abilities such as reading, writing, and calculating; and he could recall most autobiographical episodes from his past life (with the exception of those that had occurred within approximately 1 year prior to surgery[134]). His ability to form new memories, however, was severely and persistently disrupted. Throughout the many decades of his subsequent life he was able to record only a few fragments of new information, such as the assassination of President Kennedy.

H. M. has been extensively studied from April 1955 to the present in the course of investigations which reflect the increasing theoretical sophistication of neuropsychological and neuroradiological research.[30,31] It was found that H. M. is able to acquire and retain certain kinds of information under special conditions of stimulus presentation and retrieval[59] and also when learning occurs implicitly as in skill learning, priming, and conditioning.[61,220]

Magnetic resonance imaging (MRI) revealed that H. M.'s brain damage is confined to the amygdala, parahippocampal–entorhinal cortex, and the anterior hippocampus (Fig. 4–1).

Medial Diencephalic Damage: Case A. B.

Studies of chronic alcoholics with the Wernicke-Korsakoff syndrome have shown that damage within limbic diencephalic structures such as the mammillary bodies, the mediodorsal nucleus of the thalamus, and the medial pulvinar can result in a syndrome remarkably similar to the one found after medial temporal lobe damage. An example of diencephalic amnesia is provided by case A. B.[114]

Ten years after a bilateral infarct sustained at the age of 66 years in the region of the mediodorsal diencephalon (Fig. 4–2), A. B. still had the appearance of a jovial and respectable professor of medicine. However, a few minutes of conversation would be sufficient to reveal that he was completely unable to retain new information and that he had to be constantly prompted by his patient and caring wife. Asked about the current year, he always responded with the year of his infarct; asked to repeat a brief story of less than 100 words that had just been told to him, he could not accurately retrieve even one item of information. Similarly, he was totally unable to reproduce a complex figure (Rey-Osterrieth Figure) which he had just copied without error 2 minutes before (see Fig. 48.6 in Markowitsch[106]). However, A. B. still had above average intelligence (as measured by IQ), high motivation, and excellent attentive functions as shown by his digit span of seven. His concept formation ability was above average and he was able to recall street names where he had lived as a child. He also could name former teachers and relatives such as aunts and uncles from his youth. However, when asked about events related to current news, he was unable to recall anything that had happened since his brain damage and occasionally would confabulate. As an

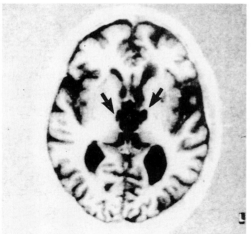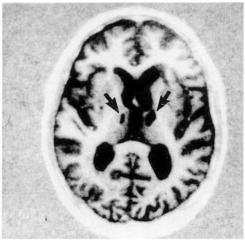

FIGURE 4–2. T1-weighted MRI scans of patient A. B. with medial diencephalic damage (arrows). The extent of the right and left lesion in the polar region of both thalami is shown in axial sections of the brain. The damage pattern can be considered typical for infarcts in the territory of the polar ("premammillary") thalamic artery/arteries and includes the mediodorsal thalamic nucleus as well as portions of the mammillothalamic tract and the anterior/inferior thalamic peduncle. The lesion is larger on the left than on the right side.

example, in 1991 he was asked whether anything special had happened recently with respect to East–West relations (e.g., falling of the Berlin Wall in Germany). He said that he was not a keen observer of the political scenery and that there was nothing special: "Just the always occurring minor quarrels between Germany and France."

A. B.'s severe anterograde amnesia prevented him from reflecting on his memory problems. When asked about his memory he judged it as "good." When asked in more detail whether he could mention problems in certain areas of his memory, he responded that he had problems in remembering his dreams and in repeating jokes. A psychologist who had worked with him for a long time remarked that he once stated, "I have no memory at all, isn't that terrible?" but immediately thereafter had forgotten this statement and its consequences.

In the course of further investigations, we found that A. B. was able to acquire new perceptuomotor skills as assessed by the stylus maze and mirror drawing tasks. A. B. was also shown a series of 20 incomplete pictures (Fig. 4–3). Each of these pictures was shown in ten versions, which increased in completeness from version 1—very incomplete—to version 10—complete. The patient was asked to identify the sketched object as early in the sequence as possible. The task was administered in an identical way over four sessions. When asked, A. B. always responded that he had never done the test, but his performance improved across sessions (Fig. 4–4). It can thus be concluded that he had successfully acquired some knowledge, though this was not consciously available to him.

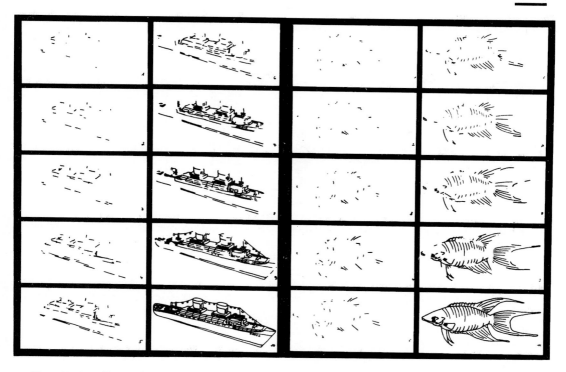

FIGURE 4–3. Examples of the *Incomplete Pictures Test*, which is used to assess priming performance in amnesic patients. Patients are shown frames 1–10, one at a time, until they can identify the object. They are then shown the same pictures to see if the point of recognition can be shifted to the more incomplete frames.

A. B.'s behavior resembled that of H. M. with the possible exception that H. M. may have had slightly more insight into his deficit. Both A. B. and H. M. share features which are typical for most patients with limbic amnesia: Both are grossly deficient in forming stable memories of new experience—that is, they have an anterograde amnesia. This anterograde amnesia is, however, selective insofar as it holds only for information that requires explicit (declarative) reference to a particular learning episode, while other—implicitly learned—information is largely preserved. There is retrograde amnesia for events that occurred shortly before the onset of the brain damage. Consolidated old memories from early youth are immune to the retrograde amnesia. Social skills and intellectual capabilities in domains other than memory are preserved.

A. B. and H. M. both represent examples of what is known as the classic limbic amnesic syndrome, which appears to be due to bilateral damage within one or more bottleneck structures of the limbic system.[187] The limbic amnesic syndrome occurs when brain damage interrupts a circuit of interconnected structures which encode, associate and retrieve recently required information and which enable its long-term storage in other parts of the brain, including unimodal and heteromodal association cortices (Chapter 1).

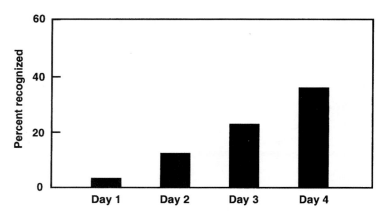

FIGURE 4–4. Priming performance of patient A. B. with midline diencephalic damage when identifying the content of incompletely presented pictures. Each of 20 pictures used was shown in ten versions from very incomplete (stage 1) to complete (stage 10). As the ten steps from incomplete to complete did not reflect equal "distances" of identification, the percentage values of subjects detecting the contents of the picture at each level were taken as reference and the patient's performance is given in relation to these reference values. (Interpretation: On day 1, A. B. detected on the average less than 10% of the information the controls had detected on day 1, but on day 4 A. B. detected nearly 40% of the information the controls had detected on day 1.)

III. MEMORY AND ITS DISORDERS

What Is Memory?

The type of memory impaired in H. M. and A. B. was described by Sinz[192] as the "learning-dependent storage of ontogenetically acquired information." This information is stored in neuronal structures so that it can be retrieved at future time points and used for adaptive behavior. The term engram is frequently used to describe the stored information and a wealth of data exist to indicate that the retrieved information need not to be identical to the original experience. Instead, modifications, adaptations, and distortions of the engram may occur, depending on the nature of subsequently stored material and on the state of the organism at the point of retrieval. These modifications also led Tulving[208] to reintroduce Semon's[184] term "ecphory" to describe the process by which retrieval cues interact with stored information so that the reconstruction of the queried information represents a complex interaction of the two.

Dudai[46] referred to Luria's[96] case of a mnemonist who remembered everything but was quite poor in structuring the information, abstracting it, and distinguishing trivial from important information. The important factor is not necessarily the storage capacity of human memory but its ability to support adaptive behaviors. Elephants and sperm whales may have brains with greater storage capacity than our own but that does not seem to have endowed these species with intellectual abilities superior to those of humans.

Subtyping Memory According to Temporal Parameters

The one unique feature of memory is its temporal dimension. This is what distinguishes it from feelings, emotions, and thoughts, which deal with the here and now. Memory can be used to travel back in time.[211] Information first is *registered* (that is, perceived via sensory channels), *encoded* (that is, further processed for identification and association), and finally *stored* in multifocal anatomical sites in the form of "engrams."

In 1870, Hering[70] (a physiologist known for his opponent-color theory, and the Hering-Breuer reflex) stated that memory unites the countless single phenomena to a whole and that without its binding power our consciousness would disintegrate into as many fragments as there are moments.[70] As H. M. exemplifies, the binding and interrelating of information along a temporal dimension is disrupted in amnesic patients. Such patients have lost the capacity to reflect on the passage of time, as shown by H. M.'s statement that "Every day is alone."

A contemporary of Hering, Ebbinghaus,[47] differentiated short-term from long-term memory. Atkinson and Shiffrin[2] introduced the further subdivisions of ultrashort, short-term (working), and long-term memory. The ultrashort (iconic or echoic) form of memory refers to a process measured in milliseconds which may, for instance, be related to the decay of the photopigments in the retina's rods and cones. Short-term memory has attracted a great deal of research, especially after Baddeley's[4] introduction of the term "working memory." Working memory refers to the active on-line holding and manipulation of information and includes the preparation of stored information for retrieval. Long-term memory refers to information which is stored off-line for periods which extend from minutes to decades.

The learning of word lists helps to distinguish short-term from long-term memory. When recalling items from a list of 12 words, for example, subjects tend to retrieve a disproportionally higher number of words that were presented at the beginning and end of the list. The greater recall of initial items is known as the primacy effect and reflects processes related to long-term memory, whereas the greater recall of late items is known as the recency effect and is more closely related to short-term memory. Short-term or working memory appears to rely on sensorial or surface encoding, while long-term memory seems to be more dependent on semantic (or deep) encoding. Certain forms of neurological damage may spare short-term but impair long-term memory (as in the case of the classic limbic amnesic syndrome), while other types of damage may lead to the converse dissociation,[117,186,201] and still others may impair both types of memory (e.g., Alzheimer's disease[201]). The existence of such dissociations illustrates the independence of short-term from long-term memory.

Limbic lesions lead to selective impairments of long-term memory whereas frontal lobe damage leads to selective impairments of working memory (Chapter 1). An interesting experiment on the distinction between short-term and long-term memory was made by Richards[160] who asked H. M. to reproduce time intervals ranging from 1 to 300 seconds. H. M. was quite accurate in estimating intervals under 20 seconds but underestimated longer ones. For example, he estimated 1 hour as equivalent to approximately 3 minutes.

Subtyping Memory According to its Contents

While the time-based subdivisions of memory are widely accepted, content-based subdivisions are more controversial.[173,197,206,211] Some of the terms used for content-based subdivisions include episodic memory, semantic memory, declarative memory, explicit and implicit memory, procedural memory, priming, and conditioning.

Squire and Zola[197] identify episodic and semantic memory as two subtypes of declarative memory, the first one dealing with personal events and the second with general facts. Tulving and Markowitsch[211] view episodic memory as an extension of semantic memory (Fig. 4–5). Episodic memory refers to specific events in one's biography. These events are embedded in time and place; they are of the type, "Yesterday I ate a snapper," and "Last August I climbed Mount Kinabalu." Episodic memory is actively *remembered*, while semantic information is only *known*: I know that Madrid is the capital of Spain and that 2^3 is 8. A term like "factual memory" would in fact be more appropriate than that of semantic memory, since "semantic" may give the mistaken impression that grammatical or vocabulary knowledge is involved.

The existence of patients with selective amnesia for either episodic or semantic memory supports their distinctiveness. For instance, patients with damage to predominantly the right frontotemporopolar region have been found to be unable to retrieve episodic events,[90] while those with corresponding damage to mainly the left hemisphere may have difficulties in retrieving semantic information.[42,106]

The category of procedural memory was identified by investigating the acquisition of motor skills. Already in 1912 Schneider[180] had noted that amnesic patients were able to learn how to solve jigsaw puzzles although they could not remember new episodes. Later it was noted that H. M. was able to learn new motor skills, such as those involved in rotor pursuit.[135] It was subsequently found that patients with the amnesias caused by limbic lesions could acquire a whole range of perceptual, motor, and strategy skills,[178,195] while patients with basal ganglia damage were severely impaired in such tasks[219]—providing evidence for a further anatomical–behavioral distinction of memory systems. Examples of procedural memory include learning to drive, ski, and play musical instruments.

Another recently rediscovered memory system (see Heilbronner[69] and Schneider[180]) is the priming system, which refers to the influence that a previously perceived stimulus has on future performance. Psychologists differentiate between perceptual and conceptual priming. In perceptual priming the stimuli are of an identical sensory structure at all phases of presentation, while in conceptual priming they only belong to the same category, or concept (e.g., fruits, when an apple had

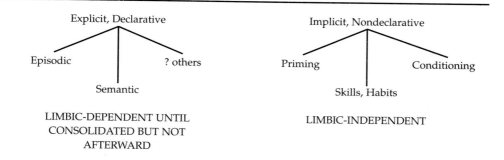

Sketch of the relations between semantic and episodic memory. Information is encoded into semantic memory independently of episodic memory, and into episodic memory "through" semantic memory. When encoded and stored, information can be retrieved from one of the two systems, or from both of them (after Fig. 1 of Tulving and Markowitsch[211]).

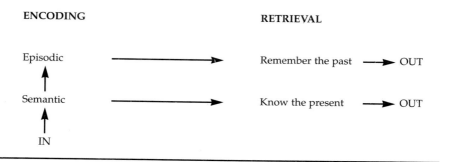

FIGURE 4–5. Content-dependent subdivisions of long-term memory.

been seen previously). In priming tests, the stimuli are not required to be learned actively. (For example, instead of being asked to "memorize" the words, the subject may just be asked to count how many "a"s they contain.) When presented again at a later time point, the previously presented stimuli are more likely to be selected or to guide subsequent performance, as in the case of stem completion or lexical decision tasks. Tulving and Schacter[212] defined priming as a process of information recognition in the absence of conscious reflection. The *Incomplete Pictures Test*, given to patient A. B. (Figs. 4–3 and 4–4), is an example of priming.

A definition or description of the various terms used in psychological memory research can be found in Table 4–1. The one most important distinction is that episodic memory is explicit in the sense that the subject is aware of its acquisition and recall whereas priming and skill learning (as well as conditioning) are implicit in the sense that the subject may have no awareness of the acquisition or even of possessing the information.[155] The former is impaired by limbic lesions but not the latter.

TABLE 4–1 Frequently Used Expressions in Neuropsychological Memory Research

REGISTRATION OF INFORMATION (*sensory organs, primary cortex, association neocortex*)
Information enters the nervous system via the sensory organs or is generated internally[77]
SHORT-TERM MEMORY/WORKING MEMORY (*parietal and prefrontal cortex*)
The on-line retention of 7 ± 2 items of information is limited to a time range of seconds to maximally a few minutes. The information is distributed in many cortical areas but the critical areas that hold it on-line seem to be situated in the parietal and dorsolateral prefontal cortex (Chapter 1)
ENCODING AND CONSOLIDATING INFORMATION (*limbic system*)
Recently acquired information is encoded in association cortex and transferred to the limbic system where it is evaluated for relevance, subjected to further associations (including multimodal binding), integrated with preexisting information, and engaged in a process that will lead to consolidation (Chapter 1)
STORAGE OF INFORMATION (*cerebral cortex*)
The "engrams" are represented in a distributed form within unimodal, heteromodal, and paralimbic areas. Components of the limbic system (such as the hippocampus and entorhinal cortex) are necessary for binding. There may be a hemispheric asymmetry such that the left hemisphere stores primarily verbal or general knowledge (i.e., semantic information) and the right primarily nonverbal or autobiographical (i.e., episodic) information
RETRIEVAL/ECPHORY OF INFORMATION (*prefrontotemporopolar network*)
Information retrieval (or ecphory) seems to depend on triggering mechanisms which originate in portions of the prefrontal and the anterior temporal cortex. However, based on the retrograde amnesia that is seen in patients such as H. M., some authors conclude that the critical role of the limbic system extends to the process of retrieval as well (Chapter 1)

TIME-DEPENDENT FORMS OF MEMORY	
Sensory memory ("iconic," "echoic" memory)	The retaining of information for milliseconds, based on the input along sensory channels
Short-term memory, working memory attention	The on-line holding of very limited amounts of information (5–7 items) for a very restricted time (up to a few minutes at most)
Long-term memory	Principally lifelong retention of information

CONTENT-DEPENDENT FORMS OF MEMORY	
Episodic memory	The storage of single events which can be traced back with respect to time and place of occurrence and emotional valence
Knowledge system	The storage of general facts

(continued)

IV. THE ANATOMICAL SUBSTRATES OF MEMORY

Amnesias occur after a wide range of disease conditions (Table 4–2). This fact alone implies that memory is not controlled by a single center in the brain but, instead, by a distributed network (Chapter 1). Furthermore, memory is also dependent on a large number of sensory, perceptual, attentive, emotional, and motivational processes, each with its own anatomical substrates. Chow's[27] caveats with respect to deficits caused by brain lesions should be remembered here: First, if a brain lesion fails to affect a learning task, it cannot be stated that this part of the brain does not participate in that function. Second, if the lesion does influence performance of the task, it does not necessarily mean that it is the only neural structure involved. The

TABLE 4–1—Continued

Declarative memory	Episodic and semantic memories are collectively known as declarative memory
Explicit memory	Memory which requires the conscious recollection of the episode. Sometimes used also for facts and then taken as synonym for declarative memory
Implicit memory	Memory which is independent from conscious recollection; memory is inferred indirectly through a faster or better performance on certain tasks
Procedural memory	Learning of perceptuomotor skills, and the acquisition of rules and sequences. This is a type of implicit memory
Priming	The influence on performance of previously presented (but not consciously identified) information. This is another type of implicit memory
MISCELLANEOUS TERMS	
Engram	Hypothetical memory trace
Ecphory	Ecphory refers to the process wherein retrieval cues interact with stored information so that an image or a representation of the desired information becomes activated
Forgetting	The loss of information available for explicit recall or recognition. Usually processes of *decay* are assumed to exist
Free recall	Voluntary recall of learned information without external help or cuing
Cued recall	Recall with the help of superficial (first letter) or deep (category of word) cues
Recognition	Identification of the previously presented stimulus in a list containing a large number of similar stimuli
Amnesia	Originally, the term meant a complete, "global" loss of memory. In recent times the term is frequently also used to indicate fractionated memory impairments
Anterograde amnesia	The inability to acquire new information for long-term storage and retrieval
Retrograde amnesia	The inability to retrieve information that had been stored prior to the onset of the amnesia
Amnesic snydrome	Global memory loss in explicit (declarative, episodic) domains as exemplified by patient H. M.

aim of ablation methods to clarify the functions of the damaged area is never fully attainable, for it is based on observations in patients who no longer have the region of the brain one wishes to study. These challenges can be addressed by integrating results derived from focal lesions with those based on functional imaging.

Implicit Learning

Processes of implicit memory, such as priming and procedural learning, are processed differently from episodic information. Numerous investigations have addressed the possible biological representation of implicit learning. With the excep-

Table 4–2 Overview of Patient Groups in Whom Severe Global Amnesic Disorders
May Be Prominent

Etiology	Most Common Lesion Sites
Closed head injury	Temporal pole, orbitofrontal cortex, fornix
Cerebral infarctions, ruptured aneurysms, aneurysm surgery	Bilateral lesions in hippocampus, medial temporal lobe, and limbic nuclei of the thalamus (posterior cerebral artery) or in orbitofrontal cortex and basal forebrain (anterior communicating artery)
Intracranial tumors	Limbic thalamus (glioblastoma), medial temporal lobe (sphenoid wing meningioma), or posterior cingulate gyrus (lipoma)
Viral infections (e.g., herpes simplex encephalitis)	Hippocampus and nearly all components of the limbic and paralimbic cortex
Avitaminoses (e.g., B_1 deficiency)	Limbic thalamus, mammillary bodies (as in Korsakoff's disease)
Neurotoxin exposure (e.g., trimethylin intoxication)	Hippocampal complex
Temporal lobe epilepsy	Hippocampus and medial temporal lobe
Degenerative diseases of the CNS (e.g., Alzheimer's or Pick's disease)	Hippocampus, entorhinal cortex and amygdala
Anoxia or hypoxia (e.g., after a heart attack or drowning)	Hippocampus (CA1 sector)
Drugs such as anticholinergics, β-adrenergic blockers, benzodiazepines	Limbic system
Electroconvulsive therapy	Probably limbic system
Transient global amnesia	Usually limbic structures in medial temporal lobe when an etiology is found
Paraneoplastic limbic encephalitis	Limbic structures in medial temporal lobe

tion of fear conditioning, which has been related to the amygdala,[143,161] implicit learning seems to be mediated by nonlimbic structures. These may be neocortical or may be found in the cerebellum and the basal ganglia.

While results from earlier research suggested that visual priming may just be processed within peristriate unimodal sensory cortex, more recent results obtained with functional imaging methods, evoked potentials, and the investigation of patients with focal brain damage indicate a more distributed representation which includes heteromodal association areas of the temporal and parietal cortex as well.[48,62,144,174,183,203] Procedural memory may be processed predominantly within regions of the cerebellum and the basal ganglia, perhaps with the additional participation of dorsolateral frontal cortex.[89,137,206,219] For example, impairment of procedural memories (as tested by tasks such as the reading of mirror image words or rotor-pursuit tracking) was observed in patients with Parkinson's disease and Huntington's disease.[3,45,108,193]

Short-term (Working) Memory

Numerous experiments using monkeys, cats, and rats have reported that bilateral damage to the prefrontal cortex interferes with the short-term storage (on-line holding) of information and that neurons in this region display working memory related firing.[121,122] More recently, evoked potential recordings and functional imaging techniques have confirmed the dominant role of dorsolateral prefrontal regions for working memory in the human brain.[26,32] Functional imaging experiments suggest that dorsolateral and ventrolateral portions of the prefrontal cortex contribute to both spatial and non-spatial working memory.[150] Animal experiments, however, suggest that dorsal prefrontal cortex may be more closely related to spatial working memory whereas ventral prefrontal cortex may be more closely related to working memory for objects.

Some reports found that parietal regions are also implicated in short-term memory.[26,32] Evidence for quite selective deficits in short-term but not in long-term memory can be found in several reports of patients with circumscribed unilateral parietal lesions.[216,168,185,97] Markowitsch and co-workers,[117] for example, had studied a 44-year-old left handed patient after removal of a circumscribed left hemispheric tumor centered in the angular gyrus and in the subcortical white matter of the left parietal lobe (Fig. 4–6). The patient had a distinct and persistent working memory impairment, but preserved long-term explicit memory, as shown by a preserved primacy effect in the presence of an impaired recency effect. That is, when given a word list, he was able to reproduce the first, but not the last, words of this list.

In summary, short-term (or working) memory is a predominantly attentional function under the control of a fronto-parietal network whereas long-term explicit (or episodic) memory is under the control of a limbic network. (See Chapters 1 and 3 for further discussion.)

Brain Regions Relevant to Episodic (Declarative, Explicit) Memory

Hebb[68] proposed that newly acquired information reverberates in a neural circuit before being transferred into long-term storage. Such circuits for encoding and consolidating information (see Table 4–1 for terminology) include regions of the limbic system, especially the hippocampo-entorhinal complex, as their critical components.[218]

The hippocampal region, the amygdala, paralimbic cortices, certain medial and anterior thalamic nuclei, the mammillary bodies, other hypothalamic nuclei, the basal forebrain, the ventral striatum, and interconnecting fiber systems are the major components of the limbic system.[109,145,151] (Fig. 4–7).

There are two interacting circuits within the limbic system: the Papez circuit,[151]

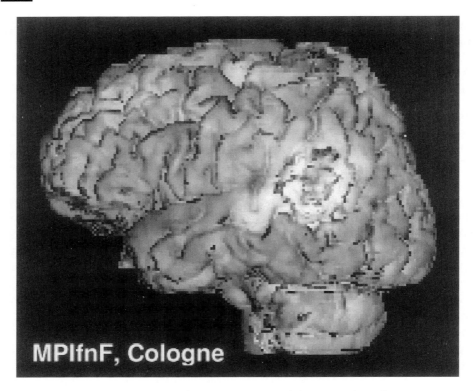

FIGURE 4–6. Three-dimensional reconstruction of brain surface from postoperative T1-weighted MRI datasets. Shape and size of the tumor were defined by increased ^{11}C-methionine uptake measured with position emission tomography (PET). MPIfnF, Max-Planck-Institut für Neurologische Forschung, Cologne.

centered around the hippocampus, and the basolateral limbic circuit (amygdaloid circuit).[172] Papez[151] considered the circuit he had described as principally engaged in the analysis of emotions, but subsequent work showed that it plays a critical role in the transfer of information into long-term memory.[108] The amygdaloid circuit is more closely related to emotional processing but is also relevant for encoding the emotional valence of experiences. It includes the amygdala, the mediodorsal thalamic nucleus, and associated paralimbic regions such as the parolfactory gyrus of the subcallosal region, the temporal pole, the insula, the orbitofrontal cortex, and interconnecting fibers such as the ventral amygdalofugal pathway, the anterior thalamic peduncle, and the diagonal band.

Bilateral damage to structures situated within the limbic system, especially within components of the Papez circuit, is usually followed by severe memory disturbances—a fact which led researchers to speculate that amnesia might arise from an interruption of interconnections within the Papez circuit or from a disconnection between limbic structures necessary for consolidation and neocortical structures necessary for storage.[217] Each component of the limbic system influences the processes of declarative/explicit/episodic memory (Chapter 1). However, the

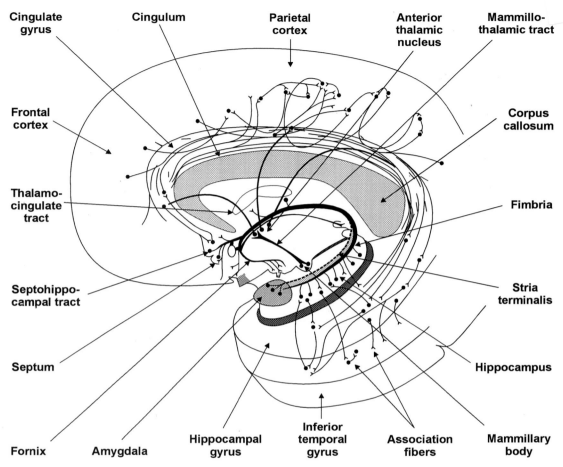

Cingulate gyrus
Cingulum
Parietal cortex
Anterior thalamic nucleus
Mammillo-thalamic tract
Frontal cortex
Corpus callosum
Thalamo-cingulate tract
Fimbria
Septohippo-campal tract
Stria terminalis
Septum
Hippocampus
Fornix
Amygdala
Hippocampal gyrus
Inferior temporal gyrus
Association fibers
Mammillary body

FIGURE 4–7. The major pathways of the limbic system. (Modified after Fig. 3 of Kahn and Crosby.[80])

hippocampo-entorhinal complex and the limbic nuclei of the thalamus have the most critical relationship to this function (Fig. 4–8). Thus, human case reports have shown that bilateral damage to the region of the medial thalamus or the hippo-campo–entorhinal region will regularly result in severe and persistent amnesia—that is, in an inability to form new stable memories that are accessible to explicit recall. (See the two case descriptions given in Section II.)

Bilateral damage to the amygdaloid region may induce the Klüver-Bucy syndrome,[87] which is characterized (originally in the monkey, but later in man as well[93,205]) by the following symptom complex: agnosia, amnesia, hypersexuality, hyperorality, hyperphagia, tameness/placidity, and hypermetamorphosis. These behavioral changes encompass the functions of emotion and drive rather than memory. However, since information encoding is also dependent on emotional content, damage to the amygdala would be expected to have detrimental effects on memory.

This has been shown in patients with selective bilateral amygdala damage as part of Urbach-Wiethe disease. The patients were presented stories containing emotionally charged items and asked to recall the detail. They were significantly impaired because they could not show the preferential encoding of emotionally laden versus neutral items.[18,113]

Lesions in the basal forebrain may also disturb memory processing.[36] The patient described by Cramon and co-workers[36] had a lesion in the (medial) septal region. She was hypersensitive to emotional material and—as a consequence of this hypersensitivity—was unable to properly abstract and encode material for later reproduction. Aside from the medial septal nucleus, other structures of the basal forebrain such as the diagonal band of Broca and the basal nucleus of Meynert have also been found to be of importance for long-term memory.[37,155] In the majority of reported cases, the memory deteriorations after damage to these structures seem to be less severe and enduring than those after hippocampo–entorhinal or diencephalic damage.[43,155,198] Personality disturbances and tendencies to confabulate are quite common after basal forebrain damage, however.[35]

Damage to the fiber pathways of the limbic system can also cause amnesia.[63,102] A right-handed patient of average intelligence, for example, sustained damage to the fornix during the removal of a tumor and developed major anterograde amnesia for both verbal and nonverbal material.[21] But his attention, concentration, and working memory abilities were preserved, as were his cognitive flexibility, procedural memory, and priming. Figure 4–9 shows his performance in reading mirror-image words, a task of procedural memory.

The similarity between the amnesic conditions arising after bilateral damage to medial temporal and medial diencephalic structures led Squire and associates[196] to conclude that these structures might be components of a common memory system and to speak of "medial temporal–diencephalic amnesia."[156] While this seems likely, there may also be regional functional specializations. Patients with bilateral diencephalic damage, for example, have less awareness of their memory than those with medial temporal lobe damage. [30,73,102,114,136] They also demonstrate a greater tendency to confabulate [30,73,99,102,114,136,215] and have a larger span of retrograde amnesia. [74,99,102,215]

Encoding and Consolidation

As defined in Table 4–1, the processes of encoding and of consolidation are frequently separated on the assumption that the consolidation process follows and leads to a deeper sort of encoding. However, not all authorities in this field adhere to this view. Cermak[25] considers consolidation as principally part of encoding—mainly because there is no strong evidence for a differential involvement of limbic structures in one process but not the other.

There are, however, case reports which suggest a possible dissociation. One is that of O'Connor and colleagues,[147] who described a patient with temporal lobe epilepsy and paraneoplastic limbic encephalitis. This patient retained information for hours to days but thereafter manifested disproportionally high rates of forgetting. Another is the patient of Kapur and co-workers[83] with temporal lobe epilepsy,

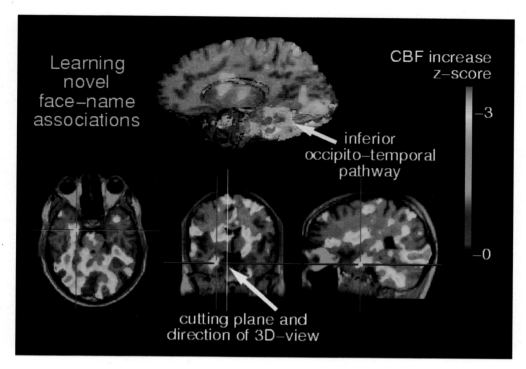

Learning
novel
face–name
associations

CBF increase
z–score

−3

−0

inferior
occipito–temporal
pathway

cutting plane and
direction of 3D–view

FIGURE 4–8. ^{15}O-PET-MRI coregistration images of brain activation during a face–name association learning task. Three orthogonal cuts (transaxial, coronal, and sagittal) through the activated right amygdalohippocampal region are shown in the bottom row. Above, activation of the inferior occipitotemporal pathway is shown. Bottom row shows the medial temporal (amygdalohippocampal) activation focus. Task design: In a preparatory phase, a series of faces was presented together with the associated names. These faces were then shown again in random order, and names had to be identified from a selection of four until a criterion of 40% correct responses was reached. During the imaging, ten randomly selected faces from the previously presented series were shown again and the correct name had to be identified. The reference condition consisted of presentation of other faces for gender identification. CBF, cerebral blood flow. (Courtesy of Prof. Dr. Karl Herholz, University of Cologne and Max-Planck-Institute for Neurological Research, Cologne, Germany).

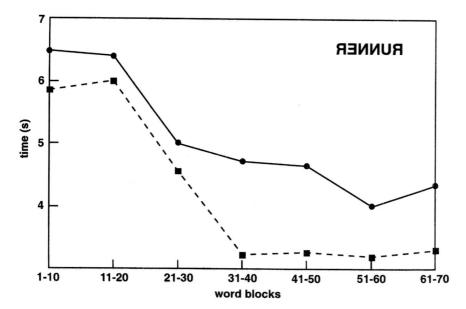

FIGURE 4–9. Unimpaired learning performance of a patient with major anterograde amnesia in a procedural memory task (mirror-image reading of words). The top line gives his results when seeing mirror-image written words of defined length for the first time, and the bottom line gives his faster performance when seeing the words a second time. (After data from Calabrese and colleagues.[20])

who showed normal long-term memory encoding and recall for many days but was unable to recall learned information 40 days later. These reports suggest that initial encoding into long-term memory and the subsequent process of more stable consolidation (or retention) may be dissociable.

Another patient of this kind was studied by Markowitsch and co-workers.[118] This 30 year-old university-educated woman had a severe amnesia after a whiplash trauma. There was no specific brain injury detectable with static and functional imaging methods, but she had persistent hearing problems after the injury. She was quite superior in intelligence and in verbal and visuospatial functions (e.g., she gained the highest possible score of 136 in the *General Memory Index* of the revised *Wechsler Memory Scale*), but she had a *Delayed Recall Index* below the lowest score (<50) because of the complete fading of her memories within 30–120 minutes.

These examples indicate that there may be quite different biological substrates for initial encoding into episodic (explicit) memory and the subsequent consolidation/retention of the information. Memory traces are likely to become more robust over time and to become increasingly more resistant to decay as they become consolidated. The biological substrates of consolidation remain to be elucidated.

Storage of Information

The tremendous volume of information that needs to be acquired during a lifetime becomes accommodated within distributed cerebral cortical networks.[48,124,222] The way in which memories are stored or represented in the brain is still a riddle. Though there is a lot of evidence pointing to changes in synaptic morphology, protein synthesis, and gene expression,[1,5,52,223] the way in which these alterations sustain lifelong engrams remains to be clarified.[162,181] Swain and associates[202] suggested that vascular, glial, and neuronal changes might all work together in engram production and that memory formation might be considered a special case of brain adaptation which might be more readily identifiable in psychological than in physiological terms.

The most frequently formulated proposal is that information is stored throughout association cortex but that the limbic system has a critical role in binding this information during storage and perhaps also retrieval (Chapter 1).

Retrieval of Information

Results from functional imaging studies point to a strong and very consistent activation of left prefrontal cortical structures during the encoding and of right prefrontal cortex during the retrieval process.[56,209,211] This finding was largely unexpected given investigations in animals and patients with focal lesions. Jetter and co-workers[76] had found that patients with prefrontal (but not posterior cortical) damage were disproportionally impaired in retrieving information after a long (1 day) delay period under free recall conditions, but they were indistinguishable from patients with other lesion locations under cued recall and recognition conditions (cf. Table 4–1 for terminology)—that is, when they did not need to mentally organize the retrieval of the stored information (Fig. 4–10).

Retrograde amnesia refers to the inability to retrieve information that had been stored prior to the onset of the amnesia-causing lesion (or event). The term is used in at least two ways: For one it refers to information which is no longer accessible because it is permanently lost. This may for instance be the case in patients with Alzheimer's disease.[108] Secondly, the term refers to an inability to (explicitly) retrieve stored information which nevertheless may still exist in the brain. This inability may occur after certain types of focal brain damage,[106] but it can also be found in cases with psychogenic[107] or "functional amnesia."[41] The possibility that retrograde amnesia represents an inability to access existing "engrams" was emphasized by Benson and Geschwind,[11] who showed a "shrinkage" of the time span encompassed by the retrograde amnesia during the recovery phase of amnesic patients.

Patients with functional amnesia frequently have retrograde amnesia for their whole past life and therefore differ from patients with the more typical form of retrograde amnesia, where the most recent experiences are also the most difficult to recall.[106] The typical time-graded retrograde amnesia is usually observed in patients after head trauma[167] and in patients with medial temporal[126,158] or medial diencephalic[73,126] brain damage. For these patients with "medial temporal–diencephalic amnesia" the severity and duration of retrograde amnesia are quite variable and the same type of lesion may sometimes lead to extensive[73] or no retrograde amnesia.[84]

Traditional accounts of amnesia had led to the assumption that retrograde amnesia should always be accompanied by anterograde amnesia. However, in the

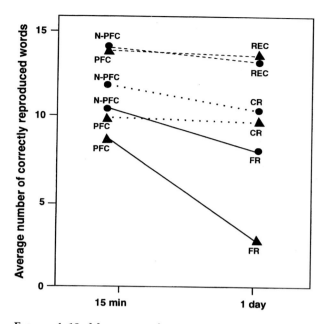

FIGURE 4–10. Memory performance of patient groups with prefrontal (PFC) or posterior cortical damage (N-PFC) under conditions of free recall (FR), cued recall (CR), and recognition (REC). (Data from Jetter and associates.[76])

1980s clinical reports described patients who manifested pure retrograde amnesia in the absence of equivalent anterograde amnesia.[105] The type of brain damage was quite diverse and these patients did not help to identify the brain areas critical for memory retrieval. In the 1990s a more precise and consistent demarcation became possible.[20,82,90,112,115,146] These findings led to the conclusion that inferolateral prefrontal and temporopolar regions play an important role in the retrieval of old memories, and that the right hemisphere is more critical for retrieving episodic (autobiographical) information, whereas the left hemisphere is more critical for retrieving stored general knowledge (semantic memories).[55,106,107,209,210]

Figure 4–11 shows the frontotemporal structures that may be involved in the retrieval of old memories (ecphory). The prefrontal contribution in this process of ecphory may involve the willed initiation and mobilization of the relevant networks,[106,107] the selection of information among competing alternatives, and possibly the postretrieval monitoring processes. The temporopolar regions, through their limbic connections, may coordinate access to engrams encoded within association cortices. As was shown by several studies, selective damage to either the prefrontal or the temporal component of this network is insufficient to cause permanent disruption of the retrieval process. Enduring and severe retrograde amnesia usually requires bilateral damage to both components.[90,203] (That is, there needs to be minor right hemisphere and major left temporofrontal damage for patients with predominantly semantic retrograde amnesia, and minor left and major right hemispheric damage in patients with predominantly episodic retrograde amnesia.)

While some authors have attributed a critical role also to the hippocampo–

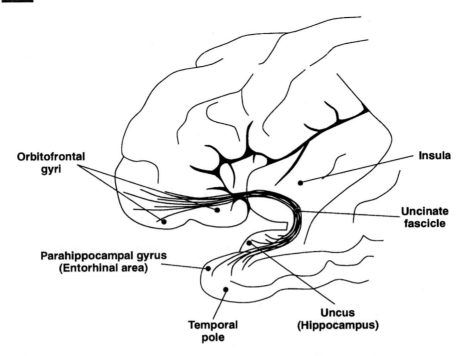

FIGURE 4–11. Schematic view of the anterior lateral half of the human cerebral cortex. The brain regions discussed as central for ecphory are delineated.

entorhinal regions in declarative long-term memory retrieval,[142,158] others have found pure retrograde amnesia can occur after temporofrontal damage without an identifiable lesion in the mesial temporal areas.[82,90,112] This finding indicates that hippocampal damage may not be necessary for the emergence of selective retrograde amnesia. Nevertheless, it should be emphasized again that there is a surprising clinical similarity between the pure retrograde amnesia of temporoprefrontal damage and that of patients with psychogenic amnesias,[107] raising major questions about the biological substrates of this syndrome.

The Memory Network

The foregoing review shows that explicit/declarative/episodic memory processing is dependent on distributed neural networks, containing limbic as well as nonlimbic components, as shown in Figure 4–12.[17,60,129,130,132] Neither modular nor holographic models seem to fit the brain's way of handling information. Neither do Lashley's principles of "equipotentiality" and "mass action," which led him to conclude that there is no specific brain locus at all for memory.[91,92]

Nevertheless one has to keep in mind the influence of functional plasticity.[75,81,103,119] For example, frontal, cingulate, thalamic, and hippocampal lesions, which cause major and persistent postsurgical performance deficits in rats, have a

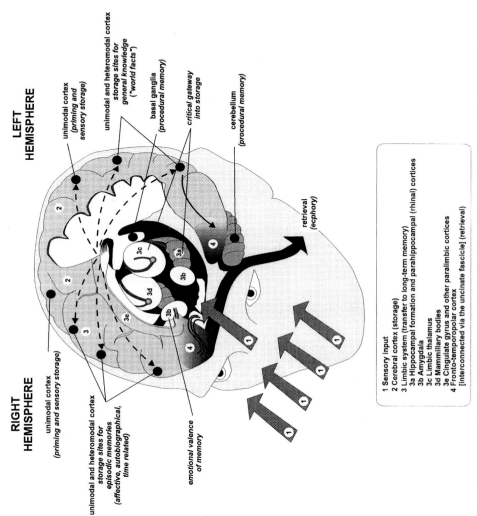

RIGHT
HEMISPHERE

unimodal cortex
(priming and sensory storage)

unimodal and heteromodal cortex
storage sites for
*episodic memories
(affective, autobiographical,
time related)*

*emotional valence
of memory*

LEFT
HEMISPHERE

unimodal cortex
*(priming and
sensory storage)*

unimodal and heteromodal cortex
storage sites for
general knowledge
("world facts")

basal ganglia
(procedural memory)

*critical gateway
into storage*

cerebellum
(procedural memory)

retrieval
(ecphory)

1 Sensory input
2 Cerebral cortex (storage)
3 Limbic system (transfer to long-term memory)
3a Hippocampal formation and parahippocampal (rhinal) cortices
3b Amygdala
3c Limbic thalamus
3d Mammillary bodies
3e Cingulate gyrus and other paralimbic cortices
4 Fronto-temporopolar cortex
[interconnected via the uncinate fascicle] (retrieval)

FIGURE 4–12. Sketch of the brain structures implicated in long-term information processing.

much less severe effect if the rat is overtrained.[119] Thus, some degree of latent equipotentiality may exist in the brain.

V. AMNESIA SYNDROMES

Global Amnesias (Core Amnesic Syndromes)

Global amnesias have already been illustrated in the beginning with the cases of H. M. and A. B. They are characterized by

1. Anterograde amnesia for all explicit memory functions.
2. Retrograde amnesia for nonconsolidated information, according to Ribot's[159] law, so information closer to the time of brain damage is more inaccessible while more remote information is more likely to be preserved.
3. Preservation of semantic knowledge.
4. Relative preservation of some types of implicit learning.
5. Preservation of sensory, perceptual, attentive, language and motor skills.

This type of amnesia is almost *always* associated with bilateral lesions in the limbic system.

Disconnection Amnesias

Focal cortical damage may lead to amnesic conditions which are restricted to certain modalities or to specific materials.[38,153] Prosopagnosia, for example, may be interpreted as a defect of visual recognition for faces (Chapter 7). Selective anterograde amnesias for the visual and tactile modalities were described by Ross[163,164]. A disconnection between visual cortex and the medial temporal lobe was assumed to be the cause for the visual amnesia. In the three patients with unilateral tactile memory loss a lesion location in the medial temporal lobe contralateral to the involved hand was hypothesized, presumably leading to a tactile–limbic disconnection. In fact, severe tactual and visual memory deficits can be detected in monkeys after combined removal of medial temporal lobe structures and after lesions which interrupt the flow of modality-specific information into the limbic system.[140,141]

Other material-specific memory disorders included amnesias for color, where the brain damage is usually found in parietal and temporal regions of the neocortex, sometimes also reaching into the occipital regions.[38] Topographical amnesia, an inability to remember the spatial location of an object, is another phenomenon found after posterior lesions in the convergence zone of the temporal, parietal, and occipital lobes.[39] Verbal anomias and semantic amnesias involve deficits in retrieving names of objects,[85] describing verbs,[24] recalling the characteristic features of living objects (animals),[191,53] and retrieving the names of familiar people.[157]

Furthermore, lesions in the angular gyrus or the occipitoparietal border may selectively affect memory for number facts and may lead to acalculia, dyscalculia, and anarithmetria).[28,29,65,128,165] However, these types of deficits are usually attributed to spatial neglect, aphasia, and agnosia rather than "amnesia" (Chapters 1, 3, 5, and 7).

Transient Global Amnesia

Transient global amnesia (TGA) undoubtedly has many etiologies. Transient Global Amnesia has a short duration (<24 hours) and appears late in adulthood.[71,104] It is characterized by a major amnesia which goes mainly in the anterograde, but also in retrograde, direction.[67] Not all cases of TGA can be linked to a specific neuroanatomical lesion. However, in the vast majority of cases where such a correlation can be made, the dysfunction has involved the medial temporolimbic regions of the brain.

Most TGA patients are around 60 years old. Onset prior to the age of 40 years is rare. Though it was initially assumed that attacks rarely recur, a more thorough screening of relevant data indicates that many patients experience more than one event.[22,58,101] Risk factors include high blood pressure, coronary heart disease, previous strokes or transient ischaemic attacks, migraine, hyperlipidemia, smoking, diabetes, and peripheral vascular diseases.[22,57,58,71,72,74] Schmidtke and Ehmsen[177] emphasized that TGA most likely does not represent a type of migraine aura or migraine equivalent. Instead, they suggested that there may be an inherited brain state disposing to different states of paroxysmal dysregulation, including migraine and TGA. Thus individuals susceptible to migraine may also be susceptible to TGA. An investigation using diffusion-weighted MRI revealed cellular edema in the anterior temporal lobe during TGA.[200] This finding, together with a related one of Zorzon and co-workers,[224] supports the spreading depression hypothesis, which Olesen and Jörgensen[149] had introduced as an explanation for some cases of TGA.

The precipitants of TGA include physical and psychic factors. Caplan[22] listed the following: *1)* emotional stress, *2)* pain, *3)* angiography, *4)* sexual intercourse, *5)* physical activity, *6)* immersion in cold water, *7)* hot bath or shower, *8)* driving or riding in a motor vehicle. This list shows that various stressors and hemodynamic challenges can lead to TGA.

The three most common correlates of TGA include migraine, temporal lobe epilepsy, and ischemia in the posterior cerebral artery distribution. All three causes involve medial temporal lobe structures. The regions of decreased cerebral perfusion (revealed with SPECT [single photon emission computed tomography] or PET [positron emission tomography]) during the TGA period are usually located in the temporal lobes and the diencephalon but may extend to cortical and striatal regions as well.[50,179] The TGA episodes are neuropsychologically quite uniform. There are anterograde and retrograde components to the amnesia. As the patient recovers, the retrograde amnesia shrinks and then totally disappears just as the patient gains his ability to retain new information. Following the ictus, the patient is left with a permanent island of memory loss for the period encompassed by the TGA episode. During the ictus, the patient repetitively asks questions about his or her plight, identity, and location in ways that indicate an acute awareness of the amnesia.

Several reports noted a continuing prefrontal hypometabolism in patients with TGA.[7,64] Others reported a hypometabolism in the hippocampi and thalami 20 days after the attack.[169]

Functional Amnesias

De Renzi and co-workers[42] used the term "functional amnesia" to define amnesias with poorly defined neurological substrates. The spectrum of antecedents includes minor head trauma, psychiatric disorders, depression, stress, and chronic fatigue syndrome. That psychic shock may result in amnesia has been known for a long time,[15,138] and the manifestations of post-traumatic stress disorder (PTSD) frequently involve memory disturbances.[9,127,190] While many of these conditions are transient in nature or affect memory to only a minor degree, others may interfere with the recall of all autobiographical information[116] or may lead to both retrograde and anterograde amnesia.[120]

Minor head injury (without identifiable structural brain damage) has been associated with a major retrograde amnesia for autobiographic memory. Barbarotto and colleagues[6] described a woman who slipped and fell in her office. She had been on the floor for about 15–20 minutes when she was found. No brain damage was detected; nevertheless the patient was retrogradely amnesic even half a year after the event. She had a pure retrograde amnesia. However, she made implicit use of information she was unable to recall. The authors describe a personality pattern compatible with conversion hysteria.

A similar case is that of a 26-year-old farmer who was hit by a tractor, but whose brain imaging was largely negative.[40] The only exception was a slight hypometabolism in the posterior temporal lobes. The patient had been hypoxic for a short time and showed retrograde amnesia and abnormally fast forgetting. The retrograde amnesia encompassed biographical information from his whole life as well as semantic knowledge acquired at school and through newspapers and television. Furthermore, following motor car accidents two patients with negative MRI, SPECT, and PET developed selective retrograde amnesias for autobiographical and public events even years after the accident.[41,42] Together these cases—and a number of additional ones[110]—suggest that major and enduring retrograde amnesia may occur after putative head injury even in the absence of demonstratable lesions by neurodiagnostic procedures. Changes in metabolism, hormonal state, and receptor function in memory sensitive regions of the brain have been invoked to explain this state of affairs.[107,110,127]

Dramatic loss of autobiographical information has also been described in association with hysteric states, poriomania and multiple personalities, and it has a peak incidence in the third decade of life.[105] The term "psychogenic amnesia" is commonly used to designate these conditions. Sometimes it is difficult to distinguish this symptom picture from that of malingering.[6,152,213] Cases with psychogenic amnesia show some common features: a weak, underdeveloped personality, a problematic childhood or youth, and the appearance of emotionally negative events such as sexual abuse[123,175] during early life. The amnesia may be interpreted as a mechanism for blocking awareness of previous traumatic events.[107]

Numerous case descriptions of patients with (likely) psychogenic amnesia have been reported. Markowitsch and associates[116] investigated a 37-year-old man with a persistent fugue. He remained unsure of his relationship to family members and changed a number of personality traits. While having been an avid car driver prior to the fugue, he became quite hesitant to enter a car thereafter, lost his asthma, gained substantially in body weight, and changed his profession. Regional cerebral blood flow was measured in an autobiographic memory paradigm. Significant biographical events from the patient's past (which had been obtained from his wife and relatives) were transformed into sentences and presented to the patient for imagery during PET scanning. Results revealed a mainly left-hemispheric activation instead of the usual right-hemispheric one found with the same paradigm by Fink and colleagues.[55] This result suggests that he might indeed have been unable to recall his own past, processing this information as new and unrelated to his person.

Markowitsch and associates[120] described a patient who at the age of 4 had witnessed a man burn to death and then at the age of 23 had a fire in his house. Immediately following this second exposure to a fire, the patient developed anterograde amnesia and a retrograde amnesia covering a period of 6 years. Conventional neurodiagnostic tests (MRI, electroencephalogram [EEG], cerebrospinal fluid [CSF]) did not show any abnormalities. However, PET results demonstrated a severe reduction of glucose metabolism, especially in the memory-related temporal and diencephalic regions of the brain. His amnesic condition persisted for months but improved thereafter as his brain metabolism returned to normal levels after 1 year. Even then his long-term memory was quite poor, so he remained unable to return to his former job.

The neurology of psychogenic amnesia is poorly understood. Psychological stress can conceivably alter the structure and function of mediotemporal limbic areas, perhaps through the mediation of stress-related hormones (glucocorticoids).[14,95,98,110,111,120,170,194] For example, patients with post-traumatic stress disorder (PTSD) are vulnerable to become depressed and to manifest memory disturbances.[12,54,86,127,189] The release of endogenous stress-related hormones is altered (dysregulated) in PTSD and this abnormality may result in altered neural function.[14,95,98,110,170,194,214]

Some studies point to hippocampal volume reductions in association with stress.[66,199] It was suggested that massive and prolonged stress might induce changes in regions with a high density of glucocorticoid receptors such as the anterior and medial temporal lobe.[95,170] In animals it was shown that stress enhances hippocampal long term depression[221] and blocks long-term potentiation.[44] Teicher and colleagues[204] found that early physical or sexual abuse hinders the development of the limbic system and may therefore induce a predisposition for the outbreak of stress-related amnesia syndromes (Chapter 9).

Distorted Memory and Paramnesias

As reviewed in Chapter 8, epileptic conditions of medial temporal lobe or prefrontal origin can lead to persistent memory deficits[8,78,79,147,176] and can also result in very specific memory distortions such as powerful feelings of déjà vu (illusion of familiarity) or jamais vu (illusion of unfamiliarity).[133]

Special syndromes of distorted memory include Capgras's syndrome,[23] reduplicative paramnesia[188] and related phenomena such as Frégoli's syndrome[33] and intermetamorphosis.[34] Patients with Capgras's syndrome have the delusional belief that family members and friends have been replaced by impostors.[131] The patients confabulate extensively in order to rationalize their delusional distortion of reality. The most frequent type of neurological concomitant of Capgras's syndrome takes the form of a partial or recovering limbic lesion superimposed on frontal lobe damage, especially in the right hemisphere.[100,131] Additional examples of Capgras's syndrome can be found in Brugger and colleagues[16] and O'Connor and co-workers.[148] The case of Brugger and associates[16] in fact had a Doppelgänger syndrome, implying that the patient himself believed he had been replaced by an identical other. The belief that a person can take over the appearance of another one is Frégoli's syndrome.[33] The belief that things or persons can mutually exchange their appearance or identity is intermetamorphosis.[34]

Patients with reduplicative paramnesia are convinced that a person, a place, or an object exists in duplicate. Pick[154] described a form of memory disturbance in which a locus or a person is reduplicated. One of his patients believed in the existence of two exactly identical clinics with two clinic heads of the same name. Another one believed that there were two identical clinics with partly the same patients who were taken care of by the same professor and his co-workers. Pick[154] considered a disturbed sense of familiarity as a possible cause of the phenomenon. The patients would be unable to associate the present situation with a previously experienced and familiar one, so the present situation would be given a different identity.

VI. MEMORY REHABILITATION

The rehabilitation of memory is one of the greatest challenges for clinical neuroscience. While animal research has provided evidence for extensive brain plasticity,[13,139] the relevance of this knowledge to human amnesia and its recovery remains unclear.

Approaches to treatment range from pharmacological interventions[125,171] to behavioral therapy.[10,207] Nootropics and other cognition-enhancing drugs have up to now resulted in improvements for only very limited time periods and may have side effects, especially when given to demented patients. Memory training has also been used, either alone or coupled to psychotherapy and drug treatment.[51,166]

An example of potentially successful therapy in a 54-year-old patient who became severely amnesic after a heart attack is reported by Calabrese and Markowitsch.[19] Following 18 months of training with multiple modalities, the patient returned to work. In the absence of a controlled study, however, the precise contribution of this training to his recovery could not be determined. The generalization and stability of strategies acquired during memory training is the most important aim for all kinds of therapy.[88] The cognitive rehabilitation of amnesia is still in its infancy, but this state of affairs should elicit more research rather than pessimism.

VII. OVERVIEW

Memory is not a unitary phenomenon. The distinction between short-term and long-term memory is securely established. Limbic lesions lead to a characteristic amnesia with preserved short-term or working memory but impaired long-term memory. Short-term memory is an attentional function quite independent of the limbic system. Memory can further be divided into the capacities for remembering old information and for acquiring new information. The impairment of the former leads to retrograde amnesia and of the latter leads to anterograde amnesia.

Patients with memory impairment usually do not show either a total obliteration of previously learned information or a total inability to acquire new information. Very old consolidated memories (related to childhood events or the meaning of words) almost always escape the retrograde amnesia due to limbic lesions. The ability to drive cars, to learn to avoid painful stimulations, or to know basic information about social facts is also preserved after damage to the limbic system.

Different neurobiological substrates can be delineated for remembering the temporal and spatial details of personal experience (episodic memory), stable facts about the world (semantic memory), and motor–perceptual skills (procedural memory, priming). Some of these processes (such as episodic memory) are explicit whereas others are implicit (as in priming) and may operate even without full awareness.

A network of numerous brain regions is involved in information acquisition, on-line holding, transfer to long-term memory (encoding, storage and consolidation), and retrieval (or ecphory). All information is initially encoded in relevant primary and association cortices. The on-line (attentional) holding of information in short-term memory is coordinated by parietal and frontal cortices. Long-term encoding (and in part also retrieval) is coordinated by the limbic system. The actual memory engrams are widely distributed in limbic and neocortical areas. Prefrontotemporopolar regions contribute to the retrieval or ecphory of information with the two hemispheres participating differently with respect to the content of the information. The prefrontal cortex further participates in providing the contextual integration that is necessary for episodic memories. A schematic summary of the involved regions is given in Figure 4–12.

The study of memory distortion,[49,131–133] false memories,[94] and stress-related amnesias provides an interesting avenue for unraveling the neural bases of memory and the etiologies of unusual memory disorders. The presently available methodologies in neuroimaging and neuropsychology allow a more refined description of brain–behavior interactions and may have implications for the selection of memory retraining strategies. The various forms of neuroplasticity will eventually provide clues to mechanisms that may lead to successful memory recovery after brain damage.

I thank the patients whose case descriptions are included in this chapter and the colleagues who referred these patients to me or collaborated in their examination. M.-M. Mesulam did a tremendous job editing and improving the content of this chapter. I am also grateful to Eva Böcker and Margot Rengstorf for technical and secretarial assistance. The preparation of this chapter was supported in part by the Deutsche Forschungsgemeinschaft (German Research Council; Ma 795/25 and 26).

References

1. Abel, T, Martin, K C, Bartsch, D and Kandel, E R: Memory suppressor genes: inhibitory constraints on the storage of long-term memory. Science 279:338–341, 1998.
2. Atkinson, R C and Shiffrin, R M: Human memory: a proposed system and its control processes. In Spence, K W and Spence, J T (Eds.): The Psychology of Learning and Motivation. Academic Press, New York, 1968, pp. 89–195.
3. Bäckman, L, Robins-Wahlin, T-B, Lundin, A, Ginovart, N and Farde, L: Cognitive deficits in Huntington's disease are predicted by dopaminergic PET markers and brain volumes. Brain 120:2207–2217, 1997.
4. Baddeley, A D: Working memory. Science 255:556–559, 1992.
5. Bailey, C H and Kandel, E R: Molecular and structural mechanisms underlying long-term memory. In Gazzaniga, M S (Ed.): The Cognitive Neurosciences. MIT Press, Cambridge, MA, 1995, pp. 19–36.
6. Barbarotto, R, Laiacona, M and Cocchini, G: A case of simulated, psychogenic or focal pure retrograde amnesia: did an entire life become unconscious? Neuropsychologia 34: 575–585, 1996.
7. Baron, J C, Petit-Taboué, C, Le Doze, F, Desgranges, B, Ravenel, N and Marchal, G: Right frontal cortex hypometabolism in transient global amnesia. Brain 117:545–552, 1994.
8. Barr, W B: Examining the right temporal lobe's role in nonverbal memory. Brain Cogn 35: 26–41, 1997.
9. Barrett, D H, Green, M L, Morris, R, Giles, W H and Croft, J B: Cognitive functioning and posttraumatic stress disorder. Am J Psychiatry 153:1492–1494, 1996.
10. Berg, I A: Memory Rehabilitation for Closed-Head Injured Patients. University of Groningen, Groningen, 1993.
11. Benson, D F and Geschwind, N: Shrinking retrograde amnesia. J Neurol Neurosurg Psychiatry 30:539–544, 1967.
12. Bleich, A, Koslowsky, M, Dolev, A and Lerer, B: Post-traumatic stress disorder and depression. Br J Psychiatry 170:479–482, 1997.
13. Bonhoeffer, K: Die akuten Geisteskrankheiten der Gewohnheitstrinker. Fischer, Jena, 1901.
14. Bremner, J D, Randall, P, Scott, T M, Bronen, R A, Seibyl, J P, Southwick, S M, Delane, Y R C, McCarthy, G, Charney, D S and Innis, R B: MRI-based measurement of hippocampal volume in patients with combat-related posttraumatic stress disorder. Am J Psychiatry 152:973–981, 1995.
15. Breuer, J and Freud, S: Studien über Hysterie. Deuticke, Wien, 1895.

16. Brugger, P, Regard, M and Landis, T: Unilaterally felt "presences": the neuropsychiatry of one's invisible Doppelgänger. Neuropsychiat Neuropsychol Behav Neurol 9:114–122, 1996.

17. Bullmore, E T, Rabe-Hesketh, S, Morris, R G, Williams, S C R, Gregory, L, Gray, J A and Brammer, M J: Functional magnetic resonance image analysis of a large-scale neurocognitive network. Neuroimage 4:16–33, 1996.

18. Cahill, L, Babinsky, R, Markowitsch, H J and McGaugh, J L: Involvement of the amygdaloid complex in emotional memory. Nature 377:295–296, 1995.

19. Calabrese, P and Markowitsch, H J: Recovery of mnestic functions after hypoxic brain damage. Int J Rehabil Health 1:247–260, 1995.

20. Calabrese, P, Markowitsch, H J, Durwen, H F, Widlitzek, B, Haupts, M, Holinka, B and Gehlen, W: Right temporofrontal cortex as critical locus for the ecphory of old episodic memories. J Neurol Neurosurg Psychiatry 61:304–310, 1996.

21. Calabrese, P, Markowitsch, H J, Harders, A G, Scholz, A and Gehlen, W: Fornix damage and memory: a case report. Cortex 31:555–564, 1995.

22. Caplan, L R: Transient global amnesia: characteristic features and overview. In Markowitsch, H J (Ed.): Transient Global Amnesia and Related Disorders. Hogrefe, Toronto, 1990, pp. 15–27.

23. Capgras, J and Reboul-Lachaux, J: L'illusion des "sosies" dans un délir systématisé chronique. Bull Soc Clin Med Ment 2:6–16, 1923.

24. Caramazza, A and Hillis, A E: Lexical organization of nouns and verbs in the brain. Nature 349:788–790, 1991.

25. Cermak, L S: A positive approach to viewing processing deficit theories of amnesia. Memory 5:89–98, 1997.

26. Chao, L L and Knight, R T: Prefrontal and posterior cortical activation during auditory memory. Cogn Brain Res 4:27–37, 1996.

27. Chow, K L: Effects of ablation. In Quarton, G C, Melnechuk, T and Schmitt, F O (Eds.): The Neurosciences. Rockefeller University Press, New York, 1967, pp. 705–713.

28. Cohen, L and Dehaene, S: Amnesia for arithmetic facts: a single case study. Brain Lang 47:214–232, 1994.

29. Cohen, L, Dehaene, S and Verstichel, P: Number words and number non-words. A case of deep dyslexia extending to arabic numerals. Brain 117:267–279, 1994.

30. Corkin, S: Lasting consequences of bilateral medial temporal lobectomy: clinical course and experimental findings in H.M. Sem Neurol 4:249–259, 1984.

31. Corkin, S, Amaral, D G, Gonzalez, R G, Johnson, K A and Hyman, B T: H. M.'s medial temporal lobe lesion: findings from magnetic resonance imaging. J Neurosci 17:3964–3979, 1997.

32. Coull, J T, Frith, C D, Frackowiak, R S J and Grasby, P M: A fronto-parietal network for rapid visual information processing: a PET study of sustained attention and working memory. Neuropsychologia 34:1085–1095, 1996.

33. Courbon, P and Fail, G: Syndrome "d'illusion de Frégoli" et schizophrenie. Bull Soc Clin Méd Ment 15:121–124, 1927.

34. Courbon, P and Tusques, J: L'illusion d'intermetamorphose et de charme. Annal Med Psychol 90:401–406, 1932.

35. Cramon, D Y von and Markowitsch, H J: The septum and human memory. In Numan R (Ed.): The Behavioral Neuroscience of the Septal Area. Springer, New York, 2000.

36. Cramon, D Y von, Markowitsch, H J and Schuri, U: The possible contribution of the septal region to memory. Neuropsychologia 31:1159–1180, 1993.

37. Damasio, A R, Graf-Radford, N R, Eslinger, P J, Damasio, H and Kassell, N: Amnesia following basal forebrain lesions. Arch Neurol 42:263–271, 1985.

38. De Renzi, E: Memory disorders following focal neocortical damage. Philos Trans R Soc Lond Biol 298:73–83, 1982.

39. De Renzi, E: Disorders of Space: Exploration and Cognition. Wiley, Chichester, 1982.

40. De Renzi, E and Lucchelli, F: Dense retrograde amnesia, intact learning capability and abnormal forgetting rate: a consolidation deficit? Cortex 29:449–466, 1993.

41. De Renzi, E, Lucchelli, F, Muggia, S and Spinnler, H: Persistent retrograde amnesia following a minor head trauma. Cortex 31:531–542, 1995.

42. De Renzi, E, Lucchelli, F, Muggia, S and Spinnler, H: Is memory without anatomical damage tantamount to a psychogenic deficit? The case of pure retrograde amnesia. Neuropsychologia 35:781–794, 1997.

43. D'Esposito, M, Alexander, M P, Fischer, R, McGlinchey-Berroth, R and O'Connor, M: Recovery of memory and executive function following anterior communicating artery aneurysm rupture. J Int Neuropsychol Soc 2:565–570, 1996.

44. Diamond, D M and Rose, G M: Stress impairs LTP and hippocampal-dependent memory. Ann NY Acad Sci 746:411–414, 1994.

45. Dubois, B and Pillon, B: Cognitive deficits in Parkinson's disease. J Neurol 244:2–8, 1997.

46. Dudai, Y: How big is human memory, or on being just useful enough. Learning and Memory 3:341–365, 1997.

47. Ebbinghaus, H: Über das Gedächtnis. Duncker & Humblot, Leipzig, 1885.

48. Eichenbaum, H: To cortex: thanks for the memories. Neuron 19:481–484, 1997.

49. Estes, W K: Processes of memory loss, recovery, and distortion. Psychol Rev 104:148–169, 1997.

50. Eustache, F, Desgranges, B, Petit-Taboué, M C, Sayette, V de la, Piot, V, Sablé, C, Marchal, G and Baron, J-C: Transient global amnesia: implicit/explicit memory dissociation and PET assessment of brain perfusion and oxygen metabolism in the acute stage. J Neurol Neurosurg Psychiatry 63:357–367, 1997.

51. Ewald, K: Computer Assisted Mnemonic Strategy Acquisition and Tailored Memory Training Approaches: A Study with Brain Injured Individuals. Logos Verlag, Berlin, 1997.

52. Fagnou, D D and Tuchek, J M: The biochemistry of learning and memory. Mol Cell Biochem 149/150:279–286, 1995.

53. Farah, M J, McCullen, P A and Meyer, M: Can recognition of living things be selectively impaired. Neuropsychologia 29:185–193, 1990.

54. Fawzi, M C S, Murphy, E, Pham, T, Lin, L, Poole, C and Mollica, R F: The validity of screening for post-traumatic stress disorder and major depression among Vietnamese former political prisoners. Acta Psychiatr Scand 95:87–93, 1997.

55. Fink, G R, Markowitsch, H J, Reinkemeier, M, Bruckbauer, T, Kessler, J and Heiss, W-D: A PET-study of autobiographical memory recognition. J Neurosci 16:4275–82, 1996.

56. Fletcher, P C, Frith, C D and Rugg, M D: The functional neuroanatomy of episodic memory. Trends Neurosci 20:213–218, 1997.

57. Frederiks, J A M: Transient global amnesia: an amnesic TIA. In Markowitsch, H J (Ed.): Transient Global Amnesia and Related Disorders. Huber, Toronto, 1990, pp. 28–47.

58. Frederiks, J A M: Transient global amnesia. Clin Neurol Neurosurg 95:265–283, 1993.

59. Freed, D M and Corkin, S: Rate of forgetting in H.M.: 6-months recognition. Behav Neurosci 102: 823–827, 1988.

60. Fuster, J M: Network memory. Trends Neurosci 20: 451–459, 1997.

61. Gabrieli, J, Corkin, S, Mickel, S F and Growdon, J H: Intact acquisition and long-term retention of mirror-tracing skill in Alzheimer's disease and in global amnesia. Behav Neurosci 107:899–910, 1993.

62. Gabrieli, J D, Fleischman, D A, Keane, M M, Reminger, S L and Morrell, F: Double dissociation between memory systems underlying explicit and implicit memory in the human brain. Psychol Sci 6:76–82, 1995.

63. Gaffan, D and Gaffan, E A: Amnesia in man following transection of the fornix: a review. Brain 114:2611–2618, 1991.

64. Goldenberg, G, Podreka, I, Pfaffelmeyer, N, Wessely, P and Deecke, L: Thalamic ischemia in transient global amnesia: a SPECT Study. Neurology 41:1748–1752, 1991.

65. Grafman, J, Passafiume, D, Faglioni P and Boller, F: Calculation disturbances in adults with focal hemispheric damage. Cortex 18:37–50, 1982.
66. Gurvits, T V, Shenton, M E, Hokama, H, Ohta, H, Lasko, N B, Gilbertson, M W, Orr, S P, Knis, R, Jolesz, F A, McCarley, R W and Pitman, R K: Magnetic resonance imaging study of hippocampal volume in chronic, combat-related posttraumatic stress disorder. Biol Psychiatry 40:1091–1099, 1996.
67. Härting, C and Markowitsch, H J: Different degrees of impairment in recall/recognition and anterograde/retrograde memory performance in a transient global amnesic case. Neurocase 2:45–49, 1996.
68. Hebb, D O: The Organization of Behavior. Wiley, New York, 1949.
69. Heilbronner, K: Zur klinisch-psychologischen Untersuchungstechnik. Monatsschr Psychiat Neurol 17:115–132, 1904/05.
70. Hering, E: Ueber das Gedächtnis als eine allgemeine Funktion der organisierten Materie. Vortrag gehalten in der feierlichen Sitzung der Kaiserlichen Akademie der Wissenschaften in Wien am XXX. Mai MDCCCLXX. (3. Aufl.). Akademische Verlagsgesellschaft, Leipzig, 1921.
71. Hodges, J R: Transient Amnesia: Clinical and Neuropsychological Aspects. Saunders, London, 1991.
72. Hodges, J R: Unraveling the enigma of transient global amnesia. Ann of Neurol 43:151–153, 1998.
73. Hodges, J R and McCarthy, R A: Autobiographical amnesia resulting from bilateral paramedian thalamic infarction. Brain 116:921–940, 1993.
74. Hodges, J R and Warlow, C P: The aetiology of transient global amnesia. A case-control study of 114 cases with prospective follow-up. Brain 113:639–657, 1990.
75. Irle, E: Lesions size and recovery of function: some new perspectives. Brain Res Rev 12:307–320, 1987.
76. Jetter, J, Poser, U, Freeman, R B Jr and Markowitsch, H J: A verbal long term memory deficit in frontal lobe damaged patients. Cortex 22:229–242, 1986.
77. Johnson, M K and Raye, K L: Reality monitoring. Psychol Rev 88:67–85, 1981.
78. Jokeit, H, Ebner, A, Holthausen, H, Markowitsch, H J, Moch, A, Pannek, H, Schulz, R and Tuxhorn, I: Individual prediction of change in delayed recall of prose passages after left-sided anterior temporal lobectomy. Neurology 49:481–487, 1997.
79. Jokeit, H, Seitz, R, Markowitsch, H J, Neumann, N, Ebner, A and Witte, O W: Prefrontal asymmetric interictal glucose hypometabolism and cognitive impairment in patients with temporal lobe epilepsy. Brain 120:2283–2294, 1997.
80. Kahn, E A and Crosby, E C: Korsakoff's syndrome associated with surgical lesions involving the mammillary bodies. Neurology 22:117–125, 1972.
81. Kapur, N: Paradoxical functional facilitation in brain-behaviour research: a critical review. Brain 119:1775–1790, 1996.
82. Kapur, N, Ellison, D, Smith, M P, McLelland, D L and Burrows, E H: Focal retrograde amnesia following bilateral temporal lobe pathology. Brain 115:73–85, 1992.
83. Kapur, N, Millar, J, Colbourn, C, Abbott, P, Kennedy, P and Docherty, T: Very long-term amnesia in association with temporal lobe epilepsy: evidence for multiple-stage consolidation processes. Brain Cogn 35:58–70, 1997.
84. Kapur, N, Thompson, S, Cook, P, Lang, D and Brice, J: Anterograde but not retrograde memory loss following combined mammillary body and medial thalamic lesions. Neuropsychologia 34:1–8, 1996.
85. Kay, J and Ellis, A: A cognitive neuropsychological case study of anomia. Brain 110:613–629, 1987.
86. Kessler, R C: The effects of stressful life events on depression. Annu Rev Psychol 48:191–214, 1997.
87. Klüver, H and Bucy, P C: "Psychic blindness" and other symptoms following bilateral temporal lobectomy in rhesus monkeys. Am J Physiol 119:352–353, 1937.

88. Knight, R G and Andrewes, D G: The assessment and remediation of memory disordered patients. NZ J Psychol 13:53–62, 1984.

89. Knowlton, B J, Mangels, J A and Squire, L R: A neostriatal habit—learning system in humans. Science 273:1399–1402, 1996.

90. Kroll, N E A, Markowitsch, H J, Knight, R and von Cramon, D Y: Retrieval of old memories—the temporo-frontal hypothesis. Brain 120:1377–1399, 1997.

91. Lashley, K S: Brain Mechanisms and Intelligence. University of Chicago Press, Chicago, 1929.

92. Lashley, K S: In search of the engram. Soc Exp Biol Symp 4:454–482, 1950.

93. Lilly, R, Cummings, J L, Benson, D F and Frankel, M: The human Klüver-Bucy syndrome. Neurology 33:1141–1145, 1983.

94. Loftus, E F: Creating false memories. Sci Am 277:70–75, 1998.

95. Lupien, S J and McEwen, B S: The acute effects of corticosteroids on cognition: integration of animal and human model studies. Brain Res Rev 24:1–27, 1997.

96. Luria, A R: The Mind of a Mnemonist. J. Cape, London, 1968.

97. Maeshima, S, Uematsu, Y, Ozaki, F, Fujita, K, Nakai, K, Itakura, T and Komai, N: Impairment of short-term memory in left hemispheric traumatic brain injuries. Brain Inj 11: 279–286, 1997.

98. Magarinos, A M, Verdugo, J M G and McEwen, B S: Chronic stress alters synaptic terminal structure in hippocampus. Proc Natl Acad Sci USA 94:14002–14008, 1997.

99. Mair, W G P, Warrington, E K and Weiskrantz, L: Memory disorder in Korsakoff psychosis. A neuropathological and neuropsychological investigation of two cases. Brain 102: 749–783, 1979.

100. Malloy, P, Cimino, C and Westlake, R: Differential diagnosis of primary and secondary Capgras delusions. Neuropsychiat Neuropsychol Behav Neurol 5:83–96, 1992.

101. Markowitsch, H J: Transient global amnesia. Neurosci Biobehav Rev 7:35–43, 1983.

102. Markowitsch, H J: Diencephalic amnesia: a reorientation towards tracts? Brain Res Rev 13:351–370, 1988.

103. Markowitsch, H J: Individual differences in memory performance and the brain. In Markowitsch, H J (Ed.): Information Processing by the Brain. H. Huber, Toronto, 1988, pp. 125–148.

104. Markowitsch, H J (Ed.): Transient Global Amnesia and Related Disorders. Hogrefe & Huber, Toronto, 1990.

105. Markowitsch, H J: Intellectual Functions and the Brain. An Historical Perspective. Hogrefe & Huber, Toronto, 1992.

106. Markowitsch, H J: Which brain regions are critically involved in the retrieval of old episodic memory? Brain Res Rev 21:117–127, 1995.

107. Markowitsch, H J: Retrograde amnesia: similarities between organic and psychogenic forms. Neurol Psychiat Brain Res 4:1–8, 1996.

108. Markowitsch, H J: The biological bases of memory. In Tröster, AI (Ed.): Memory in Neurodegenerative Disease: Biological, Cognitive and Clinical Perspective. Cambridge University Press, New York, 1998, pp. 140–153.

109. Markowitsch, H J: The limbic system. In Wilson, R and Keil, F (Eds.): The MIT Encyclopedia of Cognitive Science. MIT Press, Cambridge, MA, 1999, pp. 472–475.

110. Markowitsch, H J: Functional neuroimaging correlates of functional amnesia. Memory, in press, 1999.

111. Markowitsch, H J, Calabrese, P, Fink, G R, Durwen, H F, Kessler, J, Härting, C, König, M, Mirzaian, E B, Heiss, W-D, Heuser, L and Gehlen, W: Impaired episodic memory retrieval in a case of probable psychogenic amnesia. Psychiatr Res Neuroimag Sect 74: 119–126, 1997.

112. Markowitsch, H J, Calabrese, P, Haupts, M, Durwen, H F, Liess, J and Gehlen, W: Searching for the anatomical basis of retrograde amnesia. J Clin Exp Neuropsychol 15: 947–967, 1993.

113. Markowitsch, H J, Calabrese, P, Würker, M, Durwen, H F, Kessler, J, Babinsky, R, Brechtelsbauer, D, Heuser, L and Gehlen, W: The amygdala's contribution to memory—A PET-study on two patients with Urbach-Wiethe disease. Neuroreport 5:1349–1352, 1994.

114. Markowitsch, H J, von Cramon, D Y and Schuri, U: Mnestic performance profile of a bilateral diencephalic infarct patient with preserved intelligence and severe amnesic disturbances. J Clin Exp Neuropsychol 15:627–652, 1993.

115. Markowitsch, H J and Ewald, K: Right-hemispheric fronto-temporal injury leading to severe autobiographical retrograde and moderate anterograde episodic amnesia. Neurol Psychiatr Brain Res 5:71–78, 1997.

116. Markowitsch, H J, Fink, G R, Thöne, A I M, Kessler, J and Heiss, W-D: Persistent psychogenic amnesia with a PET-proven organic basis. Cognit Neuropsychiatr 2:135–158, 1997.

117. Markowitsch, H J, Kalbe, E, Kessler, J, von Stockhausen, H-M, Ghaemi, M and Heiss, W-D: Short-term memory deficit after focal parietal damage. J Clin Exp Neuropsychol, in press, 1999.

118. Markowitsch, H J, Kessler, J, Kalbe, E and Herholz, K: Functional amnesia and memory consolidation. A case of persistent anterograde amnesia with rapid forgetting following whiplash injury. Neurocase 5:189–200, 1999.

119. Markowitsch, H J, Kessler, J and Streicher, M: Consequences of serial cortical, hippocampal, and thalamic lesions and of different lengths of overtraining on the acquisition and retention of learning tasks. Behav Neurosci 99:233–256, 1985.

120. Markowitsch, H J, Kessler, J, Van der Ven, C, Weber-Luxenburger, G and Heiss, W-D: Psychic trauma causing grossly reduced brain metabolism and cognitive deterioration. Neuropsychologia 36:77–82, 1998.

121. Markowitsch, H J and Pritzel, M: Comparative analysis of prefrontal learning functions in rats, cats, and monkeys. Psychol Bull 84:817–837, 1977.

122. Markowitsch, H J and Pritzel, M: Single unit activity in cat prefrontal and posterior cortex during performance of spatial reversal tasks. Brain Res 149:53–76, 1978.

123. Markowitsch, H J, Thiel, A, Kessler, J and Heiss, W-D: Ecphorizing semi-conscious episodic information via the right temporopolar cortex—a PET study. Neurocase 3:445–449, 1997.

124. Markowitsch, H J and Tulving, E: Cognitive processing in cerebral cortical sulci. Neuroreport 6:413–418, 1995.

125. Marx, J: Searching for drugs that combat Alzheimer's. Science 273:50–53, 1996.

126. Mayes, A R, Daum, I, Markowitsch, H J and Sauter, B: The relationship between retrograde and anterograde amnesia in patients with typical global amnesia. Cortex 33:197–217, 1997.

127. McGrath, J: Cognitive impairment associated with post-traumatic stress disorder and minor head injury: a case report. Neuropsychol Rehab 7:231–239, 1997.

128. McNeil, J E and Warrington, E: A dissociation between addition and subtraction with written calculation. Neuropsychologia 32:717–728, 1994.

129. Mesulam, M-M: Large-scale neurocognitive networks and distributed processing for attention, language, and memory. Ann Neurol 28:597–613, 1990.

130. Mesulam, M-M: Neurocognitive networks and selectively distributed processing. Rev Neurol 150:564–569, 1994.

131. Mesulam, M-M: Notes on the cerebral topography of memory and memory distortion: a neurologist's perspective. In Schacter, D L (Ed.): Memory Distortion. Harvard University Press, Cambridge, MA, 1995, pp. 379–385.

132. Mesulam, M-M: From sensation to cognition. Brain 121:1013–1052, 1998.

133. Mesulam, M-M: Neural substrates of behavior: the effects of focal brain lesions upon mental state. In Nicoli, A (Ed.): The Harvard Guide to Psychiatry, 2nd Ed. Harvard University Press, Cambridge, MA, 1999, pp. 101–133.

134. Milner, B: Amnesia following operation on the temporal lobes. In Whitty, C W M and Zangwill, O L (Eds.): Amnesia. Butterworth, London, 1966, pp. 109–133.

135. Milner, B: Memory and the medial temporal regions of the brain. In Pribram, K H and Broadbent, D E (Eds.): Biology of Memory. Academic Press, New York, 1970, pp. 29–50.

136. Milner, B, Corkin, S and Teuber, H L: Further analysis of the hippocampal amnesic syndrome: fourteen year follow-up study of H.M. Neuropsychologia 6:215–234, 1968.

137. Molinari, M, Leggio, M G, Solida, A, Ciorra, R, Misciagna, S, Silveri, M C and Petrosini, L: Cerebellum and procedural learning: evidence from focal cerebellar lesions. Brain 120: 1753–1762, 1997.

138. Monakow, C von: Die Lokalisation im Grosshirn und der Abbau der Funktion durch kortikale Herde. Bergmann, Wiesbaden, 1914.

139. Munk H: Ueber die Functionen der Grosshirnrinde. Hirschwald, Berlin, 1881.

140. Murray, A and Mishkin, M: Severe tactual memory deficits in monkeys after combined removal of the amygdala and hippocampus. Brain Res 270:340–344, 1983.

141. Murray, A and Mishkin, M: Severe tactual as well as visual memory deficits follow combined removal of the amygdala and hippocampus in monkeys. J Neurosci 4:2565–2580, 1984.

142. Nadel, L and Moscovitch, M: Memory consolidation, retrograde amnesia and the hippocampal complex. Curr Opin Neurobiol 7:217–227, 1997.

143. Nader, K and LeDoux, J E: Is it time to invoke multiple fear learning systems in the amygdala? Trends Cogn Sci 1:241–246, 1997.

144. Nielsen-Bohlman, L, Ciranni, M, Shimamura, A P and Knight, R T: Impaired word-stem priming in patients with temporal-occipital lesions. Neuropsychologia 35:1087–1092, 1997.

145. Nieuwenhuys, R, Voogt, J and van Huizen, C: The Human Central Nervous System. A Synopsis and Atlas, 3rd Ed. Springer, Berlin, 1988.

146. O'Connor, M, Butters, N, Miliotis, P, Eslinger, P and Cermak, L S: The dissociation of anterograde and retrograde amnesia in a patient with Herpes encephalitis. J Clin Exp Neuropsychol 14:159–178, 1992.

147. O'Connor, M, Sieggreen, M A, Ahern, G, Schomer, D and Mesulam, M: Accelerated forgetting in association with temporal lobe epilepsy and paraneoplastic encephalitis. Brain Cogn 35:71–84, 1997.

148. O'Connor, M, Walbridge, M, Sandson, T and Alexander, M: A neuropsychological analysis of Capgras syndrome. Neuropsychiat Neuropsychol Behav Neurol 9:265–271, 1996.

149. Olesen, J and Jörgensen, M B: Leao's spreading depression in the hippocampus explains transient global amnesia. Acta Neurol Scand 73:219–220, 1986.

150. Owen, A M: Cognitive planning in humans: neuropsychological, neuroanatomical and neuropharmacological perspectives. Progr Neurobiol 53:431–450, 1997.

151. Papez, J W: A proposed mechanism of emotion. Archs Neurol Psychiat 38:725–743, 1937.

152. Parwatikar, S D: Medicolegal aspects of TGA. In Markowitsch, H J (Ed.): Transient Global Amnesia and Related Disorders. Hogrefe & Huber, Toronto, 1990, pp. 191–205.

153. Perrine, K, Gershengorn, J, Brown, E R, Choi, I S, Luciano, D J and Devinsky, O: Material-specific memory in the intracarotid amobarbital procedure. Neurology 43:706–711, 1993.

154. Pick, A: Clinical studies: III. On reduplicative paramnesia. Brain 26:260–267, 1903.

155. Rajaram, S: Basal forebrain amnesia. Neurocase 3:405–415, 1997.

156. Reber, P J, Stark, CEL and Squire, L R: Cortical areas supporting category learning identified using functional MRI. Proc Natl Acad Sci USA 95:747–750, 1998.

157. Reinkemeier, M, Markowitsch, H J, Rauch, B and Kessler, J: Memory systems for people's names: a case study of a patient with deficits in recalling, but not learning people's names. Neuropsychologia 35:677–684, 1997.

158. Rempel-Clower, N L, Zola-Morgan, S, Squire, L R and Amaral, D G: Three cases of enduring memory impairment after bilateral damage limited to the hippocampal formation. J Neurosci 16:5233–5255, 1996.

159. Ribot, T: Diseases of Memory. D. Appleton, New York, 1882.
160. Richards, W: Time reproductions by H.M. Acta Psychol 37:279–282, 1973.
161. Rogan, M T, Stäubli, U V and LeDoux, J E: Fear conditioning induces associative long-term potentiation in the amygala. Nature 390:604–607, 1997.
162. Romijn, H: About the origin of consciousness. A new, multidisciplinary perspective on the relationship between brain and mind. Proc Kon Ned Akad Wetensch 100:181–267, 1997.
163. Ross, E D: Sensory-specific and fractional disorders of recent memory. I. Isolated loss of visual recent memory. Arch Neurol 37:193–200, 1980.
164. Ross, E D: Sensory-specific and fractional disorders of recent memory. II. Unilateral loss of tactile recent memory. Arch Neurol 37:267–272, 1980.
165. Rosselli, M and Ardila, A: Calculation deficits in patients with right and left hemisphere damage. Neuropsychologia 27:607–617,1989.
166. Ruff, R L, Baser, C A, Johnston, J W, Marshall, L F, Klauber, S K, Klauber, M R and Minter, M: Neuropsychological rehabilitation: an experimental study with head-injured patients. J Head Trauma Rehab 4:20–36, 1989.
167. Russell, W R: The Traumatic Amnesias. Oxford University Press, Oxford, 1971.
168. Saffran, E M and Marin, O S M: Immediate memory for word lists and sentences in a patient with deficient auditory short-term memory. Brain Lang 2:420–433, 1975.
169. Sakashita, Y, Sugimoto, T, Taki, S and Matsuda, H: Abnormal cerebral blood flow following transient global amnesia. J Neurol Neurosurg Psychiatry 56:1327, 1993.
170. Sapolsky, R M: Stress, glucocorticoids, and damage to the nervous system: the current state of confusion. Stress 1:1–19, 1996.
171. Sarter, M, Bruno, J P, Givens, B, Moore, H, McGaugh, J and McMahon, K: Neuronal mechanisms mediating drug-induced cognition enhancement: cognitive activity as a necessary intervening variable. Cogn Brain Res 3:329–343, 1996.
172. Sarter, M and Markowitsch, H J: The amygdala's role in human mnemonic processing. Cortex 21:7–24, 1985.
173. Schacter, D L: Multiple forms of memory in humans and animals. In Weinberger, N M, McGaugh, J L and Lynch, G (Eds.): Memory Systems of the Brain. Guilford Press, New York, 1985, pp. 351–379.
174. Schacter, D L and Buckner, R L: Priming and the brain. Neuron 20:185–195, 1998.
175. Schacter, D L, Koutstall, W and Norman, K A: Can cognitive neuroscience illuminate the nature of traumatic childhood memories? Curr Opin Neurobiol 6:207–214, 1996.
176. Schmidt, D and Shorvon, S: The epilepsies. In Brandt, T, Caplan, L R, Dichgans, J, Diener, H C and Kennard, C (Eds.): Neurological Disorders. Course and Treatment. Academic Press, San Diego, 1996, pp. 159–181.
177. Schmidtke, K and Ehmsen, L: Transient global amnesia and migraine: a case control study. Eur Neurol 40:9–14, 1998.
178. Schmidtke, K, Handschuh, R and Vollmer, H: Cognitive procedural learning in amnesia. Brain Cogn 32:441–467, 1997.
179. Schmidtke, K, Reinhardt, M and Krause, T: Cerebral perfusion during transient global amnesia: findings with HMPAO SPECT. J Nucl Med 39:155–159, 1998.
180. Schneider, K: Über einige klinisch-psychologische Untersuchungsmethoden und ihre Ergebnisse. Zugleich ein Beitrag zur Psychopathologie der Korsakowschen Psychose. Z Neurol Psychiat 8:553–615, 1912.
181. Schuman, E M: Synapse specificity and long-term information storage. Neuron 18:339–342, 1997.
182. Scoville, W B and Milner, B: Loss of recent memory after bilateral hippocampal lesions. J Neurol Neurosurg Psychiatry 20:11–21, 1957.
183. Seeck, M, Mainwaring, N, Cosgrove, M D, Blume, H, Dubuisson, D, Mesulam, M M and Schomer, D L: Neurophysiologic correlates of implicit face memory in intracranial visual evoked potentials. Neurology 49:1312–1316, 1997.

184. Semon, R: Die Mneme als erhaltendes Prinzip im Wechsel des organischen Geschehens. Wilhelm Engelmann, Leipzig, 1904.

185. Shallice, T: Neuropsychological research and the fractionation of memory systems. In Nilsson, L G (Ed.): Perspectives on Memory Research. Erlbaum, Hillsdale, NJ, 1979, pp. 257–277.

186. Shallice, T and Warrington, E K: Independent functioning of the verbal memory stores: a neuropsychological study. Q J Exp Psychol 22:261–273, 1970.

187. Shaw, C-M and Alvord, E C Jr: Neuropathology of the limbic system. Neuroimag Clin N Am 7:101–142, 1997.

188. Signer, S F: Capgras syndrome and delusions of reduplication in neurologic disorders. Neuropsychiat Neuropsychol Behav Neurol 5:138–142, 1992.

189. Silove, D, Sinnerbrink, I, Field, A, Manicavasagar, V and Steel, Z: Anxiety, depression and PTSD in asylum-seekers: association with pre-migration trauma and post-migration stressors. Br J Psychiatry 170:351–357, 1997.

190. Silver, J M, Rattok, J and Anderson, K: Post-traumatic stress disorder and traumatic brain injury. Neurocase 3:151–157, 1997.

191. Silveri, M C, Daniele, A, Giustolisi, L and Gainotti, G: Dissociation between knowledge of living and nonliving things in dementia of the Alzheimer type. Neurology 41:545–546, 1991.

192. Sinz, R: Neurobiologie und Gedächtnis. VEB, Berlin, 1979.

193. Solveri, P, Brown, R G, Jahanashi, M, Caraceni, T and Marsden, C D: Learning manual pursuit tracking skills in patients with Parkinson's disease. Brain 120:1325–1337, 1997.

194. Southwick, S M, Morgan, III A, Nicolaou, A L and Charney, D S: Consistency of memory for combat-related traumatic events in veterans of Operation Desert Storm. Am J Psychiatry 154:173–177, 1997.

195. Squire, L R and Frambach, M: Cognitive skill learning in amnesia. Psychobiology 18: 109–117, 1990.

196. Squire, L R, Knowlton, B and Musen, G: The structure and organization of memory. Annu Rev Psychol 44:453–495, 1993.

197. Squire, L R and Zola, S M: Structure and function of declarative and nondeclarative memory systems. Proc Natl Acad Sci USA 93:13515–13522, 1996.

198. Stabell, K E and Magnoes, B: Neuropsychological course after surgery for intracranial aneurysms. A prospective study and a critical review. Scand J Psychol 38:127–137, 1997.

199. Stein, M B, Koverola, C, Hanna, C, Torchia, M G and McClarty, B: Hippocampal volume in women victimized by childhood sexual abuse. Psychol Med 27:951–959, 1997.

200. Strupp, M, Brüning, R, Wu, R H, Deimling, M, Reiser, M and Brandt, T: Diffusion-weighted MRI in transient global amnesia. Elevated signal intensity in the left mesial temporal lobe in 7 of 10 patients. Ann Neurol 43:164–170, 1998.

201. Sullivan, E V and Sagar, H J: Double dissociation of short-term and long-term memory for nonverbal material in Parkinson's disease and global amnesia. A further analysis. Brain 114:893–906, 1991.

202. Swain, R A, Armstrong, K E, Comery, T A, Humphreys, A G, Jones, T A, Kleim, J A and Greenough, W T: Speculations on the fidelity of memories stored in synaptic connections. In Schacter, DL (Ed.): Memory Distortion. Harvard University Press, Cambridge, MA, 1995, pp. 274–297.

203. Swick, D and Knight, R T: Contributions of right inferior temporal-occipital cortex to visual word and non-word priming. Neuroreport 7:11–16, 1995.

204. Teicher, M H, Glod, C A, Surrey, J and Swett, C: Early childhood abuse and limbic system ratings in adult psychiatric outpatients. J Neuropsychiatry Clin Neurosci 5:301–306, 1993.

205. Terzian, H and Dalle Ore, G: Syndrome of Klüver and Bucy. Reproduced in man by bilateral removal of the temporal lobes. Neurology 5:373–381, 1955.

206. Thompson, R F and Kim, J J: Memory systems in the brain and localization of memory. Proc Natl Acad Sci USA 93:13428–13444, 1996.
207. Thöne, A I T: Memory rehabilitation—recent developments and future directions. Restor Neurol Neurosci 9:125–140, 1996.
208. Tulving, E: Elements of episodic memory. Oxford University Press, Oxford, 1983.
209. Tulving, E, Kapur, S, Craik, F I M, Moscovitch, M and Houle, S: Hemispheric encoding/retrieval asymmetry in episodic memory: positron emission tomography findings. Proc Natl Acad Sci USA 91:2016–2020, 1994.
210. Tulving, E, Kapur, S, Markowitsch, H J, Craik, G, Habib, R and Houle, S: Neuroanatomical correlates of retrieval in episodic memory: auditory sentence recognition. Proc Natl Acad Sci USA 91:2012–2015, 1994.
211. Tulving, E and Markowitsch, H J: Episodic and declarative memory: role of the hippocampus. Hippocampus 8:198–204, 1998.
212. Tulving, E and Schacter, D L: Priming and human memory systems. Science 247:301–306, 1990.
213. Turner, M: Malingering. Br J Psychiatry 171:409–411, 1997.
214. van der Kolk, B A: The psychobiology of posttraumatic stress disorder. J Clin Psychiatry 58(Suppl 9):16–24, 1997.
215. Vargha-Khadem, F, Gadian, D G, Watkins, K E, Connelly, A, Van Paeschen, W and Mishkin, M: Differential effects of early hippocampal pathology on episodic and semantic memory. Science 277:376–380, 1997.
216. Warrington, E K, Logue, V and Pratt, R T C: The anatomical localisation of selective impairment of auditory verbal short-term memory. Neuropsychologia 9:377–387, 1971.
217. Warrington, E K and Weiskrantz, L: Amnesia: a disconnection syndrome? Neuropsychologia 20:233–248, 1982.
218. Wiebe, S P, Stäubli, U V and Ambros-Ingerson, J: Short-term reverberant memory model of hippocampal field CA3. Hippocampus 7:656–665, 1997.
219. Wise, S P: The role of the basal ganglia in procedural memory. Semin Neurosci 8:39–46, 1996.
220. Woodruff-Pak, D S: Eyeblink classical conditioning in H.M.: Delay and trace paradigms. Behav Neurosci 107:911–925, 1993.
221. Xu, L, Anwyl, R and Rowan, M J: Behavioural stress facilitates the induction of long-term depression in the hippocampus. Nature 387:497–500, 1997.
222. Yeterian, E H and Pandya, D N: Architectonic features of the primate brain: implications for information processing and behavior. In Markowitsch, H J (Ed.): Information Processing by the Brain. Huber, Toronto, 1988, pp. 7–38.
223. Yin, J C P and Tully, T: CREB and the formation of long-term memory. Curr Opin Neurobiol 6:264–268, 1996.
224. Zorzon, M, Longo, R, Mase, R, Biasutti, E, Vitrani, B and Cazzato, G: Proton magnetic resonance spectroscopy during transient global amnesia. J Neurol Sci 156:78–82, 1998.

5

Aphasia and the Neural Basis of Language

Antonio R. Damasio and Hanna Damasio

I. Introduction

The investigation of the neural basis of language occupies a unique place in the history of both neurology and neuroscience. It is fair to say that neurology began in earnest about a century and a half ago, around the study of language, and that what we now call neuroscience can be traced to that same effort. In this chapter, we take this dual status of language into account. We discuss language from the perspective of both neurology and neuroscience, mindful of the significance of language for both clinical practice and neuroscientific progress.

Although much has been learned about the neural basis of language in the past few decades, it is important to note that the results of the 19th-century studies were in every sense remarkable, especially considering that the investigators did not yet have a theory to guide them and that the available methods were the all too simple predecessors of the current lesion method and of contemporary experimental neuropsychology. Our neurological forerunners deserve immense credit for establishing a number of incontrovertible facts: (1) that the left cerebral hemisphere is usually dominant for language; (2) that language and handedness are linked; and (3) that two particular brain regions, those named after Broca and Wernicke, have a prominent role in language processing.

It is true, however, that the very discovery and dissemination of those hard facts had an unexpected negative consequence: the temporary suspension of the effort to map the language brain, and, no less importantly, of the effort to reinterpret the existing map in accordance with progressively updated views on brain function. The cartoon of the key brain structures required to receive and produce language—Broca's and Wernicke's areas, bridged by the arcuate fasciculus—was so attractive that the evidence in favor of a more varied and complex neural account was all but ignored. The view that Broca's and Wernicke's areas are *the* language centers pervades most textbooks and monographs to our day. Surprisingly, some modern workers in cognitive science and linguistics continue to use this outdated and literally phrenological view to provide a neural counterpart for their otherwise entirely unphrenological models of thought and language.

Over the past decade, with the availability of structural magnetic resonance and three-dimensional (3-D) reconstructions of the human brain, the human lesion method has gained power and made way for a new wave of cognitive experiments. The results that followed showed that language processing is not dependent on Wernicke's and Broca's areas alone, but depends, rather, on many neural sites linked as systems and working in concert. For instance, it has become clear that several regions in higher-order left temporal and left prefrontal/premotor cortices are engaged by language processing,[27,29,47] and do so in a selective manner—certain aspects of the linguistic process are more linked to some regions than to others. By the same token, it has also shown that structures in left basal ganglia, thalamus, and supplementary motor area are also engaged in language processing.[21,48,84]

Recent functional imaging studies have also provided support for this dynamic systems view. For instance, Raichle and colleagues and Frackowiak and colleagues have shown that visual word processing activates left occipital and temporal cortices outside of Wernicke's area.[38,51,91,126] We and others have shown that several areas in left temporal pole and left inferotemporal cortex are consistently activated by naming entities belonging to different conceptual categories,[33,74] and that tasks requiring the manipulation of concepts and related words activate nonclassic language areas in left temporal cortices.[73]

Additional evidence in support of the view that the language brain is not confined to the classical aphasia producing areas has come from the use of electrophysiological techniques. Especially valuable data have come from studies in which the exposed cerebral cortex of patients undergoing surgery for the treatment of seizures is exposed. The cortex can be either electrically stimulated at a particular point—with the consequence that local function is transiently inactivated—or the exposed cerebral cortex can be recorded locally within a small region, as electrical potentials are evoked by a task. Although an epileptic brain cannot be expected to be in every respect like a standard normal brain, and although some caution is required in the interpretation of the results, no other approach in living humans can reach such a degree of structural directness and functional immediacy.

This approach, which was pioneered by the Canadian neurosurgeon Wilder Penfield, has been progressively refined and has yielded several important new results. For instance, George Ojemann has shown convincingly that varied regions of left temporal cortex, outside of the classic language areas, are actively engaged by a host of language tasks.[87] More recently, a set of especially intriguing results came from the work of McCarthy and Nobre, who found that a fairly circumscribed sector of anterior and medial left temporal cortex is consistently engaged in word processing tasks.[85] Others, namely Barry Gordon and his colleagues, have reported comparable findings focusing on a region they called "basal temporal language area."[69,71]

The past few decades have thus brought forth a remarkable amount of evidence on the basis of which the classic view is being modernized. In this chapter we review some of the evidence from the perspective of lesion studies of aphasia, the central neurological condition in which language is impaired.

II. THE APHASIAS

The term "aphasia" denotes a disturbance of language processing caused by dysfunction in specific brain regions. The disturbance can compromise the comprehension of language, the formulation of language, or both. Aphasia consists of a breakdown in the two-way translation process that establishes a correspondence between thoughts and language. Patients with aphasia are not able to translate, with reasonable fidelity, the nonverbal images which constitute thought into the symbols and grammatical relationships which constitute language. In most instances of aphasia, the inverse process is also defective, so once a word or sentence is heard the patient cannot construct the nonverbal images which correspond to the meaning behind the language.

The essence of aphasia is thus a disorder of linguistic processing. Aphasia is not a disorder of perception. Deafness, even when it is caused by damage in the central nervous system, precludes language comprehension through the auditory channel but does not impair language comprehension through vision or touch. Aphasia is also not a disorder of movement. For instance, dysarthria, which is caused by incoordinated speech movements, distorts the articulation of speech sounds but does not compromise the formulation of language. No less importantly, aphasia is not a result of disordered thought processes. The disorder of thought that characterizes schizophrenia is not an aphasia, and, in effect, the intact language devices of schizophrenic patients often render quite faithfully the underlying distorted thought process.

Aphasia is not the exclusive province of auditory-based languages such as English. Users of languages based on visuomotor signs such as American Sign Language can also become aphasic. Aphasia may affect the written code of any language, auditorily based, such as in English, or based on ideograms, as is the case in some Asian languages.

Aphasia can affect varied aspects of language processing, namely: (1) *syntax* (which pertains to the grammatical structure of sentences); (2) the *lexicon* (which concerns the words available in any language to denote particular meanings); and, (3) the *morphology* of words (which concerns how individual speech sounds, known as *phonemes*, are combined to form *morphemes*, which are the base for the unique structure of a word). Often, several or even all of these aspects of language are compromised in the same patient, although the emphasis does vary—in one patient the major problem may be constructing meaningful sentences, coupled with a mild defect in selecting words; in another patient the inability to assemble a sentence according to grammar may be the main defect. The different combination of aphasia signs gives rise to different aphasia syndromes (see Table 5–1).

Aphasia can be caused by most neurological diseases, provided the language processing areas of the cerebral hemispheres are involved. Most aphasias are caused by head injury, stroke, degenerative dementias such as Alzheimer's disease, and cerebral tumors. Stroke alone causes about 100,000 new cases of aphasia every year in the United States, and head injury probably causes at least twice as many. The results are often devastating. Aphasia not only disrupts communication but any

TABLE 5–1 Principal Aphasia Syndromes*

	Speech	Comprehension	Repetition	Other Signs	Localization
Broca's	Nonfluent; sparse; effortful; melodically flat	+	−	Right hemiparesis (arm > leg); patient is aware of defect, may be depressed	Left frontal (lower posterior)
Wernicke's	Fluent; abundant; well articulated; melodic	−	−	No motor signs; patient may be agitated, euphoric, or paranoid	Left temporal (posterior and superior)
Conduction	Fluent with some articulatory defects	+	−	Often none; patient may have sensory loss or weakness in right arm; right facial weakness may be seen	Left supramarginal gyrus; or left auditory cortex and insula
Global	Scarce, monosyllables and stereotypes	−	−	Right hemiplegia, but may present *without* hemiplegia	If with hemiplegia, large left perisylvian lesion / Without hemiplegia: separate frontal and temporoparietal lesions
Transcortical motor	Nonfluent	+	+		Anterior or superior to Broca's region; may involve part of Broca's area
Transcortical sensory	Fluent, scant	−	+		Posterior or inferior to Wernicke's area
Atypical ("basal ganglia")	Dysarthric but often fluent	−	−/+	Right hemiparesis (arm > leg)	Head of caudate nucleus; anterior limb of capsule
Atypical ("thalamus")	Fluent, may be logorrheic	−	+	Attentional and memory defects in acute phase	Anterolateral thalamus

*+ Intact or largely preserved; − Impaired.

ability whose final performance depends on the use of internal speech. Decision-making, creativity, and the ability to perform calculations are often compromised because of a primary language defect, although, in and of themselves, these abilities are in good part independent of language.

Because the human left hemisphere is frequently dominant for language in both right-handers and left-handers, the lesions that cause aphasia are usually located in the left cerebral hemisphere. The distribution of cerebral dominance for language as far as handedness is concerned is asymmetric. Virtually all right-handers show left cerebral dominance for language (the few that do not develop aphasia following right hemisphere lesions, in a rare condition known as "crossed" aphasia). Most left-handers (more than two-thirds) also show left cerebral dominance for language. The left-handers that do not, develop aphasia following lesions in either hemisphere (see Figure 5–1).

Because the signs and symptoms that characterize aphasia are generally caused by circumscribed brain dysfunction, the aphasias have been used as a valuable diagnostic tool in the localization of lesions and as a natural window on the functions of the human neurophysiology. For this reason, aphasia has become an important topic not only in neurology and neurosurgery, neuropsychology and speech pathology, but also in basic neuroscience, linguistics, and the cognitive sciences. A review of the current status of research on the aphasias provides the best bridge between the results of clinical neurology and those of contemporary neuroscience.

Broca's Aphasia

The patient's speech is labored and usually slow: Pauses between words are more frequent than words themselves. The melodic modulation that characterizes normal speech is lacking, a characteristic that, in combination with the reduction in number of words, defines this speech pattern as nonfluent. Yet, the patients manage to communicate verbally with some success. The selection of words is often correct, especially in the case of words for entities (nouns), and less so in words that stand for actions (verbs) and relationships (so called grammatical words such as conjunctions). Patients with classical Broca's aphasia have a defect in verbatim sentence repetition. The patients understand the meaning of a sentence, but they are unable to repeat the words in the sentence, usually to their own puzzlement. Most patients with Broca's aphasia also have some weakness in the right arm and right side of the face.

Patients with classical Broca's aphasia have agrammatism, a defect characterized by the inability to organize words in sentences that accord with grammatical rules and by improper use or lack of use of grammatical morphemes. The grammatical morphemes are small words such as conjunctions (*and, or, if, but*), prepositions (*to, from*) and auxiliary verbs or so-called bound inflectional affixes used as verb endings to signify tense (e.g., *-ed*, in the past tense lov*ed*; e.g., *-ing* in the gerund danc*ing*) or person (e.g., *-s* in dances). The agrammatic defect is behind the telegraphic aspect of utterances such as "Go I home tomorrow" (instead of "I will go home tomorrow") in which the canonical word order for English is violated and the auxiliary

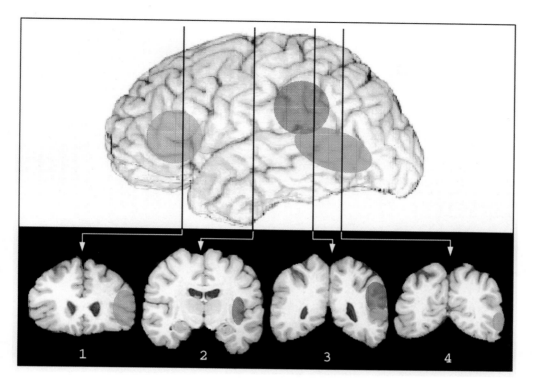

FIGURE 5–1. The top panel shows a lateral view of a human left cerebral hemisphere reconstructed in three dimensions from magnetic resonance data, using Brainvox. The three areas of the cerebral cortex highlighted with crosshatching correspond to the three main regions of the left hemisphere whose damage causes aphasia. The regions are, respectively, Broca's area, in the left frontal operculum; Wernicke's area, in the left lateral and posterior temporal cortex; and the general area of the supramarginal gyrus in the lower parietal operculum.

The lower panel shows four coronal sections depicting the typical subcortical extensions of the lesions which cause aphasia. Sections 1, 3, and 4 run through the three regions named above. Section 2 depicts the involvement of a region of the cerebral cortex which is not visible on the cortical surface: the insula. The lesions which cause conduction aphasia occasionally extend from the supramarginal gyrus and primary auditory cortices toward the insula, thus encompassing this region.

Damage to the first and second regions is typically associated with Broca's and Wernicke's aphasias. Damage to the third region is commonly associated with conduction aphasia.

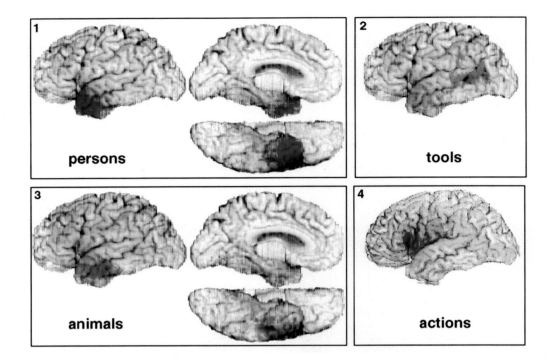

Figure 5–2. Panels 1–4 reveal the regions of maximal overlap for lesions associated, respectively, with impairments in the naming of persons *(1)*, manipulable tools *(2)*, animals *(3)*, and actions *(4)*. The overlap was obtained using the Map 3 technique, which is based on the three-dimensional spatial superposition of lesions. The regions of maximal overlap are all located within the left cerebral hemisphere. As far as naming unique persons, manipulable tools, and animals is concerned, the critical regions are either entirely outside of the classical language areas, or, in the case of manipulable tools, partially overlapping. As far as the naming of actions is concerned, there is superposition with Broca's area.

verb is dropped. Some of the agrammatic difficulties noted in language production can also be found in language comprehension. Broca's aphasics have difficulty recognizing the meaning of "reversible" passive sentences such as "The girl was kissed by the boy," in which girl and boy are equally likely to be the recipient of the action, but have little problem in assigning correct meaning to a "nonreversible" passive such as "The apple was eaten by the girl," or to the active sentence "The girl kissed the boy."[12,14,18,43,50,60,97,98]

Patients with Broca's aphasia typically manifest some degree of naming impairment, but recently it has been shown that the severity of this deficit may vary to a large extent depending on the grammatical category to which the words being retrieved belong. Specifically, these patients frequently have considerably more difficulty with the retrieval of verbs than with the retrieval of nouns. We have shown that lesions in and near Broca's area impair retrieval of verbs while sparing retrieval of nouns.[27] In this study, we found that lesions in the left frontal operculum, involving both prefrontal and premotor cortex and underlying white matter, were associated with defective retrieval of verbs and normal retrieval of nouns. Similar findings have been reported by other investigators.[34,78] These findings are also in keeping with a number of other investigations. For example, Goodglass and colleagues compared syntactic constructions between agrammatic (usually Broca's) aphasics and conduction aphasics.[46] Consistent with previous studies of this type,[72,77,81] the authors found that agrammatic aphasics had a preponderance of nouns over verbs in running speech and in single-constituent utterances. This finding is consistent with other studies reporting noun–verb discrepancies in word repetition[59] and written word retrieval.[19]

Patients with classical Broca's aphasia distort the production of speech sounds (phonemes) and omit or add phonetic features that do not belong in the proper articulation of a given phoneme. An example is the misproduction of /b/ for /p/, which differ only in the temporal alignment of their articulatory components, a phenomenon known as "phonetic disintegration."[13,68] Curiously, Broca's aphasics also have difficulty discriminating closely related phonemes (such as /b/ for /p/) although the recognition of morphemes is unaffected.[13]

In classical Broca's aphasia there is extensive damage involving Broca's area: the combination of BA44 and 45 in the inferior left frontal gyrus, the surrounding frontal areas (the external aspect of BA6, BA8, 9, 10, 47, and 46), and the underlying white matter and the subjacent basal ganglia.[30,64,83]

Patients in whom damage is restricted to Broca's area alone and to immediately subjacent white matter without involvement of the surrounding cortical areas and basal ganglia do not develop classical Broca's aphasia. They have a mild and transient aphasia that has been referred to as "Broca's area aphasia."[70,79] Even more restricted damage to Broca's area or to the underlying white matter causes a disturbance of speech without true language defect which is known as "aphemia."[102,113]

The structures usually damaged in Broca's aphasia and in Broca's area aphasia are part of a neural system involved in both the assembly of phonemes into words and the assembly of words into sentences—that is, the temporal ordering of linguistic components. We have suggested that this system is concerned with the relational aspects of language, which include the grammatical structure of sentences and the proper use of grammatical morphemes and verbs. The other cortical components of the system are located in external left frontal cortices (BA47, 46, 9), in the interconnected left parietal cortices (BA40, 39, 7), and in the sensorimotor cortices above the sylvian fissure between Broca's and Wernicke's regions (the lower sector of BA3, 1, 2, and 4). The critical subcortical component is in the left basal ganglia and includes the head of the caudate nucleus and the putamen.

Wernicke's Aphasia

Patients with Wernicke's aphasia resemble those with classical Broca's aphasia in the defective repetition of sentences, the defective assembly of phonemes, and the defective naming: In every other aspect they are quite different. First, the speech of Wernicke's aphasics is "fluent"—that is, effortless, melodic, and produced at normal or faster than normal rates. Second, because of frequent errors in phoneme choice and word choice the content of speech may be unintelligible. Third, Wernicke's aphasics have difficulty comprehending the sentences they hear. Fourth, patients with Wernicke's aphasia rarely have any motor impairment. This last characteristic poses a significant problem for the unforewarned because the diagnosis must be established on the basis of speech performance with no help from other neurological signs such as weakness or sensory loss.

Patients with severe Wernicke aphasia's and a premorbid anxious personality may become agitated and develop paranoid ideation, perhaps because of their combined inability to understand speech of others and to have their own speech understood. In rare instances they may become suicidal or homicidal. Curiously, depression is less common in Wernicke's than in Broca's aphasics.

Wernicke's aphasics have great difficulty with the mere selection of the words that accurately represent their intended meaning. This is the source of naming errors. The wrong words the patients end up selecting instead of the intended one are often related by meaning, as in "headman" for "president." (This is known as a "verbal" or "semantic paraphasia."). Patients frequently resort to generic terms such as "thing" and "stuff" as substitutes for the word they are unable to conjure up. Incidentally, the term "paraphasia" refers to any substitution of an erroneous individual sound [phoneme] or entire word for the intended and correct one.

Patients with Wernicke's aphasia have no difficulty with the production of individual sounds, but they often shift the order in which sounds and sound clusters are produced, and they can add or delete sounds in a way that distorts the phonemic plan of an intended word—for example, "trable" for table; "pymarid" for pyramid. This defect gives rise to "phonemic paraphasias." When phoneme shifts occur frequently and in close temporal proximity, the words become unintelligible and constitute neologisms (neologistic paraphasias) rather than legitimate words—for example, "hipidomateous" for hippopotamus.

Wernicke's aphasia is usually caused by damage to the posterior sector of the left auditory association cortex (BA22). Often there is involvement of BA37, 39 and 40, or all three.[30,64,66,83,105–107]

Although damage to Wernicke's area disrupts auditory comprehension, Wernicke's area should not be seen as the center in which auditory comprehension takes place (Chapter 1). We see it as a processor of speech sounds which recruits auditory inputs to be mapped as words, and to be used subsequently to evoke concepts. Auditory comprehension in the proper sense occurs later in a chain of events initiated in Wernicke area, when the concepts that are pertinently associated with a given word's records become activated and attended. The process of auditory comprehension involves numerous cerebral cortices of varied sensory modalities as well as higher-order cortices distributed over parietal, temporal, and frontal regions. Wernicke's area should also not be seen as a center for word selection. Once a word is selected for possible use in an utterance, Wernicke's area is part of the system needed to implement its constituent speech sounds, in the form of internal auditory and kinesthetic representations which support the upcoming vocalization.

Conduction Aphasia

Patients with conduction aphasia can comprehend simple sentences and produce intelligible sentences. They cannot, however, repeat sentences *verbatim*, they cannot assemble phonemes effectively (and thus produce many phonemic paraphasias), and they cannot name objects correctly in confrontation naming tasks. Conduction aphasia shares with Broca's and Wernicke's an inability to repeat, a defective assembly of phonemes, and defective naming. The relatively preserved speech production and auditory comprehension distinguish conduction aphasia from Broca's and Wernicke's aphasia. Other than for right facial weakness, motor signs are absent. Although its distinctiveness was in doubt, conduction aphasia is now well established as an individual aphasia.[10,30,64,83,96]

Conduction aphasia is caused by damage in one of two regions: (*1*) left BA40 (supramarginal gyrus), with or without extension to the white matter underneath the posterior insula, or (*2*) the left primary auditory cortices (BA41 and 42), the insula, and the underlying white matter. In either variant most of BA22 is spared. There is no evidence that conduction aphasia can be caused by pure white matter disconnection as proposed by Wernicke,[125] although the damage does compromise white matter and destroy feedforward and feedback projections which conjoin temporal, parietal, and frontal cortices.[40] Such a connectional system, as it traverses underneath the angular and supramarginal gyri, constitutes the classical arcuate fasciculus, damage to which was originally linked to this aphasia.[42] This seems to be part of the system required to assemble phonemes into morphemes, an operation necessary for the vocalization of a word perceived auditorily or generated internally, in the mind's ear.

Global Aphasia

Global aphasics have an almost complete loss of the ability to comprehend language or formulate speech, thus combining the features of Broca's and Wernicke's aphasias. Deliberate speech, also known as "propositional" speech, is reduced to a few words and sentences. The same stereotypical word may be used repeatedly in a vain attempt to communicate an idea. Some nondeliberate ("automatic") speech is preserved. The only effective aspect of verbal communication in these patients consists of stock expletives—for example, "Goddamn it"—which are used appropriately and with normal phonemic, phonetic, and inflectional structures. Other "automatic" speech routines, such as counting or reciting the days of the week, are often intact, and so is the ability to sing parts of previously learned melodies and their lyrics. Auditory comprehension is limited to a small number of nouns, verbs, and idioms. Patients with global aphasia do not comprehend grammatically elaborate sentences and cannot recognize grammatical words.

Global aphasia is usually accompanied by a weakness in the right side of the face and right hemiplegia. The presence or absence of hemiplegia is an important clue to the localization of brain damage. When hemiplegia is present ("classic global aphasia") the damage is in (1) the anterior language region (as in Broca's aphasia); (2) the entire basal ganglia region, (3) the insula and auditory cortices (as in conduction aphasia), and (4) the posterior language region (as in Wernicke's aphasia). This large degree of damage is caused by a large infarct in the region supplied by the middle cerebral artery.[30] Global aphasics with such lesions are severely aphasic from the outset and show little or no improvement of their aphasia or motor defect. When global aphasics have transient hemiparesis or no weakness at all ("global aphasia without hemiplegia"), the damage is usually divided by two regions: one frontal and the other parietotemporal. The pattern of damage spares several motor, sensory, and language-related structures[114,120] and the patients tend to recover. Such double lesions may result from an embolic stroke or brain metastases.

Another group of patients with global aphasia shows only dominant frontal lobe damage with extension into insula and basal ganglia but leaving temporal and parietal regions entirely intact. In the chronic stage most of these patients become severe Broca's aphasics rather than global aphasics.[30,64,83]

The Transcortical Aphasias

Little new has been uncovered regarding the transcortical aphasias, which are distinguished from all others above by normal sentence repetition. The "motor" variant usually occurs with damage in the left frontal cortices above and in front of Broca area, although there may be substantial damage to Broca's area itself and sufficient damage to left supplementary motor area can, on occasion, present as transcortical motor aphasia.[30] The "sensory" variant occurs with lesions in temporal or parietal cortices in the surround of Wernicke area.[30]

III. Language Impairments Following Damage Outside Classical Language Territories

Atypical Aphasias Following Subcortical Damage

All the classical aphasia types are caused by lesions in the cerebral cortex or in subjacent white-matter pathways. However, it is now clear that following nonhemorrhagic infarction of the left basal ganglia (a set of large gray nuclei that is often regarded as a purely motor structure), a peculiar aphasia ensues. The syndrome does not fit in the established diagnostic categories and is thus "atypical." It combines signs of Wernicke's aphasia, such as defective auditory comprehension, with signs suggestive of other aphasias such as dysarthria and hemiparesis.[4,15,21,39,84] The lesions involve the head of the left caudate nucleus and the nearby white matter in the anterior limb of the internal capsule. Lesions in the remainder of the left caudate nucleus (the body and tail of this structure) or in the putamen (the other principal component of the basal ganglia) do not cause aphasia. Lesions of the equivalent structures of the nondominant hemisphere also do not cause aphasia.[21] Sequential computed tomography (CT) studies suggest that the cerebral cortex does not suffer structural damage[32] and the available postmortem verification supports that assumption.[7]

The placement of these lesions in a special territory of vascular supply (that of the lenticular arteries) points to a particular mechanism of stroke: The occlusion of the middle cerebral artery stem blocks the smaller lenticular branches which arise out of it and leads to infarction in the terminal and noncollateralized vascular bed of those branches. The overlying cerebral cortex does not develop a concomitant infarction because its patent collateral supply is capable of bypassing the occlusion and resupplying the cortex.[31]

These findings established the region of the left head of the caudate and surrounding white matter as relevant to language processing. This region is interconnected with the auditory cortex and with cortices related to movement, memory, decision-making, and emotion.[3,44,127] It plays a central role in habit-learning. Our hypothesis is that it is part of a network necessary for the *automatic* processing of frequently used sentence structures.

Evidence from nonhemorrhagic infarctions also confirms that some thalamic nuclei in the left hemisphere are necessary for the implementation of speech and language, as previously hypothesized by Penfield.[2,48,80,89] Damage to the anterolateral nuclei seems necessary for the appearance of aphasia, which is characterized by fluent speech (the speech may be so fluent that it has been described as logorrhea) and normal repetition.[48] Damage to other nuclei of the dominant side and to nuclei of the nondominant thalamus are associated with somatosensory defects, attentional defects, and memory impairment, but not with disorders of speech and language.

Language Impairments Following Mesial Frontal Damage

Some frontal cortices located in the internal (mesial) cerebral surface of the left hemisphere (including the supplementary motor area and the anterior cingulate) play an important role in the initiation and maintenance of speech.[30,67,89] They also play a role in attention and emotion and can thus influence many higher functions. Damage in these areas does not cause aphasia per se but rather varied degrees of "akinesia" (a difficulty with the initiation of movement), and "mutism," a complete absence of speech that is rarely seen in true aphasia in any but its inaugural stages. The akinetic–mute patients fail to communicate *both* by word and by gestures or facial expressions. Their drive to communicate is no longer present. Upon recovery they describe a peculiar experience: The range and resonance of thought processes was reduced and their will to speak was preempted. (Note again, that on rare occasions damage to supplementary motor area can present as transcortical motor aphasia.)

Language Impairments Following Damage to the Left Temporal Cortices

Damage to the anterior and inferotemporal cortices had not been associated with language impairment. Recent studies, however, reveal unequivocally that damage to *left* temporal cortices in BA21, 20, and 38 causes severe impairments of word retrieval without any accompanying grammatical or phonemic/phonetic difficulty— that is, such lesions cause "pure naming defects".[29,33,116] The finding is especially exciting because of its linguistic specificity. It appears that when the damage is confined to the left temporal pole (BA38), patients have a defect in the retrieval of "proper nouns" (the unique names of unique places and persons) but not in the retrieval of "common nouns" (the names for nonunique objects).[33,108,116] When the lesions involve the cortices of the left BA21 and 20, the defect encompasses *both* a retrieval of proper nouns and of common nouns. The evidence uncovered so far also indicates that retrieval of other word categories (verbs, adjectives, grammatical words) is not compromised.[27,29] Thus, these findings suggest that the left anterior temporal cortices contain neural systems which hold the key to *accessing words* that go with objects, places, or persons, but not words that stand for qualities of those entities, or their actions or relationships. Note that the defect is one of *accessing* the means to implement words and is not a loss of the "representation" of those words. The evidence does not mean that nouns are in a certain brain place—only that certain brain places must be intact in order for them to be re-evoked. The neurological conditions which damage these areas and cause such naming defects include not only stroke, head injury, and herpes encephalitis but also selective degenerative processes such as Alzheimer's and Pick's disease.[6,24,49,75,104] These new findings are in agreement with Ojemann's report that naming is disrupted by electrical stimulation of these same cortices.[86] Moreover, they are related to an intriguing new entity, progressive aphasia, which is discussed below.

Progressive Aphasia

"Progressive aphasia" is defined as a progressive deterioration in speech and language, with an insidious onset and in the relative absence of decline in other aspects of cognition.[76,124] Several neuropathologic substrates have been associated with this condition, including, in approximate decreasing order of frequency, Pick's disease, focal spongiform degeneration, and Alzheimer's disease. The purity of the language impairment is probably not present in the majority of progressive aphasics, in whom careful testing may eventually reveal cognitive impairments in nonlanguage domains. Nonetheless, affected patients do manifest a disturbance in speech and language that is out of proportion to other cognitive defects and that remains a predominant sign as the disease courses (Chapter 10). Progressive aphasia has been associated primarily with dysfunction of the left temporal lobe.[49,65]

IV. Sign Language Aphasia

One of the new developments in the field of aphasia has been the discovery of aphasia in relation to a nonauditory-based language, American Sign Language (ASL). Bellugi and Klima have shown unequivocally that deaf individuals can become aphasic in ASL as a result of focal brain damage in the *left* hemisphere.[9] Deaf signers with right hemisphere lesions, however, develop neuropsychological manifestations of right hemisphere damage (e.g., visual neglect, constructional apraxia) but not sign language aphasia. This suggests that nonauditory-based languages are as linked to the left hemisphere as auditory based ones and that the left hemisphere may be genetically endowed for language independently of the sensory channel of acquisition and processing.

V. The Role of Nondominant Hemisphere Cortices in Language

It has long been recognized that right hemisphere cortices are the likely source of the residual "automatic" utterances exhibited by global aphasics. It is also suspected that right hemisphere cortices support some aspects of recovery in severe aphasics. In addition, however, it is now well recognized that right hemisphere damage impairs a language ability known as "discourse," which refers to the skill with which one can organize a narrative—that is, tell a story, make a joke, write a letter.[41] Right hemisphere damage also impairs the ability to appreciate a story or get the point of a joke. Following right hemisphere lesions, there are also marked changes in "prosody," an ability which refers to the inflections, stresses, and melody of speech that can provide words and sentences with meanings that go beyond their basic dictionary.[94,118] Consider, as an example, how the sentence "You are a bad boy" can have radically different meanings depending on whether the inflection reveals the speaker as irate, or quietly concerned, or as an ironical observer. In short, the right hemisphere cortices are not concerned with the core phonetic, lexical, and grammatical processes whose impairment hallmarks aphasia. But they contribute critical aspects of normal language processing: automated idioms, prosody, and discourse (Chapters 1, 2, 6).

VI. APHASIA MANAGEMENT

It is well acknowledged that classifications of biological phenomena are as much a help as a hindrance. The classification of aphasias is no exception, and the available systems have been criticized either for their theoretical assumptions or practical imperfections. The major problem with classifications, especially syndrome classifications, lies with their use in research, because exemplars of syndromes are usually not entirely comparable in terms of constituent signs. It is justifiable, however, to use syndromes as a means to communicate among investigators and clinicians. In this chapter, we have retained a classical syndromatic classification.

From the standpoint of assessment, it is clear that standardized neuropsychological measures are indispensable for studying and managing aphasia. Accepted diagnostic tools include the *Boston Diagnostic Aphasia Examination* (known as the *BDAE*);[45] Iowa's *Neurosensory Center Examination of Aphasia* or *NCCEA*,[112] and its offspring the *Multilingual Aphasia Examination* or *MAE*;[11] and the *Western Battery of Aphasia*,[61] which evolved from the *Boston* examination. These batteries use validated neuropsychological tasks to probe a broad range of speech and language abilities (Chapter 2). On the basis of the performance profile they help produce, it is possible to establish a diagnosis and a treatment plan. Other useful instruments include the *Porch Index of Communicative Ability (PICA)*,[93] the *Functional Communication Profile (FCP)*,[99] and the *Communicative Ability in Daily Living Test*, which measure pragmatic aspects of communication.[55]

Following damage, the brain and its impaired functions tend to show some degree of spontaneous recovery, assuming the cause of damage is removed. But when the altered speech and language of an aphasic are left to their own devices, the degree of improvement is limited. The fact that therapeutic intervention is beneficial is now generally accepted.[8] The outcome of treatment depends largely on the underlying disease, on the profile of aphasia signs, and on their severity. Other factors do influence the result, however. For example, premorbid intelligence and communication skills is an important factor—creative ability and rich vocabularies are generally helpful in recovery. The presence and degree of nonlanguage cognitive defects—for instance, the presence of major visual or auditory defects, or of defects in attention and memory—are critical factors in the efficacy of rehabilitation). Pre- and postmorbid emotional balance is another important factor. Depression reduces the incentive to learn compensatory strategies, while a positive personal attitude and strong family support help overcome the frustrations of the teaching sessions. In brief, the success of the therapeutic intervention depends on the individual premorbid characteristics of each patient, on the type and severity of language and nonlanguage defects, on emotional status, and on human support.

In aphasia caused by focal and nonprogressive disease processes, including stroke and head injury, the maximal recovery seems to occur in the first 3 months following onset.[20,37,63,92,100,119,121] Holland and her colleagues have suggested that this period of maximal recovery may actually be as short as 2 months.[56,57,88]

The mechanisms which permit recovery are not clear, but several investigators have struggled with the problem. Kertesz has summarized the neural factors that may account for recovery from the cognitive defects associated with focal brain injury as follows: (1) presence of intact ipsilateral cortical structures physiologically and anatomically connected to the damaged structures, (2) presence of intact contralateral homologous cortical areas, and (3) presence of intact subcortical systems hierarchically and physiologically related to the damaged structures.[62]

Rubens[95] has suggested that some spontaneous recovery from aphasia appears due to the reversal of physiological changes caused directly by stroke. These include lessening of edema; reestablishment of premorbid neurotransmitter activity; reabsorption of blood in hemorrhagic lesions; and recovery from diaschisis.

There is no standard approach to the treatment of aphasia. Each patient needs a customized program tailored to the linguistic, neuropsychologic, and personal factors discussed earlier. The best treatment plans result from collaborations among speech pathologists, neuropsychologists, and neurologists. Although patients with severe impairments of auditory comprehension or poor speech output generally have a less good prognosis than patients with partial defects, there are techniques that can help all patients. Some special techniques include melodic intonation therapy,[1] which relies on the ability to handle musical tones as opposed to speech sounds and is helpful in patients with poorly articulated speech; syntax training programs for patients with agrammatism;[52] and Visual Action Therapy,[53] the Sentence Level Auditory Comprehension Treatment Program,[82] and Visual Communication Therapy,[41] which are helpful to severe global aphasics.

VII. OVERVIEW

In the foregoing sections of this chapter we have presented a number of findings relating a variety of language processes to a host of neural structures and operations. In an attempt to provide a perspective to interpret those findings, we will present briefly a framework for discussing the neural basis of concepts and words.

We and others have presented evidence that the retrieval of knowledge for concrete entities from different conceptual categories depends on partially segregated neural systems.[5,17,22,24,28,35,54,101,109,111,115,122,123] These findings have clarified further the neural correlates of knowledge retrieval, and here we outline our notion of how the neural circuitry subserving retrieval of conceptual and lexical knowledge operates.

We believe that neural sites crucial for knowledge retrieval are instrumental in generating the recall of separate items of knowledge whose collection effectively denotes the concept of a given entity. The neural sites operate as catalysts for retrieving the multidimensional aspects of knowledge which are necessary and sufficient for the mental representation of the concept of an entity. The retrieval of those separate aspects of knowledge occurs in a temporally correlated fashion. Nonetheless, as far as neural tissue is concerned, the retrieval takes place in a spatially segregated manner.[16] In a sense, the relevant neural sites can be said to contain conceptual knowledge, but it is important to emphasize that the explicit mental representation of concepts does not occur at those sites because of the *dispositional* nature of the records that maintain the knowledge (see later). Thus, the sites should not be seen as centers for conceptual knowledge. Rather, each site should be seen as part of a multicomponent system, each containing circuitry necessary for the process of optical concept retrieval. We do not believe that these neural sites contain either facsimile representations of entities or lexicographic definitions of the concepts for entities.

According to the theoretical framework we have been using with regard to the neural substrates of learning, memory, and sensorimotor processing,[23–26] we assume that conceptual knowledge is held in "dispositional" form (nonexplicit, nonmapped), in higher-order association cortices and subcortical nuclei, within circuitry with convergence–divergence connectional properties. The dispositional knowledge coded in convergence–divergence zones can be made explicit (in mapped form) in early sensory cortices as well as in motor structures. The recall of knowledge pertinent to a particular concept requires the activation of multiple convergence–divergence sites, which, in turn, direct the reconstruction of the explicit images which comprise the concept in the pertinent early sensory cortices. The activation of early sensory cortices is essential for the conscious processing of a concept to occur, although activation of the primary cortices within the set of early sensory cortices is not required.

In this perspective, we suggest that insofar as retrieval of conceptual and lexical knowledge is concerned, there are critical neural regions which play an *intermediary* or *mediational* role. Let us consider further the case of concept retrieval. When a stimulus depicting a given entity (say, a hammer) is shown to a subject, and the visual properties of that stimulus are processed, an intermediary region becomes active and promotes the explicit sensorimotor representation of knowledge pertaining to the hammer, which occurs in certain early sensory cortices and motor structures. For instance, sensory images would represent the typical action of the tool in space, its typical relationship to the hand and to other objects, the typical somatosensory and motor patterns associated with the handling of the tool, the sound characteristics associated with the tool's operation, and so on. The evocation of some part of the potentially large number of such images, over a brief lapse of time and in varied sensorimotor cortices, would constitute the conceptual evocation for the given tool. When a concept from another category is evoked—say, that of an animal or of a person—different intermediary regions would be engaged. This would provide the neural basis for the types of category-specific recognition impairments that have been reported in a number of lesion studies (as discussed in the section on temporal lobe damage, for instance), and for the category-related neural segregation that has been hinted at in recent functional imaging work.[33,73,90] However, the intermediary regions for conceptual knowledge retrieval do *not* contain in explicit form the concepts for various concrete entities, such as tools, persons, or animals.

Let us consider now the case of retrieval of lexical knowledge—specifically, the retrieval of a particular word that denotes a concrete entity. Again, we have suggested that certain neural regions play an intermediary or mediational role. For example, when the concept of a given tool (take a hammer again as an example) is evoked (based on the activation of regions which support pertinent conceptual knowledge and promote its explicit representation in sensorimotor terms, as described earlier), an intermediary region becomes active and promotes (in the appropriate sensorimotor structures) the explicit representation of phonemic knowledge pertaining to the word form which denotes the given tool. The process can operate in reverse to link word-form information to conceptual knowledge. Thus, one can go from the concept to the word form (as in seeing a picture of a hammer and retrieving the word "hammer") or from the word form to the concept (as in hearing "hammer" and retrieving the varied images of what a hammer is). In keeping with our comments on concept retrieval, we do not believe that the intermediary regions for lexical retrieval contain the names for entities in explicit form. Rather, they hold knowledge about how to reconstruct a certain pattern (e.g., the phonemic structure of a given word) in "explicit" form, within the appropriate sensorimotor structures. When concepts from differing categories are evoked—say, those of persons or those of animals—intermediary regions different from those related to word-form retrieval for the "tools" category are engaged (see Fig. 5–2).

Here we do not address the issue of the possible microstructure of the intermediary regions for conceptual and lexical knowledge retrieval. It is very important to reiterate, however, that we do not envision these regions as rigid "modules" or "centers." We see their structure and operation as flexible and modifiable by learning. An individual's learning experience of concepts of a similar kind (e.g., concepts of manipulable tools), or of the names for those concepts, leads to the recruitment, within the available neural architecture, of a critical set of spatially linked microcircuits. We presume that there is nothing random about the anatomical placement of the region within which the microcircuits are recruited for a certain range of items. The anatomical placement is, rather, the one best suited to permit the most effective preferential interaction, by means of feedforward and feedback projections, between the regions of cerebral cortex which subtend perception and represent explicitly the images which define pertinent conceptual knowledge and those required to represent explicitly the word-form knowledge which subserves the names for concrete entities. The number of microcircuits recruited to operate as intermediaries for a certain range of concepts or names would vary with the learning experience, and we would expect normal individuals to develop, under similar conditions, a similar type of large-scale architecture. We would also predict ample individual variation of microcircuitry within each key region and would expect that at different times the same individual would engage the same macroregions, but not necessarily the same microcircuitry within them.

Our working hypothesis is that there are two overriding reasons why retrieval of concepts or of names for different kinds of entities are correlated with different neural sites. One pertains to the overall physical characteristics of the entity in question, which has determined the sort of sensorimotor mapping generated during interactions between an organism and the entity as it was learned. The other pertains to the fine physical characteristics and contextual linkages of an entity, which permitted the mapping of unique items such as familiar persons. For instance, the multiple sensory channels (somatosensory, visual) and the hand motor patterns which are inherent in the conceptual description of the manipulable tool lead to the preferential recruitment, for the role of intermediary region, of a sector of cortex capable of receiving such multiple sensory signals and spatially close to regions involved in the processing of visual motion and hand motion.[36]

In short, intermediary systems process preferentially certain physical characteristics and contexts of entities. Because entities within a given conceptual category tend to share more of those characteristics than entities outside of it,[58,103,110,117] lesions at a particular site are more likely to impair the recognition of stimuli from that category rather than another. The situation is much the same in regard to the retrieval of lexical knowledge, for which we have suggested that principles similar to those articulated here have determined the placements of *lexical* intermediary regions.[33,116]

This work was supported by National Institute of Neurological Diseases and Stroke NINCDS grant PO1 NS19632.

REFERENCES

1. Albert, M L, Sparks, R and Helm, N: Melodic intonation therapy for aphasia. Arch Neurol 29:130–131, 1973.
2. Alexander, M P, and Loverme, S R Jr: Aphasia after left hemispheric intracerebral hemorrhage. Neurology 30:1193–1202, 1980.
3. Alexander, G E, Delong, M R and Strick, P L: Parallel organization of functionally segregated circuits linking basal ganglia and cortex. Annu Rev Neurosci 9:357–381, 1986.
4. Aran, D M, Rose, D F, Rekate, H L and Whitaker, H A: Acquired capsular/striatal aphasia in childhood. Arch Neurol 40:614–617, 1983.
5. Arguin, M, Bud, D and Dubek, G: Shape integration for visual object recognition and its implication in category-specific visual agnosia. Vis Cogni 3:221–275, 1996.
6. Arnold, S E, Hyman, B T, Flory, J, Damasio, A R and Van Hoesen, G W: The topographical neuroanatomical distribution of neurofibrillary tangles and neuritic plaques in the cerebral cortex of patients with Alzheimer's disease. Cereb Cortex 1:103–116, 1991.
7. Barat, M, Mazaux, J M, Bioulac, B, Giroire, J M, Vital, C and Arne, L: Troubles du langage de type aphasique et lesions putamino-caudees. Rev Neurol (Paris) 137(5):343–356, 1981.
8. Basso, A, Capitani, E and Vignolo, L: Influence of rehabilitation on language skills in aphasic patient: a controlled study. Arch Neurol 36:190–196, 1979.
9. Bellugi, V, Poizner, H and Klima, E S: Sign Language aphasia. Hum Neurobiol 2:155–170, 1983.
10. Benson, D F, Sheremata, W A, Bourchard, R, Segarra, J M, Price, D L and Geschwind, N: Conduction aphasia: a clinicopathological study. Arch Neurol 38:339–346, 1973.
11. Benton, A L and Hamsher, K: Multilingual Aphasia Examination. Iowa City: University of Iowa, 1983.
12. Berndt, R and Caramazza, A: A redefinition of the syndrome of Broca's aphasia: Implications for a neuropsychological model of language. Appl Psycholing 1:225–278, 1980.
13. Blumstein, S E, Cooper, W E, Zurif, E B and Caramazza, A: The perception and production of voice-onset time in aphasia. Neuropsychologia 15:371–383, 1977.
14. Bradley, D C, Garrett, M E and Zurif, E B: Syntactic deficits in Broca's aphasia. In CAPLAN, D (Ed.): Biological studies of mental processes. MIT Press, Cambridge, MA, 1980, pp. 269–286.

15. Brunner, R J, Kornhuber, H H, Seemuller, E, Suger, G and Wallesch, C W: Basal ganglia participation in language pathology. Brain Lang 16:281–299, 1982.
16. Buchel, C, Price, C and Friston, K: A multimodal language region in the ventral visual pathway. Nature 394:272–277, 1998.
17. Bunn, E M, Tyler, L K and Moss, H E: Category-specific semantic deficits: the role of familiarity and property type reexamined. Neuropsychology 12:367–379, 1998.
18. Caplan, D and Futter, F: Assignment of thematic roles to nouns in sentence comprehension by an agrammatic patient. Brain Lang 27:117–134, 1986.
19. Caramazza, A and Hillis, A: Lexical organization of nouns and verbs in the brain. Nature 349:788–790, 1991.
20. Culton, G: Spontaneous recovery from aphasia. J Speech Hear Disord 12:825–832, 1969.
21. Damasio, A, Damasio, H, Rizzo, M, Varney, N and Gersh, F: Aphasia with non-hemorrhagic lesions in the basal ganglia and internal capsule. Arch Neurol 39:15–20, 1982.
22. Damasio, A R: Time-locked multiregional retroactivation: a systems-level proposal for the neural substrates of recall and recognition. Cognition 33:25–62, 1989.
23. Damasio, A R: Concepts in the brain. Mind Lang 4:24–28, 1989.
24. Damasio, A R: Category-related recognition defects as a clue to the neural substrates of knowledge. Trends Neurosci 13:95–98, 1990.
25. Damasio, A R and Damasio, H: Cortical systems underlying knowledge retrieval: Evidence from human lesion studies. In Poggio, T A and Glaser, D A (Eds.): Exploring brain functions: models in neuroscience. Wiley, New York, 1993, pp. 233–248.
26. Damasio, A R and Damasio, H: Cortical systems for retrieval of concrete knowledge: The convergence zone framework. In Koch, C (Ed.): Large-scale neuronal theories of the brain. MIT Press, Cambridge, MA, 1994, pp. 61–74.
27. Damasio, A R and Tranel, D: Nouns and verbs are retrieved with differently distributed neural systems. Proc Natl Acad Sci U S A 90:4957–4960, 1993.
28. Damasio, A R, Damasio, H and Van Hoesen, G W: Prosopagnosia: anatomic basis and behavioral mechanisms. Neurology 32:331–341, 1982.
29. Damasio, A R, Damasio, H, Tranel, D and Brandt, J P: Neural regionalization of knowledge access. Symposia on Quantitative Biology, Vol. 55. Cold Spring Harbor Laboratory Press, 1990, pp. 1039–1047.
30. Damasio H: Anatomical and neuroimaging contributions to the study of aphasia. In Goodglass, H (Ed.): Handbook of Neuropsychology, Vol. 1. Language. Elsevier, Amsterdam, 1987, pp. 3–46.
31. Damasio, H and Damasio, A: Lesion Analysis in Neuropsychology, Oxford University Press, New York, 1989.
32. Damasio, H, Eslinger, P and Adams, H P: Aphasia following basal ganglia lesions: new evidence. Semin Neurol 4:151–161, 1984.
33. Damasio, H, Grabowski, T J, Tranel, D, Hichwa, R D and Damasio, A R: A neural basis for lexical retrieval. Nature 380:499–505, 1996.
34. Daniele, A, Giustolisi, L, Silveri, M C, Colosimo, C and Gainotti, G: Evidence for a possible neuroanatomical basis for lexical processing of nouns and verbs. Neuropsychologia 32:1325–1341, 1994.
35. De Renzi, E and Lucchelli, F: Are semantic systems separately represented in the brain? The case of living category impairment. Cortex 30:3–25, 1994.
36. Decenty, J, Perani, D, Jeannerod, M, Bettinardi, V, Tadary, B, Woods, R, Mazziotta, J and Fazio, F: Mapping motor representations with positron emission tomography. Nature 371: 600–602, 1994.
37. Demeurisse, G, Demol, O, Derouck, M, de Beuckelaer, R, Coekaerts, M J and Capon, A: Quantitative study of the rate of recovery from aphasia due to ischemic stroke. Stroke 11:455–460, 1980.
38. Frith, C D, Friston, K J, Liddle, P F and Frackowiak, R S J: A PET study of word finding. Neuropsychologia 29:1137–1148, 1991.

39. Fromm, D, Holland, A L, Swindell, C S and Reinmuth, O M: Various consequences of subcortical stroke. Arch Neurol 42:943–950, 1985.

40. Galaburda, A M and Pandya, D N: The intrinsic architectonic and connectional organization of the superior temporal region of the rhesus monkey. J Comp Neurol 221:169–84, 1983.

41. Gardner, H, Brownell, H H, Wapner, W and Michelow, D: Missing the point: the role of the right hemisphere in the processing of complex linguistic materials. In Perecman, E (Ed.): Cognitive processing in the right hemisphere. Academic Press, New York, 1983, pp. 169–191.

42. Geschwind, N: Disconnexion syndromes in animals and man. Brain 88:237–294, 1965.

43. Gleason, J B, Goodglass, H, Green, E, Ackerman, N and Hyde, M R: The retrieval of syntax in Broca's aphasia. Brain Lang 2:451–471, 1975.

44. Goldman-Rakic, P: Topography of cognition: parallel distributed networks in primate association cortex. Annu Rev Neurosci 11:137–156, 1988.

45. Goodglass, H and Kaplan, E: The assessment of aphasia and related disorders. Philadelphia: Lea and Febiger, 1972 (2nd Ed. 1982).

46. Goodglass, H, Christiansen, J A and Gallagher, R E: Syntactic constructions used by agrammatic speakers: comparison with conduction aphasics and normals. Neuropsychology 8:598–613, 1994.

47. Goodglass, H, Wingfield, A, Hyde, M R and Theurkauf, J: Category specific dissociations in naming and recognition by aphasic patients. Cortex 22:87–102, 1986.

48. Graff-Radford, N, Damasio, H, Yamada, T, Eslinger, P and Damasio, A: Nonhemorrhagic thalamic infarctions: clinical, neurophysiological and electrophysiological findings in four anatomical groups defined by CT. Brain 108:485–516, 1985.

49. Graff-Radford, N R, Damasio, A R, Hyman, B T, Hart, M N, Tranel, D, Damasio, H, Van Hoesen, G W and Revai, K: Progressive aphasia in a patient with Pick's disease: a neuropsychological, radiologic and anatomic study. Neurology 40:620–626, 1990.

50. Grodzinsky, Y: The syntactic characterization of agrammatism. Cognition 16:99–120, 1984.

51. Habib, M, Démonet, J-F and Frackowiak, R:Neuroanatomic cognitive du langage: contribution de l'imagerie fonctionnelle cérébrale. Rev Neurol (Paris) 152:249–260, 1996.

52. Helm-Estabrooks, N and Ramsberger, G: Treatment of agrammatism in six long-term aphasic patients. Br J Disord Commun 21:39–45, 1986.

53. Helm-Estabrooks, N, Fitzpatrick, P and Barresi, B: Visual action therapy for global aphasia. J Speech Hear Disord 47:385–389, 1982.

54. Hillis, A E and Caramazza, A: Category-specific naming and comprehension impairment: a double dissociation. Brain 114:2081–2094, 1991.

55. Holland, A L: Communication Abilities in Daily Living. University Park Press, Baltimore, 1980.

56. Holland, A L: Recovery in aphasia. In Boller, F and Grafman, J (Eds.): Handbook of Neuropsychology, Vol. 2. Elsevier, Amsterdam, 1989, pp. 83–90.

57. Holland, A L, Fromm, D, Greenhouse, J B and Swindell, C S: Predictors of language restitution following stroke: a multivariate analysis. J Speech Hear Res 32:232–238, 1990.

58. Humphreys, G W, Riddoch, M J and Price, C J: Top-down processes in object identification: evidence from experimental psychology, neuropsychology and functional anatomy. Philos Trans R Soc Lond Biol, 352:1275–1282, 1997.

59. Katz, R B and Goodglass, H: Deep dysphasia: analysis of a rate type of repetition disorder. Brain Lang 39:153–185, 1990.

60. Kean, M L: The linguistic interpretation of aphasic syndromes: agrammatism in Broca's aphasia, an example. Cognition 5:9–46, 1977.

61. Kertesz, A: Aphasia and Associated Disorders. Grune & Stratton, New York, 1979.

62. Kertesz, A: Recovery and treatment. In Heilman, K M and Valenstein, E (Eds.): Clinical Neuropsychology, 3rd Ed. Oxford University Press, New York, 1993, pp. 647–674.

63. Kertesz, A and McCabe, P: Recovery patterns and prognosis in aphasia. Brain 100:1–18, 1977.
64. Kertesz, A, Harlock, W and Coates, R: Computer tomographic localization, lesion size, and prognosia in aphasia and nonverbal impairment. Brain Lang 8:34–50, 1979.
65. Kertesz, A, Hudson, L, Mackenzie, I R and Munoz, D G: The pathology and nosology of primary progressive aphasia. Neurology 44:2065–2072, 1994.
66. Knopman, D S, Selnes, O A, Niccum, N and Rubens, A B: Recovery of naming in aphasia: relationship to fluency, comprehension and CT findings. Neurology 34:1461–1470, 1984.
67. Laplane, D, Talsirach, J and Meininger, V: Clinical consequences of corticectomies involving the supplementary motor area in man. J Neurol Sci 34:301–314, 1977.
68. Lecours, A R and Lhermitte, F: The "pure form" of the phonetic disintegration syndrome (pure anarthria): anatomo-clinical report of a historical case. Brain Lang 3:88–113, 1976.
69. Lesser, R and Gordon, B: Electrical stimulation and language. J Clin Neuropscyhol 11: 191–204, 1994.
70. Levine, D N and Mohr, J P: Language after bilateral cerebral infarctions: role of the minor hemisphere in speech. Neurology 29:927–938, 1979.
71. Luders, H, Lesser, R P, Hahn, J, Dinner, D S, Morris, H H, Wyllie, E and Godoy, J: Basal temporal language area. Brain 114:743–754, 1991.
72. Marin, O S M, Saffran, E M and Schwartz, M F: Dissociations of language in aphasia: implications for normal functions. Ann N Y Acad Sci 280:868–884, 1976.
73. Martin, A, Wiggs, C L, Ungerleider, L G and Haxby, J V: Neural correlates of category-specific knowledge. Nature 379:649–652, 1996.
74. Mazoyer, B M, Tzourio, N, Frak, V, Syrota, A, Murayama, N, Levrier, O, Salamon, G, Dehaene, S, Cohen, L and Mehler, J: The cortical representation of speech. J Cog Neurosci 5:467–479, 1993.
75. McCarthy, R A and Warrington, E K: Evidence for modality-specific meaning systems in the brain. Nature 334:428–430, 1988.
76. Mesulam, M-M: Slowly progressive aphasia without generalized dementia. Ann Neurol 11:592–598, 1982.
77. Miceli, G, Mazzucchi, A, Menn, L and Goodglass, H: Contrasting cases of Italian agrammatic aphasia without comprehension disorder. Brain Lang 19:65–97, 1983.
78. Miozzo, A, Soardi, S and Cappa, S F: Pure anomia with spared action naming due to a left temporal lesion. Neuropsychologia 32:1101–1109, 1994.
79. Mohr, J P, Pessin, M S, Finkelstein, S, Funkenstein, H H, Duncan, G W and Davis, K R: Broca's aphasia: pathologic and clinical. Neurology 28:311–324, 1978.
80. Mohr, J P, Watters, W C and Duncan, G W: Thalamic hemorrhage and aphasia. Brain Lang 2:3–17, 1975.
81. Myerson, R and Goodglass, H: Transformational grammars of three agrammatic patients. Lang Speech 15:40–50, 1972.
82. Naeser, M: A sentence level auditory comprehension (SLAC) treatment program for adult aphasics with language comprehension deficits. Arch Phys Med Rehabil 67:393–399, 1986.
83. Naeser, M A, and Hayward, R W: Lesion localization in aphasia with cranial computed tomography and the Boston Diagnostic Aphasia Exam. Neurology 28:545–551, 1978.
84. Naeser, M A, Alexander, M P, Helm-Estabrooks, N, Levine, H L, Laughlin, S A and Geschwind, N: Aphasia with predominantly subcortical lesion sites. Arch Neurol 39:2–14, 1982.
85. Nobre, A C, Allison, T and McCarthy, G: Word recognition in the human inferior temporal lobe. Nature 372:260–263, 1994.
86. Ojemann, G A: Brain organization for language from the perspective of electrical stimulation mapping. Behav Brain Sci 189:230, 1983.
87. Ojemann, G A: Cortical organization of language. J Neurosci 11:2281–2287, 1991.
88. Pashek, G V and Holland, A L: Evolution of aphasia in the first year post onset. Cortex 24:411–423, 1988.

89. Penfield, W and Roberts, L: Speech and Brain Mechanisms. Princeton University Press, Princeton, NJ, 1959.

90. Perani, D, Cappa, S F, Bettinardi, V, Bressi, S, Gorno-Tempini, M, Matarrese, M and Fazio, F: Different neual systems for the recognition of animals and man-made tools. Neuroreport 6:1637–1641, 1995.

91. Petersen, S E, Fox, T P, Posner, M I, Mintun, M and Raichle, M E: Positron emission tomographic studies of the cortical anatomy of single-word processing. Nature 331:585–589, 1988.

92. Pickersgill, M N and Lincoln, N B: Prognostic indicators and the pattern of recovery of communication in aphasic stroke patients. J Neurol Neurosurg Psychiatry 46:130–139, 1983.

93. Porch, B E: Porch Index of Communicative Ability. Consulting Psychologists Press, Palo Alto, CA, 1971.

94. Ross, E D and Mesulam, M-M: Dominant language functions of the right hemispheres? Prosody and emotional gesturing. Arch Neurol 36:144–148, 1979.

95. Rubens, A: The role of changes within the central nervous system during recovery from aphasia. In Sullivan, M A and Kommers, M S (Eds.): Rationale for Adult Aphasia Therapy. University of Nebraska Medical Center, Lincoln, NE, 1977, pp. 28–43.

96. Rubens, A and Selnes, O: Aphasia with insular cortex infarction. Proceedings of the Academy of Aphasia Meeting, Nashville, 1986.

97. Saffran, E M, Schwartz, M F and Marin, O S M: The word order problem in agrammatism. II. Production. Brain Lang 10:263–280, 1980.

98. Saffran, E M, Schwartz, M F and Marin, O S M: Evidence from aphasia: isolating the components of a production model. In Butterworth, B (Ed.): Language Production. Academic Press, London, 1980, pp. 221–241.

99. Sarno, M T: The Functional Communication Profile. New York University Press, New York, 1969.

100. Sarno, M T and Levita, E: Natural courses of recovery in severe aphasia. Arch Phys Med Rehabil 52:175–178, 1971.

101. Sartori, G, Job, R, Miozzo, M, Zago, S and Marchiori, G: Category-specific form-knowledge deficit in a patient with herpes simplex virus encephalitis. J Clin Exp Neuropsychol 15:280–299, 1993.

102. Schiff, H B, Alexander, M P, Naeser, M A and Galaburda, A M: Aphemia: clinic-anatomic correlations. Arch Neurol 40:720–727, 1983.

103. Schlaghecken, F: On processing BEASTS and BIRDS: an event-related potential study on the representation of taxonomic structure. Brain Lang 64:53–82, 1998.

104. Schwartz, M F, Marin, O S M and Saffran, E M: Dissociations of language function in dementia: a case study. Brain Lang 7:277–306, 1979.

105. Selnes, O A, Knopman, D S, Niccum, N and Rubens, A B: The critical role of Wernicke's area in sentence repetition. Arch Neurol 17:549–557, 1985.

106. Selnes, O A, Knopman, D S, Niccum, N, Rubens, A B and Larson, D: Computed tomographic scan correlates of auditory comprehension deficits in aphasia: a prospective recovery study. Arch Neurol 13:558–566, 1983.

107. Selnes, O A, Niccum, N, Knopman, D S and Rubens, A B: Recovery of single word comprehension: CT scan correlates. Brain Lang 21:72–84, 1984.

108. Semenza, C and Zettin, M: Evidence from aphasia for the role of proper names as pure referring expressions. Nature 342: 678–679, 1989.

109. Silveri, M C and Gainotti, G B: Interaction between vision and language in category specific semantic access impairment. Cognit Neuropsychol 5:677–709, 1988.

110. Small, S L, Hart, J, Nguyen, T and Gordon, B: Distributed representations of semantic knowledge in the brain. Brain 118:441–453, 1995.

111. Spitzer, M, Kischka, U, Guckel, F, Bellemann, M E, Kammer, T, Seyyedi, S, Weisbrod,

M, Schwartz, A and Brix, G: Functional magnetic resonance imaging of category-specific cortical activation: evidence for semantic maps. Cognit Brain Res 6:309–319, 1998.

112. Spreen, O and Benton, A L: Neurosensory Center Comprehension Examination for Aphasia, 2nd Ed. University of Victoria, Victoria, British Columbia, 1977.

113. Tonkonogy, J and Goodglass, H: Language function, foot of the third frontal gyrus, and rolandic operculum. Arch Neurol 38:486–490, 1981.

114. Tranel, D, Biller, J, Damasio, H, Adams, H and Cornell, S: Global aphasia without hemiparesis. Arch Neurol 44:304–308, 1987.

115. Tranel, D, Damasio, H and Damasio, A R: A neural basis for the retrieval of conceptual knowledge. Neuropsychologia 35:1319–1327, 1997.

116. Tranel, D, Damasio, H and Damasio, A R: On the neurology of naming. In Goodglass, H and Wingfield, A (Eds.): Anomia: Neuroanatomical and Cognitive Correlates. Academic Press, New York, 1997, pp. 67–92.

117. Tranel, D, Logan, C G, Frank, R J and Damasio, A R: Explaining category-related effects in the retrieval of conceptual and lexical knowledge for concrete entities: operationalization and analysis of factors. Neuropsychologia 35:1329–1339, 1997.

118. Tucker, D M, Watson, R T and Heilman, K B:Affective discrimination and evocation in patients with right parietal disease. Neurology 17:947–950, 1977.

119. Vignolo, A: Evolution of aphasia and language rehabilitation: a retrospective exploratory study. Cortex 1:344–367, 1964.

120. Vignolo, L A, Boccardi, E and Caverni, L: Unexpected CT scan findings in global aphasia. Cortex 22:55–69, 1986.

121. Wade, D T, Hewer, R L, David, R M and Enderby, P M: Aphasia after stroke: natural history and associated deficits. J Neuol Neurosurg Psychiatry 49:11–16, 1986.

122. Warrington, E K and McCarthy, R A: Multiple meaning systems in the brain: a case for visual semantics. Neuropsychologia 32:1465–1473, 1994.

123. Warrington, E K and Shallice, T: Category specific semantic impairments. Brain 107:829–853, 1984.

124. Weintraub, S, Rubin, N P and Mesulam, M-M: Primary progressive aphasia: longitudinal course, neuropsychological profile, and language features. Arch Neurol 47:1329–1335, 1990.

125. Wernicke, C: Der aphasische symptomencomplex. Cohn and Weigert, Breslau, 1874.

126. Wise, R, Chollet, F, Hadar, U, Friston, K, Hoffner, E and Frackowiak, R: Distribution of cortical neural networks involved in word comprehension and word retrieval. Brain 114:1803–1817, 1991.

127. Yeterian, E H and Van Hoesen, G W: Cortico-striate projections in the rhesus monkey. I. The organization of certain cortico-caudite projections. Brain Res 139: 43–63, 1978.

6

Affective Prosody and the Aprosodias

Elliott D. Ross

I. Introduction

Following the seminal discoveries of Broca[18] and Wernicke[106] that focal left hemisphere lesions may cause profound deficits of language, neurological studies of human communication have, for the most part, focused on left hemisphere injury and resultant aphasias. These studies have led to the widely held belief that the left hemisphere has an overall dominant role in human language and behavior.[3,7,84] However, over the last 25 years, considerable evidence has emerged to support the concept that communication functions are subserved by both hemispheres.[13–15,17,36,40,47,51–53,70,72,80,84,88,93,97,98,105] This chapter focuses on the dominant contributions of the right hemisphere to human language, specifically the affective–prosodic and gestural aspects of communication. Other potential right hemisphere functions, such as inference, decoding of thematic content and intent, connotation (nonstandard word meaning), and the comprehension of nonliteral phrases and complex linguistic relationships,[20,21,43,99,101,103,108] will not be covered.

Communication through the medium of language is based on four major constituents: lexicon (vocabulary), syntax (grammar), prosody, and kinesics. The smallest articulated feature of language is known as a segment, which is closely aligned to the syllable.[57,59] Segments are the primary phonetic building blocks for words, which form the lexicon. Words, in turn, are concatenated according to grammatical relationships into phrases and sentences. These features of language, also known as the linguistic or propositional elements, are severely impaired by focal left brain injury. The ensuing combinations of language disturbances give rise to the various aphasic syndromes reviewed in Chapter 5.[7]

Prosody and kinesics constitute the paralinguistic elements of language and play an equally prominent role in the organization of human communication and discourse.[10] The right hemisphere appears to exert a major influence on the organization of these paralinguistic functions. Prosody is a suprasegmental feature of language that conveys information beyond that transmitted by word choice and word order alone.[10,28,57,66,98,100] The acoustic features associated with prosody include pitch, intonation, melody, cadence, loudness, timbre, tempo, stress, accent, and timing of pauses.[27,28,41,57–59] Modulation of prosodic elements appears to precede the emergence of phonetic segmentation during the early acquisition and development of human language.[27,62]

Kinesics refers to limb, body, and facial movements that normally accompany discourse and serve to modulate the verbal message being communicated.[26] Movements that are used to express mutually agreed-upon symbols, such as the "V" for victory, are classified as pantomime since they convey specific semantic information, whereas movements used to color, emphasize, and embellish speech are classified as gestures.[26,56] Spontaneous kinesic activity associated with discourse usually represents a mixture of gestures and pantomime.

II. Neurology of Prosody

The first systematic inquiry into the neurology of prosody was initiated by Monrad-Krohn.[65,66] During World War II he cared for a native Norwegian woman who sustained a shrapnel wound to the left frontal area, causing an acute Broca's aphasia. The woman made an excellent recovery except for a lingering alteration in her normal accent; this caused her great emotional distress during the Nazi occupation since she was consistently mistaken for being German and was, consequently, socially ostracized. Her speech was reported to have preserved melody, as evidenced by her ability to sing, intone, and emote. The acquired foreign accent was due to an altered application of stresses and pauses to the articulatory-line.

Based on this patient and others, Monrad-Krohn[65] divided prosody into four basic types. "Intrinsic" (linguistic) prosody is used to clarify the meaning of a sentence by the proper distribution of intonation, stresses, and pauses, which are equivalent to the application of commas, colons, semicolons, periods, and question marks in written language. Examples include raising instead of lowering the intonation contour at the end of a sentence to indicate a question and changing the stress and pausal pattern to clarify potentially ambiguous semantic or syntactic information. For instance *"The **Red**coats have arrived"* (British regulars) versus *"The red . . . **coats** have arrived"* (red-colored coats) or *"A man . . . and a **woman** dressed in formal attire . . . came to party"* (only the woman was wearing formal clothes) versus *"A **man** and **woman** . . . dressed in formal attire . . . came to the party"* (both were dressed in formal clothes).[28,98,100] Dialectal and idiosyncratic prosody are also to some degree subsumed by the term "intrinsic prosody" and refer to regional and individual differences in enunciation, pronunciation, stresses, and pausal patterns of speech. "Intellectual" prosody imparts attitudinal information to discourse and may drastically influence meaning. For example, if the sentence *"He is clever"* is emphatically stressed on **"is,"** it becomes a resounding acknowledgment of the person's ability, whereas if the emphatic stress resides on **"clever"** with a marked rise in intonation, sarcasm becomes apparent. "Emotional" prosody inserts moods and emotions, such as happiness, sadness, fear, and anger, into speech. The term "affective prosody" refers to the combination of attitudinal and emotional prosody. When coupled with gestures, affective prosody imparts vitality to discourse and greatly influences the content and impact of the message. If a statement contains an affective–prosodic intent that is at variance with its literal meaning, the former usually takes precedence in the interpretation of the message both in adults and to a lesser degree in children.[1,9,14,32,64] For example, if the sentence *"I had a really great day"* is spoken with an ironic tone of voice, it will be understood as communicating an intent opposite to its linguistic meaning. The paralinguistic features of language, as exemplified by affective prosody, may thus play an even more important role in human communication than the exact choice of words.[10] "Inarticulate" prosody refers to the use of certain paralinguistic elements, such as grunts and sighs, to embellish discourse.

Monrad-Krohn[66] also described various clinical disorders of prosody. "Dysprosody" is a change in voice quality that in some patients gives rise to a foreign accent syndrome. It is encountered primarily in patients who have recovered from nonfluent aphasias and is, therefore, usually associated with left hemisphere lesions. Dysprosody impairs the articulatory aspects of speech related to enunciation, pronunciation, and intonation but may leave affective prosody relatively intact. "Aprosody" denotes a constriction in the modulation of intonation that is commonly encountered in Parkinson's disease as part of the bradykinesia, masked facies, and hypophonia. "Hyperprosody" refers to the excessive use of prosody. This phenomenon is often observed in mania or in some patients with Broca's aphasia who have very few words at their disposal but use those words with excessive prosodic variation to communicate emotional distress. Monrad-Krohn predicted that disorders of prosodic comprehension should be encountered in brain-damaged patients. However, he did not assign any special role for the right hemisphere in modulating prosody.

III. NEUROLOGY OF KINESICS

Disturbances in the production and comprehension of pantomime have been firmly linked to left brain damage.[23,33,35,42,45,50,91] Goodglass and Kaplan[50] proposed that aphasics with comprehension deficits would have problems comprehending pantomime whereas nonfluent aphasics with preserved comprehension would have problems producing pantomime because of ideomotor apraxia. Other investigators, however, have failed to show such a tight correlation between pantomime disturbances and specific linguistic deficits.[23,35,42]

The neurology of gestures has not been studied in much detail. Anecdotal reports have mentioned that gestural activity is often preserved in aphasic patients.[26,56] Ross and Mesulam[84] observed that lesions of the right frontal operculum may not only cause loss of spontaneous affective prosody but also loss of spontaneous gestural activity in the face and limbs even in the absence of ideomotor apraxia. They suggested that gesture (as opposed to pantomime) is dominantly modulated by the right hemisphere. Since then a number of studies have lent further support to this hypothesis by showing that the right hemisphere is not only specialized for producing gestures but also for comprehending their meaning.[6,11,12,16,24,34,51,72]

IV. THE APROSODIAS

A series of clinical studies have shown that focal damage to the right hemisphere selectively impairs the production, comprehension, and repetition of affective prosody without disrupting the propositional elements of language.[14,15,30,51–53,72,84,88,97] Although Hughlings-Jackson[56] had suggested over a hundred years ago that the right hemisphere may have a dominant role in communicating emotion, the first modern study of affective prosody was not published until 1975—by Heilman and co-workers.[53] They assessed the ability of patients with unilateral retro-Rolandic lesions to recognize the affective content of otherwise linguistically neutral statements spoken with various emotional intonations. Right brain-damaged patients were markedly impaired on the task when compared to normals or left brain-damaged patients, some of whom were mildly aphasic. In a follow-up study, Tucker and associates[97] found that right but not left hemisphere lesions impaired the ability to insert affective variation into verbally neutral sentences both on request and on a repetition task.

In 1979, Ross and Mesulam[84] described two patients with infarctions involving the right anterior supraSylvian region as documented by computed tomographic (CT) imaging. Neither patient was aphasic or apraxic. However, they could not insert affect into their voice or produce spontaneous gestures during discourse. These changes in behavior caused them to experience significant psychosocial difficulties.[73,76,84] One patient was a school teacher who could no longer discipline her class because she was unable to project anger in her voice and gestures to let the children know she was displeased with them. The second patient was a retired physician whose wife eventually sought divorce because he no longer spoke to her in solicitous tones and was perceived as being "nasty." Both patients were able to interpret affective displays in others and reported the ability to feel and experience emotions inwardly. Based on these patients and previous publications by Heilman and co-workers,[53,97] it was hypothesized that the right hemisphere plays a dominant role in modulating affective prosody and gestures and that the functional–anatomic organization of these aspects of language in the right hemisphere is analogous to the functional–anatomic organization of propositional language in the left hemisphere.

The anatomic organization of affective prosody and gesture was further investigated by Ross[72] in ten patients with focal right brain damage. The patients were examined at the bedside for specific deficits in processing affective prosody as described below in Section V. Specific patterns of deficits were encountered that appeared analogous to the functional–anatomic patterns of aphasic deficits[7] observed after focal brain damage in the left hemisphere. The various syndromes of impaired affective communication were called "**aprosodias**" and the same modifiers as those used in the aphasias[7] were applied for classification purposes (Table 6–1). The val-

TABLE 6-1 Classification of the Aprosodia*

Type of Aprosodia	AFFECTIVE PROSODY			GESTURES	
	Spontaneous	Repetition	Comprehension	Spontaneous	Comprehension
Motor	Poor	Poor	Good	Poor	Good
Sensory	Good	Poor	Poor	Good	Poor
Conduction	Good	Poor	Good	Good	Good
Global	Poor	Poor	Poor	Poor	Poor
Transcortical motor	Poor	Good	Good	Poor	Good
Transcortical sensory	Good	Good	Poor	Good	Poor
Agesic	Good	Good	Good	Good	Poor
Mixed transcortical	Poor	Good	Poor	Poor	Poor

*Agestic aprosodia has recently been described by Bowers and Heilman.[16] Motor, sensory, global, and transcortical sensory aprosodias have good anatomical correlation with lesions in the left hemisphere known to cause analogous aphasias.

idation of this classification was supported by a subsequent study by Gorelick and Ross[51] in which the investigators classified the aprosodic deficits based on audiotape recordings without knowing the CT location of the lesions and mapped the CT lesions without knowing the results of the clinical classifications. This study also found that the incidence of aprosodia following right brain damage was equal to that of aphasia following left brain damage, thus underscoring that the aprosodias are common rather than esoteric syndromes.

Most recently, Ross and co-workers[85] studied 15 patients under the age of 72 years with unilateral ischemic infarctions of the right hemisphere that were predominantly cortical in distribution based on magnetic resonance imaging (MRI) scans. The patients were examined 3–6 weeks after suffering a stroke and classified into those with normal versus impaired spontaneous affective prosody and those with normal versus impaired comprehension of affective prosody in a manner that parallels the classification of aphasic patients on the basis of fluency and comprehension.[7] The distribution of each cortical lesion was overlapped on a template of the right hemisphere as shown in Figure 6–1. Patients with impaired spontaneous affective prosody had lesions involving (but not confined to) the posterior–inferior frontal lobe which included the pars opercularis and triangularis, a region similar in location to Broca's area in the left hemisphere. All patients with impaired comprehension of affective prosody had cortical lesions involving (but not confined to) the posterior–superior temporal lobe, a region similar in location to Wernicke's area in the left hemisphere. This finding is in agreement with three other studies in the literature reporting that comprehension of affective prosody depends on the integrity of the right posterior temporoparietal operculum.[30,36,95] Although many of the patients had extensions of their predominantly cortical lesions to involve deep ganglionic structures, no consistent functional–anatomic relationships were found to support the suggestion that aprosodic deficits were predominantly due to subcortical involvement.[22]

Thus, current evidence supports the hypothesis that the functional–anatomic

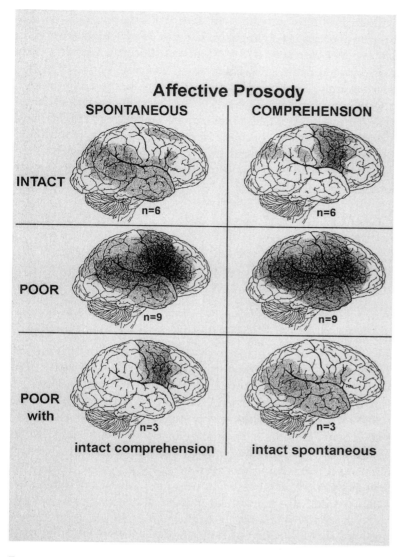

FIGURE 6–1. Cortical distribution of ischemic strokes observed on magnetic resonance imaging (MRI) scan in 15 right brain-damaged patients sorted by affective-prosodic performance.[85]

correlates of the aprosodias in the right hemisphere are analogous, in a general sense, to the functional–anatomic correlates of propositional language in the left hemisphere. Frontal opercular lesions are likely to impair the spontaneous production of affective prosody whereas posterior temporoparietal lesions are likely to impair comprehension of affective prosody. However, functional–anatomic relationships that do not fit this pattern have been encountered in elderly patients.[85] It is important to keep in mind that equally aberrant patterns of language dysfunction have also been described in elderly patients with left hemisphere lesions causing aphasias.[4,25,54,69] Subcortical lesions involving basal ganglionic structures in the right hemisphere may also produce aprosodias[51,72,82,109] just as subcortical lesions in the left hemisphere may produce aphasias.[2,29,67] There have been case reports of crossed aprosodia in which a strongly right-handed patient becomes aprosodic but not aphasic following a left hemisphere stroke,[78] similar to cases of crossed aphasia in which a strongly right-handed patient becomes aphasic following a right hemisphere stroke. Acquired aprosodias in children[5,96] and developmental disorders of affective prosody associated with early right brain damage[63,102,104] have been reported. These syndromes tend to be comparable to the syndromes of acquired aphasia and developmental dyslexia in children.

V. CLINICAL EXAMINATION OF AFFECTIVE PROSODY AND GESTURE

Clinicians can readily incorporate into their bedside examination an assessment for aprosodia similar to an assessment for aphasia.[72]

Production of Spontaneous Affective Prosody and Gesturing

During the interview observations are made to ascertain whether the patient imparts affect into spontaneous conversation through gestures and prosody. One should ask emotionally loaded questions about current illness and past experiences. Attention should be directed to the modulation of intonation, rather than to changes in loudness, to determine if emotional coloring is present in the patient's discourse and if it fits the verbal content. Patients with right hemisphere lesions may display inappropriate verbal jocularity ("dry humor") concerning their neurological deficits that should be differentiated from impairments in affective prosody. Elements of intrinsic (linguistic) prosody, such as stresses, pauses, and simple modulation of intonation, such as the terminal rise in pitch to indicate a question, may be preserved in a patient who is otherwise unable to produce affective prosody. Patients with impaired comprehension of affective prosody may produce prolific but inappropriate affective prosody similar to aphasic patients who have fluent but paraphasic speech. These patients may appear inappropriately euphoric regardless of the topic under discussion.

Repetition of Affective Prosody

A declarative sentence, free of emotional words, is produced by the examiner using a happy, sad, tearful, disinterested, angry, or surprised tone of voice. The examiner immediately asks the patient to repeat the sentence with the same affective intonation. Performance should be judged on how well the patient imitates the affective tone of the examiner. Raising or lowering the overall loudness of the voice, slightly raising the voice at the end of a statement to indicate a question rather than surprise, or producing the incorrect affective tone should be marked as errors.

Comprehension of Affective Prosody

The examiner utters a declarative statement, free of emotional words, using different affective intonations and asks the patient to either name the underlying emotion or identify it from a list containing five choices. The examiner stands behind the patient during this assessment to avoid giving the patient visual clues through gestural behaviors.

Comprehension of Gestures

This is accomplished by standing in front of the patient and conveying a particular affective state or attitude using only gestural activity involving the face and limbs. The patient is requested to either verbally identify the emotion or, if necessary, choose the correct answer from a list of five choices.

VI. HEMISPHERIC LATERALIZATION OF AFFECTIVE PROSODY AND CALLOSAL INTEGRATION OF LANGUAGE FUNCTIONS

The terms "dominant" and "lateralized" brain functions are often used interchangeably in the literature although they have overlapping but different neurological implications.[88] A brain function is considered dominant if a unilateral lesion produces a behavioral deficit that subtends both sides of space,[37,38] a criterion easily met by the various aphasic and aprosodic syndromes. For a function to be strongly lateralized, however, it must also be shown that the behavioral deficit does not occur following lesions of the opposite hemisphere. In this regard, soon after his initial discovery that damage to the left third frontal convolution caused loss of articulate speech,[18] Broca[19] reported that similar lesions in the right hemisphere did not impair articulate speech, thus establishing that articulation was a dominant and lateralized function of the left hemisphere.[60] The extent to which affective prosody is lateralized has been more difficult to establish. Some authors have incorrectly assumed that all prosodic systems, including intinsic, affective, and dialectal, are modulated exclusively by the right hemisphere without realizing that the neurological literature makes such claims only for affective prosody.[74,89] However, some publications[22,31,88,90,92] have reported considerable disturbances in the production and comprehension of affective prosody after left brain injury, suggesting that the control of affective prosody may not be as strongly lateralized as that of propositional language.

De Bleser and Poeck,[31] for example, reported loss of affective prosody following left hemisphere lesions. They examined prosodic intonation in global aphasics whose speech output was restricted to one or two recurring syllables. They found stereotypic rather than modulated intonations, bringing into question the validity of Hughlings-Jackson's[56] observation that severely aphasic patients are able to communicate intent through heightened emotional modulation of otherwise impoverished speech. Furthermore, Schlanger and colleagues[90] found that aphasic patients with left hemisphere injury could not decode affective prosody, an observation that ran counter to the original studies by Heilman and co-workers.[53] This discrepancy is most likely attributable to differences in the clinical populations studied. Heilman and associates[53] assessed patients with relatively preserved comprehension whereas Schlanger and colleagues[90] assessed patients with severe deficits in verbal comprehension. In fact, Seron and co-workers[91] reported a significant positive correlation between comprehension of affective prosody and comprehension of propositional language in aphasic patients, suggesting that left hemisphere lesions which impair comprehension may also impair the decoding of affective prosody. However, other explanations for these discrepant findings are possible.[74,88]

The production of speech is likely to entail considerable interhemispheric interaction in order to ensure that the articulatory–verbal and affective–prosodic elements achieve behavioral unification and temporal coherence.[82,94] As a paralinguistic feature of speech, affective prosody is, per force, embedded into and carried by the articulatory line.[28,44] For example, if a speaker wishes to express surprise when uttering a simple sentence such as *"He is clever,"* the right hemisphere must be appraised by the left hemisphere of the words that will be articulated and their cadence so that it can correctly insert the intended affective–prosodic intonation into the intended articulatory line. One could also envision, however, that the intended intonation requirements for affective signaling by the right hemisphere could alter the left hemisphere's articulatory timing. When producing a sarcastic or emphatic statement, it is often necessary to prolong certain phonetic units to give correct attitudinal cues; for example—*"I* **rrree***ally like it."*[10] In either case, a left hemisphere lesion could disrupt the higher order linkage of affective prosody with the propositional aspects of speech, indirectly causing disruption of affective–prosodic functions.

This possibility was recently explored by Ross and co-workers[88] in a series of patients with right and left brain damage due to ischemic infarction defined by MRI scan. The patients were tested by using utterances in which various emotions were carried either by words, or a repeated monosyllable (*"ba ba ba ba ba ba"*) or an asyllabic articulation (*"aaaaaahhhh"*). In patients with left brain damage, reducing the verbal–articulatory demands caused a significant improvement in the ability to comprehend and repeat affective prosody whereas the similar maneuver in patients with right brain damage led to either no improvement or worsening of their performance. More importantly, the affective–prosodic deficits in patients with left brain damage were not correlated to the presence, severity, and type of aphasic deficit(s) or the distribution of the cortical aspects of the lesions. In fact, there were a number of patients who were not aphasic but still had impairments in affective prosody. Based on functional–anatomic assessment, lesions involving the deep white matter adjacent to the anterior body of the corpus callosum best predicted affective–prosodic disturbances following left brain damage.[85,88] These findings suggest that the most likely mechanism underlying affective–prosodic deficits following left brain damage is loss of callosal integration of the language functions represented in each hemisphere. They also sustain the hypothesis that affective prosody is a dominant and lateralized function of the right hemisphere and lend strong support to the research by Blonder and associates[8] and Bowers and colleagues[14,15] suggesting that injury to the right hemisphere causes loss of affective–communicative representations as the neural basis for the aprosodias, similar to left brain damage causing loss of lexical–syntactic representations as the neural basis for the aphasias.

VII. Aprosodias in Tone Languages

In English the most salient acoustic strategy for imparting affect in speech is through the modulation of pitch over time to produce intonation contours.[80,93] Since English is not a tone language, this use of pitch does not alter lexical referents.[79] However, over half the world's population communicates using tone languages, such as Mandarin Chinese, Taiwanese, and Thai. In tone languages, specific and often brief intonation contours (tones) that are linked to the articulated segments of speech form the basis of word meaning (Fig. 6–2). Thus, an important issue to address is whether the neurology and acoustical underpinning of affective prosody in tone languages is different from English.

Hughes and associates,[55] using a bedside assessment of affective prosody in a series of Mandarin-speaking patients with focal damage to the right hemisphere, observed various types of aprosodias with functional–anatomic correlations similar to those seen in English-speaking patients.[72] Furthermore, these patients did not display alterations in their ability to either produce or interpret meaning-relevant tonal modulations, in contrast to patients with aphasic deficits due to focal lesions of the left hemisphere.[46,68] In a series of investigations using computer-assisted techniques, Edmondson,[39] Ross,[79–81] and colleagues explored the acoustic underpinnings of affective prosody in native speakers of English and various tone languages. They found that speakers of tone languages use different acoustical strategies to signal affect in speech because of the need to preserve tone contrasts, which is essential for word meaning.[79,81] The acoustic profiles of Taiwanese patients with right hemisphere lesions and motor types of aprosodias were, thus, distinctly different from English-speaking patients with similar types of aprosodias.[39,80] These findings sug-

Mandarin Character	Phoneme/Tone		English Meaning
媽	ma	—	mother
麻	ma	╱	numb(ness)
馬	ma	∨	horse
罵	ma	╲	[curse]

FIGURE 6–2. Changes in word meaning due to changes of intonation in Mandarin Chinese.

gest that it is the behavioral goal rather than the innate ability of each hemisphere to control a certain set of acoustical features that drives the lateralization of communicative functions.

VIII. APROSODIAS, DISPLAY BEHAVIORS, AND EMOTIONAL EXPERIENCE

As reviewed in Chapter 1 and elsewhere,[48,49,61,77,83,110] the limbic system, especially the amygdala, functions as a nodal point in a distributed neuroanatomic network for the experiential aspects of emotions, emotional cognition, and the modulation of species-specific emotional displays such as laughing, crying, fear, and anger. Lesions associated with aprosodias rarely involve limbic structures. Affective prosody is organized predominantly at the level of the neocortex as part of the language-related neurocognitive networks.[51,72,77,85] It is a graded and variable behavior under volitional control, as opposed to species-specific emotional displays which are stereotypic, brief, all-or-none phenomena. Patients with motor or global aprosodia with extremely flat affect may occasionally have sudden displays of sadness, laughter, or anger when discussing personal situations that evoke emotional memories.[51,72,86,87] These emotional displays tend to be all-or-none, uncontrollable, and socially embarrassing, giving them the quality of pathological regulation of affect, similar to behaviors observed in patients with pseudobulbar palsy.[7,71,107] The changes in affective behaviors associated with the aprosodias may also lead to various discrepancies between mood and demeanor. For example, severely depressed patients with motor aprosodia may exhibit a flat affective demeanor even when discussing highly emotional issues, such as suicide.[86,87] Consequently, verbal reports of emotional distress in these patients can easily be discounted by both clinicians and family members. When evaluating and managing patients with right hemisphere damage, the clinician must always consider the possibility that profound dissociations may occur between feeling and affect and that observed behaviors may not be indicative of the patient's underlying mood state.

This work was supported in part by grants to the author from the Merit Review Board, Department of Veterans Affairs, Washington, DC, and the EJLB Foundation, Montreal, Canada.

REFERENCES

1. Ackerman, B P: Form and function in children's understanding of ironic utterances. J Exp Child Psychol 35:487–508, 1983.
2. Alexander, M P and LoVerme, S R: Aphasia after left hemispheric intracerebral hemorrhage. Neurology 30:1193–1202, 1980.
3. Ardila, A and Ostrosky-Solis, F: The right hemisphere and behavior. In Ardila, A and Osrtrosky-Solis F (Eds.): The Right Hemisphere: Neurology and Neuropsychology. Gordon and Breach: New York, 1984, pp. 3–49.

4. Basso, A, Capitani, E, Laiacona and M, Luzzati, C: Factors influencing type and severity of aphasia. Cortex 16:631–636, 1980.
5. Bell, W L, Davis, D L, Morgan-Fisher, A and Ross E D: Acquired aprosodias in children. J Child Neurol 5:19–26, 1989.
6. Benowitz, L I, Bear, D M, Rosenthal, R, Mesulam, M M, Zaidel, E and Sperry, R W: Hemispheric specialization in nonverbal communication. Cortex 19:5–14, 1983.
7. Benson, D F: Aphasia, Alexia and Agraphia. Churchill Livingston, Edinburgh, 1979.
8. Blonder, L X, Bowers, D and Heilman, K M: The role of the right hemisphere in emotional communication. Brain 114:1115–1127, 1991.
9. Bolinger, D (Ed.): Intonation. Penguin Press, Hardmondsworth, 1972.
10. Bolinger, D: Language: The Loaded Weapon. Longman Group, London, 1980.
11. Borod, J C, Koff, E, Lorch, M P and Nicholas, M: Channels of emotional communication in patients with unilateral brain damage. Arch Neurol 42:345–348, 1985.
12. Borod, J C, Koff, E, Perlman, M, Lorch, M P and Nicholas, M: The expression and perception of facial emotion in focal lesion patients. Neuropsychologia 24:169–180, 1986.
13. Bottini, G, Corcoran, R, Sterzi R, Paulesu E, Schenone P, Scarpa P, Frackowiak R S, and Frith C D: The role of the right hemisphere in the interpretation of figurative aspects of language: a positron emission tomography activation study. Brain 117:1241–1253, 1994.
14. Bowers, D, Bauer, R M and Heilman, K M: The nonverbal affect lexicon: theoretical perspectives from neuropsychological studies of affect perception. Neuropsychology 7:433–444, 1993.
15. Bowers, D, Coslett, H B, Bauer, R M, Speedie, L J and Heilman K M: Comprehension of emotional prosody following unilateral hemispheric lesions: processing defect versus distraction defect. Neuropsychologia 25:317–328, 1987.
16. Bowers, D and Heilman, K M: Dissociation between the processing of affective and non-affective faces: a case study. J Clin Neuropsychol 6:367–379, 1984.
17. Bradshaw, C, Hodge, C, Smith, M, Bragdon, A and Hickins, S: Localization of receptive prosody in the right hemisphere: evidence from intraoperative mapping and functional neuroimaging. J Int Neuropsychol Soc 3:1, 1996.
18. Broca, P: Remarques sur le siege de la faculte du langage articule, suives d'une observation d'aphemie. Bull Soc Anthropol Paris 6:330–337, 1861 (translated in von Bonin G: The Cerebral Cortex. Thomas, Springfield, 1960).
19. Broca, P: Du siege de la faculte du langage articule. Bull Soc Anthropol, Paris 6:337–393, 1865.
20. Brownell, H H, Potter, H H and Bihrle, A: Inference deficits in right brain-damaged patients. Brain Lang 29:310–321, 1986.
21. Brownell, H H, Potter, H H, Michelow, D and Gardner, H: Sensitivity to lexical denotation and connotation in brain-damaged patients: a double dissociation? Brain Lang 22:253–265, 1984.
22. Cancelliere, A E B and Kertesz, A: Lesion localization in acquired deficits of emotional expression and comprehension. Brain Cogn 13:133–147, 1990.
23. Cicone, M, Wapner, W, Foldi, N, Zurif, E and Gardner, H: The relationship between gesture and language in aphasic communication. Brain Lang 8:324–349, 1979.
24. Cicone, M, Wapner, W and Gardner, H: Sensitivity to emotional expressions and situations in organic patients. Cortex 16:145–158, 1980.
25. Coppens, P: Why are Wernicke's aphasia patients older than Broca's? A critical review of the hypotheses. Aphasiology 5:279–290, 1991.
26. Critchley, M: The Language of Gesture. Edward Arnold, London, 1939.
27. Crystal, D: Non-segmental phonology in language acquisition: review of the issues. Lingua 32:1–45, 1973.
28. Crystal, D: The English Tone of Voice. St. Martin's Press, New York, 1975.
29. Damasio, A R, Damasio, H, Rizzo, M, Varney, N and Gersch, F: Aphasia with nonhemorrhagic lesions in the basal ganglia and internal capsule. Arch Neurol 39:15–20. 1982.

30. Darby, D G: Sensory aprosodia: a clinical clue to lesions of the inferior division of the right middle cerebral artery? Neurology 34:567–572, 1993.

31. De Bleser, R and Poeck, K: Analysis of prosody in the spontaneous speech of patients with CV-recurring utterances. Cortex 21:405–416, 1985.

32. De Groot, A: Structural linguistics and syntactic laws. Word 5:1–12, 1949.

33. De Renzi, E, Motti, F and Nichelli, P: Imitating gestures. A quantitative approach to ideomotor apraxia. Arch Neurol 37:6–10, 1980.

34. DeKosky, S T, Heilman, K M, Bowers, D and Valenstein, E: Recognition and discrimination of emotional faces and pictures. Brain Lang 9:206–214, 1980.

35. Delis, D, Foldi, N S, Hambe, S, Gardner, H and Zurif, E: A note on temporal relations between language and gestures. Brain Lang 8:350–354, 1979.

36. Denes, G, Caldognetto, E M, Semenza, C, Vagges, K and Zettin, M: Discrimination and identification of emotions in human voice by brain damaged subjects. Acta Neurol Scand 69:154–162, 1984.

37. Denny-Brown, D and Banker, B Q: Amorphosynthesis from left parietal lesion. Arch Neurol Psychiatry 71:302–313, 1954.

38. Denny-Brown, D, Meyer, J S and Horenstein, S: The significance of perceptual rivalry resulting from parietal lesion. Brain 75:433–471, 1952.

39. Edmondson, J A, Ross, E D, Chan, J L and Seibert, G B: The effect of right brain damage on acoustical measures of affective prosody in Taiwanese patients. J Phonetics 15:219–233, 1987.

40. Ehlers, L and Dalby, M: Appreciation of emotional expressions in the visual and auditory modality in normal and brain-damaged patients. Acta Neurol Scand 76:251–256, 1987.

41. Emmorey, K: The neurologic substrates for the prosodic aspects of speech. Brain Lang 30:305–320, 1987.

42. Feyereisen, P and Seron, X: Nonverbal communication and aphasia: a review (in 2 parts; I. Comprehension, II. Expression). Brain Lang 16:191–212, 213–236, 1982.

43. Foldi, N C: Appreciation of pragmatic interpretations of indirect commands: comparison of right and left brain-damaged patients. Brain Lang 31:88–108, 1987.

44. Fry, D B: Prosodic phenomena. In Malberg, B (Ed.): Manual of Phonetics. North-Holland Press, Amsterdam, 1968, pp. 365–410.

45. Gainotti, G and Lemmo, M: Comprehension of symbolic gestures in aphasia. Brain Lang 3:451–460, 1976.

46. Gandour, J and Dardarananda, R: Identification of tonal contrasts in Thai aphasic patients. Brain Lang 18:98–114, 1983.

47. George, M S, Parekh, P I, Rosinsky, N, Ketter, T A, Kimbrell, T A, Heilman, K M, Herscovitch, P and Post, R M: Understanding emotional prosody activates right hemisphere regions. Arch Neurol 53:665–670, 1996.

48. Gloor, P: Experiential phenomena of temporal lobe epilepsy: facts and hypothesis. Brain 113:1673–1694, 1990.

49. Gloor, P, Olivier, A, Quesney, L F, Andermann, F and Horowitz, S: The role of the limbic system in experiential phenomena of temporal lobe epilepsy. Ann Neurol 12:129–144, 1982.

50. Goodglass, H and Kaplan, E: Disturbance of gesture and pantomime in aphasia. Brain 86:703–720, 1963.

51. Gorelick, P B and Ross, E D: The aprosodias: further functional-anatomic evidence for the organization of affective language in the right hemisphere. J Neurol Neurosurg Psychiatry 50:553–560, 1987.

52. Heilman, K M, Bowers, D, Speedie, L and Coslett, H B: Comprehension of affective and nonaffective speech. Neurology 34:917–921, 1984.

53. Heilman, K M, Scholes, R and Watson, R T: Auditory affective agnosia: disturbed comprehension of affective speech. J Neurol Neurosurg Psychiatry 38:69–72, 1975.

54. Holland, A L and Barlett, C L: Some differential effects of age on stroke-produced aphasia. In Ulatowska, H K (Ed.): The Aging Brain: Communication in the Elderly. College-Hill Press: San Diego, CA, 1985, pp. 141–155.

55. Hughes, C P, Chan, J L and Su, M S: Aprosodia in Chinese patients with right cerebral hemisphere lesions. Arch Neurol 40:732–736, 1983.

56. Hughlings-Jackson, J: On affections of speech from diseases of the brain. Brain 38:106–174, 1915.

57. Kent, R D and Read, C: The Acoustic Analysis of Speech. Singular Publishing Group, San Diego, CA, 1992.

58. Kent, R D and Rosenbeck, J C: Prosodic disturbances and neurologic lesion. Brain Lang 15:259–291, 1982.

59. Ladefoged, P: A Course in Phonetics. Harcourt Brace Jovanich, New York, 1975.

60. Lecours, A R and Lhermitte, F: Historical review: from Franz Gall to Pierre Marie. In Lecours, A R, Lhermitte, F and Bryans, B (Eds.): Aphasiology. Bailliere Tindall, London, 1983, pp. 12–14.

61. LeDoux, J E: Emotion and the amygdala. In Aggleton, J P (Ed.): The Amygdala: Neurobiological Aspects of Emotion, Memory, and Mental Dysfunction. Wiley-Liss, New York, 1992, pp. 339–351.

62. Lewis, A: Infant Speech: A Study of the Beginings of Language. Harcourt Brace, New York, 1936.

63. Manoach, D S, Sandson, T A and Weintraub, S: The developmental social-emotional processing disorder is associated with right hemisphere abnormalities. Neuropsychiat Neuropsychol Behav Neurol 8:99–105, 1995.

64. Mehrabian, A and Weiner, M: Decoding of inconsistent communications. J Pers Soc Psychol 6:109–114, 1967

65. Monrad-Krohn, GH: Dysprosdy or altered 'melody of language'. Brain 70: 405–415, 1948.

66. Monrad-Krohn, G H: The third element of speech: prosody and its disorders. In Halpern, L (Ed.): Problems in Dynamic Neurology. Hebrew University Press, Jerusalem, 1963, pp. 101–118.

67. Naeser, M A, Alexander, M P, Helm-Estabrooks, N, Levine, H L, Laughlin, S A and Geschwind, N: Aphasia with predominantly subcortical lesion sites: description of three capsular/putaminal aphasia syndromes. Arch Neurol 39:2–14, 1982.

68. Naeser, M A and Chan, S W: Case study of a Chinese aphasic with the Boston Diagnostic Aphasia exam. Neuropsychologia 18:389–410, 1983.

69. Obler, L, Albert, M, Goodglass, H and Benson, D F: Aphasia type and aging. Brain Lang 6:318–322, 1978.

70. Pihan, H, Altenmuller, E and Ackermann, H: The cortical processing of perceived emotion: a DC-potential study on affective speech prosody. Neuroreport 8:623–627, 1997.

71. Poeck, K: Pathophysiology of emotional disorders associated with brain damage. In Vinken, P J and Bruyn, G W (Eds.): Handbook of Clinical Neurology, Vol 3. North-Holland Publishing, Amsterdam, 1969, pp. 343–367.

72. Ross, E D: The Aprosodias: functional-anatomic organization of the affective components of language in the right hemisphere. Arch Neurol 38:561–569, 1981.

73. Ross, E D: The divided self. The Sciences 22:8–12, 1982.

74. Ross, E D: Prosody and brain lateralization: fact vs fancy or is it all just semantics? Arch Neurol 45:338–339, 1988.

75. Ross, E D: Hemispheric specialization for emotions, affective aspects of language and communication and the cognitive control of display behaviors in humans. Prog Brain Res 107:583–594, 1996.

76. Ross, E D: Right hemisphere syndromes and the neurology of emotions. In Schacter, S C and Devinsky, O (Eds.): Behavioral Neurology and the Legacy of Norman Geschwind. Raven Press, New York, 1997, pp. 183–194.

77. Ross, E D: Cortical representation of the emotions. In Trimble, M R and Cummings, J L (Eds.): Contemporary Behavioral Neurology. Butterworth-Heineman, Boston, 1997, pp. 107–126.

78. Ross, E D, Anderson, B and Morgan-Fisher, A: Crossed aprosodia in strongly dextral patients. Arch Neurol 46:206–209, 1989.

79. Ross, E D, Edmondson and J, Seibert, G B: The effect of affect on various acoustic measures of prosody in tone and non-tone languages: a comparison based on computer analysis of voice. J Phonetics 14:283–302, 1986.

80. Ross, E D, Edmondson, J A, Seibert, G B and Homan, R W: Acoustic analysis of affective prosody during right-sided Wada test: a within-subjects verification of the right hemisphere's role in language. Brain Lang 33:128–145, 1987.

81. Ross, E D, Edmondson, J A, Seibert, G B and Chan, J-L: Affective exploitation of tone in Taiwanese: an acoustical study of "tone latitude." J Phonetics 20:441–456, 1992.

82. Ross, E D, Harney, J H, de Lacoste, C and Purdy, P. How the brain integrates affective and propositional language into a unified brain function. Hypotheses based on clinicopathological correlations. Arch Neurol 38:745–748, 1981.

83. Ross, E D, Homan, R W and Buck, R: Differential hemispheric lateralization of primary and social emotions: Implications for developing a comprehensive neurology for emotion, repression, and the subconscious. Neuropsychiat Neuropsychol Behav Neurol 7:1–19, 1994.

84. Ross, E D and Mesulam, M-M: Dominant language functions of the right hemisphere?: prosody and emotional gesturing. Arch Neurol 36:144–148, 1979.

85. Ross, E D, Orbelo, D M, Burgard, M and Hansel, S: Functional-anatomic correlates of aprosodic deficits in patients with right brain damage. Neurology 50(Suppl 4):A363, 1998.

86. Ross, E D and Rush, A J: Diagnosis and neuroanatomical correlates of depression in brain-damaged patients: Implications for a neurology of depression. Arch Gen Psychiatry 38:1344–1354, 1981.

87. Ross, E D and Stewart, R: Pathological display of affect in patients with depression and right focal brain damage: an alternative mechanism. J Nerv Ment Dis 175:165–172, 1987.

88. Ross, E D, Thompson, R D and Yenkosky, J P: Lateralization of affective prosody in brain and the callosal integration of hemispheric language functions. Brain Lang 56:27–54, 1997.

89. Ryalls, J: Concerning right hemisphere dominance for affective language. Arch Neurol 45:337–338, 1988.

90. Schlanger, B B, Schlanger, P and Gerstmann, L J: The perception of emotionally toned sentences by right hemisphere-damaged and aphasic subjects. Brain Lang 3:396–403, 1976.

91. Seron, X, Van der Kaa, M A, Remitz, A and Van der Linden, M: Pantomime interpretation and aphasia. Neuropsychologia 17:661–668, 1979.

92. Seron, X, Van der Kaa, M A, Van der Linden, M, Remits, A and Feyereisen, P: Decoding paralinguistic signals: effect of semantic and prosodic cues on aphasic comprehension. J Commun Disord 15:223–231, 1982.

93. Shapiro, B and Danly, M: The role of the right hemisphere in the control of speech prosody in propositional and affective contexts. Brain Lang 25:19–36, 1985.

94. Speedie, L J, Coslett, B and Heilman, K M: Repetition of affective prosody in mixed transcortical aphasia. Arch Neurol 41:268–270, 1984.

95. Starkstein, S E, Federoff, J P, Price, T R, Leiguarda, R C and Robinson, R G: Neuropsychological and neuroradiological correlates of emotional prosody comprehension. Neurology 44:515–522, 1994.

96. Trauner, D A, Ballantyne, A, Friedland, S and Chase, C: Disorders of affective and linguistic prosody in children after early brain damage. Ann Neurol 39:361–367, 1996.

97. Tucker, D M, Watson, R T and Heilman, K M: Discrimination and evocation of affectively intoned speech in patients with right parietal disease. Neurology 27:947–950, 1977.

98. Van Lancker, D: Cerebral lateralization of pitch cues in the linguistic signal. Int J Hum Commun 13:201–277, 1980.

99. Van Lancker, D: The neurology of proverbs. Behavioral Neurol 3:169–187, 1990.

100. Van Lancker, D, Canter, G J and Terbeek, D: Disambiguation of ditropic sentences: acoustic and phonetic cues. J Speech Hearing Res 24:330–335, 1981.

101. Van Lancker, D and Kempler, D: Comprehension of familiar phrases by left- but not right hemisphere damaged patients. Brain Lang 32:256–277, 1987.

102. Voeller, KKS: Right hemisphere deficit syndrome in children. Am J Psychol 143:1004–1009, 1986.

103. Wapner, W, Hamby, S and Gardner, H: The role of the right hemisphere in the apprehension of complex linguistic materials. Brain Lang 14:15–33, 1981.

104. Weintraub, S and Mesulam, M-M: Developmental learning disabilities of the right hemisphere: emotional, interpersonal, and cognitive components. Arch Neurol 40:463–468, 1983.

105. Weintraub, S, Mesulam, M-M and Kramer, L: Disturbances in prosody. Arch Neurol 38:742–744, 1981.

106. Wernicke, C: Der aphasische Symptomencomplex. Eine psychologische Studie auf anatomischer Basis. Cohn & Weigert, Breslau, 1874 (translated in Eggert GH: Wernicke's Works on Aphasia: Sourcebook and Review. Mouton, The Hague, 1977).

107. Wilson, SAK: Some problems in neurology. II. Pathological laughing and crying. J Neurol Psychopathol 4:299–333, 1924.

108. Winner, E and Gardner, H: The comprehension of metaphor in brain-damaged patients. Brain 100:717–729, 1977.

109. Wolfe, G I and Ross, E D: Sensory aprosodia with left hemiparesis from subcortical infarction. Right hemisphere analogue of sensory-type aphasia with right hemiparesis? Arch Neurol 44:661–671, 1987.

110. Zola-Morgan, S, Squire, L R, Alvarez-Royo, P and Clower, R P: Independence of memory functions and emotional behavior: separate contributions of the hippocampal formation and the amygdala. Hippocampus 1:207–220, 1991.

7

Disorders of Complex Visual Processing

Antonio R. Damasio, Daniel Tranel, and Matthew Rizzo

Disorders of visual processing are one of the frequent consequences of neurologic disorders involving the cerebral hemispheres. These disorders can be evaluated at the bedside on the basis of history and neurologic exam, but the comprehensive appraisal of the defects requires neuropsychologic, neuro-ophthalmologic, and neuroimaging techniques. In this chapter, we review those disorders that are important either because of their frequency or because of their scientific implications.[49,52]

I. Disorders of Pattern Recognition

Visual Agnosias

The neuropsychologist Hans-Lukas Teuber is credited with a definition of agnosia. In his words, agnosia is "a normal percept stripped of its meanings"[173]—a definition that remains lapidary and applies well to what Lissauer designated as visual "associative" agnosias.[118] (The definition does not apply to Lissauer's visual "apperceptive" agnosias since visual perception is manifestly abnormal in "apperceptive" agnosias.) A current definition of visual agnosias, well in keeping with Teuber's words, could read as follows: a disorder of cognition and behavior *confined to the visual realm*, in which an *alert, attentive, intelligent, and nonaphasic* patient who has normal visual perception gives evidence of *not knowing the meaning* of visual stimuli, that is, of *not recognizing* visual stimuli. We shall begin by examining the components of this definition.

The statement that the deficit pertains to the visual realm reminds us that agnosias usually occur in relation to one sensory modality, leaving recognition intact in other channels. Visual and auditory agnosias are the most dramatic and frequent. They are also, from the standpoint of cognitive and behavioral neurology, the most revealing. Alertness, intelligence, and intact command of language are prerequisites for the diagnosis of agnosia. A disturbance of attention precludes both the normal perception and the normal cognitive search process that are necessary for the attribution of meaning and recognition. Likewise, a severe disturbance of intellect (e.g., in a syndrome of dementia) impairs this process. It is especially important to note the latter requisite, because in the past, as exemplified in the work of the German neurologist Bay,[17] there was an attempt to explain agnosia as the consequence of dementia combined with decayed perception. At first glance, a patient with visual agnosia may appear demented, because the magnitude of the defect impairs a normal appraisal of the environment, but careful evaluation reveals that intellect is not compromised. Likewise, a patient with primary dementia may develop signs of visual agnosia. The point remains that the two functional processes are independent.

Let us now turn to the criterion of normal perception present in the definition. This issue is complicated, because the practical distinction between perception and recognition does not have a clear neurophysiologic counterpart and because it is difficult to determine whether a patient perceives stimuli as well as the examiner does. However, although perception and recognition are part of a continuum, we believe that it is possible to identify, both behaviorally and neurophysiologically, some components of the process that are mostly related to perception and some that are mostly related to recognition.

The painstaking search for supporting evidence of satisfactory perception should proceed in the following way. First, because most patients with visual agnosia are not aphasic, the examiner should try to obtain a substantial verbal description of what the patient sees. A fairly accurate description of stimuli in terms of shapes, number, position, and distribution in space should help establish whether the basics of visual perception are impaired or normal. Such features as definition of contour and sense of depth should also be investigated, and verbal descriptions should be obtained. A statement by the patient to the effect that vision is "blurred" or "foggy" is generally not compatible with the diagnosis of visual associative agnosia but does not exclude the diagnosis. Further confirmation of the patient's ability to perceive normally should come from procedures such as copying a drawing of an object or matching an actual object with the appropriate drawing or photograph of a similar object.

Patients affected by true visual agnosia—agnosia of the associative type—will perform normally in all of these procedures. They will also be able to draw or describe the major details of the stimuli, with the exception of color, in that visual field: This is because some patients with visual agnosia also have achromatopsia, an impairment of color perception caused by central nervous system damage, as discussed in the next section of this chapter. The combination of defects is due to the contiguity of the lesions that cause both impairments. In contrast, patients with so-called visual apperceptive agnosia fail in their ability both to copy a drawing and to match visual stimuli; usually, they complain of unclear vision. They may or may not have achromatopsia.

As far as agnosia is concerned, the observations of a behavioral neurologist or neuropsychologist should be aimed at establishing whether the patient's perceptual state is compatible with *seeing* an object and yet not knowing the meaning of it. For patients who offer a detailed description of the visual structure of the object, who can copy it and match it with another—that is, who behave in relation to the object in much the same manner as the observer—the answer is affirmative. But from a theoretical standpoint, the observer should be aware of the following: (1) The patient may have fine disturbances of perception not detectable by this form of testing, and such possible disturbances may actually contribute to the recognition defect; and (2) the fact that the patient behaves as if he or she *sees* the object does not guarantee that all cerebral structures involved in the recognition process have access to the information gathered in visual perception. In other words, by a mechanism of disconnection, the patient could see with one part of the brain and yet not have another crucial brain area gain access to perceived information.

The final criterion in the definition of agnosia pertains to the inability to arrive at the meaning of (to recognize) the stimuli. Once again, the first means to establish that the patient no longer recognizes a stimulus is verbal inquiry. Most patients with agnosia will actually state that they do not know what a given object is. The examiner should make sure, however, that the statement does not reflect an inability to *name* the object, as opposed to an inability to *recognize* the object. A patient who cannot recognize an object will not be able to name it either, but the converse is not true. When the disturbance affects naming only, patients will still be able to know what the object is and what it is used for, and they often have an appropriate affective reaction to the object. That can be established by inquiring about the use and functional category of the object or by having the patient produce responses pertinent to the object both by manipulating it or by choosing logically connected items from a multiple choice display. In other words, once the examiner suspects or is told by the patient that a stimulus cannot be recognized, both verbal and nonverbal analyses are necessary in order to establish whether the defect is one of naming or of recognition.

We must emphasize that the distinction between knowing and naming is crucial and that it is often missed in the clinical evaluation of patients. The error goes both ways. Anomic patients are often classified as agnosic and agnosic patients are often classified as anomic. This common error can result from incomplete observation, but more often than not it occurs because the distinction between naming and knowing is improperly drawn in the examiner's mind. It is clear that comprehensive knowledge of the world, as possessed by normal humans, includes both nonverbal and verbal components. However, it is also true that most stimuli in the environment can be known adequately by nonverbal means alone—that is, they can be properly recognized without appeal to a verbal memory. Examples of this are readily available in everyday life. One is often introduced to new human faces, socially or through the media, that one can later recognize at a strictly nonverbal level but that one is entirely unable to name, either because the verbal tag of that face was never learned or because it was learned but quickly forgotten. In the animal world, it is clear that high-level recognition of individual stimuli and of complex configurations of visual stimuli can be achieved without any intervening verbal mediation. The clinical analysis of visual agnosia, then, is aimed at establishing the presence of a *nonverbal recognition defect* and at eliminating the possibility that what poses as impaired recognition is impaired verbal communication. Finally, it should be noted that visual recognition defects are generally accompanied by visual learning defects.

Prosopagnosia

The word "prosopagnosia" derives from the Greek *prosopon* (face) and *gnosis* (knowledge) and was introduced by Bodamer.[32] As the term implies, prosopagnosia is a visual agnosia hallmarked by an inability to recognize previously known human faces (the retrograde defect) and to learn new ones (the anterograde defect). The onset often involves the sudden realization that the well-known face of a relative can no longer be recognized visually and appears entirely unfamiliar. Yet the voice easily gives away the identity of the unrecognized face, as do a variety of clues such as body build, attire, movements, and posture. The use of such strategies highlights the remarkable preservation of recognition through other channels, generally auditory, as well as the intactness of intellectual means to formulate intelligent guesses about the environment.

The notion that the deficit in prosopagnosia is limited to human faces is erroneous; the defect is usually of a greater magnitude. For example, a farmer will no longer be able to recognize his cows individually and a bird-watcher will no longer identify different species of birds; in other words, patients with prosopagnosia also fail to recognize stimuli that, as do faces, belong to a group containing numerous, visually "ambiguous" stimuli. We define visually "ambiguous" stimuli operationally as stimuli that share the same type of subcomponents, that are arranged in the same way, and that can be distinguished only by relatively minor differences of shape or size of subcomponents. Human faces form groups of visually "ambiguous" stimuli, with numerous members. The specific recognition of those members is a social necessity, and the survival value of this seemingly trivial ability is incalculable. On a different level of importance, automobiles or a collection of dresses in a closet also constitute groups of visually "ambiguous" stimuli, in the sense that recognition of each separate one depends on relatively minor distinguishing features.

Patients with prosopagnosia can recognize any object in the environment provided the examiner does not require a recognition of the specific object within the group (e.g., when the examiner does not inquire into the historic relation between that specific object and the patient). Thus, patients are able to recognize a pencil, or an article of furniture, or a car, as, respectively, pencils, furniture, and cars; but they cannot decide whether such an article belongs to them or not, or who the specific manufacturer of a given car is. In other words, these patients can perform a *generic recognition*, which shows that they still possess the knowledge of the class to which a stimulus belongs. The identification of a *specific member* within the generic class eludes these patients, however. Nowhere is this dissociation more clear than with human faces. Patients with prosopagnosia are unable to recognize previously known faces, including their own. Yet they do know that a face is a face, and they can generally point to, or name, without difficulty, the eyes, ears, nose, or mouth of the examiner, or those in their own reflection in a mirror. Testing for such an ability will immediately assure the examiner that the patient's perception of both the whole and the parts of a facial stimulus is intact and that the real defect lies in the appropriate evocation of associated information—that is, that it lies in a failure to activate contextual memory. Prosopagnosic patients are generally able to perform complex perceptual tasks such as the Benton and Van Allen[25] test of unfamiliar facial discrimination. Many patients with severe disturbances of visuospatial performance do not, however, have prosopagnosia. [127,138] In most instances, prosopagnosia is a defect of visually triggered memory, one in which the memories pertinent to a given visual stimulus fail to be evoked, thus blocking the activation of the multimodal memory traces on which the matrix of recognition is built. Patients with prosopagnosia can evoke those multimodal traces without difficulty when a different sensory channel is used. Thus, the patient who fails to recognize his wife visually will easily do so when she speaks and makes herself known acoustically. Such an experiment indicates the intactness of multimodal memory records. Resorting to an arbitrary and necessarily crude distinction between perception and recognition, we would say that the defect in most instances of associative agnosias occurs beyond the early stages of perception but before the stage of multimodal memory activation on which recognition depends. In the model of facial recognition we have proposed, we presume that the dysfunction responsible for prosopagnosia (1) interferes with activation of records pertinent to the face or (2) destroys those records.[53] Depending on the exact placement of the lesion in each case, it is possible that either of the mechanisms is responsible for the defect. (For discusion of theoretical framework aimed at accounting for such disorders, see references 49 and 52.)

The studies of Hecaen and Angelergues[87] and of Meadows,[126] based on clinical data alone, raised the possibility that prosopagnosia was preferentially linked to right hemisphere lesions. Analysis of the pathologic material published in the literature (Table 7–1) and of our own experience with structural imaging suggests that most cases of prosopagnosia in which the defect endures beyond the acute period prove to have bilateral lesions.[11,20,34,38,45,53,79,87,89,118,149,198] The lesions compromise either the inferior and mesial visual association cortices in the lingual and fusiform gyri or their subjacent white matter. We have noted that those lesions are approximately symmetric from the functional point of view; that is, they involve equivalent portions of the central visual pathways in the left and right hemispheres (Fig. 7–1). Bilateral lesions located exclusively in the superior visual association cortices do not cause prosopagnosia, although the inferiorly located lesions can extend into parts of the superior visual association cortex in some patients (in which case patients may have disturbances in addition to agnosia).

It is apparent that patients with right hemispherectomy can recognize familiar faces[54] and that split-brain patients have little difficulty recognizing faces presented tachistoscopically to each of their hemifields.[116] The value of human facial recognition is such that the process appears to be represented in both hemispheres. But we have postulated that the mechanism for facial learning and recognition should be different in each hemisphere,[53] and there is some evidence to support that con-

TABLE 7–1 Pathologic Correlates of Prosopagnosia*

	Left Hemisphere	Right Hemisphere
Wilbrand (1982)[197]	The white matter of the entire occipital lobe is destroyed. The cortical component is located between 1st and 2nd occipital gyri	Damage to fusiform gyrus, cuneus (posterior portion) and cortex of calcarine fissure
Heidenhain (1927)[89]	Damage to striate cortex. Lesion extends anteriorly into mesial and inferior portions of the occipital lobe. Third occipital gyrus is destroyed, too. Lingual gyrus as well as inferior lip of calcarine cortex is involved	Design of lesion is identical to the left side, but damage is more at the occipital pole
Pevzner et al. (1962)[149]	The core of the lesion is in angular gyrus, but damage extends into occipitoparietal sulcus	Lower lip of calcarine fissure
Gloning et al. (1970)[79]	Damage to lingual and fusiform gyri. There is involvement of optic radiations and extension into occipital pole	Fusiform and lingual gyri. Lesion extends into supramarginal gyrus and involves optic radiations
Lhermitte et al. (1972)[118]	Cortex of fusiform gyrus. Lesion extends into occipital horn	Fusiform and lingual gyri, predominantly the latter. Lesion extends into inferior lip of calcarine fissure and into hippocampus
Benson et al. (1974)[20]	Brunt of damage is in parahippocampal cortex and anterior third of fusiform gyrus. Lesion extends to posterior periventricular white matter and to cingulate gyrus (lesion is much larger on the left)	Cyst in fusiform gyrus
Cohn et al. (1977)[45]	Case 1: upper and lower lip of calcarine fissure (spares polar portion of area). Caudal portion of hippocampal gyrus. Fusiform and lingual gyri Case 2: all of lingual and fusiform gyrus (the lesion is much larger than on the right)	Upper and lower lip of calcarine fissure all the way to occipital pole. Lower portion of cingulate gyrus and precuneus. Caudal portion of hippocampal gyrus. Fusiform gyrus Lingual and fusiform gyri close to the pole of the occipital lobe
Hecaen and Angelergues (1962)[87]	Glioblastoma extending to mesial occipital region through the splenium of the corpus callosum	Invasion in parietotemporo-occipital region
Arseni and Botez (1965)[11]	Spongioblastoma invading the posterior half of fusiform and lingual gyri, and splenium of the corpus callosum.	The tumor occupied the posterior portion of the centrum ovale, in the temporo-occipital junction, level of the splenium
Bornstein (1965)[34]		

Note: Reviews on prosopagnosia often include one postmortem case of neoplasm by Bornstein. However, the autopsy description of that particular case is not published. To complicate matters Bornstein has commented elsewhere (1965)[34] on an additional tumor case about which no postmortem details are available. It is known, however, that both cases had primary involvement of the left hemisphere.

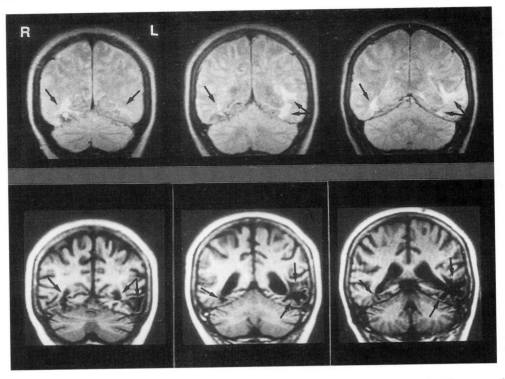

FIGURE 7–1. Magnetic resonance imaging (MRI) of a patient with prosopagnosia. The coronal slices in the top row were obtained with a spin echo technique. These are two areas of infarction, one in each hemisphere, indicated by the bright white signal (black arrows). Both involve inferior visual association cortex, in the occipitotemporal region. The corresponding coronal slices in the lower row were obtained with an inversion recovery technique.

cept.[75,168] Moreover, we have seen patients who develop face recognition defects following either right or left lesions alone. The patients with right hemisphere damage usually have large lesions involving ventral and dorsal aspects of the visual system. Their prosopagnosia is often incomplete—they recognize some faces from photographs and do especially poorly in real-time face recognition. Patients with posterior left hemisphere lesions can develop a condition we have termed "deep prosopagnosia" in which faces are recognized at the level of the group to which they belong (e.g., politician, actor) but not at the level of unique identity.

From the pathologic standpoint, most cases of prosopagnosia are caused by cerebrovascular accidents, generally from occlusion of branches of the posterior cerebral arteries due to emboli. In some cases, the lesions occur on different occasions and may be separated by months or years. Patients who already have an upper quadrantic visual field defect, hemiachromatopsia, or alexia on the basis of a unilateral occipitotemporal lesion may suddenly develop a second, contralateral lesion, that renders them agnosic and severely handicapped. In a small number of cases, prosopagnosia is due to cerebral tumors, especially gliomas, which can originate in one hemisphere and traverse to the opposite side through the splenium of the corpus callosum. Prosopagnosia can occur as an ictal phenomenon related to a bilateral epileptic focus or to a unilateral focus with momentary spreading to the opposite hemisphere.[4]

Patients with defective visual perception, such as those described subsequently in the section on Bálint's syndrome, often appear not to recognize objects and faces and can thus be misdiagnosed as agnosic. Their disorder is primarily perceptual.

II. Other Disorders of Face Processing

Facial Emotion

Many patients with prosopagnosia, despite their inability to identify familiar faces, have relatively or entirely spared recognition of facial expressions of emotion.[179] This profile is most common in patients with a relatively pure "associative" form of face agnosia—that is, in whom the face identity-recognition impairment occurs in the absence of any major deficits in visual perception—and is strongly associated with bilateral damage to higher-order visual association cortices in the occipitotemporal region.[179] The reverse dissociation—impaired recognition of emotional facial expressions with normal recognition of face identity—has also been described,[2,3,41,200] and given that this latter profile is associated with a different neuroanatomical correlate (bilateral amygdala damage), the findings together constitute a double dissociation from both anatomical and behavioral perspectives. These findings suggest that the neural systems subserving the processing of face identity and facial expressions of emotion are anatomically distinct, at least in part. Neurophysiological studies in humans[73] and monkeys[86,148,193] have also supported this notion, as have recent functional imaging studies.[10,39,132,169,170,196]

Social Knowledge

Studies in laboratory animals have provided consistent evidence that the amygdala is important in social behaviors, especially those related to fear and aggression. In humans, though, the specific role of the amygdala in social behavior has not been well studied. To begin to address this issue, we conducted a study in which we investigated the ability of subjects with bilateral amygdala damage to perform certain social judgments; specifically, we asked them to rate the extent to which unfamiliar faces looked approachable and trustworthy.[1] We found that subjects with bilateral amygdala damage were impaired in this capacity, supporting the notion that the human amygdala is critical for accurate social judgments of strangers, based on their facial appearance.

We have interpreted the findings from this study as suggesting that the human amygdala triggers socially and emotionally relevant information in response to visual stimuli. The role of the amygdala appears to be primarily important for social judgments of faces that are normally interpreted as highly unapproachable and untrustworthy, a finding consistent with the documented role of the amygdala in processing threatening and aversive stimuli.

Nonconscious Recognition of Familiar Faces in Prosopagnosia

We have used a psychophysiological index (skin conductance) to explore whether prosopagnosic subjects, despite their profound inability to recognize familiar faces at conscious level, might nonetheless produce some evidence that they can discriminate well-known faces from faces of strangers.[177,178] Skin conductance responses (SCRs) were recorded while subjects sat and viewed a series of face stimuli. The stimulus sets included some faces that ought to have been well known to the subjects (e.g., family members, themselves, famous persons; we refer to these as *targets*), mixed in random order with faces the subjects had never seen before (*nontargets*). Subjects with prosopagnosia produced significantly larger-amplitude SCRs to target faces compared to nontargets. This occurred in three separate experiments: one in which target faces were family members and friends, one in which targets were famous individuals (movie stars, politicians), and one in which the targets were faces of persons with whom the subject had had considerable exposure after the onset of their condition but not before. In sum, prosopagnosic subjects produced clear evidence of nonconscious discrimination of facial stimuli they could not otherwise recognize and for which even a remote sense of familiarity was lacking. These findings suggest that some part of the physiological process of face recognition remains intact in the subjects, although the results of this process are unavailable to consciousness. The fact that the subjects were able to produce SCR discrimination of faces to which they had been exposed only after the onset of their condition is particularly intriguing, as it suggests that the neural operations responsible for the formation and maintenance of new "face records" can proceed independently from conscious influence.

Other paradigms have also yielded evidence of nonconscious or "covert" face recognition in prosopagnosic subjects. Bauer,[15,16] for example, presented prosopagnosics with either correct or incorrect face-name pairs, and found that subjects produced larger-amplitude SCRs to the correct pairs (an effect that also obtains in normal individuals). Rizzo and colleagues[157] showed that prosopagnosic subjects produced different scanpath patterns for familiar faces compared to unfamiliar ones. de Haan,[61,62] using a reaction time paradigm in which a prosopagnosic subject had to decide whether two photographs "matched" (were of the same individual) or did not match (were of different individuals), found that reaction time was systematically faster for familiar faces compared to unfamiliar ones.

A Double Dissociation Between Conscious and Nonconscious Face Recognition

Stimuli with strong affective valence and "signal value" produce large-amplitude SCRs in normal subjects.[183] In a series of studies of brain-damaged subjects with bilateral damage to ventromedial prefrontal cortices, however, we found that the subjects were remarkably impaired in their ability to generate SCRs to highly potent "signal" stimuli, such as nudes and mutilation scenes.[56,57] We have interpreted this outcome as reflecting an impairment of somatic marker activation,[18] by which we mean defective activation of bodily states that would normally accompany the perception of emotionally arousing stimuli. The somatic marker framework has been elaborated in detail elsewhere.[48] In brief, the theory posits that "marker" signals arising from bioregulatory processes (including those which express themselves in emotions and feelings) are key influences guiding behavior, especially in social situations. The markers, which can be either overt or covert, are critical for normal reasoning and decision-making.

The somatic marker hypothesis predicts that somatic marker activation (indexed by SCRs) should occur in relationship to perceiving highly familiar faces given that such stimuli have a high degree of personal relevance, familiarity, and overall signal value.[177,178,183] Following this rationale, we predicted that subjects with ventromedial prefrontal lesions would show defective electrodermal responses to familiar faces, as they do for other emotionally laden visual stimuli. This prediction has received empirical support.[180] Specifically, we found that four subjects with bilateral ventromedial prefrontal lesions failed to generate SCRs to pictures of familiar faces derived from either the retrograde or anterograde compartments. This occurred despite the fact that the ventromedial subjects have normal overt (conscious) recognition of the faces. Together with previous findings in prosopagnosic subjects, who demonstrate impaired conscious face recognition but normal nonconscious recognition, these results constitute a behavioral and anatomical "double dissociation" between overt and covert face recognition. The findings indicate that the neural systems that process the somatic-based valence, or what could be termed the "emotional significance" of stimuli, are separate from the systems that process the factual information associated with those same stimuli.

Visual Object Agnosia

Visual object agnosia occurs in two distinct forms. One form one might call "general" visual object agnosia; the other is "category-specific" visual object agnosia.

Patients with "general" visual object agnosia are behaviorally and anatomically distinct from those with prosopagnosia. In addition to prosopagnosia, these patients have an inability to recognize even the generic class to which an object belongs. Those patients are unable to know that a face is a face or that a car is a car. They may also have a defect of visual naming, which, in the presence of intact auditory and tactile naming, is traditionally known as "optic aphasia" (Freund's[72] rarely used term). Such patients are almost invariably alexic. Unlike patients with prosopagnosia, some patients with object agnosia may suddenly "unblock" their agnosia and either name or describe the use of an object when it is moved or rotated slowly. Because of the effect of movement upon performance, this defect has been called "static visual agnosia."[35]

Some patients with visual object agnosia complain of "unclear," "blurred" vision, and they probably have a selective defect of low to middle spatial frequency vision that especially impairs appreciation of static, low-contrast stimuli but that may leave intact the vision of moving, high-contrast stimuli. Those patients certainly do not fit the diagnosis of visual agnosia in the associative sense, as we defined it here. In some patients, provided they have stable lesions, the perceptual impairment may diminish and a truly associative type of agnosia may thus appear.

General visual object agnosia is associated with comparable but more extensive damage than prosopagnosia (bilateral lesions in the ventral and mesial parts of occipitotemporal visual areas that often extend dorsally and laterally). It is possible that polar and lateral occipital lesions may be sufficient, in the absence of mesial occipitotemporal damage, but there is insufficient evidence at this point.

Category-specific visual object agnosia occurs when patients have difficulties with identification of objects within a given category—for instance, manipulable tools—but are otherwise capable of recognizing most objects. In a recent study of a large number of patients with lesions of the telencephalon, we have shown that certain sites of damage are especially likely to produce category-specific recognition defects.[182,183] Visual object agnosia for manipulable objects is especially well defined and associated with damage to a territory of posterior and lateral temporal cortex in the vicinity of the human homologue of area MT (Fig. 7–2).

Cortical Blindness and Anton's Syndrome

Severe bilateral damage to visual cortices and to optic radiations may obliterate vision entirely. This dramatic condition is commonly accompanied by the denial of blindness (Anton's syndrome). The condition known as Anton's syndrome was not described in Anton's 1899 paper,[6] which dealt with denial of somatosensory defects,[102] but the eponym is traditionally used in connection with denial of blindness. In many cases, both the blindness and its denial are transient. A phenomenon related to this condition is "blindsight," in which a blind patient remains capable of pointing, with considerable success, to a point of light flashed in his inoperative field of vision. We have interpreted these situations to be a result of the patients having intact visually related parietal cortices, intact superior colliculi, and intact pathways connecting the latter to the former via the pulvinar. The engagement of the retinas and superior colliculi by the presence of an object would provide the parietal cortices with signals indicative of the usual situation of looking and seeing and thus provide the basis for the subsequent misinterpretation that characterizes Anton's syndrome and blindsight.

Pure Alexia

Pure alexia, otherwise known as alexia-without-agraphia or "wordblindness," is also a disorder of visual pattern recognition. The reading of most words and of sentences is severely impaired. In many patients even the reading of single letters is defective. Patients with pure alexia are able to *see* the sentences, words, or letters that they are unable to read. This is easily demonstrated by showing that patients can copy what they cannot read. In most instances in spite of quadrantanopic or

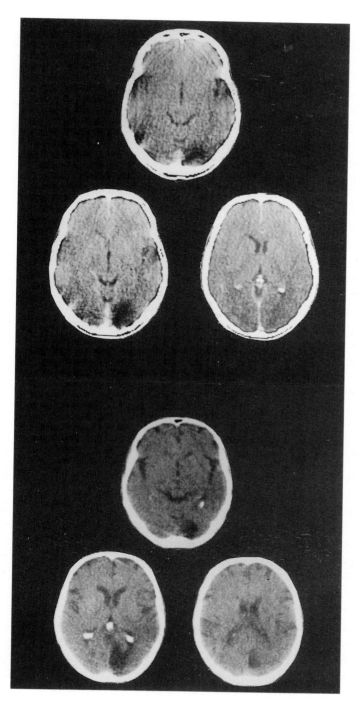

FIGURE 7–2. Top: A CT scan of a patient with left hemiachromatopsia. The lesion involves the polar and mesial visual cortex, located below the calcarine fissure in the right hemisphere.

Bottom: This CT scan is that of a patient with left hemianopia—that is, with an entire blind left field. Note that the lesion encompasses an additional cut which involves the primary visual cortex and, of necessity, the optic radiations traveling toward it.

hemianopic field defects, the patient has normal visual acuity and has normal recognition of nonverbal visual stimuli. Patients with pure alexia cannot recognize words, probably because they are unable to evoke the appropriate associated material when confronted with those words. Thus, a phenomenon of agnosia can probably explain many cases of pure alexia (Chapter 1).

Any lesion capable of disconnecting both visual association cortices from the dominant, language-related, temporoparietal cortices will cause pure alexia. In most instances a lesion in the corpus callosum or in its outflow, in either hemisphere, achieves an interhemispheric disconnection (of right-to-left visual information), whereas an additional lesion in the left occipital lobe achieves an intrahemispheric disconnection (from left visual association cortex to left language cortex). In some cases, the lesion in the left occipital lobe actually prevents the arrival of visual information in the visual cortex. (Such cases have a right homonymous hemianopia, a common but not necessary accompaniment of pure alexia). In many cases, a single lesion strategically located in what we have termed the left paraventricular area (the region behind, beneath, and under the occipital horn) can cause both types of disconnection by damaging pathways en route from the callosum and pathways en route from the left visual association cortex. Déjérine's[66] original case of a patient with pure alexia had the prototype of that lesion. (See Damasio and Damasio[51] for additional anatomic details and Chapter 5 for additional discussion on alexia). It should be noted that patients with other forms of alexia (e.g., alexia-with-agraphia) may fail to read owing to different mechanisms that are related to aphasia rather than agnosia. Some patients with alexia can also have visual agnosia when an additional lesion is present in the right hemisphere.[20,51]

Disorders of Topographic (Spatial) Orientation

A variety of disorders fall under this designation. The acquired inability to locate a public building in a city, to find one's room at home, and to describe either verbally or by means of a map how to get to a specific room or place have been classified under this heading. Some patients develop such deficits on the basis of unilateral hemispatial neglect or on the basis of a global amnestic syndrome (chapters 3 and 4). In this chapter, we do not deal with these causes, but we do focus on disorders of topographic orientation, which are based on the mechanisms of agnosia.

Such defects are likely to reflect an impairment of visuospatial memory, and the kinship to the visual agnosias is apparent. When confronted by a given architectural or topographic detail, these patients can no longer conjure previously stored memories that would help them establish their bearings and plan their route to the desired destination. The complex operations involved in topographic orientation are likely to involve a variety of structures in both inferior and superior visual association cortices with a special contribution from the right occipitoparietal region. The limited literature on the subject supports this view. Hecaen and Angelergues[87] noted that the defect is strongly associated with either bilateral posterior lesions or with right posterior lesions and also remarked that, in either case, the disturbance is infrequent.

The ability to learn new topographic routes after focal brain lesions certainly depends on yet another type of process. It has been our experience that patients with bilateral lesions of the visual system, both superiorly and inferiorly, have difficulty in learning new topographic information. The inability to learn how to get back to the room in the novel hospital environment is often seen. Patients with prosopagnosia are certainly disturbed in this regard.[155] Studies based on patients with well-localized lesions are not available.

Semmes and associates[167] developed a laboratory technique to study route learning disturbances in which patients were asked to follow a route depicted in a map. The patients could not read the map visually or tactually (with either hand). The impairment was strongly associated with parietal lesions and clearly independent from the mode in which the map was presented. The results highlight the supramodal nature of route learning and its functional association with a brain structure in which visual and somatosensory information can interact. Ratcliff and Newcombe,[155] using a similar task, noted that only patients with bilateral posterior lesions performed defectively. Bowen and associates[36] found that patients with parkinsonism, who presumably had active bilateral dysfunction of the neostriatum, also were defective in this task. Patients with parkinsonism whose signs predominated in the left side (whose dysfunction was more marked in the right striatum) performed more poorly.

A different but perhaps related impairment, that of geographic orientation, denotes the inability to identify cities in a map or to construct a map of a country or a state. This appears to be a far more frequent defect and is seen in patients with both bilateral and unilateral posterior cerebral lesions.[26,87] In Benton and Van Allen's test, a map of the United States is presented and the subject is asked to point to the places where major cities or states are supposed to be. Patients with neglect characteristically fail this test, either by not supplying the location of cities in one of the halves of the map or by displacing them eastward or westward of their true locations. The performance of these patients may reflect the presence of hemispatial neglect (Chapter 3).

Recent studies using functional neuroimaging have contributed to our understanding of visual recognition and topographic orientation. Using functional magnetic resonance imaging (fMRI), Kanwisher and co-workers[108] localized a "fusiform face area" that responds to faces somewhat selectively. Epstein and Kanwisher,[70] also using fMRI, found a specific area within human parahippocampal cortex that responds to places more than faces. This area, the so-called parahippocampal place area (PPA), is involved in perceiving the local visual environment, an essential component of navigation. The PPA responds selectively and automatically to passively viewed scenes and weakly to single objects. Information about the layout of local space is a critical factor for this activation. The authors proposed that the PPA represents places by encoding the geometry of the local environment.

III. DISORDERS OF COLOR PERCEPTION

In this section, we concentrate on acquired deficits of perception, the "central achromatopsias." This group of deficits can be defined as an *acquired* disorder of *color perception involving all or part of the visual field, with relative preservation of the vision of form,* caused *by focal damage of the visual association cortex* or of its subjacent white matter. The existence of these defects has been known since the last quarter of the 19th century. For historical reasons to be discussed later the concept all but vanished from clinical neurology and was only reinstated in the mid-1970s. The disorder occurs most frequently in the setting of cerebrovascular disease and is important both as a clinical sign and as an indicator of disordered physiology.

Patients with achromatopsia experience a loss of color vision in a quadrant, a hemifield, or the whole visual field. The loss of color may be complete to the point that a patient experiences only black and white or it may be partial, generally described as a "washing out" of the colors as if they were "dirty" or "dulled" yet still distinguishable as individual colors. In general, the precipitous loss of color vision is a noticeable phenomenon. One of our patients described it as if the "color of my TV screen had gone out of tune," giving way to a black and white image. Depending on the ambient lighting conditions, patients describe the affected field as "whitish" or "blackish" or merely as a collection of shades of gray. But although color is lost, the perception of forms is maintained, so patients can still see accurately in the colorless region of their visual field. Furthermore, definition of contour and the sense of depth of the colorless field are generally not compromised. In short, achromatopsia amounts to a loss of color vision with preservation of form vision. In patients in whom only a hemifield or a quadrant is affected, the disorder can be tested by moving stimuli in and out of the achromatopsic area and crossing into the area of intact color perception.[106]

Full-field achromatopsia is usually associated with visual agnosia, especially prosopagnosia. Most of the patients also have some impairment of the visual field; for example, a bilateral or unilateral upper quadrantic defect or a combination of a hemifield defect with a quadrant defect on the opposite side. In other words, patients with full-field achromatopsia come to medical attention because of (1) visual agnosia, (2) achromatopsia in the portion of the field with intact form vision, and (3) blindness for both form and color vision in the remainder of the field. Some of those patients may have pure alexia as well, and all have bilateral occipitotemporal lesions, as described for prosopagnosia.

Some patients exhibit hemiachromatopsia only. Patients with left hemiachromatopsia have a unilateral lesion in the right occipitotemporal region and usually have no other neuropsychologic defects. This is the purest form of achromatopsia and can be associated with a single lesion located inferiorly in the occipitotemporal cortex. Patients with right hemiachromatopsia have unilateral lesions of the left occipitotemporal region and may or may not have associated alexia.[51] Some of these patients have both pure alexia and blindness in the right upper quadrant. In these patients, the upper quadrant blindness results from damage to the inferior optic radiations or, on occasion, to the lower calcarine cortex; the lower quadrant achromatopsia results from damage to color processing regions located medially and ventrally in occipitotemporal cortex; and the alexia follows damage to intra- and interhemispheric visual pathways within the left occipital cortex, which connect visual association cortex with language areas. Form vision is preserved in the colorless right lower quadrant because the superior calcarine cortex and the superior contingent of optic radiations *are* intact.

In most cases of pure achromatopsia, the lesion is located in the visual association cortex of the occipitotemporal region. The lesion is usually an infarct in the territory of one of the branches of the posterior cerebral artery, often of embolic origin. The lesion is positioned in such away that both optic radiations and primary visual cortex are mostly spared (Fig. 7–2, top). Because it is far more common for the primary visual cortex or the attending optic radiations to be damaged than spared in occlusions of the posterior cerebral arteries, the occurrence of hemianopia is far more common than is that of hemiachromatopsia (Fig. 7–2, bottom). In addition, it is possible that the defect may not be brought to the attention of physicians as often or as quickly as with hemianopia.

Our current view regarding the position of the lesion that causes achromatopsia is that, as mentioned earlier, damage has to be located in the ventral part of the visual association cortex in an occipitotemporal area that encompasses the fusiform and lingual gyri. This was the location first described by Verrey[189] in a patient who developed a right hemiachromatopsia with no other defect of reading or form vision. A similar location can be surmised in the renowned patient of Déjérine[66] in whom right hemiachromatopsia was associated with alexia but not with blindness. As noted in the detailed neuropathologic study of this case by Déjérine's disciple Vialet, the primary visual cortex in the calcarine region was almost entirely spared, and the lesion was located in the inferior visual association cortex as well as in the subjacent white matter, extending into the paraventricular region.[51,191] In the cases we have studied to date, our impression is that lesions in this vicinity will cause achromatopsia provided they are located fairly posteriorly in the visual association cortex, that is, immediately below the occipital pole, under the caudal half of the calcarine cortex. By the same token, we have seen patients with lesions located more anteriorly in the visual association cortex (i.e., immediately below the rostral half or one third of the calcarine cortex) who did not have achromatopsia. Those patients had form vision defects in the periphery of the opposite upper quadrant, but they did not complain of color loss in the remainder of their intact field, nor did they exhibit color loss when tested in the color perimeter. We have, however, studied patients with lesions in the white matter of the occipitotemporal region who also developed achromatopsia, and we have seen instances of patients with achromatopsia related to superior occipital lesions. It should be clear that the exact location and range of the lesions that can cause achromatopsia remains a matter of current research.

Several neuropsychologic studies published during the 1960s had indicated an apparent preponderance of color perception defects in patients with right hemisphere lesions.[12,64,117,166] All of these studies were based on large series of patients with damage to either the right or the left hemisphere. But exact anatomic definition was lacking, and the groups were heterogenous from the pathologic standpoint. Furthermore, the defect in color perception (color "imperception," according to some of the authors) was defined on a statistical basis as a performance below that of normal subjects. In fact, few if any of these patients had real achromatopsia as defined here. Evidence from the literature on achromatopsia has not supported the notion that color processing is the specialty of the right hemisphere. Nonetheless, the right hemisphere might process color differently than the left, even though unilateral right hemisphere damage may not lead to clinical complaints characteristic of achromatopsia.

We have studied patients with achromatopsia who recover markedly; but we have also seen patients in whom the disturbance remains unchanged. It is reasonable to suspect that the position and extent of the lesion will play a major role in the patient's recovery. This is also a matter of current study, and it is not yet possible to make reliable predictions of outcome on the basis of available information. We suspect that the most posterior lesions in visual association cortex are the ones that cause the most permanent forms of achromatopsia.

The reason why the concept of central achromatopsia vanished from clinical neurology and is rarely mentioned in textbooks of neurology or ophthalmology deserves a special mention. The two fundamental descriptions of the phenomenon, complete with appropriate postmortem correlation, were available between 1888 and 1893. (See the articles of the ophthalmologist Verrey;[188,189] the notes by Landolt, which were included in Déjérine's[66] paper of 1892; and Vialet's[191] postmortem study of Déjérine's patient.) Other cases of achromatopsia were described, with autopsy.[121] None of these articles gained a foothold in the German and English literature of the time. Furthermore, after World War 1, when Gordon Holmes made his contribution to the understanding of the visual system based on patients with gunshot wounds, he did not cite these articles and unwittingly denied their substance. Most of Holmes's patients had dorsal occipitoparietal lesions, and none exhibited achromatopsia.[96,97] Holmes saw few if any pure occipitotemporal lesions and, in spite of his sample of patients being skewed, concluded that disorders of color perception could not be caused by focal damage of the visual cortices. His authority and the importance of his other superb observations cast a shadow on the descriptions of acquired achromatopsia. The existence of acquired achromatopsia secondary to lesions of the central nervous system was only acknowledged by Critchley,[47] in 1965, even though no pathologic correlate was proposed then. Another decade would pass before a handful of papers would revive and expand the observations of Verrey and Landolt.[5,58,82,121,147]

Application of modern computed tomographic (CT) and magnetic resonance (MR) imaging techniques has resulted in replication of Verrey's findings that cerebral color loss is associated with inferotemporal lesions affecting the fusiform and lingual gyri (e.g., Pearlman[147]; Damasio and associates;[58] Victor and co-workers;[193] Heywood and colleagues;[92]). Three-dimensional MRI reconstructions in achromatopsia show damage in the middle third of the lingual gyrus or white matter just behind the posterior tip of the lateral ventricle.[59,159] Functional neuroimaging using positron emission tomography[120] and fMRI has shown activation in comparable regions in normal subjects viewing color stimuli.

A lesion of either hemisphere can cause color loss. The color loss occurs in the contralateral visual hemifield (hemiachromatopsia or hemidyschromatopsia). Both cerebral hemispheres process color, and bilateral lesions are required for complete achromatopsia affecting the whole visual field. Some patients with hemiachromatopsia are not aware of their color vision loss,[5,111,146] but those with complete achromatopsia will generally complain of the deficit.

Hemiachromatopsia can be detected by having patients report on the appearance of color tokens moved from the ipsilateral to the contralateral hemifield. For instance, a patient may report that a red object turns grayish as it is moved into the aberrant field. Hemifield color loss is difficult to quantify with standard color tests, however, because these tests are designed for viewing within the central few degrees of vision where color vision is best. Hemiachromatopsics can score well on these tests despite having a true color deficit because of spared color vision near fixation.[159]

Color perception deficits in full-field achromatopsia of cerebral origin can be tested with standardized tests used to assess color impairments due to eye disease. Pseudoisochromatic plates such as the *American Optical Hardy-Rand Rittler*[85] and *Standard Pseudoisochromatic Plates, Part 2*[103] are useful. Patients with alexia or aphasia can perform on these tests by tracing the target patterns using their fingers without ever having to read or speak the target names. Color arrangement tests consist of color chips that can be arranged in a unique sequence and are also useful. Arrangement tests differ in the number and difficulty of the discriminations required, and the region of color space they probe, such as hue (i.e., color of the spectrum), saturation (the amount a color is mixed with gray), and brightness. The *Farnsworth-Munsell 100 Hue* evaluates hue discrimination of tokens that do not vary in luminance. A shorter version, the *D-15* test, screens for severe hue discrimination loss along protan ("red," or short wavelength cone), deutan ("green," or middle wavelength cone), or tritan (blue-yellow) dimensions. The *Lanthony New Color Test* tests hue discrimination at different saturation levels, as well as which colors are confused with grays. The *Sahlgren Saturation Test*[74] tests saturation discrimination by asking patients to separate greenish blue and bluish purple caps of varying saturation. The *Lightness Discrimination Test* consists of caps of different grays, to be ranked from dark to light.[150,190] Achromatopsic patients can show abnormal discrimination of hues and saturation[159] but normal perception of brightness.[91,159,192]

On the Nagel anomoloscope, a patient tries to match a yellow light in one test field with a mixture of yellow-green and yellow-red lights in another by varying the proportion in the mix. Normal persons rapidly find the unique proportion needed. Patients with congenital color defects or acquired cerebral achromatopsia lack a unique solution and make abnormal matches over a wide range.[97,159] The pattern of deficits on the anomoloscopic and color-sorting tasks suggests that cerebral lesions produce a spectrum of color impairments affecting the processing of signals from all cone types[88,92,159] although there may be a greater vulnerability to color loss along the tritan (B–Y) axis.[159] Another factor requiring further investigation is the role of size: Normal individuals see color less well in objects below a certain size, and this effect may be exaggerated by cerebral dyschromatopsia.

Color naming alone is not sufficiently sensitive or specific to diagnose achromatopsia. Patients with may fail to name color tokens because of color anomia or agnosia.[60,65,77,98,143] These patients cannot name colors shown to them or point to colors when they are named by others, but unlike achromatopsics, they can discriminate between colors on cap-sorting tests and pseudoisochromatic plates. Conversely, color naming may remain normal in a color-deficient field. The million colors discriminated by the visual system comprise a dozen categorical names in any language.[29] A true color deficit may not suffice to shift color percepts across the boundaries of differently named categories.

The wavelengths reaching the eye from an object depend upon its reflectance and the lighting of the scene. Yet, colors of objects appear stable over a range of environmental lighting conditions.[109,114,202] Thus, an apple looks red whether viewed under sunlight in an orchard or fluorescent light at a grocery counter. This phenomenon, referred to as color constancy, depends on neural mechanisms that compensate for the illuminant (the Retinex theory)[113] to derive the true colors of objects in a scene.[113,114] Zeki[202] speculated that impaired color constancy is the key defect in cerebral achromatopsia. If so, patients should report large shifts in the color appearance of objects under different illuminants, which they do not. Color constancy probably does not explain reports of a gray or colorless world.[58,121,126,144,159] Though it may contribute, a defect of color constancy does not adequately account for the phenomena reported cerebral achromatopsia.

Color is important for perception of objects and shape, and this aspect of color vision may be partly preserved in achromatopsia. Some patients can detect differences between different color areas with similar luminances even if they do not perceive the hues in those colors. This information can be used to detect the boundaries between regions[91,193] and may reflect residual color opponent processing in striate cortex.[192]

Using functional magnetic resonance imaging, McKeefry and Zeki[125] found evidence of distinct activation, by abstract color Mondrian patterns, of a human cortical color center they call human V4. This area occupies the lateral aspect of the collateral sulcus on the fusiform gyrus. The lingual gyrus was not activated. The human V4 contains a representation of both the superior and inferior visual fields. The authors also reported a retinotopic organization of V4 with the superior visual field represented more medially on the fusiform gyrus and the inferior field more laterally and abutting the former. They reported no evidence of a separate representation of the inferior hemifield for color in more dorsolateral regions of occipital lobe. These results appear to be consistent with clinical observations that an inferiorly placed lesion can alter color perception in both the superior and inferior visual hemifields fields contralateral to the lesion. Color is also processed outside V4, however. Based on patterns of brain brain activation to different color stimuli, Zeki and Marini[204] proposed three stages of color processing in human brain. The first depends on V1/V2 to register the presence and intensity of different wavelengths and perform "wavelength differencing." The second depends on V4 and is concerned with automatic color constancy (independent of memory). The third depends on inferior temporal and frontal cortex and is concerned with object colors. The authors believe their schema can help reconcile the low-level computational theory of Land, and the ideas of Helmholtz and Hering, which view cognitive factors such as memory and learning as essential ingredients in color perception.

IV. OTHER DISORDERS RELATED TO COLOR PROCESSING

Disorders of Color Naming

A situation entirely different from achromatopsia occurs when otherwise nonaphasic patients can experience color and can match colors according to hue but are unable to name the colors that they perceive without difficulty. An operational definition should read as follows: *failure to name colors or to point to colors* given their names, in the *absence of a demonstrable defect of color perception or of aphasia.*

In our experience all patients with a color-naming defect have a right-homonymous hemianopia and intact color perception in the left field. The other common correlate of color-naming defect is pure alexia.[51] In only one case to our knowledge has a color-naming defect been described without alexia, although right-homonymous hemianopia was present.[129]

Analysis of an extensive series of our own patients as well as review of the literature has led us to conclude that the lesion necessary for color-naming defects is located in the left hemisphere, mesially, in the transition between the occipital and temporal lobes, in a subsplenial position. The right-homonymous hemianopia, which is also present, is caused by an additional lesion either in the geniculate body, visual cortex, or optic radiations.

Regardless of the lesion that causes it, the net effect of the right field cut is to circumscribe visual information to the right visual cortex. The effect of the occipitotemporal lesion is to interfere with the ability of language areas in the left hemisphere to receive visual information related to color. It is not known whether this lesion simply disconnects color information conveyed by the corpus callosum or whether some crucial step in the processing of that information takes place in the occipitotemporal transition cortex. It should be clear, however, that other types of visual information still reach the remainder of the left visual association cortices, which explains the preservation of other aspects of visual naming.

Some authors prefer to call this disorder "color agnosia." They argue that the terms "color-naming defect" and "color anomia" fail to suggest the two-way impairment that renders patients unable to name a color and also unable to point to a color when given its name. Furthermore, they indicate that the perception of color devoid of its verbal tag corresponds to a percept without meaning—that is, an agnosia. We have some reservations about the term "color agnosia" to denote this difficulty. At any rate, the reader should know that a color-naming impairment, as described here, generally implies a two-way defect, and that the means of distinguishing a color-naming defect from achromatopsia include (1) verbal inquiry concerning the patient's experience of color, (2) testing of the ability to perform color matching, and (3) the *Ishihara* and *Farnsworth-Munsell* tests. We should note that in some patients with color anomia, especially as they recover, the magnitude of the impairment of naming colors on confrontation is greater than that of pointing to colors when given the names. This has been termed a "one-way" defect. The explanation for this dissociation is not evident, but the two tasks are cognitively different. In the condition of pointing to colors when given their names, it is possible that presentation of the color name activates bilateral hemispheric structures, directly or through auditory callosal transfer, and thus permits a more prompt auditory–visual matching in the right hemisphere. In the opposite condition, given the patient's lesions, the activation caused by color stimuli is confined to the right hemisphere alone and may be less likely to arouse pertinent verbal information.

Disorders of Color Association

An entirely different process is the ability to indicate which color is associated with a specific object using an exclusively verbal question and a verbal mode of response (e.g., requesting the patient to complete sentences such as "The color of blood is_____" or "The color of a banana is_____"). Performance of this task does not require the processing of visual information. It is reasonable to expect that patients with disturbances of the visual system will not show an impairment in such a task, whereas patients with an auditory or auditory–verbal defect may perform defectively. That is indeed the case. Although patients with aphasia do poorly in this task, patients with isolated color naming defects perform such tasks accurately.

Another type of color association task consists of asking the patient to color black and white line drawings of common objects. The patient must select the correct pencil out of an array of colored pencils and proceed with coloring. Patients with a color-naming defect may or may not fail such a task. A study we performed some years ago persuaded us that when they do fail, the failure often results from an intriguing mechanism, which consists of (1) making the correct verbal choice of which color pencil to use (i.e., "This is a banana; a banana is yellow; I'll color it yellow"), but then (2) choosing the wrong pencil because the correct choice depends on a verbal–visual match (yellow name to yellow pencil). After applying the wrong color, these patients are often puzzled by the result and may be uncertain that there is indeed an error. Analysis of this kind of performance has led us to believe that the patient switches strategies and solves part of the problem at a verbal level and another at a visual level but has no means to combine the results of both approaches.[55] Such a failure does raise the question of whether the patients still have a working concept of color and hence whether they should be considered agnosic. It has been our impression that the cognitive basis of the concept of color is fragile, being principally dependent on (1) the association of a verbal tag with a given color and (2) the association of a given color with the objects that commonly carry it (an association that must be, at least in part, verbally mediated). Thus, a functional dissociation between visual and verbal processes is likely to prevent the concomi-

tant arousal of verbal and visual memory traces on which the attribution of meaning to a normal color perception must depend. Some support for this hypothesis
comes from studies that indicate that patients with aphasia not only fail tasks involving the linguistic aspects of color but also frequently fail color-matching tasks
of a nonverbal variety.[64]

V. Disorders of Spatial Analysis

Bálint's Syndrome and Its Components

Bálint's[14] syndrome (named after the Hungarian neurologist who called attention
to this symptom complex in 1909) is one of the most striking disorders of spatial
analysis. The eponym should be reserved for those cases that present all three major
components: *visual disorientation* (also known as simultanagnosia), *optic ataxia* (deficit of visually guided reaching), and *ocular apraxia* (deficit of visual scanning). Both
visual disorientation and optic ataxia can occur by themselves. To the best of our
knowledge ocular apraxia is always accompanied by either optic ataxia or visual
disorientation. The patients may have visual field defects (when they do, they consist of inferior quadrant cuts), but these are not necessary for the appearance of
Bálint's syndrome. We have seen several cases of patients in whom the visual fields
were intact. An operational definition of Bálint's syndrome would be as follows:
an *acquired* disturbance of the *ability to perceive the visual field as a whole*, resulting in
the *unpredictable perception and recognition of only parts of it (simultanagnosia)*; which
is accompanied by an *impairment of target pointing under visual guidance (optic ataxia)*
and an *inability to shift gaze at will toward new visual stimuli (ocular apraxia)*.

The essence of the syndrome, visual disorientation (simultanagnosia), is subjective. The patient becomes unable to grasp the whole field of vision in its entirety
and appears to see clearly in only a small fraction of the panorama, outside of
which vision is described as hazy. But to complicate matters this fragment of useful
field (usually a part of the macular representation) is not stable and moves errati-
cally from quadrant to quadrant. This often happens in the absence of a true visual
field cut, although some patients may also have inferior visual field defects. As a
result of this disturbance, patients commonly fail to detect and orient to new stimuli
that may appear in the periphery of the visual field, except when, by chance, fixation is directed toward the new stimulus. Also as a result of this defect, an object
that is clearly seen at a given moment may suddenly disappear from view as the
fixation shifts. Patients often complain about objects vanishing from the scene they
are inspecting. This is also why the patients are not able to report more than one
or two components of the visual field at any one time. The term "simultanagosia"
refers to this feature. The defect can be easily tested by asking for the description
of a large array of objects or people in front of the patient or by requesting the
description of a complex scene. The Cookie Theft picture from the *Boston Diagnostic
Aphasia Examination*[81] is an excellent means of deciding whether or not the patient
can cope with the rapid analysis of a visual scene.

Some patients with visual disorientation complain that moving objects are especially difficult to perceive, and we have noted that these patients fail to acknowledge the presence of an object moving about in the visual field. Such a defect, the converse of "visual–static agnosia" mentioned in the section on pattern recognition, indicates the likelihood that the perception of movement is handled separately from that of static stimuli. It is important to note, however, that the patient reported by Zihl and associates[207] as having a "selective" disturbance of movement vision also had visual disorientation, optic ataxia, and astereopsis (see below).

The second component of the syndrome is optic ataxia. The defect consists of an inability to point accurately to a target, under visual guidance. Patients with optic ataxia have no difficulty pointing with precision to targets in their own body or garments using somatosensory information. Nor to they have difficulty pointing to the source of sounds. But under visual guidance there is marked difficulty, especially in reaching toward small targets and in finger pointing. The error may be as small as half an inch, and the mispointing is generally not accompanied by tremor. Optic ataxia, also known as visuomotor ataxia, can be found in isolation, in both upper limbs, and in patients who are recovering from Bálint's syndrome and no longer have visual disorientation or significant ocular apraxia.[30,50] Optic ataxia can also be seen in the absence of visual disorientation or ocular apraxia, unilaterally, in the field opposite the affected hand.[160]

Ocular apraxia consists of the inability to direct gaze voluntarily toward a new stimulus that has appeared in the periphery of the visual field. In other words, whereas a normal individual will easily produce a quick saccade toward a new interesting stimulus that has appeared in the periphery of the visual field, a patient with ocular apraxia will not be able to produce this saccade even when alerted verbally that a stimulus has indeed entered his visual field. Or, if a saccade does take place, it may be directed inaccurately and not bring the new stimulus into the fovea. Patients probably fail to see anything that is not brought or maintained in optimal central vision. In his original description, Bálint referred to ocular apraxia as "psychic gaze paralysis." Gordon Holmes called it "spasm of fixation."

The appearance of the full Bálint's syndrome is, in our experience, strongly related to bilateral damage of the occipitoparietal region. More often than not, the lesions are the result of infarctions in the border zone (watershed) between the anterior and posterior cerebral artery territories. Sudden and severe hypotension is perhaps the main cause of this type of cerebrovascular accident. Most of the patients who come to medical attention with Bálint's syndrome are elderly individuals who are especially vulnerable to systemic blood pressure drop and who may already have reduction of useful vision due to glaucoma, cataract, macular degeneration, or cognitive disorders as in Alzheimer's disease. In the vascular cases, the lesions are often quite symmetric, but they may be of different sizes. Thus, the presence of Bálint's syndrome in a patient with cerebrovascular disease usually indicates a type of stroke different from the one that causes the agnosias or pure alexia. Whereas the lesions in the agnosias are ventral (occipitotemporal), those in Bálint's syndrome tend to be more dorsal (occipitoparietal). Bálint's syndrome can also be caused by bilateral metastases in the occipitoparietal region, even when asymmetrically placed (Fig. 7–3).

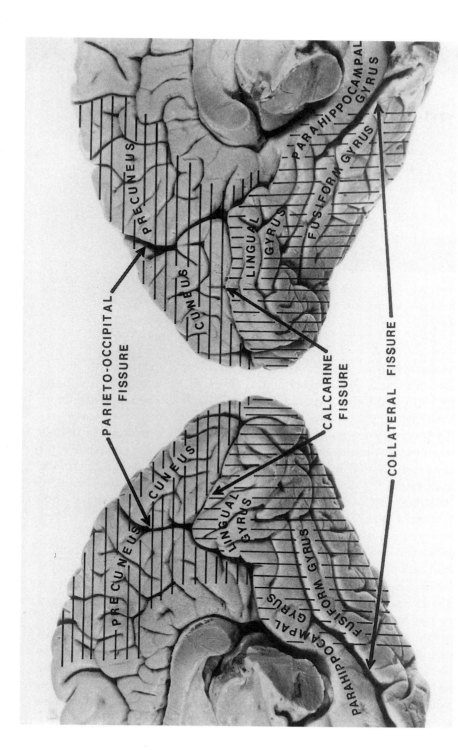

FIGURE 7-3. Mesial view of the posterior part of a human brain, showing major sulci and gyri. Patients with visual agnosia (including prosopagnosia) have bilateral lesions in structures of the occipitotemporal region (vertical hatching) comprising the lingual, fusiform, and parahippocampal gyri. Patients with Bálint's syndrome have bilateral lesions in the occipitoparietal region (horizontal hatching), which is composed of the cuneus and precuneus. Unilateral lesions of the left occipitotemporal region often produce the syndrome of pure alexia (in patients with left cerebral dominance for language, provided that connections of the corpus callosum are also damaged).

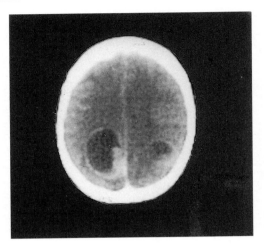

FIGURE 7–4. A CT scan of a patient with Bálint's syndrome caused by bilateral metastases from carcinoma. Note that the metastases involve functionally comparable areas in the occipitoparietal region.

When the entire syndrome is present some involvement (either medially or dorsally) of Brodmann's[40] area (BA) 7 is common, although the adjoining BA19 and sometimes part of BA39 are also involved.[105] In some patients, the lesions are more extensive and may encompass white matter or cortex in the lower occipital or occipitotemporal region. In such patients severe visual field defects or an additional agnosia may complicate the presentation. In general, the lesions responsible for Bálint's syndrome are located in the occipitoparietal sector of the visual cortex. Ratcliff and co-workers[154,155] obtained results compatible with these notions in an experimental task requiring patients to touch stimuli presented in a perimeter while maintaining fixation of gaze. The authors found that patients with posterior lesions of either hemisphere performed defectively in this task and that a visual field defect was not a significant correlate.

Cursory observation of patients with Bálint's syndrome may often give the examiner the false impression of dealing with a case of visual agnosia. (Some patients with so-called apperceptive agnosia may have had Bálint's syndrome.) This may occur when the patients report that they *see* but do not *know* what the stimulus is. This may happen with any stimulus, including human faces, and often occurs with reading material. The consequence is that these patients are often mislabeled as agnosic and alexic. It is necessary to take pains to introduce the stimuli in the effective portion of the visual field and to show that the patient's real recognition performance is, in fact, preserved under certain conditions of stimulus presentation.

We have now seen instances of patients with visual disorientation (simultanagnosia) in isolation—that is, without optic ataxia. In these intriguing cases of defective spatial analysis, the patients claim not to see objects that they can point to accurately. It is possible, in those instances, that there is enough visual information to permit appropriate guidance of the hand and fingers but that the patient is unable to synthesize a visual field into a coherent whole. Patients with visual disorientation alone have bilateral lesions confirmed to the supracalcarine cortex, thus sparing the adjoining parietal cortex (Fig. 7–4).

The contrast between the lesions that cause the full Bálint's syndrome (occipitoparietal) and those that cause visual disorientation alone (superior-occipital) suggests that these two regions may have different roles in spatial analysis and visuomotor performance. Both human data[50] and animal experiments[80,83,130,131,133,134,199] suggest that the parietal lobe, especially BA7, contains a visuomotor center capable of directing gaze toward interesting new stimuli that appear in panoramic vision and of guiding hand movements toward visual targets (Chapter 3). The superior occipital cortex (striate and peristriate), however, appears to contain structures and contribute to the structuring of the visual field as a whole.

Disturbances of Stereo Vision (Stereopsis)

"Stereopsis" is the *ability to discriminate depth on the basis of binocular visual information.* Because of the physical separation of the eyes, the two-dimensional projections of three-dimensional objects occupy slightly different positions on the right and left retinas. This horizontal disparity is the source of stereopsis. Stereopsis does not depend on *monocular* cues of depth derived from image contours, texture, apparent size of familiar objects, interposition of near and far, linear perspectives, or monocular parallax.

The first step in the testing of stereopsis consists of ensuring that the patient has adequate visual acuity and that the ocular alignment is correct. (The latter may be assessed with orthoptic techniques such as the four-diopter baseout prism and the *Wirth four-dot* tests.) Full-field stereopsis can be tested with standard handheld tests of stereovision, available commercially. Such tests include the *TNO anaglyphs* (Lameris Instrumenten), which require red-green glasses, and the *Titmus* (Titmus Optical Company) and *Randot* (Stereo Optical Company) stereotests, which use polarized glasses and printed materials. Testing of stereopsis within quadrants is a difficult task that should only be undertaken in a laboratory equipped with a tachistoscope.

Carmon and Bechtoldt[42] and Benton and Hecaen[24] postulated that the right hemisphere was dominant for stereopsis. Brain-damaged patients were asked to localize random-letter stereograms to one quadrant of a background field. Performance appeared especially impaired and response time prolonged in patients with damage to the right hemisphere. But the exact cerebral localization of the lesions was not known and the age, type, and size of lesions were not considered. Several patients had malignant tumors and intracerebral hematomas, which could have increased intracranial pressure and affected brain function in a nonfocal manner. Support for the hypothesis that stereopsis could be preferentially related to right hemisphere processing also came from a study in normal individuals in which random-dot stereograms were presented tachistoscopically, and performance in the left hemifield proved superior. In contrast, Julesz and associates found markedly different results in normal subjects, in whom the left and right visual fields showed equivalent stereoptic ability.[107] These results indicate that both hemispheres are capable of processing stereopsis. However, Julesz did find a significant difference between upper and lower visual fields.[107] Interestingly, Gazzaniga and co-workers[76] found that stereopsis was preserved after complete callosal lesions, except when the chiasm was also split. This finding indicates the existence of stereoptic ability in each hemisphere.

The visual cortex has both monocular and binocular cells.[30,31] Direct electrophysiologic evidence in the cat and monkey shows that many cells in striate and prestriate cortex respond to binocular stimuli. Animals deprived of binocular stimuli at a critical age develop predominantly monocular cortex.[69,99,104] Neuropsychological and electrophysiologic studies show that humans also have binocular and monocular visual cortices.[115] The use of random-dot stereograms has enabled researchers to study stereopsis and confirmed the need to postulate a central processing mechanism for this function.[104] Random-dot stereograms consist of two nearly identical computer-generated stereopairs composed of black dots. They differ in that a group of these random elements, in the shape of a geometric form, has been shifted in precise fashion with respect to the identical random sequence in the other member of the stereopair. When viewed stereoscopically (one array presented to each eye), a form such as a square is seen above or below the random background. Levels of brightness, spatial and temporal disparity, order of presentation, object size, stimulus familiarity, and area of retinal stimulation influence performance.[106,161,196]

Information from animal studies is limited but does confirm that stereopsis depends on central processing and that neurons related to stereopsis are localized at a high level in the hierarchy of the visual system. Along central visual pathways, there is no known binocular interaction prior to area 17.[153] Hubel and Wiesel[100] found that binocular disparity units are found in area 18 and beyond in the macaque, but not in area 17. Four kinds of neurons involved in stereopsis were isolated in the macaque.[100]

Current research in this area is aimed at discovering the neuroanatomic sites of damage associated with astereopsis and learning whether or not unilateral lesions can impair stereopsis. The elucidation of the phenomenon could lead to a better understanding of amblyopia in children with strabismus, who are deprived of stereoscopic stimuli during critical phases of brain development. Syndromes of monofixation and stereoblindness in individuals with normal peripheral visual apparatus could also be better understood. Testing stereopsis is crucial in individuals with occupations dependent on binocular depth discrimination, such as airline piloting, and can be used with advantage in the evaluation of patients with visual disorders caused by focal lesions of the central visual system.

Cerebral Akinetopsia

Akinetopsia is an acquired defect of motion processing caused by acquired cerebral lesions. As motion cues serve many purposes,[135] a range of deficits can result, from defective smooth-pursuit eye movements to trouble perceiving motion-defined objects (structure-from-motion or kinetic depth). The deficits are most often reported with damage around the angular gyrus, parietal-temporo-occipital, and parieto-occipital regions and may be part of a more pervasive disturbance (as in Bálint's syndrome or Alzheimer's disease).

Zihl and colleagues[206] reported an instance of cerebral akinetopsia in patient L. M., who had a severe, persistent disturbance of movement vision following damage to the posterior hemispheres that was probably caused by venous sinus thrombosis. Patient L. M. could see movement in slowly moving targets, but targets moving at greater than 10 to 14° per second seemed to materialize at successive positions with no movement in between. Her smooth ocular pursuit of moving targets broke down at 8° per second and she could not even follow the trajectory of her own finger if it moved "too fast." L. M. underestimated the speed of faster moving targets and showed breakdown of the ø mechanism, which allows us to perceive apparent motion between successive pictures in an animation sequence. Also, she had reduced perception of motion aftereffects, the spiral aftereffect elicited no sense of motion-in-depth, and she reported seeing changes in position but not movement in depth when a target was moved toward and away from her. Static binocular stereoacuity and manual reaction times to visual targets were also somewhat impaired.

However, L. M. reportedly had good static visual acuity, normal perception of temporal flicker of a light presented at several locations in the visual fields, normal visual evoked potentials in response to contrast-reversing checkerboard stimuli, normal perception of tactile and acoustic motion, accurate localization of visual targets by saccadic eye movements, no visual field defect for form or luminance, and no neglect of visual targets flashed simultaneously in both hemifields. Relative preservation of face and object recognition, reading, and color vision distinguished L. M. from patient's such as Verrey's, with damage in ventromesial visual association cortices, located below the calcarine fissure in the occipital lobe and in adjacent inferotemporal regions. Zeki[203] labeled L. M.'s deficit "cerebral akinetopsia" in analogy to the term "cerebral achromatopsia" used to describe acquired cerebral color processing defects.

The report of L. M. sparked new research activity aimed at identifying the cerebral substrates for motion perception. The lesions reported in L. M.[207] and in subsequent patients with motion perception deficits often include structures in an occipito-temporoparietal and a parieto-occipital location (e.g, Thurston and colleagues,[174] Vaina;[186] Vaina and co-workers;[187] Beckers and Hömberg;[19] Morrow and Sharpe;[133] Plant and associates[151,152]). The dorsolateral lesions reported in these cases overlap the localizations provided by functional neuroimaging studies for a human motion processing region.[176,195] These cortical areas include BA19 and adjacent BA37. Judging by criteria of myelogenesis,[71] myeloarchitecture, and callosal connections, part of these areas may resemble monkey's area MT[8,44] also known as V5.[68,201]

Area MT (V5) occupies the posterior wall of the superior temporal sulcus[9,68] and receives a preponderance of M-pathway (broad band) inputs from striate (area V1) and early extrastriate areas (e.g., V2).[124] Area MT contains a large proportion of neurons that are sensitive to stimulus direction, speed, orientation, and binocular disparity,[7,13,123,124,128] are active during perceptual decisions on these properties,[162] and probably contribute to motion direction discrimination[140] and even shape-from-motion perception.[165]

Area MT processes different types of motion.[6,205] First-order motion refers to a change in luminance over space and time, as when a shadow passes over the ground. Second order motion perception requires a more complex mechanism sensitive to absolute change in contrast, not just luminance.[43,95] Area MT may also process third order (pattern-tracking) motion that is attention dependent.[94] The human brain should follow a similar organization, and motion deficits in a few well-documented human cases are comparable to those in the monkey, although motion deficits in humans appear to last much longer.[152,187,207]

Ibotenic acid lesions of MT in monkey produce a relatively selective deficit for motion perception in the contralateral visual hemifield[122,139,140,142,145,165] that recovers to prelesion levels within a few weeks. The deficits in patient L. M., however, have endured for almost two decades.[13,90,171,206] This could be due to lower selectivity of human lesions, which occur by chance and involve white matter and probably several functional areas (and are not created through controlled application of a selective cytotoxin such as ibotenic acid), rather than due to interspecies differences.

Mounting evidence indicates that lesions in dorsolateral visual association cortices thought to contain an area MT homolog can impair the perception of surface-from-motion (SFM)[158,186] and cause selective failure of visual processing of motion-defined form.[156] Three-dimensional SFM is encoded by area MT neurons[37] and seems to involve the occipital and parietal cortex more than simpler types of motion discrimination. Orban and associates[141] used passive viewing tasks with functional MRI to show that visual motion regions (including MT/V5 and parietal regions) in humans respond more to 3D motion than to 2D motion. Participation of MT/V5 was predicted from experiments in monkeys showing that MT/V5 neurons are tuned to the direction of speed gradients corresponding to direction of tilt;[122,198] spatial properties of the antagonistic surround are crucial.[122,198]

Testing for motion perception deficits requires use of stimuli that minimize inferences of movement from noticeable changes in the visual scene, the way we infer movement of the moon over the sky. We use computer generated animation sequences known as random dot cinematograms (RDC). The RDCs present a motion signal amid spatially random background noise and allow variation of spatial displacement and temporal intervals at programmable exposure durations. The RDCs can be used to test different aspects of motion processing (e.g., speed or direction discrimination, shape-from-motion) that can be affected with cerebral lesions. Motion processing deficits can also be assessed by measuring a patient's ability to track moving targets with ocular smooth pursuit, but failure on this task could due to defective motor control rather than to a true motion perception deficit.

Use of RCD has shown that L. M. perceives global coherent ("first order") motion and can discriminate direction of movement, but this ability fails at moderate levels of background visual noise.[158] L. M. can perceive 2D shape and 3D structure from first-order motion, but these abilities break down at moderate levels of moving and stationary noise. However, L. M. also has trouble perceiving 2D shapes defined by nonmotion signals including "on" and "off" transients, dynamic and static binocular disparity, and static texture cues. These findings highlight the role of the visual association cortex in extracting salient information from noise and do not support the idea that visual motion is localized to a single area of the brain or that motion blindness can occur in isolation. The observation in L. M. that lesions of the dorsolateral pathways can affect object recognition whether the cues that define the object are moving or static is incompatible with the strong hypothesis that shape and object perception and recognition are exclusive property of the ventral visual, or "what" pathway.

Human motion processing deficits have been reported in patients with lesions in structures outside those usually associated with a human area MT homolog. Severe deficits of motion perception can occur with lesions in parietal insula[137] and midline cerebellum,[136] compatible with the idea that many areas of the brain respond to visual motion.[69] Also, the homologies between motion processing areas in monkey and human may not be a close as they once appeared.

Human and monkey extrastriate cortex appear to be organized differently at, or beyond, V3A and V4.[67,175] Van Oostende and associates[187] used functional MRI to identify the kinetic occipital region (KO), a motion area that differs in function and location and from other motion processing areas and has not yet been identified in monkeys. The KO is located posterior to MT/V5 and is activated selectively by kinetic contours. Recent studies of human brain activity showed surprisingly little involvement of human MT/V5 in discriminations of motion direction[46] and speed.[141] Yet, parietal regions are active, together with a supposed human area V3A and a ventral (lingual) area, suggesting discrimination performance for simple motion is mediated more by occipitotemporal regions than previously suspected.

The inferior temporal area in the macaque contains neurons that respond to shapes independently of cue types (of static texture, luminance, and relative motion, i.e., cues that are processed in ventral and dorsal visual pathways[163]) and may be responsible for cue-invariant coding of boundaries and edges.[163] Damage to such a mechanism could affect perception of shapes defined by moving or static stimulus cues and help explain the strong correlations between impairments of SFM and complex stationary patterns found in a recent study of motion processing in Alzheimer's disease (AD). Discussion of movement processing deficits in AD has centered on stage of disease and the selectivity and locus of neuropathological changes from retina to visual association cortex (e.g., Gilmore and co-workers;[78] Hinton and associates;[93] Kurylo and colleagues;[112] Sathian;[164] Silverman and Feldon[172]). Most motion processing deficits that we know of are caused by cerebrovascular disease.

Other Disorders of Spatial Analysis

The ability to judge the directional orientation of lines has been the object of several experimental studies and is a useful test of visual abilities in neurologic patients (Chapter 2). In the *Judgment of Line Orientation* test,[27] the patient is presented with pairs of lines placed in a given angle and requested to point to similarly oriented lines in a different array. Defective performance on this test is strongly correlated with right posterior lesions.[28] We believe that right occipitoparietal lesions are probably the best correlate of such defects.

The ability to discriminate unfamiliar faces is another process that is dependent on intact visual perception. The widespread use of Benton and Van Allen's *Facial Recognition* test has shown that impaired performance is strongly associated with right hemisphere damage, especially postrolandic, but also with left hemisphere damage in patients with fluent, postrolandic aphasias.[84] Incidentally, the well-entrenched title of the test may be misleading because the task calls for a matching of unfamiliar faces on the basis of a visual discrimination performance, and not on the basis of recognition. As noted earlier, prosopagnosic patients can pass this test.

VI. DISTURBANCES OF CONSTRUCTIONAL ABILITY

Impairments in the ability to construct a copy of a visually presented model by means of assembling blocks or by drawing are generally known as "constructional apraxia," a term introduced by Kleist.[110] The term is commonly used but the fact that the disorder bears no relation to Liepmann's definition of apraxias has given rise to some confusion. We prefer to define these impairments as disturbances of "visuoconstructive ability" or "constructional ability" rather than as apraxias.

The performance of construction tasks presupposes normal visual acuity, the ability to perceive the several elements of the model as well as their spatial relationship, and finally adequate motor ability. Failure in any of these elementary prerequisites can lead to impairment in these tasks so that the constructional abilities of such patients cannot be tested meaningfully.

There are numerous ways of testing for visuoconstructive ability. Using paper and pencil, the examiner can test two-dimensional constructions by requiring that line drawings be copied. In a variation on these tasks, the examiner may request the drawing of a simple object from memory (e.g., a house, a clock, or a face) or may ask for the copy of a line model using small sticks or matches. The testing of three-dimensional construction requires an appropriate set of models and of separate building components. Benton's *Three Dimensional Praxis Test* is a well-standardized example.[28] The block design subtest of the *Wechsler Adult Intelligence Scale* is commonly used to assess constructional abilities.

Although Kleist was convinced that a disturbance of constructional ability was caused by left parietal damage, numerous studies have now confirmed that both left and right parietal lesions can cause a defect (Chapter 2). In our experience, lesions of the left parietal region are less likely to lead to constructional defects than are lesions of the right. Furthermore, defects caused by lesions of the right parietal region tend to be different in degree and in nature. The disturbance is more profound and quite often there is a characteristic neglect of the left side of the elements being copied, assuming that the patient can copy anything at all.[21,23,63]

Most patients with constructional defects caused by a left hemisphere lesion tend to be aphasic as well. The aphasia is of the fluent type, generally associated with postrolandic lesions.[22] It is possible that the presence of a linguistic defect can contribute to the disturbance, although it is equally probable that the lesions more frequently associated with constructional praxis are located closer to the language cortices of the left hemisphere and thus determine an association of symptoms on the basis of anatomic contiguity.

The types of tasks and the degree of difficulty of the tasks that have been used in studies of visuoconstructive ability are extremely varied. Obviously, two-dimensional and three-dimensional models pose different degrees of difficulty, as does copying from actual models versus copying from graphic representations of those models. These differences underscore the difficulty in comparing the results of various studies and the potential for discrepancy and controversy.

From the practical perspective of diagnosis, a marked deficit of constructional ability is a useful indicator of parietal dysfunction.

VII. Disturbance of the Ability to Dress

Numerous neurologic patients are unable to don a shirt or a coat properly, even when the specific garment is handed to them. The symptom, generally known as dressing apraxia, is perhaps most frequent in patients with dementia or confusion, although patients with clear sensorium and preserved intellect can show the symptom as well. (Much the same reservations that apply to the term "constructional apraxia" apply to "dressing apraxia.") In those with focal lesions, the impairment is generally seen in the setting of left-sided neglect or Bálint's syndrome—that is, in patients with right occipitoparietal or bilateral occipitoparietal lesions. But we must emphasize that we have never seen dressing apraxia in isolation.

A variety of mechanisms account for the impairment. For instance, patients with left-sided motor neglect will fail to swing a jacket around their backs, in a leftward direction, and will not orient the left arm toward the opening of the sleeve. Sensory neglect of the left hemispace, even in the absence of motor neglect or hemiparesis, may lead to a similar result. Patients with simultanagnosia and optic ataxia, however, maintain all the automatic motions related to dressing and yet are unable to coordinate the orientation of the garment in relation to the body. When patients attempt a corrective action under visual guidance, their visuomotor impairment often does not permit a successful movement.

In theory, it seems possible that a somatosensory feedback defect, in the absence of paralysis, could lead to an impairment in dressing. But we have never seen a patient who fit that specification.

VIII. Concluding Remarks

The involvement of vision-related cortices by neurological diseases results in a large variety of disorders of complex visual processing, as reviewed in the text here. Acquaintance with the clinical profiles of these disorders is important for clinicians faced with diagnostic problems and equally important for rehabilitation professionals concerned with managing the recovery process of neurological patients. Last but not least, the disorders of complex visual processing reviewed here continue to contribute to our understanding of brain-behavior relationships, either by posing new questions for investigation or by offering an opportunity to test hypotheses generated by fundamental studies.

This work was supported by National Institute of Neurological Diseases and Stroke (NINCDS) grant PO1 NS19632.

REFERENCES

1. Adolphs, R, Tranel, D and Damasio, A R: The human amygdala in social judgment. Nature 393:470–474, 1998.
2. Adolphs, R, Tranel, D, Damasio, H and Damasio, A R: Impaired recognition of emotion in facial expressions following bilateral damage to the human amygdala. Nature 372:669–672, 1994.
3. Adolphs, R, Tranel, D, Damasio, H and Damasio, A R: Fear and the human amygdala. J Neurosci 15:5879–5891, 1995.
4. Agnetti, V, Carreras, M, Pinna, L and Rosati, G: Ictal prosopagnosia and epileptogenic damage of the dominant hemisphere: a case history. Cortex 14:50–57, 1978.
5. Albert, M L, Reches, A and Silverberg, R: Hemianopic colour blindness. J Neurol Neurosurg Psychiatry 38:546–549, 1975.
6. Albright, T D: Direction and orientation selectivity of neurons in visual area MT of the macaque. J Neurophysiol 52:1106–1130, 1984.
7. Albright, T D: Form-cue invariant motion processing in primate visual center. Science 255: 1141–1143, 1992.
8. Allman, J M: Evolution of the visual system in early primates. In: Sprague J, Epstein A N, (Eds.) Progress in Psychology, Physiology, and Psychiatry, Academic Press, New York; 1–53, 1977.
9. Allman, J M and Kaas, J H: A representation of the visual field in the caudal third of the middle temporal gyrus of the owl monkey (*Aotus trivirgatus*). Brain Res 31: 85–105, 1971.
10. Andreasen, N C, O'Leary, D S, Arndt, S, Cizadlo, T, Hurtig, R, Rezai, K, Watkins, G L, Ponto, L B and Hichwa, R D: Neural substrates of facial recognition. J Neuropsychiatry Clin Neurosci 8:139–146, 1996.
11. Arseni, C and Botez, M: Consideraciones sobre un caso de agnosia de las fisonomias. Rev Neuropsiquiatr 3:157–160, 1965.
12. Assal, G, Eisert, H G and Hecaen, H: Analyse des resultats du Farnsworth D15 chez 155 nialades atteints de lesions hemispheriques droites ou gauches. Acta Neurologica et Psychiatrica Belgica 69:705–717, 1969.
13. Baker, C L Jr, Hess, R F and Zihl, J: Residual motion perception in a 'motion-blind' patient, assessed with limited-lifetime random dot stimuli. J Neurosci 2: 454–461, 1991.
14. Bálint, R: Seelenlahmung des "Schauens", optische Ataxie, raumliche Storung der Aufmerksamkeit. Monatsschr Psychiat Neurol 25:51–81, 1909.
15. Bauer, R M: Autonomic recognition of names and faces in prosopagnosia: a neuropsychological application of the Guilty Knowledge Test. Neuropsychologia 22:457–469, 1984.
16. Bauer, R M and Verfaellie, M: Electrodermal discrimination of familiar but not unfamiliar faces in prosopagnosia. Brain Cogn 8:240–252, 1988.
17. Bay, E: Disturbances of visual perception and their examination. Brain 76:515–550, 1953.

18. Bechara, A, Damasio, A R and Tranel, D: Decision-making and the somatic marker hypothesis. In Gazzaniga, M (Ed.): The Cognitive Neurosicences, 2nd Ed. MIT Press, Cambridge, MA; in press.

19. Beckers, G and Hömberg, V: Cerebral visual motion blindness: transitory akinetopsia induced by transcraial magnetic stimulation of human area V5. Proc R Soc Lond Biol 249: 173–178, 1992.

20. Benson, D F, Segarra, J and Albert, M L: Visual agnosia-prosopagnosia. Arch Neurol 30: 307–310, 1974.

21. Benton, A L: Constructional apraxia and the minor hemisphere. Confin Neurol 29:1–16, 1967.

22. Benton, A L: Visuoconstructive disability in patients with cerebral disease: its relationship to side of lesion and aphasic disorder. Doc Ophthalmol 34:67–76, 1973.

23. Benton, A L and Fogel, M L: Three-dimensional constructional praxis. Arch Neurol 7: 347–354, 1962.

24. Benton, A L and Hecaen, H: Stereoscopic vision in patients with unilateral cerebral disease. Neurology 20:1084–1088, 1970.

25. Benton, A L and Van Allen, M W: Impairment in facial recognition in patients with cerebral disease. Cortex 4:344–358, 1968.

26. Benton, A L, Levin, H S and Van Allen, M W: Geographic orientation in patients with unilateral cerebral disease. Neuropsychologia 12:183–191, 1974.

27. Benton, A L, Varney, N R and Hamsher, K: Visuospatial judgment: A clinical test. Arch Neurol 35:364–367, 1978.

28. Benton, A L, Hamsher, K, Varney, N R and Spreen, O: Contributions to Neuropsychological Assessment. Oxford University Press, New York, 1983.

29. Berlin, B and Kay, P: Basic Color Terms. University of California Press, Berkeley, 1969.

30. Blake, R and Cormack, R: Psychophysical evidence for a monocular visual cortex in stereoblind humans. Science 203:274–275, 1979.

31. Blake, R and Levinson, E: Spatial properties of binocular neurons in the human visual system. Exp Brain Res 27:221–232, 1977.

32. Bodamer, J: Die Prosop-Agnosie. Arch Psychiatr Nervenkr 179:6–54, 1947.

33. Boller, F, Cole, M, Kim, Y, Mack, J L and Patawaran, C: Optic ataxia: Clinical radiological correlations with the EMI scan. J Neurol Neurosurg Psychiatry 38:954–958, 1975.

34. Bornstein, B: Prosopagnosia. 8th Int Congr Neurol Proc 3:157–160, 1965.

35. Botez, M I: Two visual systems in clinical neurology: readaptive role of the primitive system in visual agnosic patients. Eur Neurol 13:101–122, 1975.

36. Bowen, F P, Hoehn, M M and Yahr, M D: Parkinsonism: alterations in spatial orientation as determined by a route-walking test. Neuropsychologia 10:355–361, 1972.

37. Bradley, D C, Chang, G C and Andersen, R A: Encoding of three-dimensional structure-from-motion by primate area MT neurons (letter). Nature 392: 714–717, 1998.

38. Brazis, P W, Biller, J and Fine, M: Central achromatopsia. Neurology 31:920–921, 1981.

39. Breiter, H C, Etcoff, N L, Whalen, P H, Kennedy, W A, Rauch, S L, Buckner, R L, Strauss, M M, Hyman, S E and Rosen, B R: Response and habituation of the human amygdala during visual processing of facial expression. Neuron 17:875–887, 1996.

40. Brodmann, K: Vergleichende lokalisationslehre der grosshirnrinde in ihren prinzipien dargestellt auf grund des zellenbaues. J. A. Barth, Leipzig, 1909.

41. Calder, A J, Young, A W, Rowland, D, Perrett, D I, Hodges, J R and Etcoff, N L: Facial emotion recognition after bilateral amygdala damage: differentially severe impairement of fear. Cognit Neuropsychol 13:699–745, 1996.

42. Carmon, A and Bechtoldt, H P: Dominance of the right cerebral hemisphere for stereopsis. Neuropsychologia 7:29–39, 1969.

43. Chubb, C and Sperling, G: Drift-balanced random stimuli: a general basis for studying non-Fourier motion perception. J Opt Soc Am [A], 5:1986–2007, 1988.

44. Clarke, S and Miklossy, J: Occipital cortex in man: organization of callosal connections, related myelo- and cytoarchitecture, and putative boundaries of functional visual areas. J Comp Neurol 298: 188–214, 1990.

45. Cohn, R, Neumann, M S and Wood, D H: Prosopagnosia: a clinicopathological study. Ann Neurol 1: 177–182, 1977.

46. Cornette, L, Dupont, P, Rosier, A, Sunaert, S, Van Hecke, P, Michiels, J, Mortelmans, L and Orban, G A: Human brain regions involved in direction discrimination. J Neurophysiol 79:2749–2765, 1998.

47. Critchley, M: Acquired anomalies of colour perception of central origin. Brain 88:711–724, 1965.

48. Damasio, A R: Descartes' Error: Emotion, reason, and the Human Brain. Grosset/Putnam, New York, 1994.

49. Damasio, A R: Time-locked multiregional retroactivation: a systems level proposal for the neural substrates of recall and recognition. Cognition 33:25–62, 1989.

50. Damasio, A R and Benton, A L: Impairment of hand movements under visual guidance. Neurology 29:170–178, 1979.

51. Damasio, A R and Damasio H: Anatomical basis of pure alexia. Neurology 33:1573–1583, 1983.

52. Damasio, A R and Damasio, H: Cortical systems for retrieval of concrete knowledge: the convergence zone framework. In Koch, C (Ed.): Large-Scale Neuronal Theories of the Brain. MIT Press, Cambridge, MA, 1994, pp. 61–74.

53. Damasio, A R, Damasio, H and Van Hoesen, G W: Prosopagnosia: anatomic basis and behavioral mechanisms. Neurology 32:331–341, 1982.

54. Damasio, A R, Lima, P A and Damasio, H: Nervous function after right hemispherectomy. Neurology (Minneapolis) 25:89–93, 1975.

55. Damasio, A R, McKee, J and Damasio, H: Determinants of performance in color anomia. Brain Lang 7:74–85, 1979.

56. Damasio, A R, Tranel, D and Damasio, H: Individuals with sociopathic behavior caused by frontal damage fail to respond autonomically to social stimuli. Behav Brain Res 41:81–94, 1990.

57. Damasio, A R, Tranel, D and Damasio, H: Somatic markers and the guidance of behavior: Theory and preliminary testing. In Levin, H S, Eisenberg, H M, and Benton, A L (Ed.): Frontal Lobe Function and Dysfunction. Oxford Univeristy Press, New York, 1991, pp. 217–229.

58. Damasio, A R, Yamada, T, Damasio, H, Corbet, J and Mckee, J: Central achromatopsia: Behavioral, anatomic and physiologic aspects. Neurology 30:1064–1071, 1980.

59. Damasio, H and Frank R: Three-dimensional in vivo mapping of brain lesions in humans. Arch Neurol 49:137–143, 1992.

60. Davidoff, J B and Ostergaard, A L: Color anomia resulting from weakened short-term color memory. Brain 107:415–431, 1984.

61. De Haan, E H F, Young, A and Newcombe, F: Face recognition without awareness. Cognit Neuropsychol 4:385–415, 1987b.

62. De Haan, E H F, Young, A and Newcombe, F: Faces interfere with name classification in a prosopagnosic patient. Cortex 23:309–316, 1987a.

63. De Renzi, E and Faglioni, P: The relationship between visuospatial impairment and constructional apraxia. Cortex 3:327–342, 1967.

64. De Renzi, E and Spinnler, H: Impaired performance on color tasks in patients with hemispheric damage. Cortex 3:194–216, 1967.

65. De Vreese, L P: Two systems for color-naming defects: verbal disconnection versus color imagery disorder. Neuropsychologia 29:1–18, 1991.

66. Déjerine, J: Contribution a l'étude anatomo-pathologique et clinique des differentes varietés de cecité verbale. Memoires Societé Biologique 4:61–90, 1892.

67. Deyoe, E A, Hockfield, S, Garren, H and Van Essen, D C: Antibody labeling of functional

subdivisions in visual cortex: cat-301 immunoreactivity in striate and extrastriate cortex of the macaque monkey. Vis Neurosci 5:67–81, 1990.

68. Dubner, R and Zeki, S M. Response properties and receptive fields of cells in an anatomically defined region of the superior temporal sulcus in the monkey. Brain Res 35:528–532, 1971.

69. Dupont, P, Orban, G A, De Bruyn, B, Verbruggen, A and Mortelmans, L: Many areas in the human brain respond to visual motion. J Neurophysiol 72:1420–1424, 1994.

70. Epstein, R and Kanwisher, N: A cortical representation of the local visual environment. Nature 392:598–601, 1998.

71. Flechsig, P: Developmental (myelogenetic) localisation of the cerebral cortex in the human subject. Lancet 2:1027–1029, 1901.

72. Freund, S: Zur ueber optische aphasie and seelenblindheit. Arch Psychiatr Nervenkr 20: 276–297, 371–416, 1889.

73. Fried, I, Mateer, C, Ojemann, G, Wohns, R and Fedio, P: Organization of visuospatial functions in human cortex. Brain 105:349–371, 1982.

74. Frisen, L and Kalm, P: Sahlgren's saturation test for detecting and grading acquired dyschromatopsia. Am J Ophthalmol 92:252–258, 1981.

75. Gazzaniga, M S and Smylie, C S: Facial recognition and brain asymmetries: clues to underlying mechanisms. Ann Neurol 13:537–540, 1984.

76. Gazzaniga, M S, Bogen, J E and Sperry, R W: Observations on visual perception after disconnexion of the cerebral hemispheres in man. Brain 88:221–236, 1965.

77. Geschwind, N and Fusillo, M: Color-naming defects in association with alexia. Arch Neurol 15:137–146, 1966.

78. Gilmore, G C, Wenk, H E, Naylor, L A and Koss, E: Motion perception and Alzheimer's disease. J Gerontol 49:52–57, 1994.

79. Gloning, I, Gloning, K, Jellinger, K and Quatember, R: A case of "prosopagnosia" with necropsy findings. Neuropsychologia 8:199–204, 1970.

80. Goldberg, M E and Robinson D L: Visual mechanisms underlying gaze: function of the cerebral cortex. In Baker, R. and Berthoz, A. (Eds.): Control of Gaze by Brain Stem Neurons, Developments in Neuroscience, Vol. 1. Biomedical Press, Elsevier North-Holland, 1977, pp. 469–476.

81. Goodglass, H and Kaplan, E: The Assessment of Aphasia and Related Disorders. Lea & Febiger, Philadelphia, 1972.

82. Green, G J and Lessell, S: Acquired cerebral dyschromatopsia. Arch Ophthalmol 95:121–128, 1977.

83. Haaxma, R and Kuypers, H G J M: Intrahemispheric cortical connexions and visual guidance of hand and finger movements in the rhesus monkey. Brain 98:239–260, 1975.

84. Hamsher, K, Levin, H S and Benton, A L: Facial recognition in patients with focal brain lesions. Arch Neurol 36:837–839, 1979.

85. Hardy, L H, Rand, G and Rittler, M C: AO-HRR pseudoisochromatic plates, 2nd Ed. American Optical, Chicago 1957.

86. Hasselmo, M E, Rolls, E T and Baylis, G C: The role of expression and identity in the face-selective responses of neurons in the temporal visual cortex of the monkey. Behav Brain Res 32:203–218, 1989.

87. Hecaen, H and Angelergues, R: Agnosia for faces (prosopagnosia). Arch Neurol 7:92–100, 1962.

88. Hecaen, H and De Ajuriaguerra, J: Bálint's syndrome (psychic paralysis of visual fixation) and its minor forms. Brain 77:373–400, 1954.

89. Heidenhain, A: Beitrag zur Kenntnis der Seelenblindheit. Monattschr Psychiatr Neurol 66:61–116, 1927.

90. Hess, R H, Baker C L Jr and Zihl, J: The 'motion-blind' patient: low level spatial and temporal filters. J Neurosci 9:1628–1640, 1989.

91. Heywood, C A, Cowey, A and Newcombe, F: Chromatic discrimination in a cortically blind observer. Eur J Neurosci 3:802–812, 1991.

92. Heywood, C A, Wilson, B and Cowey, A L: A case of cortical colour "blindness" with relatively intact achromatic discrimination. J Neurol Neurosurg Psychiatry 50:22–29, 1987.

93. Hinton, D R, Sadun, A A, Blanks, J C and Miller, C A: Optic-nerve degeneration in Alzheimer's disease. N Engl J Med 315: 485–487, 1986.

94. Ho, C E: Letter recognition reveals pathways of second-order and third-order motion. Proc Natl Acad Sci USA 95:400–404, 1998.

95. Hof, P R, Bouras, C, Constantinidis, J and Morrison, J H: Selective disconnection of specific visual association pathways in cases of Alzheimer's disease presenting with Bálint's syndrome. J Neuropathol Exp Neurol 49: 168–184, 1990.

96. Holmes, G: Disturbances of visual orientation. Br J Ophthalmol 2:449–486, 506–516, 1918.

97. Holmes, G: Disturbances of spatial orientation and visual attention with loss of stereoscopic vision. Arch Neurol Psychiatry 1:385, 1919.

98. Holmes, G: Pure word blindness. Folia Psychiatr Neurol Neurochir Neerl 53:279–288, 1950.

99. Hubel, D H and Wiesel, T N: Receptive fields and functional architecture in two non-striate visual areas (18 and 19) of the cat. J Neurophysiol 28:229–289, 1965.

100. Hubel, D H and Wiesel, T N: Cells sensitive to binocular depth in area 18 of the Macaque monkey cortex. Nature 225:41–42, 1970.

101. Hubel, D H and Wiesel, T N: Sequence regularity and geometry of orientation columns in the monkey striate cortex. J Comp Neurol 158:267–294, 1974.

102. Hubel, D H and Wiesel, T N: Laminar and columnar distribution of geniculocortical fibers in the Macaque monkey. J Comp Neurol 146:421–450, 1982.

103. Ichikawa, K, Ichikawa, H and Tanabe, S: Detection of acquired color vision defects by standard pseudoisochromatic plates, part 2. Doc Ophthalmol Proc 46:133–140, 1987.

104. Julesz, B: Binocular depth perception without familiarity cues. Science 145:356–362, 1964.

105. Julesz, B: Foundations of Cyclopean Perception. University of Chicago Press, Chicago, 1971.

106. Julesz, B and Spivack, G H: Stereopsis based on vernier acuity clues alone. Science 157: 563–565, 1967.

107. Julesz, B, Breitmeyer, B and Kropfl, W: Binocular disparity dependent upper lower hemifield anisotropy and left right hemifield isotropy as revealed by dynamic randon dot stereograms. Perception 5:129–141, 1976.

108. Kanwisher, N, McDermott, J and Chun, M M: The fusiform face area: a module in human extrastriate cortex specialized for face perception. J Neurosci 17:4302–4311, 1997.

109. Kennard, C, Lawden, M, Morland, A B and Ruddock, K H: Color identification and color constancy are impaired in a patient with incomplete achromatopsia associated with prestriate lesions. Proc R Soc Lond Biol 260:169–175, 1995.

110. Kleist, K: Kriegsverletzungen des Gehirns in ihrer Bedutung Fur die Hirnlokalisation und Hirnpathologie. In Von Schjerning, 0 (Ed.): Handbuch der Arztlichen Erfahrung im Weltkriege, Vol. 4. Barth, Leipzig, 1923.

111. Kölmel, H W: Pure homonymous hemiachromatopsia: findings with neuro-ophthalmologic examination and imaging procedures. Eur Arch Psychiatr Neurot Sci 237: 237–243, 1998.

112. Kurylo, D D, Corkin, S and Rizzo, J F: Greater relative impairment of object recognition than of visuospatial abilities in Alzheimer's disease. Neuropsychology 10: 74–81, 1986.

113. Land, E H: Recent advances in retinex theory. Vision Res 26:7–21, 1986.

114. Land, E H, Hubel, D H, Livingstone, M S, Perry, S H and Burns, M M: Color-generating interactions across the corpus callosum. Nature 303:616–618, 1983.

115. Lennerstrand, G: Binocular interaction studied with visual evoked responses (VEF) in humans with normal or impaired binocular vision. Acta Ophthalmol 56:628–637, 1978.

116. Levy, J, Trevarthen, C and Sperry, R W: Perception of bilateral chimeric figures following hemispheric disconnection. Brain 95:61–78, 1972.

117. Lhermitte, F, Chain, F, Aron, D, Leblanc, M and Jouty, O: Les troubles de la vision des couleurs dans les lesions posterieures du cerveau. Rev Neurol (Paris) 121:5–29, 1969.

118. Lhermitte, J, Chain, F, Escourolle, R, Ducarne, B and Pillon, B: Etude anatomo-clinique d'un cas de prosopagnosie. Rev Neurol 126:329–346, 1972.

119. Lissauer, H: Ein fall von Seelenblindheit nebst einem Beitrag zur Theorie derselben. Arch Psychiatr Nervenkr 21:22–70, 1890.

120. Lueck, C J, Zeki, S, Friston, K J, Deiber, M P, Cope, P, Cunningham, V J, Lammertsma, A A, Kennard, C and Frackowiak, R S: The color center in the cerebral cortex of man. Nature 340:386–389, 1989.

121. Mackay, G and Dunlop, J C: The cerebral lesions in a case of complete acquired colourblindness. Scott Med Surg J 5:503–512, 1899.

122. Marcar, V L and Cowey, A: The effect of removing superior temporal cortical motion areas in the macaque monkey: II. Motion discrimination using random dot displays. Eur J Neurosci 4:1228–1238, 1992.

123. Maunsell, J H R and Van Essen, D C: Functional properties of neurons in middle temporal visual area of the macaque monkey. 1. Selectivity for stimulus direction, speed, and orientation. J Neurophysiol 49:1127–1147, 1983.

124. Maunsell, J H R and Van Essen, D C: Functional properties of neurons in middle temporal visual area of the macaque monkey. 11. Binocular interactions and sensitivity to binocular disparity. J Neurophysiol 49:1148–1167, 1983.

125. McKeefry, D J and Zeki, S: The position and topography of the human colour centre as revealed by functional magnetic resonance imaging. Brain 120:2229–2242, 1997.

126. Meadows, J C: The anatomical basis of prosopagnosia. J Neurol Neurosurg Psychiatry 37:489–501, 1974.

127. Meier, M J and French, L A: Lateralized deficits in complex visual discrimination and bilateral transfer of reminiscence following unilateral temporal lobectomy. Neuropsychologia 3:261–272, 1965.

128. Mikami, A, Newsome, W T and Wurtz, R H: Motion selectivity in macaque visual cortex. I. Mechanisms of direction and speed selectivity in extrastriate area MT. J Neurophysiol 55: 1308–1327, 1986.

129. Mohr, J P, Leicester, J, Stoddard, L T and Sidman, M: Right hemianopia with memory and color deficits in circumscribed left posterior cerebral artery territory infarction. Neurology 21:1104–1113, 1971.

130. Moll, L and Kuypers, H: Role of premotor cortical areas and VL nucleus in visual guidance of relatively independent hand and finger movements in monkeys. Exp Brain Res 23 (Suppl): 142, 1975.

131. Moll, L and Kuypers, H G J M: Premotor cortical albations in monkeys: Contralateral changes in visually guided reaching behavior. Science 198:317–319, 1977.

132. Morris, J S, Frith, C D, Perrett, D I, Rowland, D, Young, A W, Calder, A J and Dolan, R J: A differential neural response in the human amygdala to fearful and happy facial expressions. Nature 383:812–815, 1996.

133. Morrow, M J and Sharpe, J A: Retinotopic and directional deficits of smooth pursuit initiation after posterior cerebral hemispheric lesions. Neurology 43:595–608, 1993.

134. Mountcastle, V B, Lynch, J C and Georgopoulos, A: Posterior parietal association cortex of the monkey: command functions for operations within extrapersonal space. J Neurophysiol 38:871–908, 1975.

135. Nakayama, K: Biological image motion processing: a review (Review). Vision Res 25: 625–660, 1985.

136. Nawrot, M and Rizzo, M: Motion perception deficits from midline cerebellar lesions in human. Vision Res 35:723–731, 1994.

137. Nawrot, M, Rizzo, M and Damasio, H: Motion perception in humans with focal cerebral lesions. ARVO Abstract, 34:1231, 1993.

138. Newcombe, F and Russell, W R: Dissociated visual perceptual and spatial deficits in focal lesions of the right hemisphere. J Neurol Neurosurg Psychiatry 32: 73–81, 1969.

139. Newsome, W T and Paré, E B: A selective impairment of motion perception following lesions of the middle temporal area (MT). J Neurosci 8: 2201–2211, 1988.

140. Newsome, W T, Wurtz, R H, Dursteler, M R and Mikami, A: Deficits in visual motion processing following ibotenic acid lesions of the middle temporal visual area of the macaque monkey. J Neurosci 5:825–840, 1985.

141. Orban, G A, Sunaert, S, Todd, J, Van Hecke, P and Marchal, G: 3D structure from motion displays activate human MT/V5 and parietal motion areas (abstract). Investi Ophthalmol Vis Sci 39 (Suppl):S905, 1998.

142. Orban, G A, Dupont, P, De Bruyn, B, Vogels, R, Vanderberghe, R and Mortelmans, L: A motion area in human visual cortex. Proc Natl Acad Sci USA 92:993–997, 1995.

143. Oxbury, J M, Oxbury, S M and Humphrey, N K: Varieties of color anomia. Brain 92: 847–860,1969.

144. Pallis, C A: Impaired identification of faces and places with agnosia for colors. J Neurol Neurosurg Psychiatry 18:218–224, 1955.

145. Pasternak, T and Merigan, W H: Motion perception following lesions of the superior temporal sulcus in the monkey. Cereb Cortex 4: 247–259, 1994.

146. Paulson, H L, Galetta, S L, Grossman, M and Alavi, A: Hemiachromatopsia of unilateral occipitotemporal infarcts. Am J Ophthalmol 118:518–523, 1994.

147. Pearlman, A L, Birch, J and Meadows, J C: Cerebral color blindness: an acquired defect in hue discrimination. Ann Neurol 5:253–261, 1979.

148. Perrett, D I, Rolls, E T and Caan, W: Visual neurons responsive to faces in the monkey temporal cortex. Exp Brain Res 47:329–342, 1982.

149. Pevzner, S, Bornstein, B and Loewenthal, M: Prosopagnosia. J Neurol Neurosurg Psychiatry 25:336–338, 1962.

150. Pinkers, A and Verriest, G: Results of a shortened lightness discrimination test. In Verriest, G (Ed.) Colour Vision Deficiences VIII. Dordrecht, Mirtinus Nijhoof/Dr.W. Junk, The Netherlands, 1987, pp. 163–166.

151. Plant, G T and Nakayama, K: The characteristics of residual motion perception in the hemifield contralateral to lateral occipital lesions in humans. Brain 116:1337–1353, 1993.

152. Plant, G T, Laxer, K D, Barbar, N M, Schiffman, J S and Makayama, K. Impaired visual motion perception in the contralateral hemifield following unilateral posterior cerebral lesions in humans. Brain 116:1303–1335, 1993.

153. Poggio, G R: Central neural mechanisms in vision. In Mountcastle, V D (Ed.): Medical Physiology, Vol. 1. CV Mosby, St. Louis, 1980, pp. 573–579.

154. Ratcliff, G and Davies-Jones, G A B: Defective visual localization in focal brain wounds. Brain 95:49–60, 1972.

155. Ratcliff, G and Newcombe, F: Spatial orientation in man: effects of left, right and bilateral posterior lesions. J Neurol Neurosurg Psychiatry 36:448–454, 1973.

156. Regan, D, Giaschi, D, Sharpe, J A and Hong, X H: Visual processing of motion-defined form: selective failure in patients with parietotemporal lesions. J Neurosci 12: 2198–2210, 1992.

157. Rizzo, M, Hurtig, R and Damasio, A R: The role of scanpaths in facial learning and recognition. Ann Neurol 22:41–45, 1987.

158. Rizzo, M, Nawrot, M and Zih, J: Motion and shape perception in cerebral akinetopsia. Brain 118:1105–1128, 1995.

159. Rizzo, M, Smith, V, Pokorny, J and Damasio, A R: Color perception profiles in central achromatopsia. Neurology 43:995–1001, 1993.

160. Rondot, P and De Recondo, J: Ataxie optique: trouble de la coordination visuo-motrice. Brain Res 71:367–375, 1974.

161. Ross, J: Stereopsis by binocular delay. Nature 248:363–364, 1973.
162. Salzman, C D and Newsome, W T: Neural mechanisms for forming a perceptual decision. Science 264:231–237, 1994.
163. Sàry, G, Vogels, R, Kovacs, G and Orban, G A: Responses of monkey inferior temporal neurons to luminance-, motion-, and texture-defined gratings. J Neurophysiol 73:1341–1354, 1995.
164. Sathian, K: Motion perception in Alzheimer's disease (letter; comment). Neurology 1995; 45: 1633–1634. Comment on: Neurology 1994; 44: 1814–1818.
165. Schiller, P H: The effects of V4 and middle temporal (MT) area lesions on visual performance in the rhesus monkey. Vis Neurosci 10:717–746, 1993.
166. Scotti, G and Spinnler, H: Colour imperception in unilateral hemisphere-damaged patients. J Neurol Neurosurg Psychiatry 33:22–28, 1970.
167. Semmes, J, Weinstein, S, Ghent, L and Teuber, H L: Spatial orientation in man: 1. Analysis by locus of lesion. J Psychol 39:227–244, 1955.
168. Sergent, J and Bindra, D: Differential hemispheric processing of faces: methodological considerations and reinterpretation. Psychol Bull 89:541–554, 1981.
169. Sergent, J and Signoret, J L: Functional and anatomical decomposition of face processing: evidence from prosopagnosia and PET study of normal subjects. Philos Trans R Soc Lond Biol 335:55–61, 1992.
170. Sergent, J, Ohta, S and MacDonald, B: Functional neuroanatomy of face and object processing: a positron emission tomography study. Brain 115:15–36, 1992.
171. Shipp, S, De Jong, B M, Zihl, J, Frackowiak, R S J and Zeki, S: The brain activity related to residual motion vision in a patient with bilateral lesions of V5. Brain 117:1023–1038, 1994.
172. Silverman, S E and Feldon, S E: Motion perception in Alzheimer's disease (letter; comment). Neurology 45:1634–5, 1995. Comment in: Neurology 44:1814–1818, 1994.
173. Teuber, H L: Alteration of perception and memory in man. In Weiskrantz, L (Ed.): Analysis of Behavioral Change. Harper and Row, New York, 1968, pp. 274–328.
174. Thurston, S E, Leigh, R J, Crawford, T, Thompson, A and Kennard, C: Two distinct deficits of visual tracking caused by unilateral lesions of cerebral cortex in humans. Ann Neurol 23:266–273, 1988.
175. Tootell, R B, Mendola, J D, Hadjikhani, N K, Ledden, P J, Liu, A K, Reppas, J B, Sereno, M I and Dale, A M: Functional analysis of V3A and related areas in human visual cortex. J Neurosci 17:7060–7078, 1997.
176. Tootell, R B, Reppas, J B, Dale, A M, Look, R B, Sereno, M I, Malach, R, Brady, T J and Rosen, B R: Visual motion aftereffect in human cortical area MT revealed by functional magnetic resonance imaging. Nature 375: 139–141,1995.
177. Tranel, D and Damasio, A R: Knowledge without awareness: an autonomic index of facial recognition by prosopagnosics. Science 228:1453–1454, 1985.
178. Tranel, D and Damasio, A R: Nonconscious face recognition in patients with face agnosia. Behav Brain Res 30:235–249, 1988.
179. Tranel, D, Damasio, A R and Damasio, H: Intact recognition of facial expression, gender, and age in patients with impaired recognition of face identity. Neurology 38:690–696, 1988.
180. Tranel, D, Damasio, H and Damasio, A R: Double dissociation between overt and covert face recognition. J Cognit Neurosci 7:425–432, 1995.
181. Tranel, D, Damasio, H and Damasio, A R: A neural basis for the retrieval of conceptual knowledge. Neuropsycholgia 35:1319–1327, 1997.
182. Tranel, D, Damasio, H and Damasio, A R: On the neurology of naming. In Goodglass, H and Wingfield, A (Ed.): Anomia: Neuroanatomical and Cognitive Correlates. Academic Press, New York, 1997, pp. 67–92.
183. Tranel, D, Fowles, D C and Damasio, A R: Electrodermal discrimination of familiar and unfamiliar faces: a methodology. Psychophysiology 22:403–408, 1985.

184. Tranel, D, Logan, C G, Frank, R J and Damasio, A R: Explaining category-related effects in the retrieval of conceptual and lexical knowledge for concrete entities: operationalization and analysis of factors. Neuropsychologia 35:1329–1339, 1997.
185. Vaina, L M: Selective impairment of visual motion interpretation following lesions of the right occipito-parietal area in humans. Biol Cybern 61:347–359, 1989.
186. Vaina, L M, Lemay M, Bienfang, C D, Choi, A Y and Nakayama, K: Intact 'biological motion' and 'structure from motion' perception in a patient with impaired motion mechanisms. A case study. Vis Neurosci 5:353–369, 1990.
187. Van Oostende, S, Sunaert, S, Van Hecke, P, Marchal, G and Orban, G A: The kinetic occipital (KO) region in man: an fMRI study. Cereb Cortex 7: 690–701, 1997.
188. Verrey, D (CITED By Landolt, E): De la cecité verbale. Utrecht, 1888; and Dejerine, J: Differentes varietés de cecité verbale. Societé de Biologie (Paris) 44:64, 1892.
189. Verrey, D: Hemiachromatopsie droite absolue. Arch Ophthalmol (Paris) 8:289–300, 1888.
190. Verriest, G, Uvijls, A, Aspinall, P and Hill, A: The lightness discrimination test. Bull Soc Belge Ophtalmol 183:162–180, 1979.
191. Vialet, N: Les Centres Cerebraux de La Vision et L'Appareil Nerveux Visuel Intra-Cerebral. Faculté de Medecine de Paris, Paris, 1893.
192. Victor, J D, Maiese, K, Shapely, R, Sidtis and Gazzaniga, M: Acquired central dyschormatopsia with preservation of color discrimination. Clin Vis Sci 3:183–196, 1987.
193. Wachsmuth, E, Oram, M W and Perrett, D I: Recognition of objects and their component parts: responses of single units in the temporal cortex of the macaque. Cereb Cortex 4: 509–522, 1994.
194. Watson, J D G, Myers, R, Frackowiak, R S J, Hajnal, J V, Woods, R P, Mazziotta, J C, Shipp, S and Zeki, S: Area V5 of the human brain: evidence from a combined study using positron emission tomography and magnetic resonance imaging. Cereb Cortex 3:79–94, 1993.
195. Westheimer, G: Cooperative neural processes involved in stereoscopic acuity. Exp Brain Res 36:585–597, 1979.
196. Whalen, P J, Rauch, S L, Etcoff, N L, McInerney, S C, Lee, M B and Jenike, M A: Masked presentations of emotional facial expressions modulate amygdala activity without explicit knowledge. J Neurosci 18:411–418, 1998.
197. Wilbrand, H: Ein Fall von Seelenblindheit und Hemianopsie mit Sectionsbefund. Deutsche Z Nervenheik 2:361–387, 1892.
198. Xiao, D-K, Raiguel, S, Marcar, V and Orban, G A: The spatial distribution of the antagonistic surround of MT/V5 neurons. Cereb Cortex 7:662–677, 1997.
199. Yin, T C T and Mountcastle, V B: Visual input to the visuomotor mechanisms of the monkey's parietal lobe. Science 197:1381–1383, 1977.
200. Young, A W, Aggleton, J P, Hellawell, D J, Johnson, M, Broks, P and Hanley, J R: Face processing impairments after amygdalotomy. Brain 118:15–24, 1995.
201. Zeki, S M: Functional organization of a visual area in the posterior bank of the superior temporal sulcus of the rhesus monkey. J Physiol (Lond) 236: 549–573, 1974.
202. Zeki, S M: A century of cerebral achromatopsia. Brain 113:1727–1777, 1990.
203. Zeki, S M: Cerebral akinetopsia (visual motion blindness): a review (review). Brain 114: 811–824, 1991.
204. Zeki, S and Marini, L: Three cortical stages of colour processing in the human brain. Brain 121:1669–1685, 1998.
205. Zhou, Y X and Baker, C L: A processing stream in mamalian visual cortex neurons for non-fourier responses. Science, 261:98–101, 1993.
206. Zihl, J, Von Cramon, D and Mai, N: Selective disturbance of movement vision after bilateral brain damage. Brain 106:313–340, 1983.
207. Zihl, J, Von Cramon, D, Mai, N and Schmid, C: Disturbance of movement vision after bilateral posterior brain damage: further evidence and follow-up observations. Brain 114: 2235–2252, 1991.

8

Temporolimbic Epilepsy and Behavior

Donald L. Schomer, Margaret O'Connor, Paul Spiers,
Margitta Seeck, M.-Marsel Mesulam, and David Bear

I. Introduction

The word "epilepsy" almost invariably conjures up dramatic images of tonic–clonic convulsions, incontinence, and tongue biting with a postseizure period of confusion. However, there is a large group of patients with epilepsy lacking these features who in contrast have seizures that are associated with subtle alterations of mood, perception, cognition, comportment, endocrine balance, and autonomic function without any necessary loss of consciousness. This type of epilepsy, usually emanating from the temporal lobe and related components of the limbic system, is of great interest to behavioral neurology and neuropsychiatry.

By definition, a seizure occurs when there is an excessive, synchronous, abnormal firing pattern of neurons associated with an alteration in any sphere of neurological function. Important in this definition is the awareness that the neuronal firing pattern is both abnormal and associated with an identifiable alteration of sensory, motor, autonomic, emotional, or cognitive function. Over the course of a lifetime, the likelihood of experiencing a single seizure is estimated to be 9% for people living in the western world.[79,110,143] Epilepsy is a term used to denote recurrent seizures. Epilepsy may arise as a secondary manifestation of underlying neurological disease or in isolation, as the idiopathic manifestation of an unknown, possibly hereditary, susceptibility. The estimated prevalence of epilepsy in the western world is 0.7%, suggesting that approximately two million people in the United States are affected.[79,143]

The vast spectrum of altered behaviors displayed by epileptic patients can be divided into those that are "ictal" versus those that are "interictal." Behaviors that correlate temporally with the electrophysiological ictus (see below) are defined as "ictal." All other behaviors, which are presumed to be associated with the epilepsy but which cannot be shown to have temporal linkage to the ictus, are designated "interictal." The term "interictal" contains two major ambiguities. First, the failure to detect correlated ictal seizure activity in the electroencephalogram (EEG) does not mean that such activity is absent in the brain. Secondly, in the absence of unequivocal temporal overlap, the causal linkage between the aberrant behavior and the epilepsy is often based on conjecture.

II. Classification and Definition

Classification of the epilepsies is based on both anatomy and clinical manifestations.[34,35] If the entire cerebral cortex is affected at the onset, the seizure is called a "primary generalized seizure." If seizures occur as a result of a focal discharge in the brain, they are called "partial seizures." If a partial seizure remains localized and does not alter consciousness, it is known as a "simple partial seizure." If it spreads beyond the focal area of onset and produces an alteration in consciousness (as manifested by altered awareness, impaired responsiveness, or loss of memory for the episode) the term "complex partial seizure" is used. If a partial seizure spreads to produce generalized tonic (rigid) or clonic (rhythmic) movements, it is termed a "secondary generalized seizure." Primary and secondary generalized seizures usually impair consciousness. They may produce tonic, clonic, tonic–clonic, myoclonic (brief jerking) movements, sudden loss of tone (atonia), or an isolated alteration of consciousness (absence).

A partial seizure may be associated with complex experiences including hallucinations and feelings of fear but is still called "simple" as long as consciousness is preserved. In contrast, a patient who experiences a sudden isolated interruption of consciousness without additional psychological phenomena is said to be experiencing a "complex" partial seizure.

Temporolimbic: A Descriptive Term

The seizures of greatest interest to the behavioral neurologist are those that originate in the temporal lobe, especially within its limbic and paralimbic components. The constituents of the temporal lobe include primary auditory cortex, unimodal auditory and visual association areas, the heteromodal cortices of the parahippocampal and middle temporal gyri, the paralimbic cortices of the temporal pole, insula and entorhinal cortex, and the core limbic areas of the primary olfactory cortex, amygdala, and hippocampus (Chapter 1). The modality-specific cortices of the temporal lobe are located laterally and inferiorly whereas the limbic and paralimbic components are located in its mesial and basal parts.[4,69] The limbic and paralimbic components of the temporal lobe have widespread reciprocal connections with the hypothalamus and with nontemporal paralimbic regions in the orbitofrontal, insular, and cingulate cortices.[69]

As reviewed in Chapter 1, these temporal and nontemporal components of the limbic system have many common anatomical, neurochemical, and behavioral features. The interconnectivity may lead to a rapid spread of seizure activity from one component of the limbic system to another. Electrical activity originating in the mesial and basal parts of the temporal lobe is not readily "detected" by scalp electrodes until discharges spread to more lateral parts of the temporal lobe.[99,147,148] Therefore, standard scalp EEG recordings are unreliable in identifying the site of onset of seizures originating within the limbic system. For all these reasons, we have adopted the generic term "temporolimbic epilepsy" (TLE) to designate partial seizures emanating from any part of the temporal lobe and any part of the limbic system (temporal or not).

Approximately 60% of patients with epilepsy experience partial seizures and nearly 60% of those fit the definition of temporolimbic.[79,90] However, many patients with temporolimbic seizures probably remain undiagnosed because the only symptomatology is behavioral and because the seizures are difficult to capture by EEG.

III. ANATOMICAL PATHOPHYSIOLOGY

Partial epilepsy reflects an intermittent physiological disturbance within a well-defined neural network.[54] Many of these events can be demonstrated during the interictal period but become much more pronounced during the transition to an overt seizure.

The hallmark of the interictal condition is an intermittent focal spike and slow wave complex seen on the EEG. This event represents a summated field potential of many neurons within a spatially discrete area responding in a pathological hypersynchronous fashion.[49,54] These neurons, tested with intracellular electrodes, demonstrate massive and paroxysmal depolarization shifts of their membrane, which last for about 70 ms.[49,54] A corresponding flurry of action potentials is carried down the axon so that brief but intense high-frequency communications are established between the cell participating in the generation of the spike and cells connected to it.[49,54] Recurrent collaterals to the local interneuronal pool are also activated, leading to local inhibitory responses. This causes a membrane hyperpolarization in the epileptic focus corresponding to the slow wave potential seen on EEG. This period of hyperpolarization is associated with a 200–400 ms relative refractoriness to incoming excitatory inputs.[49,54] These electrical events are called "interictal" because they are self-limited in both time and space and are not associated with classical clinical symptoms. However, interictal physiological abnormalities may influence various aspects of neurological function. For example, the spike discharges may disrupt the pulsatile function of hypothalamic nuclei involved in gonadal regulation, leading to conditions such as polycystic ovarian disease, hypogonadotrophic hypogonadism, or other abnormalities of endocrine function.[73,86–88] The spike and slow wave potentials in the limbic system may disrupt normal processes necessary for laying down memories and can interfere with the proper linkage of experience with corresponding affective states, leading to memory impairment and psychiatric symptomology.[24,25]

Single photon emission computed tomography (SPECT)[108,109,123] and positron emission tomography (PET)[123] frequently show an intermittent or permanent area of metabolic hypoactivity in or surrounding the region of seizure focus. This hypometabolism may reflect a functional depression due to the activation of recurrent inhibitory pathways. Another possible explanation for the focal "hypometabolism" is a putative decrease in the total neuronal population within the epileptic area compared to the contralateral side.[30] In either case, these observations demonstrate that the seizure focus in TLE is intermittently or constantly in an abnormal state even during the "interictal" period.

During the ictus, the paroxysmal depolarization shift of the neuronal membrane is replaced by a continuous, prolonged membrane depolarization that lasts up to several minutes.[54] The number of neurons behaving in such a pathological fashion increases substantially over time and the area of involvement expands both by local spread and through more distant neural connections. The period of sustained spiking is defined as the "seizure." It is usually self-limited and gives way to a postictal period, characterized by profound inhibition.[54]

Graham Goddard[70,71] first described the phenomenon of "kindling" as a possible model for the evolution of seizure foci and partial epilepsy. In the kindling paradigm, electrodes placed into various structures of an animal's brain deliver weak currents that initially are too weak to trigger a seizure. However, repeated subthreshold stimulation eventually does trigger a local seizure. Further stimulation at the same level produces a self-sustaining focus and leads to the generation of seizure discharges in the absence of exogenous stimulation. Such seizures may spread and lead to secondary generalization. Throughout the process of kindling, there is a gradual reduction in the threshold of the stimulation needed to induce seizures. Long-term potentiation (LTP) is one physiological phenomenon that may underlie kindling.[71,114]

Limbic structures are the most vulnerable parts of the brain to kindling, helping to explain why TLE is such a common form of epilepsy. There may be considerable individual variability in the susceptibility to kindling. For example, baboons with an autosomally dominant inherited form of primary generalized epilepsy are easier to kindle than their nonepileptic siblings.[114] It is probable that genetic susceptibilities also play a role in the emergence of human TLE.

The phenomena of mirror and daughter foci may also be related to kindling.[124–126] In the former case, patients with an epileptogenic focal structural lesion in the temporal lobe develop an independent seizure focus in the contralateral homotopic brain region. In the case of daughter foci, nontemporal focal structural lesions appear to produce independent temporolimbic seizures ipsilateral to the structural abnormality. This explains the paradoxical, but relatively common, finding of TLE in patients with focal structural lesions in the parietal and occipital lobes.[168]

Topical anesthetics such as lidocaine, procaine, and cocaine, can elicit seizure activity selectively within components of the limbic system. In animals, intermittently administered low doses of cocaine, lidocaine, and procaine have produced phenomena similar to electrical kindling.[138a] This form of "chemical kindling" may explain why some behavioral consequences of cocaine addiction resemble the symptomatology of TLE (Chapter 9).

The critical role of limbic cortices for establishing multimodal associations and their susceptibility to kindling and LTP may help to explain why they are also the most common substrates for the emergence of "reflex epilepsy." In this condition, sensory stimuli (such as certain odors or visual stimuli) or a specific cognitive process (such as reading, imagining an event, or doing mental arithmetic) can trigger TLE. Reflex epilepsy could possibly be attributed to "psychological kindling," where the epilepsy-inducing stimulus is an endogenous pattern of neural activity rather than an exogenously administered electrical or chemical stimulation.

Case Report

C. M. was a middle-aged woman with a history of complex visual hallucinations dating back to late adolescence. She had two types of recurrent visual hallucinations. The first and more frequent was of six German soldiers in World War I attire seen in a pyramidal formation from the shoulders up. These hallucinations existed for many years. Eventually, a second type of hallucination emerged, of an elderly woman sitting in a rocking chair reminiscent of Whistler's painting of his grandmother. The woman was rocking back and forth with her arms hanging over the side of the chair. There was a small rat-like animal at the side of the chair that nibbled at her fingers. The patient felt that the image was a preview of her at an older age. The hallucinations were always experienced in the left visual field. By the time the patient reached her mid 30s, she would feel a sense of dread and doom during the majority of these events. She subsequently developed a compulsion to scratch and injure herself but only over the left side of her body and only during the hallucination.

After years of relatively ineffective medical treatment, the patient underwent a right craniotomy and had intraoperative EEG recordings in the temporal lobe and at the site of a partially thrombosed arteriovenous malformation (AVM) in the right parietal lobe. While the patient was in the operating room and fully awake, she developed the hallucination of the six German soldiers. This was associated with an electrographically sustained seizure event restricted to the right parietal region. The intense sense of dread and doom was associated with a spread of seizure activity to the right parahippocampal and hippocampal sites as well as to the right amygdala. The clinical picture and the electrophysiological findings suggest a phenomenon akin to kindling and the development of a "daughter" focus.

IV. Ictal Manifestations of TLE

Ictal manifestations of TLE are usually abrupt and transient. However, there are also instances of TLE "status" where the patient may enter a prolonged period of confusion, altered mood, or "fugue" state, while superficially appearing to be fully conscious.[189]

Ictal behaviors are driven by paroxysmal seizure activity. The type of ictal phenomenon is dependent on the anatomical site of the seizure focus and the spread of the discharge. In keeping with the numerous specializations of the temporal lobe and of the limbic system, the ictal phenomena of TLE can be divided into broad categories such as motor, sensory, autonomic, experiential, emotional, cognitive, and psychiatric. Patients may experience any combination of these symptoms depending on origin and spread. Occasionally, one of these nonmotor or experiential phenomena will be the first manifestation of the seizure and will be identified as the "aura."

Motor

Motor symptoms include automatisms such as lip smacking, straightening the hair, circular running, darting eye movements, staring, and twitching or jerking of upper or lower extremities. Head turning or visual checking, furtive scanning of the environment, or looking over the shoulder as if searching for something have all been reported and may represent, in some patients, the motor response to hallucinatory stimuli.[145] Patients sometimes spontaneously assume unusual facial expressions or body postures and may demonstrate "waxy flexibility," a condition in which a passively manipulated limb remains in the configuration and position to which it was last moved. Stuttering, slurred speech and even complete speech arrest have also been described.[5,65,77] Transient weakness or motor paresis, sometimes resulting in suddenly falling to one side, may be an ictal symptom. The distribution of the weakness may be atypical and the patient's muscle tone or reflexes may remain intact.

Sensory

Somatosensory alterations accompanying TLE include headache, focal pain, discomfort, tingling, and numbness.[28,102,134] The feeling of something crawling on or under the skin (fourmillage) has also been reported. These sensory alterations may be unilateral or bilateral and can follow almost any distribution, defying conventional innervation patterns. Dizziness and vertigo are also common. Occasionally, the sensory phenomena may encompass the genitalia and be interpreted as sexual excitation.[134]

The auditory, visual, and olfactory experiences of TLE are usually referred to as hallucinatory.[134] Visual phenomena are common and may be restricted to one visual field as in the earlier case example. Fully formed, complex images of someone standing in the doorway, of a demon, or of a godlike figure have been reported. The most complex visual hallucinations are usually associated with seizure foci in the right hemisphere. The following three phenomena have also been reported: metamorphosia (the sudden distortion of a common object or person), micropsia (the illusion that objects have become smaller and moved further away), and macropsia (the illusion that objects have become larger and moved closer to the point where they appear to be "towering over" the patient). Some patients with these experiences have compared themselves to Alice in Wonderland.

Auditory hallucinations may consist of a ringing or buzzing sound or of a voice calling the patient's name or repeating stereotyped phrases.[134] Gustatory hallucinations are usually of a metallic or foul taste. Olfactory phenomena are similarly unpleasant and include odors such as ammonia, burning rubber or garbage, a decaying or fecal odor, "as if a skunk were under my nose," or a suffocating smell of garlic.[134] Even perfumed odors are usually described as sickeningly sweet and are rarely experienced as positive.

Autonomic

Temporolimbic seizures may also have autonomic manifestations.[52,181a] Patients may experience flushing or a "hot sensation" that may be bilateral or unilateral, sometimes restricted only to the head or upper torso.[117] Piloerection and "goose flesh" may constitute the only outward manifestation of TLE. Others may complain of shortness of breath,[102] "weight" on their chest, or being unable to take a full breath. Yet other individuals may have apnea attacks with cyanosis. Cardiac symptoms reported by patients may include chest pain or a feeling that the heart has stopped, is racing, or is pounding hard.[104] Obvious and identifiable changes in cardiac rhythm are not unusual. Sinus tachycardia is the most frequently documented rhythm seen in conjunction with a seizure[111] but cases of asystole have also been reported.[104] Perhaps the most frequently reported autonomic symptom is nausea and epigastric distress.[74,121,145] This is usually experienced as a rising or sinking feeling, but has also been reported to feel like a sudden urge to throw up, as if the intestines were tied in knots. Others have described the sensation of being punched in the stomach. We have seen patients who have been investigated for years for causes of severe gastrointestinal distress before the discovery of seizure discharges time-locked to the epigastric pain. A helpful sign is a unilateral sluggish pupillary reflex or spontaneous unilateral pupillary dilatation during the experience. These changes are frequently ipsilateral to the side of the seizure focus.

Experiential

Experiential manifestations of TLE may include memory flashbacks ("I feel like I did as a child in the summer, falling into the lake"), illusions of familiarity (déjà vu or déjà vécu) or unfamiliarity (jamais vu or jamais vecu), and intense feelings of depersonalization.[27,67] Déjà vu or déjà vécu (already seen or experienced) refers to a sense that the identified event, conversation, or situation has been experienced previously. Conversely, in jamais vu or jamais vécu, patients may report that they intellectually know the place or people to be familiar but that they are unable to shake the feeling that they have never seen them and have never been there before. In an extreme case, the patient felt during a seizure that she had no past and had never existed. This experience could last for over an hour without relief and was accompanied by fear and bilateral numbness of the hands.

The sense that someone is nearby, watching over a shoulder, or outside the house (e.g., the feeling of a presence), without any accompanying visual hallucination, has also been reported.[115] Patients may be reluctant to report dissociative experiences but admit, upon questioning, that they sometimes step outside of their own body or hover above themselves and are watching their own actions from the perspective of a detached observer (autoscopy).[46]

Emotion and Affect

The emotional manifestations of TLE are most often negative in valence. The emotion occurs suddenly and unpredictably without apparent precipitant, often out of context or inappropriate to the patient's activities at the time, and generally ceases as abruptly as it began. Emotional experiences reported during temporolimbic seizures have included embarrassment;[43] sadness and sudden crying;[4] explosive laughter[94] (gelastic epilepsy) usually without the feeling of happiness; peacefulness with a sense of serenity or of "being at a oneness with the universe;"[33] and, most commonly, fear.[47] This last manifestation is typically fear of personal injury or harm from some unknown source and has been described as fear of impending doom or death (timor mortis).[134] There are frequent autonomic accompaniments, and the patient may feel compelled to escape, even from familiar surroundings. This may be the phenomenon that forms the basis for "running seizures" during which patients appear confused and run great distances before regaining composure, at which time they may find themselves in an unfamiliar place. The diagnosis of TLE needs to be entertained in patients who appear to experience idiopathic panic attacks. Spontaneous orgasm, pleasurable genital sensations, and exhibitionism have been reported in several patients.[134]

Cognitive

Forced thoughts and activities of an obsessive or compulsive nature may occasionally be seizure related. One patient with left parietotemporolimbic seizures felt compelled to engage in various motor rituals, such as touching each side of his face twice and then three times, during electrographic seizure activity. Others have engaged in self-mutilation, including orchiectomy. Prolonged confusional and fugue states have also been associated with ongoing seizure activity. Ictal discharges in TLE can affect memory and language functions.[60,77,80,96,97] Temporolimbic seizures may also give rise to the manifestations of transient global amnesia (Chapter 4). Ictal discharges in the left temporal lobe are associated with aphasic disturbances that may take the form of speech arrest.[50,53] Less frequently, however, ictal discharges can give rise to anomia, paraphasias, dysgraphias, and language comprehension deficits.

Complex Psychiatric Phenomena

Many symptoms thought to have a psychiatric etiology, may, in fact, reflect TLE-like phenomena.[64,95] For example, abnormal spike and slow wave activity from the septal region has been reported during psychotic behaviors, and limbic dysrhythmias have been correlated with episodic confusion and aggressive episodes.[24,64,106,174]

One patient who had been diagnosed as having chronic paranoid schizophrenia was recorded during episodes when she was delusional, confused, disoriented, experiencing auditory and visual hallucinations, and, occasionally, while showing intense rage with aggressive and destructive acts. Depth electrodes showed repeated paroxysmal bursts of high-amplitude multiphasic spiking activity in hippocampal and septal regions, with occasional involvement of the temporal cortex.[122] Conventional scalp leads did not detect these abnormalities.

Facilities where sophisticated EEG technology is available are rarely equipped to manage patients with severe behavioral problems. Even when studies are designed to assess psychotic patients, these individuals are usually studied during a period when they are not acutely symptomatic.[1] Consequently, there may be a subgroup of individuals with a diagnosis of idiopathic schizophrenia whose psychotic episodes may be based on temporolimbic EEG abnormalities but where this association remains undetected.

Similar considerations exist with regard to the relationship between temporolimbic epilepsy and violence. Even the widely accepted opinion that premeditated and purposeful violence cannot represent an ictal manifestation[42,44,61,62] may need to be rethought in light of the findings of profoundly complex behaviors occurring during prolonged seizures confined to limbic regions and detected by stereo electroencephalography. Although the relationship between TLE and criminal violence is difficult to investigate, the theoretical, clinical, and therapeutic implications of this question are self-evident.[167,172]

Case Report

J. V. was a 35-year-old right-handed man with spike and slow wave activity in left frontotemporal regions. In between seizures, J. V. was an even-tempered and well-mannered man who worked as a restaurant manager. However, during ictal and postictal periods, J. V. demonstrated a sudden onset of paranoia and confusion. During, and for several hours following a seizure, he would carry out complex motor activities that were typically motivated by feelings of intense fear. He suspected that others were trying to kill him. He would therefore attempt to escape, frequently climbing onto the roof in order to elude his captors. On many occasions, even during winter days, he walked around the edge of the roof of his restaurant for hours. Following one seizure, he broke down the door of a neighbor's house, entered the house, and then jumped out the second story window in a state of panic.

Anatomical Substrate of Ictal Phenomena

The diverse ictal manifestations of TLE reflect the functional and anatomic heterogeneity of the temporal lobe. Visual areas of the occipital lobe have direct connections with the fusiform, inferior temporal, and middle temporal gyri. The primary auditory cortex in the supratemporal plane receives input from the medial geniculate nucleus and is closely interconnected with adjacent auditory association areas of the superior temporal gyrus. Stimulation and ablation studies in both animals and humans have demonstrated the role of these inferior and lateral regions of the temporal lobe in auditory and visual function. More medial temporal structures belong to the limbic system and are involved in the control of learning, memory, affect, visceral tone, and hormonal balance (Chapter 1). Other cortical components of the limbic system,—for example, caudal orbitofrontal cortex, cingulate cortex, and insula—are closely interconnected with these medial temporal regions and share many related behavioral affiliations (Chapter 1). One temporal lobe (the dominant), usually the left, appears to be more involved with verbal processing, whereas the other (the nondominant) is more specialized for processing nonverbal information.[119,120,146,151]

Stimulation of the temporal lobe, especially its limbic components, has resulted in autonomic responses manifested by changes in pupillary size, lacrimation, salivation, pulse rate, blood pressure, peristalsis, micturition, uterine contractions, and penile erections.[134] Bilateral symmetric lesions of medial temporal structures has resulted in amnestic syndromes, altered aggression, hypersexuality, and changes in feeding behavior (Chapters 1 and 4).[14,66,119,120,151]

Electrographic observations indicate that simple visual stimuli or vertiginous experiences are likely to be associated with discharges in the lateral posterior temporal or parieto-occipital regions. Complex auditory hallucinations, verbal as well as musical, can be time-locked to ictal discharges in or near Heschl's gyrus.[134] Motor and sensory phenomena in temporolimbic epilepsy generally reflect spread to the primary motor or sensory cortices, although in certain motor manifestations the supplementary motor area or frontal eye fields may be implicated.

Experiential and emotional manifestations of temporolimbic epilepsy are most likely to be associated with seizure activity in the limbic regions of the temporal lobe.[67,185] These manifestations include feelings of loneliness, depression, fear, and the reexperiencing of complicated scenes, experiences, and emotions. The temporal neocortex, while frequently invaded by seizure discharges, does not appear to be a necessary substrate for these experiential events. In the one study that examined this issue systematically, only 3% of experiential, hallucinatory or emotional manifestations were associated with seizures restricted to the neocortical part of the temporal lobe.[67] In contrast, almost 42% were associated with discharges restricted to the amygdala, hippocampus, and parahippocampal gyrus. Thus, almost half of all experiential events will not be associated with seizure discharges extending into the lateral temporal neocortex. Standard scalp EEG electrodes may therefore frequently miss the electrical correlates of seizure-induced experiential phenomena. Virtually identical results regarding the pivotal role of mesial limbic structures in the production of experiential, hallucinatory, or emotional ictal manifestations were obtained by examining the effects of stimulation with intraoperative depth electrodes in an independent sample of patients.[48] It has also been suggested that experiential, emotional, and autonomic manifestations are more likely to be associated with lateralization of the seizure foci to the right hemisphere.[59]

V. Interictal (Long-term) Associations of TLE

The causal relationships between TLE and many of the brief "ictal" phenomena noted above are relatively well established. However, patients with TLE also display long-term, persistent alterations in psychiatric state, cognitive abilities, and endocrine function. Some of these alterations may reflect the consequences of the interictal abnormalities at the seizure focus and their chronic influence upon distant regions synaptically connected to the seizure focus, whereas others may reflect chance associations.[13,17,19]

Schizophreniform Psychosis

The prevalence of psychosis is greatly elevated in the population of patients with TLE compared to the general population.[57,58,178,180] As many as 10%–15% of individuals with TLE may receive a diagnosis of schizophrenia or schizophreniform psychosis.[57,160,180,188] Additional risk factors for TLE-related psychosis include left-sided seizure foci, left handedness, female gender, high frequency of seizures, younger age of onset, and visible neuropathological lesions at the seizure locus.[59,160,161,175,181]

In contrast with these well established findings of schizophreniform psychosis in patients with TLE, a number of methodologically compromised studies have reported that between 20% and 50% of patients with idiopathic schizophrenia have EEG abnormalities localized to one or both temporal lobes.[72,168,171] These results may be contaminated by the EEG dysrhythmic effects of most antipsychotic agents, which are totally eliminated from a particular patient only after several months of washout.

Although TLE patients with schizophreniform psychosis have been described as similar to patients with idiopathic schizophrenia, many studies in this area have commented on atypical phenomenological aspects of their psychosis.[136,153,160–162,167,169,176] Stereotyped hallucinatory phenomena (both auditory and visual), persecutory delusions, and ideas of reference may be present in TLE as well as in idiopathic schizophrenia. In contrast to the family histories of people with idiopathic schizophrenia, TLE patients' personal and family histories tend to be negative and the characteristic premorbid schizoid or schizotypal personality patterns are generally absent. Also, affect is usually better preserved and psychotic episodes tend to be more transient and less socially disruptive in patients with TLE. In comparison to patients with idiopathic schizophrenia, TLE patients may be better able to encapsulate their psychotic symptoms and establish interpersonal rapport.

Depression and Other Psychiatric Syndromes Associated with TLE

The incidence of depression is higher in TLE than in patients with other neurological or medical disabilities.[116,144] In some instances patients experience the sudden onset of dysphoria as part of the ictal event. Others suffer from rapidly cycling, unipolar or bipolar mood disorders that are quite disabling.[166] Studies have shown that TLE patients are at much higher risk for suicide.[6] Factors that increase susceptibility to depression in TLE include the social stigma and the disabling limitations that epilepsy imposes on functional status as well as dysfunction in brain regions involved in emotional regulation. Some studies had suggested that patients with left TLE were more prone to schizophreniform symptoms while those with right TLE were more prone to affective disturbances.[59] However, other studies have failed to demonstrate a consistent relationship between the laterality of seizures and the nature of the associated psychopathology.[127]

In addition to schizophreniform psychosis and mood disorders, interictal panic attacks, anorexia nervosa, and dissociative identity disorder (multiple personalities) have been reported in TLE.[115,158,167] From both a practical point of view and a clinical perspective, the presence of atypical features in psychosis, panic disorders, affective illness, multiple personality, and even anorexia nervosa should raise the possibility of epilepsy in the differential diagnosis.

Personality Traits

Papers published since the 1950s have emphasized the association of specific personality traits with temporolimbic epilepsy[55,89,138,176,179] (Table 8–1). These have included deepened emotionality, humorlessness, hyposexuality, anger, nascent religious interests,[41] enhanced philosophical preoccupation, paranoia, moralism, obsessional thoughts, circumstantiality, viscosity (enhanced social cohesiveness), and hypergraphia (extensive writing or drawing). Although decreased libido (hyposexuality) has been most often reported, there are also cases of TLE with marked alterations of sexual behavior, including fetishism and transvestitism. Exaggerated autonomic responses to both conditioned and unconditioned stimuli have been reported. Patients with TLE may be especially sensitive to the emotional impact of sensory experiences, perhaps because they have developed a seizure-induced enhancement of effective connectivity between cortical and limbic regions of the brain.[9,10,11,21] Patients with left-sided seizures have been described as more ideative (i.e., religious, philosophical, and paranoid) and those with right-sided seizures as more emotional.[21] A study by Perini has partially upheld this typology, emphasizing an increased incidence of depression and paranoia in left-sided TLE patients versus an increased incidence of emotionality in patients with right-sided TLE.[135]

In clinical practice, one or more of the personality traits noted above are frequently seen in patients with TLE,[180] sometimes with dramatic intensity. We have seen patients with multiple conversions from one religion to another; patients whose prodigious writing output was incorporated in voluminous diaries or rambling letters full of inconsequential detail; patients in whom deep emotions and clinging mark every office visit and telephone call; and patients whose obsessive preoccupation saturates every conversation with cosmic and philosophical significance. However, we have also seen many TLE patients in whom none of these traits was particularly conspicuous. Two issues are important to consider in relation to the association between TLE and a specific constellation of personality traits: (1) Are the traits more common in TLE? (2) Can these traits be used in the diagnosis of temporolimbic epilepsy?

A number of studies with regard to the first question have demons^
many of the personality traits noted above can also be seen in patients
from other neurological or psychiatric disorders.[51] The one exception]
pergraphia, which appears to be more common in TLE than in ot
groups.[13,129,150,179,186,187] When sent a health-related questionnaire that requireu ᴡ...
ten answers, more than 50% of patients with focal TLE responded, whereas less
than 25% of patients with focal nontemporal or generalized epilepsy did so. Furthermore, the mean number of words for the TLE group was 12 times that of the
other epileptics.[150] An additional study using patients with focal temporal lobe seizures, focal nontemporal or generalized seizures, and mixed temporal and generalized seizure disorders failed to replicate this observation, even though some of
the longest replies came from patients in the focal temporal lobe group.[83]

The compulsion to write excessively is seen in many TLE patients, including

TABLE 8–1 Characteristics Historically Attributed to Temporal Lobe Epilepsy–Geschwind's Syndrome*

Inventory Trait	Reported Clinical Observation
Emotionality	Deepening of all emotions, sustained intense affect
Elation, euphoria	Grandiosity, exhilarated mood; diagnosis of manic-depressive disease
Sadness	Discouragement, tearfulness, self-deprecation; diagnosis of depression, suicide attempts
Anger	Increased temper, irritability
Aggression	Overt hostility, rage attacks, violent crimes, murder
Altered sexual interest	Loss of libido, hyposexuality, fetishism, transvestitism, exhibitionism, hypersexual episodes
Guilt	Tendency to self-scrutiny and self-recrimination
Hypermoralism	Attention to rules with no ability to distinguish significant minor infractions; desire to punish offenders
Obesssionalism	Ritualism; orderliness; compulsive attention to detail
Circumstantiality	Loquacious, pedantic, overly detailed, peripheral
Viscosity	Stickiness, tendency to repetition
Sense of personal destiny	Events given highly charged, personalized, significance; divine guidance ascribed to many features of patient's life
Hypergraphia	Keeping extensive diaries, detailed notes; writing autobiography or novel
Religiosity	Holds deep religious beliefs, often idiosyncratic; multiple conversions, mystical states
Philosophical interest	Nascent metaphysical or moral speculations, cosmological theories
Dependence	Cosmic helplessness, "at hands of fate"; protestations of helplessness
Humorlessness	Overgeneralized ponderous concern; humor lacking or idiosyncratic
Paranoia	Suspicious, overinterpretive of motives and events; diagnosis of paranoid schizophrenia

*Adapted from Bear and Fedio,[21] with permission.

Seizure

Put a gun to your head
Slowly, pull the trigger
Click
What's that mommy?
Oh, another seizure

Suppose you never knew
If the gun is loaded
Whether every time
That little flick,
That tiny discharge in your brain
goes click
you'll come out
alive

Talk to a group
Speak to anyone
Just try to work
Never knowing
If there will be
30 clicks,
or none

Life's a struggle
Everyone knows that
Click
Try it
With this extra

Trick

Phyllis Tourse
April 16, 1982

FIGURE 8–1 Poem Written by a Patient with Temporolimbic Epilepsy

some of the best adapted and highly functioning. These patients may take creative writing courses, belong to poetry groups, or write short stories. Some of the work they produce is obsessional, ruminative, and moralistic; some of it, however, is poignant, insightful, and well written (Fig. 8–1). The life and writings of Fyodor Dostoyevsky provide the most remarkable association of TLE with great writing. It could be argued that patients with TLE do not differ from thousands of nonepileptic individuals who enjoy writing. However, it is the driven nature of the writing, its excessive quantity, and the repetitive moralistic and philosophical content that tend to be relatively characteristic of TLE.

The clustering of specific personality traits listed above should increase the index of suspicion for the presence of underlying epilepsy. However, it is also abundantly clear that the absence of these traits cannot rule out TLE and conversely that there are many individuals with one or more of these traits who do not have epilepsy.

Cognitive Changes

Patients with TLE are particularly vulnerable to disruptions of language and memory.[23,36] Some studies have also demonstrated that patients with left TLE have fixed long-term deficits on tests of verbal list learning, cued verbal recall, and semantic encoding whereas patients with right TLE may do poorly on tests of nonverbal memory.[7,38,40] A subgroup of TLE patients show a form of accelerated forgetting characterized by normal retention of new information over hours to days but an amnesia for information from more remote time periods.[96,130] This accelerated forgetting may reflect the disruptive effects of seizures on the long-term consolidation of new information. TLE may be associated with atypical patterns of hemispheric specialization, probably because of the cerebral reorganization that it induces. For example, left-handedness and right hemisphere dominance for language are more common in TLE than in the general population.

Case Report[2]

J. T. was a 42-year-old right-handed man who demonstrated an unusual memory problem in that his new learning, tested by conventional instruments, was intact whereas his memory for major personal and public events from previous months and days was not.[3,130] He performed in the above average range on traditional clinical tests of memory. In marked contrast, he could not recall major personal or public events. He did not remember the ages or school grade placements of his four children, or the death of a close friend, even though he had attended the funeral several days earlier. Clinical workup revealed frequent seizures (20–30/day) with frequent bilateral mesial temporal interictal discharges. An MRI revealed bright T2 signals in both mesial temporal regions. J. T.'s seizures were ultimately attributed to paraneoplastic limbic encephalitis. Serial testing revealed that the rate of forgetting was correlated with the frequency of observed seizures. Paraldehyde was administered rectally to decrease seizure frequency.

Initial acquisition, under the influence of paraldehyde, was slightly impaired but retention over a weeklong period of time improved as if the paraldehyde had helped to reverse the impairment of consolidation (Fig. 8–2).

Endocrine Aspects

As described in Chapter 1, limbic regions have direct and reciprocal connections with hypothalamic nuclei. Stimulation and ablation of specific amygdaloid nuclei can alter the release of luteinizing hormone (LH), follicle-stimulating hormone (FSH), thyroid-stimulating hormone (TSH), and prolactin. Furthermore, estrogen and progesterone receptors on limbic neurons can directly influence their thresholds for seizure activity. [69] Estrogen tends to have convulsant properties and progesterone has an opposite effect. Catamenial epilepsy, the premenstrual increase of seizures in women with TLE, may reflect the epileptogenic effect of high estrogen concentrations relative to those of progesterone.[86–88]

Polycystic ovarian disease, recurrent endometriosis, menstrual irregularity, infertility, and impotence have been described in patients who have temporolimbic epileptiform abnormalities on the EEG.[87] The relationships of these conditions to TLE are incompletely understood. In some of these patients, the epileptiform abnormality may cause the associated endocrinologic disturbance. In others, the altered endocrinologic state may activate epileptiform disturbances.

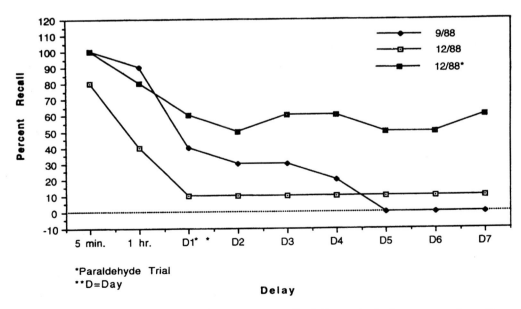

FIGURE 8–2. The y-axis represents the percent recall of 10 words during one week on three separate occasions as noted on the x-axis. Enhanced performance is observed with the administration of paraldehyde.

There are several reports of patients with abnormal EEGs and polycystic ovarian disease, amenorrhea, and hyposexuality who have remained refractory to classic endocrinologic therapy but who have responded to anticonvulsants. There are also some patients who experience better seizure control in response to therapy with progesterone. Advances in this area have immediate therapeutic implications. At the present, atypical endocrine abnormalities that remain refractory to treatment should raise the possibility of underlying TLE.

The vast majority of female patients with untreated TLE have abnormal responses to challenges with luteinizing hormone releasing hormone (LHRH).[86–88] Furthermore, TLE is also associated with abnormalities in the regulation of prolactin, FSH, and LH. Chronic hormonal changes may provide one possible mechanism for the occurrence of anorexia in some patients with epilepsy.

In addition to their well-known endocrine effects on peripheral target organs, many hypothalamic and pituitary hormones also have powerful effects on mood and behavior. The chronic influence of temporolimbic epilepsy on the endocrine milieu may therefore provide one mechanism for some of the long-term behavioral alterations in these patients.

VI. THE DIAGNOSTIC EVALUATION AND WORKUP

History and Physical Examination

Risk factors for temporolimbic epilepsy include birth complications, febrile convulsions,[142] intracranial infections, and head trauma. Why such risk factors remain dormant for many years and then suddenly trigger seizures in adolescence or early adulthood remains poorly understood. The phenomenon of kindling may play a role in this evolution as well as hormonal modulation of the seizure threshold.

A detailed history often yields important information for the diagnosis of TLE. Questions should inquire about the "ictal" and the "interictal" phenomena noted above. The history should also cover information about the endocrinological state and sexual functioning. The relationship of symptoms to the menstrual cycle, or to specific triggers suggestive of reflex epilepsy, should be explored. The clinical neurological examination should look for asymmetric skeletal development indicative of a remote cerebral injury, areas of abnormal pigmentation associated with neurofibromatosis or tuberosis sclerosis, and focal neurological deficits suggestive of an underlying structural abnormality.

EEG Studies

The EEG remains the gold standard for the diagnosis of epilepsy. The use of sphenoidal electrodes to sample the inferior temporal or orbital frontal regions and tracings obtained after a night of sleep deprivation enhance the probability of detecting an EEG abnormality[39,99,112,147,148,163,165] (Fig. 8–3). Abnormalities from posterior inferior temporal regions, the insular cortex, and the supplementary motor cortex

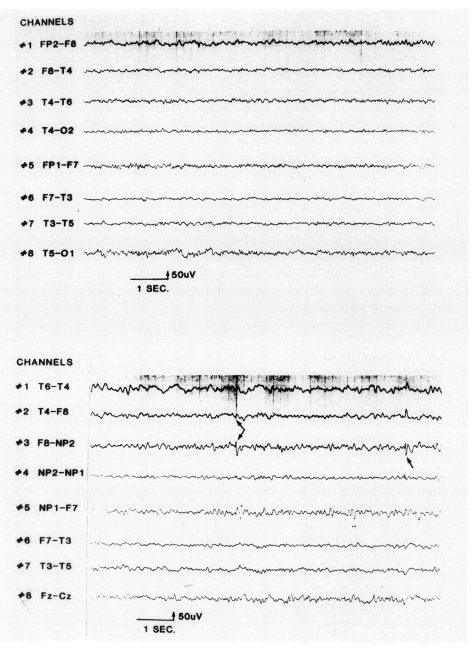

FIGURE 8–3. This is a 29-year-old female with a long history of abdominal pain associated with a feeling of fear. Multiple EEGs done over many years, including some with nasopharyngeal electrodes, were reported to be normal. This tracing was the first one done while she was symptomatic. The top tracing shows the surface scalp recording while the patient was drowsy, and it is normal. The bottom tracing shows recording from the nasopharyngeal electrodes (NP1 and NP2) as well as from the scalp. Localized spike and spike–wave complexes from the right temporal region, maximal at the right nasopharyngeal electrode, are seen (arrows). Thus, obtaining a tracing during the symptomatic phase and the use of specialized electrodes increase the yield of detection.

and the cingulate gyrus can be missed with recordings based on standard electrodes. Thus, a normal EEG does not rule out TLE. Prolonged telemetric EEG recordings or EEG tracings obtained during the episode of behavioral symptomatology can increase diagnostic yield.[26]

Invasive electroencephalography may be necessary for localizing the epileptic focus when considering surgical treatment. Electrodes may be implanted stereotactically into limbic sites and recordings can be obtained over prolonged periods of time. This allows a simultaneous recording of behavior and EEG so that the site of the behaviorally relevant seizure focus can be localized precisely for planning the surgical strategy. Subdural strip electrodes and grid arrays have also been used but are less capable of being placed in or around the deeply situated limbic regions of the brain.

Radiological Investigation

Magnetic resonance imaging, MRI, is excellent for identifying 1–2 mm lesions in the brain. Specialized imaging techniques such as the "FLAIR" sequence can help to reveal subtle abnormalities such as cortical migrational disorders.[123] Asymmetric and small hippocampi, identified by quantitative MRI morphometry, are also helpful in localizing the epileptogenic site.[93]

Functional imaging by SPECT or PET can provide additional diagnostic information.[108,109,149,123] For example, abnormalities in blood flow or metabolism may help localize the seizure focus. The ictal period can be associated with focal hypermetabolism whereas the interictal state may show an area of focal hypometabolism. Occasionally, the focal area of maximum abnormality is detected only when the values from the interictal scan are subtracted from those of the ictal one. Furthermore, image acquisition in functional MR (fMR) can be time-locked to interictal spike discharges so as to pinpoint the site of hemodynamic changes associated with spike generation.[182]

VII. TREATMENT

Medical Management

Carbamazepine, phenytoin, phenobarbital, primadone, valproate sodium, and methobarbital are the drugs that have been used most extensively for treatment of TLE. Benzodiazepines and carbonic anhydrase inhibitors are also useful for seizure control. More recently lamotrigine, gabapentin, topiramate, vigabatrin, and zonisamide have been introduced. Many of the older drugs are relatively inexpensive and their risks are better known than some of the newer drugs. Monotherapy is the preferred medical approach. Increasing the number of drugs increases the likelihood of side effects and undesirable drug interactions. However, combining drugs that behave in different biological ways from each other often improves seizure control and is referred to as rational polypharmacy. For example, phenytoin and carbamazepine work through voltage-gated sodium or calcium channels and modulate relative neuronal excitability. Benzodiazepines work primarily by modulating chloride transport so as to enhance inhibition. Still other drugs like lamotrigine work by inhibiting the release of excitatory neurotransmitters. When drugs with different mechanisms of action are combined, side effects can be minimized while improving the efficacy of seizure control.

Treatment of Behavioral and Psychiatric Symptoms

In keeping with the emphasis of this chapter, it is extremely important to distinguish ictal from interictal psychiatric symptomatology.[15,44,45,91,183] As noted previously, a frequent and important ictal psychiatric symptom is fear, which may be distinguished from an idiopathic panic attack by its briefer duration, associated olfactory, vertiginous or visual distortions, abnormal EEG and absence of a family history of panic disorder or separation anxiety.[47,78,91,183] Other important ictal psychiatric symptoms include dysphoria,[45,48,91] complex hallucinations simulating schizophrenic psychosis,[177] and ictal dissociative events such as "dreamy states" or the sense of a "doubling of consciousness" or out-of-body experience.[46,92,158,177]

Pre-ictal irritability and postictal aggression may be time-linked to seizures.[44] More recently, a mania-like state consisting of euphoria, hyperactivity, and social disinhibition has been reported in conjunction with ictal discharges originating from or spreading to the orbitofrontal cortex.[91,98,177]

When the behavioral events are time-locked to simple or complex partial seizures, treatment is directed at rigorous seizure control. Anticonvulsant medications are the primary modality for control of seizures;[137] however in cases of refractory seizures, surgical approaches to TLE achieve excellent results in appropriately selected patients.[48,91,177]

While control of ictal symptoms is often straightforward and gratifying, the treatment of persistent interictal psychiatric symptomatology is more complex and less satisfactory. Perhaps most extensively studied is the schizophreniform psychosis, as previously presented, which was first identified by Beard and Slater,[164] in patients with longstanding temporal lobe epilepsy. This condition might be better termed paranoid schizophrenia or schizoaffective disorder in modern psychiatric nomenclature, since these patients, as noted earlier, tend to have strong rather than flattened affects, significant mood swings, intense interpersonal bonds, and paranoid delusions without the other disorders of thought and are without the negative symptoms of schizophrenia.[12,61,100,177]

In this group of patients, treatment with antiepileptic medications which have been shown to stabilize mood in psychiatric studies, such as carbamazepine, valproic acid, or lamotrigine, is preferred.[91] Antipsychotic medications are frequently necessary to combat paranoid delusions but agents known to lower the seizure threshold such as many of the phenothiazines and clozapine should be avoided.[91,177] Among the traditional antipsychotics, fluphenazine and molindone appear to be the least epileptogenic. Among the atypical agents, risperidone and quetiapine show promise.[91,177]

Mood disorder, especially depression, is the most common interictal psychiatric syndrome associated with temporolimbic epilepsy.[45,90,113,116] Depression frequently includes realistic concerns about uncontrolled seizures, the stigma of epilepsy, and associated neurological deficits produced by a structural epileptogenic lesion. In addition, the cluster of interictal behavioral characteristics listed in Table 8-1, often termed Geschwind's syndrome in honor of the extraordinary American neurologist who first brought attention to alternations in the interictal behavior of many patients with TLE,[13,20,22,187] may contribute powerfully to depressive symptomotology.[45] As discussed in section V, Geschwind's syndrome[63] includes a deepening of many emotions, often resulting in religious or philosophical preoccupations; a strong moralistic sense; loss or alteration of sexual interests; and a craving for overly close interpersonal relationships.[16,22,41,63,177,186,187] These behavioral changes have been hypothesized to result from chronic epileptic activation or "kindling" within the amygdala, resulting in a suffusion of many experiences with emotional coloration.[4,8,11,38,68,75] Whether or not this view is correct, these behavioral changes can modify the personality of patients profoundly, shattering prior personal convictions and straining relations with spouses, families, and significant others.[177]

Case Report: Modified from Tisher[177]

A 33-year-old construction worker developed post-traumatic TLE. Despite good seizure control, he experienced profound depression one year following his injury. At this time, he was aware of major changes in his behavior and personality. For the first time in his life, he began to write extensively about new and bewildering philosophical concerns (hypergraphia). Not formerly religious, he now experienced the feeling that higher powers were directly controlling his life (sense of personal destiny). He underwent a change in sexual desire, leading to conflict in an intimate relationship. As his moralistic questing deepened, he was unable to enjoy his prior hobbies of hunting and fishing, not wishing to kill any living creature. He summarized the factors leading to his depression: "I can't hunt any more—all the horrors in the news make me angry—I don't know who I am—."

Treatment of such a multifaceted depression requires multiple modalities. Anticonvulsant medicines, which are mood stabilizing, are a mainstay of treatment. In particular, lamotrigine has been proposed to have unique properties as an antidepressant.[91,139,177] Treatment with the serotonin-reuptake class of antidepressants is often of value and may correct a serotonin deficiency observed in some patients with chronic TLE. Electroconvulsive therapy improves mood and often results in better seizure control.[91,164]

In our opinion, there is also an essential role for a neurologically informed type of supportive psychotherapy.[16,18,91,144] Understanding the role of temporolimbic discharges in deepening and altering emotions allows the patient and significant others to achieve perspective and develop coping strategies. Group therapy with both educational and process-oriented goals has been helpful for many patients with depression in the setting of interictal behavior changes.[48,91,177]

Surgical Treatment

Patients with TLE may consider surgery when seizures remain refractory to anticonvulsant medications and/or when the side effects of medications cannot be tolerated. Surgical candidacy requires a clear electrographic focus confined to one of the temporal lobes. Convergent data from EEG, imaging, and neuropsychological studies are important in the determination of the seizure focus.[31,32] The use of invasive electroencephalography for more intensive monitoring may be particularly helpful in this regard. Information is sought regarding the patient's psychological "readiness" for surgery, the level of expectations related to surgical outcome, the possible residual neuropsychological effects and the putative impact of the surgery on the quality of life.[32,181b] Surgery is considered when the psychosocial and medical benefits outweigh the risks of the procedure.

Surgical procedures vary across institutions. The standard resection removes 7 to 8 cm of tissue from the tip of the temporal lobe in the nondominant hemisphere and 4 to 5 cm on the dominant side.[26] Most surgeons do a tailored removal leaving in place most of the lateral neocortex and removing mesial regions, including all of the amygdala and large portions of the anterior hippocampus. A further variation, which may provide just as effective seizure control, is the selective amygdalohippocampectomy.[184] The selective amygdalohippocampectomy leads to less long-term cognitive impairment than the standard temporal lobectomy.

Surgical outcome depends upon the location of the seizure and the nature of the underlying pathology.[26] For example, 90%–95% of patients with unilateral hippocampal sclerosis may be totally seizure free following surgery.[26] Patients with clearly defined structural abnormalities that involve the anterior temporal tip or mesial temporal regions have similar success rates. When the seizure focus is in frontal and nontemporal limbic structures, surgical outcome is less successful. For surgery in the cingulate and supplementary motor cortex, good surgical outcome are in the 60%–65% range.[26]

Patients who experience a postsurgical reduction of seizure frequency often report strikingly positive changes in the quality of daily life.[118,181b] In some patients, the surgical elimination of a seizure focus also leads to a significant improvement in cognitive functions. This outcome probably reflects the liberation of the non-operated hemisphere from the spread of the seizure activity from the principal focus.

Case Report

R. O. was 36-year-old man with intractable epilepsy referred for a surgical opinion. His seizures were heralded by a sense of "not feeling well" followed by a feeling of thoracic pressure. Frequently, he had an associated thought of a specific fairy tale in which a lion ate a lamb. He had a particularly vivid visualization of the moment just before the lion was about to kill the lamb. His ictal EEG showed a focal onset (Fig. 8–4, upper left) mapped to the left temporal lobe using the LORETA technique (Fig. 8–4, upper right). The MRI revealed left hippocampal sclerosis and atrophy (Fig. 8–4, lower left). The interictal PET scan revealed left mesial decrease of FDG activity (Fig. 8–4, lower right) and MR spectroscopy revealed a decrease in the left hippocampal N-acetylaspartate (NAA)/choline ratio. He subsequently went on to a limited left temporal lobectomy and has had a marked reduction in seizure frequency.

Intracarotid Amytal Procedure (IAP) or Wada Test

The intracarotid amytal procedure (IAP) involves the selective inactivation of each cerebral hemisphere in order to determine its functional specializations.[29,82,105,107,166,173] Aphasia or amnesia following injection of Amytal (amobarbital) suggests that the inactivated hemisphere is critical for normal language or memory. If the IAP indicates severe amnesia, the surgeon becomes reluctant to remove limbic structures on that side of the brain. If the IAP produces aphasia, the surgeon should be particularly careful to avoid language cortices on that side.

Cortical Mapping

Cortical mapping procedures provide information that is used to individually tailor the boundaries of the surgical resection. This information is particularly important because patients with longstanding epilepsy often have language, cognitive, and sensorimotor functions in nontraditional locations.[80,81] Cortical mapping may allow the surgeon to remove epileptogenic tissue while preserving brain regions critical to motor and cognitive functions. Cortical maps are derived by administering small electrical currents to a variety of brain regions. The representation of function is inferred by eliciting specific sensations, movements, and cognitive impairment. For example, disrupted naming and speech hesitations indicate that language cortex is being stimulated. Functional MRI may soon replace the IAP and perhaps also corticography for identifying the regional specialization of cortical areas.

Experimental Surgical Approach

Recently, transplantation technology has introduced a potential alternative to excision therapy for TLE. For example, α aminobutyric acid (GABA)-containing cells from pig embryos have been treated with an antibody fragment that blocks their immunogenicity. These cells have been transplanted into the epileptic focus of three patients with TLE. Preliminary results have been limited but are encouraging.[157]

Postoperative Neuropsychological Effects of Surgery

There is considerable variability across patients with regard to the extent and nature of the cognitive changes that follow surgical intervention.[26,101,103,129,140,141,154,155] Group studies have shown that some patients who have undergone left temporal lobe resections experience persistent naming problems whereas other language processes such as fluency, repetition, and comprehension remain intact.[154,155] Patients with early onset epilepsy demonstrate fewer declines on tasks of naming following left temporal lobe surgery, perhaps because their brains have undergone a functional reorganization.[85,154,156,159] Cortical resections within 2 cm of identified language zones have been associated with transient anomia following surgery while resections that come within 5–7 mm of language sites may result in permanent anomia.[76,132,152]

Perhaps the most consistent postoperative finding is the verbal memory deficit seen after left temporal lobe resection.[84] Left temporal lobectomy patients have greater difficulty with the verbal retrieval of public events from the remote past than do right temporal lobectomy patients[131] whereas right temporal lobectomy patients have greater difficulty with memory for famous faces.

Behavioral and Emotional Effects of Surgery

Surgery is usually not an effective treatment for TLE-associated psychosis.[179] A small percentage of patients may even develop transient psychosis and/or depression following surgery. Increased risk of postoperative psychiatric disturbance has been associated with right-sided temporal lobectomies.[30]

Fedio and Martin found that surgery resulted in an attenuation of the features of Geschwind's syndrome. For example, patients who underwent left temporal lobectomies were less ideational than their presurgical counterparts while right temporal lobectomy patients were less emotional than patients with right TLE.[56] Right temporal lobe surgery appears to induce autonomic hypoarousal while left temporal lobe surgery leads to hyperarousal.[37,128] Patients who have undergone unilateral temporal lobe surgery are less susceptible to fear conditioning but show no difference in the ability to remember emotional words.[137]

FIGURE 8–4. Upper Left. A 26-second 20-channel EEG during the beginning of a seizure shown in a bipolar montage (electrodes named according to the 10/20 system, SP1 and SP2, are the left and right sphenoidal electrodes). Seizure onset is noted by arrow.

Upper Right. This picture is an estimation of the three-dimensional current density distribution of the electrical activity (LORETA solution) in the 2–4 Hz bandwidth. A general linear inverse solution was used in a three-spherical-circle head model. The most dominant activity is shown on horizontal slice that is 2 cm above the T3–T4–OZ plane and is indicated by the bright yellow area.

Lower Left. The area under the curves, when summated, indicates the total volumes of the left and right amygdalohippocampal structures. Note that the left sided structures are consistently smaller at all locations.

Lower Right. This is an [18]fluorodeoxy-glucose (FDG) PET image taken in the interictal state and coregistered with the two-dimensional MRI of the patient. The left image is a horizontal view, which shows a discrete left mesial and basal temporal area of hypometabolism. The image on the right is a coronal view, which shows the same area of abnormality.

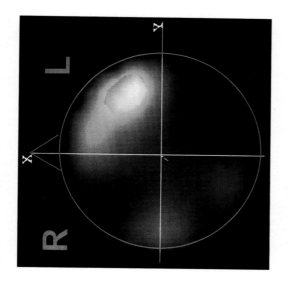

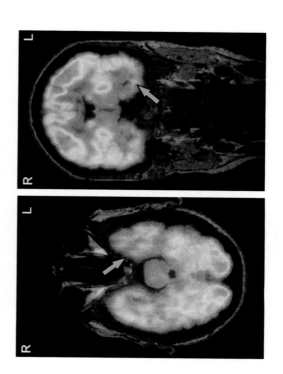

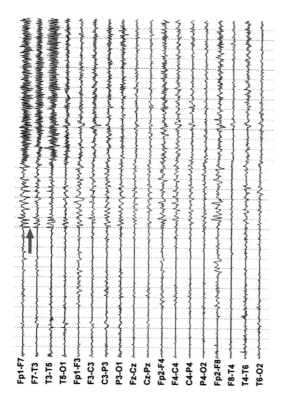

Fp1-F7
F7-T3
T3-T5
T5-O1
Fp1-F3
F3-C3
C3-P3
P3-O1
Fz-Cz
Cz-Pz
Fp2-F4
F4-C4
C4-P4
P4-O2
Fp2-F8
F8-T4
T4-T6
T6-O2

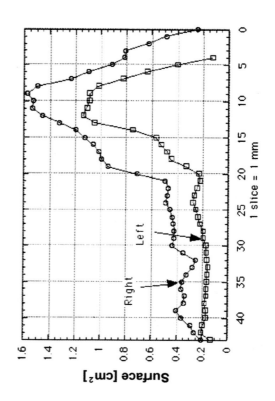

Surface [cm²]

1 slice = 1 mm

Right

Left

VIII. OVERVIEW

Epileptic discharges can trigger almost any behavior or experience associated with normal brain activity. In particular, TLE can influence the entire set of behavioral affiliations characteristic of the limbic system. In contrast to destructive limbic lesions which cause "negative" symptoms such as amnesia, hypoemotionality, and sensory–limbic disconnection syndromes (Chapters 1 and 4), TLE causes much more florid "positive" symptoms, which range from complex hallucinations to delusions, terror, and violence. The symptom complex of TLE provides excellent opportunities for increasing our understanding of limbic physiology. Furthermore, an improved approach to patients suffering from TLE by a multidisciplinary team of neurologists, psychiatrists, and neuropsychologists can lead to very effective therapeutic interventions.

REFERENCES

1. Abrams, R and Taylor, M A: Differential EEG patterns in affective disorders and schizophrenia. Arch Gen Psychiatry 36:1355–1358, 1979.
2. Aggleton, J P: The functional effects of amygdala lesions in humans: a comparison with findings from monkeys. In Aggleton, J P (Ed.): The Amygdala. Neurobiological Aspects of Emotion, Memory, and Mental Dysfunction. Wiley-Liss, New York, 1992, pp. 485–503.
3. Ahern, G, O'Connor, M, Dalmau, J, Coleman, A, Posner, J B, Schomer, D L, Herzog, A G, Kolb, D A and Mesulam, M-M: Paraneoplastic temporal lobe epilepsy with testicular neoplasm and atypical amnesia. Neurology 44:1270–1274, 1994.
4. Altshuler, L L, Devinsky, O, Post, R M and Theodore, W: Depression, anxiety and temporal lobe epilepsy. Arch Neurol 47:284–288, 1990.
5. Baratz, R and Mesulam, M-M: Adult onset stuttering treated with anticonvulsants. Arch Neurol 38:132–134, 1981.
6. Barraclough, B: Suicide and epilepsy. In Reynolds, E H and Trimble, M R (Eds.): Epilepsy and Psychiatry. Churchill Livingstone, Edinburgh, Scotland, 1981, pp. 72–76.
7. Barr, W B: Examining the right temporal lobe's role in nonverbal memory. Brain Cogn 35: 26–41, 1997.
8. Bear, D M: Interictal behavior in temporal lobe epilepsy. Possible anatomic and physiological bases. In Wada, J (Ed.): Epilepsy: Neurotransmitter Behavior and Pregnancy. Vancouver: Joint Publication of Canadian League Against Epilepsy and Western Institute on Epilepsy, 1979.
9. Bear, D M: Temporal lobe epilepsy—a syndrome of sensory-limbic hyperconnection. Cortex 15:357–384, 1979.
10. Bear, D M, Schenk, L and Benson, H: Increased autonomic responses to neutral and emotional stimuli in temporal lobe epilepsy. Am J Psychiatry, 138:843–845, 1981.
11. Bear, D M: Temporal lobe epilepsy and the Bear-Fedio personality inventory. Neurology 35:284–286, 1985.
12. Bear, D M, Levin, K and Blumer, D. Chetham, D, Ryder, J. Interictal behavior in hospitalized temporal lobe epileptics—relation to other psychiatric syndromes. J Neurol Neurosurg Psychiatry 45:481–488, 1982.
13. Bear, D M: Behavioral symptoms in temporal lobe epilepsy. Arch. Neurol. 40:467–469, 1983.
14. Bear, D: Hemispheric specialization and the neurology of emotion. Arch Neurol 40:195–202, 1983.

15. Bear, D M, Freeman, R and Greenberg, M: Psychiatric aspects of temporal lobe epilepsy. Annu Rev Psychiatry 4:190–210, 1985.

16. Bear, D, Freeman, R, Greenberg, M and Schiff, D: Psychiatric aspects of temporal lobe epilepsy. Hales, R and Frances, A (Eds.): Am Psychiatr Assoc Annu Rev. 4:190–210, 1985.

17. Bear, D: Behavioral changes in temporal lobe epilepsy: conflict, confusion, challenge. In Trimble, M R and Bolwig, T G (Eds.): Aspects of Epilepsy and Psychiatry, John Wiley, 1986.

18. Bear, D M: Organic personality syndromes. In Lazare, A (Ed.): Outpatient Psychiatry: Diagnostic and Treatment, 2nd Ed. Williams and Wilkins, Baltimore, 1989, pp. 351–360.

19. Bear, D, Hermann, B and Fogel, B: Behavior in Epilepsy. J Neuropsychiatry Clin Neurosci 1:308–311, 1989.

20. Bear, D M: Interictal behavior in temporal lobe epilepsy—-the psychiatric legacy of Norman Geschwind. In Schachter, S and Devinksy, O (Eds.): The Legacy of Norman Geschwind. Lippencott-Raven, Philadelphia, 1996, pp. 213–222.

21. Bear, D and Fedio, P: Quantitative analysis of interictal behavior in temporal lobe epilepsy. Arch Neurol 34:454–467, 1997.

22. Benson, D F: The Geschwind syndrome. Adv Neurol 55:411–421, 1991.

23. Bergin, P S, Thompson, P J, Fish, D R and Shorvon, S D: The effect of seizures on memory for recently learned material. Neurology 45:236–240, 1995.

24. Binnie, C D, Channon, S and Marston, D L: Behavioral correlates of interictal spikes. Adv Neurol 55:113–126, 1991.

25. Binnie, C D, Kasteleijn-Nolst Trenite, D G A, Smit, A M and Wilkins, A J: Interaction of epileptiform EEG discharges and cognition. Epil Res 1:239–245, 1987.

26. Blume, H and Schomer, D L: Surgical approaches to epilepsy. In Kreger, WP (Ed.): Annual Review of Medicine, Palo Alto, CA, and 1988, pp. 301–313.

27. Blume, W T, Girvin, J P and Stenerson, P: Temporal neocortical role in ictal experiential phenomena. Ann Neurol 33: 105–107, 1993.

28. Bossi, L, Munari, C, Stoffels, C, Bonis, A, Bacia, T, Talairach, J and Bancaud, J: Somatomotor manifestations in temporal lobe seizures. Epilepsia 25:70–76, 1984.

29. Branch, C, Milner, B and Rasmussen, T: Intracarotid sodium amytal for the lateralization of cerebral speech dominence. J Neurosurg 21:399–405, 1964.

30. Bruton, C J: The neuropathology of temporal lobe epilepsy. In Maudsley Monograph No 31. Oxford University Press, Oxford, England, 1988.

31. Chelune, G J: Hippocampal adequacy versus functional reserve: predicting memory functions following temporal lobectomy. Arch Clin Neuropsychol 10:413–432, 1995.

32. Chelune, G J, Naugle, R I, Hermann, B P, Barr, W B, Trenerry, M R, Loring, D W, Perrine, K, Strauss, E and Westerveld, M: Does pre-surgical IQ predict outcome after temporal lobectomy? Evidence from the Bozeman Epilepsy Consortium. Epilepsia 39:314–318, 1998.

33. Cirignotta, F, Todesco, C V and Lugaresi, E: Temporal lobe epilepsy with ecstatic seizures: so called Dostoyevsky epilepsy. Epilepsia 21:705–710, 1980.

34. Commission on the Classification and Terminology of the International League Against Epilepsy: proposal for the revised clinical and electroencephalographic classification of epileptic seizures. Epilepsia 22:489–501, 1981.

35. Commission on the Classification and Terminology of the International League Against Epilepsy: Proposal for the revised clinical and electroencephalographic classification of epileptic syndromes. Epilepsia 30:389–399, 1989.

36. Corsi, P M: Human memory and the medial temporal region of the brain. Unpublished doctoral dissertation. McGill University, 1972.

37. Davidson, R A, Fedio, P, Smith, B D, Aureille, E and Martin, A: Lateralized mediation of arousal and habituation: differential bilateral electrodermal activity in unilateral temporal lobectomy patients. Neuropsychologia 30:1053–1063, 1992.

38. Davis, M: Neurobiology of fear responses: the role of the amygdala. J Neuropsychiatry Clin Neurosci 9:382–402, 1997.

39. Declerck, A C: Interaction sleep and epilepsy. Eur Neurol 25: 117–127, 1986.

40. Delaney, R, Rosen, A, Mattson, R and Novelly R: Memory functions in focal epilepsy: a comparison of non-surgical, unilateral and frontal lobe samples. Cortex 16:103–117, 1980.

41. Dewhurst, K and Beard, A W: Sudden religious conversions in temporal lobe epilepsy. Br J Psychiatry 117:497–507, 1970.

42. Delgado-Escueta, A V, Mattson, R H, King, L, Goldensohn, E S, Speigel, H, Madsen, J, Crandall, P, Dreifuss, F and Porter, R J: The nature of aggression during epileptic seizures. N Engl J Med 305:711–716, 1981.

43. Devinsky, O, Hafler, D A and Victor, J: Embarrassment as the aura of a complex partial seizure. Neurology 32:1284–1285, 1982.

44. Devinsky, O and Bear, D: Varieties of aggressive behavior in temporal lobe epilepsy. Am J Psychiatry 141:651–656, 1984.

45. Devinsky, O and Bear, D M: Varieties of depression in epilepsy. Neuropsychiatry Neuropsychol Behav Neurol 4:49–61, 1988.

46. Devinsky, O, Putnam, F, Grafman, J, Bromfield, E and Theodore, W H: Dissociative states and epilepsy. Neurology 39:835–840, 1989.

47. Devinsky, O: Fear and epilepsy. In Canger, R, Saccheti, E, Perini, G I and Canevini, M P (Eds.): Carbamazepine: A Bridge Between Epilepsy and Psychiatric Disorders. Ciba-Geigy Edizioni Origgio, Italy, 1990, pp. 41–48.

48. Devinsky, O and Vazquez, B: Behavioral changes associated with epilepsy. Behav Neuro 11:127–149, 1993.

49. Dichter, M and Spenser, W A: Pencillin-induced interictal discharges from the cat hippoampus. I. Characteristics and topographic features. II. Mechanisms underlying origin and instruction. J Neurophysiol 32:663–687, 1969.

50. Dinner, D S, Luders, H, Lederman, R and Gretter, T E: Aphasic status epilepticus: a case report. Neurology 31:888–890, 1981.

51. Dodrill, C and Batzel, L W: Interictal behavioral features of patients with epilepsy. Epilepsia 22:S64–S76, 1986.

52. Drake, M E: Isolated ictal autonomic symptoms in complex partial seizures (letters). J Neurol Neurosurg Psychiatry 47:100–101, 1984.

53. Duchowny, M, Jayakar, P, Resnick, T, Levin, B and Alvarez, L: Posterior temporal epilepsy: electroclinical features. Ann Neurol 35:427–431, 1994.

54. Dichter, M A, Schwartzkroin, P A, Heinemann, U, MacDonald, R L and Engel, J Jr: The neurobiology of epilepsy. In Engel, J Jr and Pedley, T A (Eds.): Epilepsy: A Comprehensive Textbook. Lippincott-Raven, Philadelphia, 1998, pp. 231–512.

55. Falconer, M A: Reversibility by temporal-lobe resection of the behavioral abnormalities of temporal-lobe epilepsy. N Engl J Med 289:451–455, 1973.

56. Fedio P and Martin A: Ideative-emotive behavioral characteristics of patients following left or right temporal lobectomy. Epilepsia 24:S117–S130, 1983.

57. Flor-Henry, P: Psychosis and temporal lobe epilepsy: a controlled investigation. Epilepsia 10:363–395, 1969.

58. Flor-Henry, P: Schizophrenia-like reactions and affective psychoses associated with temporal lobe epilepsy: etiological factors. Am J Psychiatry 126:148–152, 1969.

59. Flor-Henry, P: Lateralized temporal-limbic dysfunction and psychopathology. Ann NY Acad Sci 280:777–797, 1976.

60. Gallassi, R, Morreale, A, Lorusso, S, Pazzaglia, P and Lugaresi, E: Epilepsy presenting as memory disturbances. Epilepsia 29:624–629, 1988.

61. Geschwind, N, Shader, R I, Bear, D, North, B, Levin, K and Chetham, D: Behavioral changes with temporal lobe epilepsy: assessment and treatment. J Clin Psychiatry 41:89–95, 1980.

62. Geschwind, N: Pathogenesis of behavior changes in temporal lobe epilepsy. In Ward, A A, Penry, J R and Purpura, D (Eds.): Epilepsy. Raven Press, New York, 1983, pp. 355–370.

63. Geschwind, N: Interictal behavioral changes in epilepsy. Epilepsia 24 (Suppl 1): S23–S30, 1983.

64. Gibbs, F A: Ictal and non-ictal psychiatric disorders in temporal lobe epilepsy. J Nerv Ment Dis 21:522–528, 1951.

65. Gilmore, R and Heilman, K M: Speech arrest in partial seizures: evidence of an associated language disorder. Neurology 31:1016–1019, 1981.

66. Gloor, P and Feindel, W: The temporal lobe and affective behavior. In Monniern, M (Ed.): Physiologie des Vegetativen Nerven Systems, Vol. 2. Hippokrates Verlag, Stuttgart, Germany, 1963, pp. 685–716.

67. Gloor, P, Oliver, A, Quesney, L F, Andermann, A and Horowitz, S: The role of the limbic system in experiential phenomena of temporal lobe epilepsy. Ann Neurol 12:129–144, 1982.

68. Gloor, P: Role of the amygdala in temporal lobe epilepsy. In Aggleton, J P (Ed.): The Amygdala. Neurobiological Aspects of Emotion, Memory, and Mental Dysfunction. Wiley-Liss, New York, 1992, pp. 505–538.

69. Gloor, P: (ed.): The Temporal Lobe and the Limbic System. Oxford University Press, New York, 1997.

70. Goddard, G V: Development of epileptic seizures through brain stimulation at low intensity. Nature 214:1020–1021, 1967.

71. Goddard, G V: The kindling model of epilepsy. Trends Neurosci, 275–279, 1983.

72. Goon, Y, Robinson, S and Lavy, S: Electroencephalographic changes in schizophrenic patients. Isr Ann Psychiat Relat Dis 11:99–107, 1973.

73. Gronfier, C, Luthringer, R, Follenius, M, Schaltenbrand, N, Macher, J P, Muzet, A and Brandemberger, G: Temporal relationships between pulsitile cortisol secretion and electroencephalographic activity during sleep. Electroencephal Clin Neurolphysiol 103:405–408, 1997.

74. Guerrini, R, Ferrari, A R, Battaglia, A, Salvadori, P and Bonanni, P: Occipitotemporal seizures with ictus emeticus induced by intermittent photic stimulation. Neurology 44:253–259, 1994.

75. Halgren, E, Walter, R D, Cherlow, D G and Crandall, P H: Mental phenomena evoked by electrical stimulation of the human hippocampal formation and amygdala. Brain 101:83–117, 1978.

76. Haglund, M M, Berger, M S, Shamseldin, M, Lettich, E and Ojemann, G A: Cortical localization of temporal lobe language sites in patients with gliomas. Neurosurgery 34:567–576, 1994.

77. Hamilton, N G and Matthews, T: Aphasia: the sole manifestation of focal status epilepticus. Neurology 29:745–748, 1979.

78. Harper, M and Roth, M: Temporal lobe epilepsy and the phobic anxiety-depersonalization syndrome, part I: a comparative study. Compr Psychiatry 3: 129–151, 1962.

79. Hauser, W A and Pedley, T A: Epidemiology, pathology, and genetics of epilepsy. In Engel, J Jr and Pedley, T A, (Eds.): Epilepsy: A Comprehensive Textbook. Lippincott-Raven, Philadelphia, 1998, pp. 9–230.

80. Helmsteader, C, Grunwald, K, Lehnertz, K, Gleibner, U and Elger, C E: Differential involvement of left temporolateral and temporomesial structures in verbal declarative learning and memory: evidence for temporal lobe epilepsy. Brain Cogn 35: 110–131, 1977.

81. Helmsteadter, C, Kurthen, M, Linke, D B and Elger, C E: Right hemisphere restitution of language and memory functions in right hemisphere language-dominant patients with left temporal lobe epilepsy. Brain 117: 729–734 1994.

82. Helmsteadter, C, Kurthen, M, Linke, D B and Elger, C E: Patterns of language dominance in focal left and right hemisphere epilepsies: relation to MRI findings, EEG, sex and age at onset of epilepsy. Brain Cogn 35: 110–131, 1997.

83. Hermann, B P, Whitman, S and Arntson, P: Hypergraphia in epilepsy: is there a specificity to temporal lobe epilepsy? J Neurol Neurosurg Psychiatry 46: 848–853, 1983.

84. Hermann, B P, Connell, B, Barr, W B and Wyler, A R: The utility of the Warrington Recognition Memory Test for temporal lobe epilepsy: pre- and post-operative results. J Epilepsy 8: 139–145, 1995.

85. Hermann, B P, Seidenberg, M, Haltiner, A and Wyler, A R: Relationship of age of onset, chronologic age, and adequacy of preoperative performance to verbal memory change after anterior temporal lobectomy. Epilepsia 36, 137–145, 1995.

86. Herzog, A G, Seibel, M, Schomer, D L, Vaitukatis, J L and Geschwind, N: Temporal lobe epilepsy: an extrahypothalamic pathogenesis for polycystic ovarian syndrome? Neurology 34: 1389–1393, 1984.

87. Herzog, A G, Russell, V, Vaitukatis, J L and Geschwind, N: Neuroendocrine dysfunction in temporal lobe epilepsy. Arch Neurol 39: 133–135, 1982.

88. Herzog, A G, Seibel, M, Schomer, D L, Vaitukatis, J L and Geschwind, N: Reproductive endocrine disorders in women with partial seizure of temporal lobe origin. Arch. Neurol. 43: 341–346, 1986.

89. Hill, J D: Psychiatric disorders in epilepsy. Med Press 20: 473–475, 1953.

90. Holzer, J C and Bear, D M: Epilepsy and Psychosis. Harvard Ment Health Lett, 9(12):5–6, 1993.

91. Holzer, J C and Bear, D M: Behavior in Temporal Lobe Epilepsy. In Schachter, S and Schomer, D (Eds.): Comprehensive Management and Treatment of Epilepsy. Academic Press, New York, 1998, pp. 131–148.

92. Hughlings-Jackson, J: On right or left-sided spasms at the onset of epileptic paroxysms, and on crude sensation warnings and elaborate mental states. Brain 3: 192–206, 1880.

93. Jack, C R, Sharbough, F W, Cascino, G D, Hirschorn, K A, O'Brien, P C and Marsh, W R: MRI-based hippocampal volume: correlation with temporal lobectomy. Ann Neurol 31: 138–146, 1992.

94. Jacome, D E and Risko, M: Pseudocataplexy: gelastic-atonic seizures. Neurology 34: 1381–1383, 1984.

95. Kanemoto, K, Takeuchi, J, Kawasaki, J and Kawai, I: Characteristics of temporal lobe epilepsy with mesial temporal sclerosis, with special reference to psychotic episodes. Neurology 47: 1199–1203, 1996.

96. Kapur, N, Millar, J, Colburn C, Abbott, P, Kennedy, P and Docherty, T: Very long-term amnesia in association with temporal lobe epilepsy: evidence for a multi-stage consolidation process. Brain Cogn 35: 58–70, 1997.

97. Koerner, M and Laxer, K D: Ictal speech, postictal language dysfunction, and seizure lateralization. Neurology 38: 634–636, 1988.

98. Krauthammer, C and Klerman, G L: Secondary mania. Arch Gen Psychiatry 35:1333–1339, 1978.

99. Kristensen, O and Sindrup, E H: Psychomotor epilepsy and psychosis: electroencephalographic findings. Acta Neurol Scand 57: 370–379, 1987.

100. Kristensen, O and Sindrup, E H: Psychomotor epilepsy and psychosis III: social and psychosocial correlates. Acta Neurol Scandinav 59: 1–9, 1979.

101. LaBar, K S, LeDoux, J E, Spencer, D D and Phelps, E A: Impaired fear conditioning following unilateral temporal lobectomy in humans. J Neurosci 15: 6846–6855, 1995.

102. Laplante, P, Saint-Hilaire, J M and Bouvier, G: Headache as an epileptic manifestation. Neurology 33: 1493–1495, 1983.

103. Lee, G P, Loring, D W and Thompson, J L: Construct validity of material-specific memory measures following unilateral temporal lobectomy. Psychol Ass 1: 192–197, 1989.

104. Leestma, J E, Walczak, T, Hughes, J R, Kalelkar, M B and Teas, S S: A prospective study on sudden unexpected death in epilepsy. Ann Neurol 26: 195–203, 1989.

105. Lesser, R P, Dinner, D S, Luders, H and Morris, H H: Memory for objects presented soon after intracarotid amobarbital sodium injections in patients with medically intractable complex partial seizures. Neurology 36: 895–899, 1986.

106. Lipshitz, R and Gradijan, J: Spectral evaluation of the electroencephalogram: power and

variability in chronic schizophrenics and control subjects. Psychophysiology 11: 479–490, 1974.

107. Loring, D W, Meador, K J, Lee, G P and King, D W: Amobarbital Effects and Lateralized Brain Dysfunction. Springer Verlag, New York, 1992.

108. Magistretti, P, Uren, R, Parker, T, Royal, H, Front, D and Kolodny, G: Monitoring regional blood flow by single photon emission tomography of I-123-N-isopropyl-iodamphetamine in epileptics. Ann Radiol 26: 68–71, 1983.

109. Magistretti, P, Uren, R, Schomer, D and Blume, H: Regional blood flow in ictal and interictal states in epilepsy. Eur J Nucl. Med 7: 484–485, 1982.

110. Manford, M, Hart, Y M, Sander, J W A S and Shorvon, S D: National general practice study of epilepsy (NGPSE): partial seizure patterns in a general population. Neurology 42: 1991–1917, 1992.

111. Marshall, D W, Westmoreland, B R and Sharbrough, F W: Ictal tachycardia during temporal lobe seizures. Mayo Clin Proc 58: 443–446, 1983.

112. Mattson, R H, Pratt, K L and Calverly, J R: Electroencephalogram in epileptics following sleep deprivation. Arch Neurol 13: 310–315, 1965.

113. McIntyre, M, Pritchard, P B and Lombroso, C T: Left and right temporal lobe epileptics: a controlled investigation of some psychological differences. Epilepsia 17: 377–386, 1976.

114. Wada, J A and Tsuchimachi, H: Cingulate kindling in Senegalese baboons, Papio papio. Epilepsia 36: 1142–1151, 1995.

115. Mesulam, M-M: Dissociative states with abnormal temporal lobe EEG: multiple personality and the illusion of possession. Arch Neurol 38: 176–181, 1981.

116. Mendez, M F, Cummings, J L and Benson, D R: Depression in epilepsy: significance and phenomenology. Arch Neurol 43: 766–770, 1986.

117. Metz, S A, Halter, J B, Porte, D and Robertson, R P: Autonomic epilepsy: clonidine blockade of paroxysmal catecholamine release and flushing. Ann Int Med 88: 189–193, 1978.

118. Mihara, T, Inoue, Y, Wantabe, Y, Matsuda, K, Tottori, T, Hiyoshi, T, Kubota, Y, Yagi, K and Seino, M: Improvement of quality-of-life following resective surgery for temporal lobe epilepsy: results of patient and family assessments. Jpn J Psychiatry 48: 221–229, 1994.

119. Milner, B: Visual recognition and recall after right temporal lobe excisions in man. Neuropsychologia 6: 191–209, 1968.

120. Milner, B: Disorders of learning and memory after temporal lobe lesions in man. Clin Neurosurg 19: 421–446, 1972.

121. Mitchell, W G, Greenwood, R S and Messenheimer, J A: Abdominal epilepsy: cyclic vomiting as the major symptom of simple partial seizures. Arch Neurol 40: 251–252, 1983.

122. Monroe, R R: Limbic ictus and atypical psychoses. J Nerv Ment Dis 170: 711–716, 1982.

123. Moshe, S L and Pedley, T A: Diagnostic evaluation of epilepsy. In Engle, J Jrand Pedley, T A (Eds.): A Comprehensive Evaluation. Lippincott-Raven, Philedelphia, 1998, pp. 799–1098.

124. Morrell, F: Secondary epileptogenesis in man. Arch Neurol 42: 318–335, 1985.

125. Morrell, F, Tsuri, N, Hoeppner, T J, Morgan and D, Harrison, W H: Secondary epileptogenesis in frog forebrain: effects of inhibition of protein synthesis. Can J Neurol Sci 2: 407–418, 1975.

126. Morrell, F: Physiology and histochemistry of the mirror focus: In Jasper, H H, Ward, A A and Pope, A (Eds.): Basic Mechanisms of the Epilepsies, Little, Brown, Boston, MA., 1969, pp. 357–374.

127. Naugle, R K, Rodgers, D A, Stagno, S J and Lalli, J: Unilateral temporal lobe epilepsy: an examination of the emotional and psychosocial behavior. J Epilepsy 4: 157–164, 1991.

128. Naugle, R I, Chelune, G J, Schuster, J, Luders, H and Comair, Y: Recognition memory for new words and faces before and after temporal lobectomy. Assessment 1: 373–381, 1994.

129. Nielsen, H and Kristensen, O: Personality correlates of sphenoidal EEG-foci in temporal lobe epilepsy. Acta. Neurol. Scandinav. 64; 289–300, 1981.

130. O'Connor, M, Sieggreen, M A, Ahern, G, Schomer, D L and Mesulam, M-M: Accelerated forgetting in association with temporal lobe epilepsy and paraneoplastic syndrome. Brain Cogn 35: 71–84, 1997.

131. O'Connor, M G, Greenblatt, D, Morin, M, Verfaellie, M, Doherty, R, Cahn, G and Schomer, D: Performance of temporal lobectomy patients on tests of remote memory. Poster presented at 27th Annual Meeting of the International Neuropsychological Society, Boston, 1999.

132. Ojemann, G A, Creutzfeld, O, Lettich, E and Haglund, M-M: Neurological activity in human lateral temporal cortex related to short-term verbal memory, naming and reading. Brain 111: 1383–1403, 1988.

133. Ojemann, G A: Cortical organization of language. J Neurosci 11: 2281–2287, 1991.

134. Penfield, W and Jasper, H (eds.): Epilepsy and the Functional Anatomy of the Human Brain. Little, Brown, Boston, 1954.

135. Perini, G I: Emotions and personality in complex partial seizures. Psychother Psychosom 45: 141–148, 1986.

136. Perez, M and Trimble, M R: Epileptic psychosis: diagnostic comparison with process schizophrenia. Br J Psychiatry 137: 245–249, 1980.

137. Phelps, E A, La Bar, K S and Spencer, D D: Memory for emotional words following unilateral temporal lobectomy. Brain Cogn 35: 85–109, 1997.

138. Pond, D A: Psychiatric aspects of epilepsy. J In Med Prof 3: 1441–1451, 1957.

138a. Post, R M: Lidocaine-Kindled limbic seizures: behavioral implications. In Wada, J. A. (Ed): Kindling 2, Raven Press New York. N.Y. 1981, pp. 149–160.

139. Post, R M and Udhe, T W: Anticonvulsants in nonepileptic psychosis. In Trimble, M R and Bolwig, T G (Eds.): Aspects of Epilepsy and Psychiatry. John Wiley, New York, 1986.

140. Rausch, R: Effects of temporal lobe surgery on behavior. Adv Neurol 55: 279–292, 1991.

141. Rausch, R and Babb, T: Hippocampal neuron loss and memory scores before and after temporal lobe surgery for epilepsy. Arch Neurol 50: 812–817, 1993.

142. Rasmussen, T: Relative significance of isolated infantile convulsions as a primary cause of focal epilepsy. Epilepsia 20: 395–401, 1979.

143. Robb, P: Focal epilepsy: the problem, prevalence, and contributing factors. In Purpura, D, Penry, J K and Walter, R D (Eds.): Neurosurgical Management of the Epilepsies. Raven Press, New York, 1975, pp. 11–22.

144. Robertson, M M: The organic contribution to depressive illness in patients with epilepsy. J Epilepsy 2: 189–230, 1989.

145. Robillard, A, Saint-Hilaire, J M, Mercier, R E T and Bouvier, G: The lateralizing and localizing value of adversion in epileptic seizures. Neurology 33: 1241–1242, 1983.

146. Rosenthal, L S and Fedio, P: Recognition thresholds in the central and lateral visual fields following temporal lobectomy. Cortex 11: 217–229, 1975.

147. Rovit, R L and Gloor, P: Temporal lobe epilepsy—a study using multiple basal electrodes. I. Description of method. II. Clinical EEG findings. Neurochirurgia 3: 6–19, 1960.

148. Rovit, R L, Gloor, P and Rasmussen, T: Sphenoidal electrodes in the electrographic study of patients with temporal lobe epilepsy. J Neurosurg 18: 151–158, 1961.

149. Rubin, E, Dhawan, V, Moeller, J R, Takaikawa, S, Labar, D R, Schaul, N, Barr, W B and Eidelberg, D: Cerebral metabolic topography in unilateral temporal lobe epilepsy. Neurology 45: 2212–2223, 1995.

150. Sachdev, H S and Waxman, S G: Frequency of hypergraphia in temporal lobe epilepsy: an index of interictal behaviors syndrome. J Neurol Neurosurg Psychiatry 44: 358–360, 1981.

151. Samuels, L, Butters, N and Fedio, P: Short term memory disorders following temporal lobe removals in humans. Cortex 8: 283–298, 1972.

152. Sass, K, Spencer, D D, Kim, J H, Westerveld, M, Novelly, R A and Lencz, T: Verbal memory impairment correlates with hippocampal pyramidal cell density. Neurology 40: 1694–1697, 1990.

153. Sato, M, Hikasa, N and Otsuki, S: Experimental epilepsy, psychosis, and dopamine receptor sensitivity. Biol Psychiatry 14: 537–540, 1979.

154. Saykin, A J, Stafiniak, P and Robinson, L J: Language before and after temporal lobectomy: specificity of acute changes and relationship to early risk factors. Epilepsia 36:1071–1077, 1995.

155. Sawrie, S M, Martin, R C, Gilliam, F G, Roth, D L, Faught, E and Kuniecky, R: Contribution of neuropsychological data to the prediction of temporal lobe epilepsy surgical outcome. Epilepsia 39: 319–325, 1998.

156. Schachter, S C, Bolton, A, Manoach, D, O'Connor, M, Weintraub, S, Blume, H and Schomer, D L: Handedness in patients with intractable epilepsy: correlation with side of temporal lobectomy and gender. J Epilepsy 8: 190–192, 1995.

157. Schachter, S C, Schomer, D L, Blume, H and Ives, J R: Porcine fetal gaba-producing neuronal cell transplants for human partial-onset seizures:safety and feasibility. Epilepsia 39: 67, 1998.

158. Schenk, L and Bear, D: Multiple personality and related dissociative phenomena in patients with temporal lobe epilepsy. Am J Psychiatry 138: 1311–1316, 1981.

159. Seidenberg, M, Hermann, B P, Schoefeld, J, Davies, K, Wyler, A and Dohan, F C: Reorganization of verbal memory function in early onset left temporal lobe surgery. Brain Cogn 35:132–148, 1997.

160. Sherwin, I, Peron-Magan, P, Bancaud, J, Bonis, A and Talairach, J: Prevalence of psychosis in epilepsy as a function of the laterality of the epileptogenic lesion. Arch Neurol 39:621–625, 1982.

161. Sherwin, I: Psychosis associated with epilepsy: significance of the laterality of the epileptogenic lesion. J Neurol Neurosur Psychiatry 44:83–85, 1981.

162. Sherwin, I: Differential psychiatric features in epilepsy; relationship to lesion laterality. Acta Psychiatr Scand (Suppl) 313) 92–103, 1984.

163. Sindrup, E, Thygesen, N, Kristensen, O and Alvina, J: Zygomatic electrodes: their use and value in complex partial epilepsy. Advances in Epileptology, International Symposium, p. 313–318, 1981.

164. Slater, E and Beard, A W: The schizophrenia-like psychoses of epilepsy I: psychiatric aspects. Br J Psychiatry 109: 95–150, 1963.

165. Sperling, M and Engel, J Jr: Sphenoidal electrodes. J Clin Neurophysiol 3:67–73, 1986.

166. Spiers, P A, Schomer, D L, Blume, H W, Kleefield, J, O'Reilly, G, Weintraub, S, Osborn-Shaefer, P and Mesulam, M-M: Visual neglect during intracorotid amytal testing. Neurology 40:1600–1606, 1990.

167. Stagno, S J: Psychiatric aspects of epilepsy. In Wyllie, E (Ed.): The Treatment of Epilepsy: Principles and Practice. Williams & Wilkins, Baltimore, 1996, pp. 1131–1144.

168. Stamm, J S and Rosen, S C: Learning on somesthetic discrimination and reversal tasks by monkey with epileptogenic implants in anteromedial temporal cortex. Neuropsychologia 9:185–191, 1971.

169. Stevens, J R: Interictal clinical manifestations of complex partial seizures. In Penry, J K and Daly, D D (Eds.): Advances In Neurology, Vol. 11. Raven Press, New York, 1975, pp. 85–112.

170. Stevens, J and Hermann, B P: Temporal lobe epilepsy, psychopathology, and violence: the state of the evidence. Neurology 31: 1127–1132, 1981.

171. Stevens, J R and Livermore, A: Telemetred EEG in schizophrenia: spectral analysis during abnormal behavior episodes. J Neurol Neurosurg Psychiatry 45: 385–395, 1982.

172. Stevens, J: Psychosis and epilepsy. Ann Neurol 14:347–348, 1983.

173. Strauss, E, Satz, P and Wada, J: An examination of the crowding hypothesis in epilepsy patients who have undergone the carotid amytal test. Neuropsycholgia 28:1221–1227, 1990.

174. Tarrier, N, Cooke, E C and Lader, M N: The EEG's of chronic schizophrenic patients in hospital and in the community. Electroencephal Clin Neurophysiol 44: 669–673, 1978.

175. Taylor, D: Factors influencing the occurrence of schizophrenia-like psychosis in patients with temporal lobe epilepsy. Psychol Med 5: 249–254, 1975.

176. Taylor, D C: Mental state and temporal lobe epilepsy; a correlative account of 100 patients treated surgically. Epilepsia 13: 727–765, 1972.

177. Tishler, P W, Holzer, J C, Greenberg, M, Benjamin, S, Devinsky, O and Bear, D M: Psychiatric presentations of epilepsy. Harvard Rev Psychiatry 1 (4):219–228, 1993

178. Toone, B K, Garralda, M E and Ron, M A: The psychosis of epilepsy and the functional psychoses: a clinical and phenomenological comparison. Br J Psychiatry 141: 256–261, 1982.

179. Trimble, M R: Personality disorders in epilepsy. Neurology 33:1332– 1334, 1983.

180. Trimble, M R, Ring, H A and Schmitz, B: Neuropsychiatric aspect of epilepsy. In Fogel, B S, Schiffoer, R B and Rao, S (Eds.): Neuropsychiatry. Williams and Wilkins, Baltimore. 1998, pp. 771–803.

181. Umbricht, D, Degreef, G, Barr, W B, Lieberman, J A, Pollack, S and Schaul, N: Post-ictal and chronic psychoses. Am J Psychiatry 152: 224–231, 1995.

181a. Van Buren, J M: Sensory, motor and autonomic effects of mesial temporal stimulation in man. J Neurosurg 18:273–288, 1961.

181b. Vickery, B G, Hays, R D, Graber, J, Rausch, R and Engel, J Jr, Brook, R H: A health-related quality of life instrument for patients evaluated for epilepsy surgery. Med Care 30:299–319, 1992.

182. Warach, S, Ives, J R, Schlaug, G, Patel, M, Darby, D G, Thangarji, V, Edelman, R R and Schomer, D L: EEG triggered echo-planar functional MRI in epilepsy. Neurology 90:89–93, 1996.

183. Weilberg, J P, Bear, D M and Sachs, G: Three patients with concomitant panic attacks and seizure disorder: possible clues to the neurology of anxiety. Am J Psychiatry 144: 1053–1056, 1983.

184. Wieser, H G and Yasargil, M G: Selective amygdalohippocampectomy as a surgical treatment of mesiobasal limbic epilepsy. Surg Neurol 17:445–457, 1982.

185. Wieser, H G: Depth recorded limbic seizures and psychopathology. Neurosci Biobehav Rev 7:427–440, 1983.

186. Waxman, S G and Geschwind, N: Hypergraphia in epilepsy. Neurology 24:629–638, 1974.

187. Waxman, S G and Geschwind, N: The interictal behavior syndrome of temporal lobe epilepsy. Arch Gen Psychiatry 32:1580–1588, 1975.

188. Whittman, S, Hermann, B B P and Gordon, A C: Psychopathology in Epilepsy: how great is the risk? Biol Psychiatry 19:213–216, 1984.

189. Williamson, P D, Spencer, D D, Spencer, S S, Novelly, R A and Mattson, R H: Complex partial status epilepticus: A depth-Electrode study. Ann Neurol 18:647–654, 1985.

9

Neural Substrates of Psychiatric Syndromes

Robert M. Post

I. Introduction

It is perhaps premature (but tempting) to write a chapter on the neural substrates of the various major psychiatric syndromes. In contrast to most neurological syndromes, wherein a medical history and physical examination usually lead to the diagnosis of a structural lesion that can be confirmed at autopsy (and more recently by a variety of imaging techniques), the psychiatric syndromes are by definition "functional" and, therefore, without fixed "organic lesions." Nonetheless, there is a longstanding interest in uncovering the neurobiological bases of these syndromes. The purpose of this chapter is to review the emerging information on the anatomical distribution of dysfunction in some of these syndromes and to see how this neuroanatomy fits the principles that are covered in the other chapters of this book. The goal is not to show that psychiatric diseases are based on fixed lesions but, instead, to show that they are associated with patterns of dysfunction that have neuroanatomical substrates and specificities (Fig. 9–1).

Heterogeneity and Neuroplasticity

Within the past two decades, the once impenetrable barriers of scalp and skull have yielded to a variety of anatomical and functional brain imaging techniques that promise to revolutionize the field of psychiatry much like the development of radiology did for orthopedics. Yet, the absence of a primary pathological anatomy in the major psychiatric syndromes must give us considerable pause. As in the epilepsies we are likely to encounter multiple, unstable, and evolving lesions that are nonetheless (and fortunately) amenable to intervention and amelioration with a variety of pharmacological and physiological manipulations.

Most psychiatric syndromes are characterized by waxing and waning symptoms and dysfunction. As such, their neural substrates may need to be conceptualized in terms of two components: (1) a fixed area of increased vulnerability and (2) areas

NEUROANATOMY OF EMOTION AND AFFILIATION

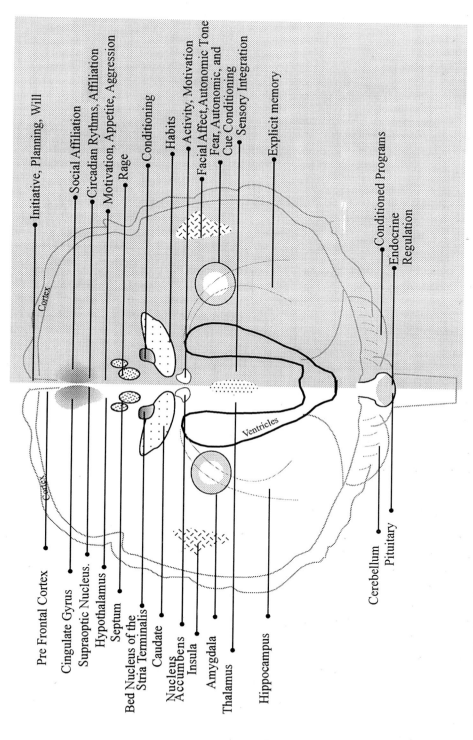

FIGURE 9–1. Provisional schematic of some areas of the brain and the putative functions they modulate as seen from a neuropsychiatric vantage point.

of more active dysfunction during periods of clinical exacerbation. The plasticity and potential treatability of the clinical symptoms suggest that the neuroanatomical substrates of these psychiatric syndromes may not take the form of traditional neuropathological lesions. The interpretation of neuroanatomical information based on neuroimaging methods requires a great deal of caution. Areas of hypofunction or hyperfunction may involve either excitatory or inhibitory pathways, and may represent either pathological processes or compensatory adaptations triggered by the pathology. Moreover, marked gender and individual differences in the processing of information as revealed by imaging techniques show that the range of normalcy is wide. One should thus not necessarily infer pathology on the basis of relatively minor deviations from customary activation patterns. These are some of the reasons why we can currently claim to have only the initial outlines of a neuroanatomy for psychiatric syndromes, although it is reasonable to predict that the next several decades will witness an explosion in this field.

Psychiatric nosology has until recently been based on clinical phenomenology. In the future, one can envision dramatic changes in illness categorization based not only on biochemistry and physiology, but also on the anatomical distribution of dysfunction. For example, within the depressive syndromes there is considerable heterogeneity. In addition to the classical presentation of depression with agitation, insomnia, anorexia, and weight loss typical of unipolar depression, there are atypical or reverse vegetative pictures (more characteristic of bipolar illness) with psychomotor retardation, hypersomnia, carbohydrate craving, and weight gain. Even within the unipolar depressive illnesses, patients present with greater or lesser degrees of anxiety, cognitive dysfunction, motor agitation, retardation, etc. At some point, it is highly likely that these clinical components of the depressive picture will, at least in part, be further resolvable on the basis of differences in anatomy and neurochemistry.

Anatomy and Biochemistry: Interactions with Gene Expression

The term "functional" has a variety of meanings in neurology and psychiatry including the older and more pejorative connotation of "not based on a real lesion." However, the demonstration of dysfunctional circuits in the obsessive-compulsive and post-traumatic stress disorders and their association with specific biochemical and pharmacological correlates have put to rest the notion that these are illnesses without neural substrates. Moreover, many psychiatric diseases have genetic bases, and thus by definition an underlying molecular biology. These genetic components can influence not only the development of the brain but also its susceptibility to certain types of stressors. Stress can affect transcription and neurotrophic factors and thus dramatically alter gene expression. Genes and experience can thus interact to influence the neuroanatomical organization of the brain. We have progressed from the realization that sensory deprivation can alter the physiology and microanatomy of visual cortex,[94] to parallel observations suggesting that experience can also alter neural systems related to more complex cognitive and emotional functions.

Schizophrenia was once considered "the graveyard of the neuropathologist," especially for neuropathologists who were looking for glial infiltrates, infarcts, and other markers found in traditional neurological illnesses. However, there are different kinds of processes, including those of programmed cell death, that may alter the central nervous system (CNS) without leaving obvious traces of fixed pathology. Virtually every cell in the entire body, including the nearly 20 billion neurons of the cerebral cortex and the twice as many glial cells, has the ability to undergo preprogrammed cell death (apoptosis). This is an exquisitely regulated process that requires cellular energy and new protein synthesis.[122]

Up to 50% of neurons in some parts of the mammalian brain may undergo apoptosis between birth and adolescence.[70,118,154] Even in the absence of apoptotic cell death, the pruning of dendrites and synapses is one of the most fundamental aspects of human CNS development and one that extends throughout much of childhood and perhaps beyond.[95] Environment and experience modulate this process. For example, stress can cause loss of dentate granule cells[84,128] and separation from the mother can double the number of neurons or glia that undergo apoptosis in the neonate,[205] while environmental enrichment can increase the ratio of progenitor cells becoming neurons rather than glia.[103] There is even unequivocal evidence that new CNS neurons can be born in adulthood.[74,103,128] Thus, neuronal, dendritic, and synaptic birth; death; differentiation; and plasticity display a delicate balance that may extend through much of the life span and that is responsive to hereditary and environmental influences via experience-dependent changes in gene expression. Perhaps Freud's much-maligned conceptualization of the death instinct may have presaged such a neuroanatomy of psychiatric illness.

Brain Imaging Tools

In the past, attempts to uncover the neural substrates of psychiatric syndromes would have been based on animal studies and on the clinical lessons learned from focal strokes, epilepsy, brain stimulation, and autopsy specimens. Today, the emphasis has shifted to structural and functional brain imaging techniques.

New behavioral activation methods can be said to offer the neuropsychological version of a cardiac stress test that can be used to uncover dysfunctional systems characteristic of specific psychiatric syndromes even when these systems appear normal at rest. It is also possible to stimulate the brain by using repeated transcranial magnetic stimulation (rTMS). In addition to its therapeutic effects, rTMS causes the firing and reversible interruption of neural circuits and allows a more active and anatomically specific probing of normal and disturbed circuits in psychiatric disease. This information may then allow a more precise anatomical targeting of rTMS for therapeutic purposes.[78,79,143]

For reasons that have been reviewed in Chapter 1, the limbic system offers a likely substrate for some of the dysfunctions associated with psychiatric syndromes. However, at each level of the CNS, including the limbic system, opposing influences balance each other. For example, the hippocampus may have generally inhibitory effects on cortisol secretion, whereas the amygdala may be more facilitatory. Within the amygdala, corticomedial versus basolateral subgroups may have opposing effects on endocrine and behavioral functions.[9,115] In fact, subdivisions of the amygdala[93,160] display a complex diversity of neurotransmitters, neuropeptides, and types of synaptic plasticity.[68,117]

In view of this complex organization, it is reasonable to expect that lesions in different areas of the limbic system could have quite different endocrine, behavioral, and neurophysiological consequences and that each of these areas may play a different role in the pathogenesis of neuropsychiatric syndromes such as panic disorder, affective illness, and schizophrenia. However, individual psychiatric syndromes also show considerable comorbidity, so they are also likely to display partially overlapping substrates in the CNS.

II. Unipolar and Bipolar Affective Disorders

Depressive and Manic Syndromes

Unipolar depression is characterized by a constellation of mood, motor, somatic, physiological, and endocrine disturbances. Signs and symptoms include depressed and anxious moods, with psychomotor agitation or retardation; impaired concentration, energy, and motivation; and inability to engage in and enjoy usually pleasurable activities including social interactions and sex. Sleep is often markedly disturbed, with a short rapid eye movement (REM) latency—a truncation of the deeper sleep stages III and IV. A paralysis of will and profound sense of guilt can lead to suicidal preoccupation. Approximately 10% of patients will die from their illness by suicide. While anorexia and weight loss are common in unipolar depression, bipolar depression may display a reverse vegetative syndrome with hypersomnia and weight gain.

According to the *Diagnostic and Statistical Manual of Mental Disorders* (Fourth Edition) (*DSM-IV*), a diagnosis of major depressive episode is made when

    A. Five (or more) of the following symptoms have been present during the same 2-week period and represent a change from previous functioning. One of these symptoms must be either #1 or #2 as listed in the next paragraph.

        (1) depressed mood most of the day, nearly every day, as indicated by either subjective report (e.g., feels sad or empty) or observation made by others (e.g., appears tearful); (2) markedly diminished interest or pleasure in all, or almost all, activities most of the day, nearly every day; (3) significant weight loss or gain without special dieting; (4) insomnia or hypersomnia nearly every day; (5) psychomotor agitation or retardation nearly every day (observable by others, not merely subjective feelings of restlessness or being slowed down); (6) fatigue or loss of energy nearly every day; (7) feelings of worthlessness or excessive or inappropriate guilt (which may be delusional) nearly every day; (8) diminished ability to think or concentrate, or indecisiveness, nearly every day; (9) recurrent thoughts

of death (not just fear of dying), or suicidal ideation with or without specific plans or attempts.

B. The symptoms cause clinically significant distress or impairment in social, occupational, or other important areas of functioning.

C. The symptoms are not due to the direct physiological effects of a substance (e.g., a drug of abuse, a medication) or a general medical condition (e.g., hypothyroidism).

D. The symptoms are not accounted for by bereavement or persist for longer than the expected 2 months for a normal grief reaction.

In hypomania and the mania of bipolar illness, nearly all of the depressive symptoms shift in the opposite direction such that the patient is energized, activated, and prone to increased social interactions to the point of intrusiveness. Guilt is replaced at times with religious fervor or delusional and grandiose schemes for great success or curing the world of its ills. There is often also increased sexuality and promiscuity, lack of judgment, inability to appreciate the negative consequences of one's acts, and even the inability to recognize oneself as ill. Mood may be either euphoric or dysphoric, with a mixture of depression, pressure of thought, agitation, and anxiety, including full-blown panic. In the most severe forms of mania, patients can be delusional, hallucinating, and as psychotic as patients with acute schizophrenia.

According to *DSM-IV*, a diagnosis of a manic episode is made when

A. There is a distinct period of abnormally and persistently elevated, expansive, or irritable mood, lasting at least 1 week (or any duration if hospitalization is necessary).

B. During the period of mood disturbance, three (or more) of the following symptoms have persisted (four if the mood is only irritable) and have been present to a significant degree:

(1) inflated self-esteem or grandiosity; (2) decreased need for sleep (e.g., feels rested after only 3 hours of sleep); (3) more talkative than usual or pressured to keep talking; (4) flight of ideas or subjective experience that thoughts are racing; (5) distractibility (i.e., attention too easily drawn to unimportant or irrelevant external stimuli); (6) increase in social, work, school, and sexual activity or psychomotor agitation; or (7) excessive involvement in pleasurable activities that have a high potential for painful consequences (e.g., engaging in unrestrained buying sprees, sexual indiscretions, or foolish business investments).

C. The mood disturbance is sufficiently severe so as to cause marked impairment in professional, interpersonal, or social activities to necessitate hospitalization to prevent harm to self or others or to cause psychotic features.

D. The symptoms are not due to the direct physiological effects of a substance (e.g., a drug of abuse, a medication, or other treatment) or a general medical condition (e.g., hyperthyroidism).

A hypomanic episode is considered present if the above symptoms last at least 4 days and are clearly different from the usual nondepressed mood, but unlike full mania, do not lead to marked impairment of function, psychotic features, or hospitalization.

Both unipolar and bipolar affective illness tend to be recurrent with an accelerating illness course—that is, longer "well intervals" between initial episodes and, in general, shorter "well" intervals with successive episodes. Early affective episodes tend to be triggered by psychosocial stresses, but later episodes eventually arise spontaneously without identifiable precipitants.[147]

Early Conceptualizations

There is a long history of postulated limbic system dysfunction in the affective disorders. This is based on the known relation of the limbic system in the control of mood, affect, and vegetative states (Chapter 1). Papez[141] and MacLean[120] have emphasized the role of the limbic system in the modulation of normal and pathological affect. This relation has been supported by stimulation and lesion studies in animals and by the presence of prominent affective disturbances in patients with temporolimbic seizures (Chapter 8).

Lateral asymmetry has also been invoked in the putative anatomical substrate of affective disorders. Flor-Henry pioneered the concept that disorders of affect were more prominently associated with dysfunction of the right temporal lobe and schizophrenia with dysfunction of the left temporal lobe.[71,72] However, more recent analyses[161] have emphasized the high incidence of depression associated with epilepsy emanating from the left temporal lobe. These data are convergent with those of Robinson,[162,163] suggesting an association of depression with strokes in the left frontal lobe and of mania with right-sided and more posterior lesions. Upon closer analysis, however, both Robinson and other groups have found that these relations are subtle and subject to complex interactions with a variety of other variables.[132] Some issues related to the neural substrate of mood and affect are reviewed in Chapters 1 and 6, where it is suggested that hemisphere asymmetries in emotional perspective may be embedded within an overall pattern of right hemisphere specialization for the control of mood and affect.

Anatomical Changes in Affective Illness

There is considerable evidence that the lateral and third ventricles are dilated when patients with affective disorders are compared to controls. However, some of the increase noted in these studies may have reflected the inconsistency in the ventricular size of the control groups rather than an increase in the ventricular size of the patient population. Moreover, several studies have reported that this dilation occurs in proportion to the degree of hypercortisolism,[102,133] raising the possibility that the putative reduction in brain substance may be reversible with termination of the depressive episode and its associated hypercortisolemia.

Magnetic resonance imaging (MRI) data on the size of the temporal lobes and two of its more important medial structures, the amygdala and hippocampus, are inconsistent. Several studies have reported a decrease in temporal lobe volume in bipolar illness,[7,88] but others have not found this effect. Sheline and colleagues[177] have reported a decrease in the size of the hippocampus as a function of the number of depressive episodes in unipolar patients. However, Ali and associates have observed the converse relation in bipolar patients whereby those with the largest hippocampal size paradoxically had the greatest cognitive impairments and higher illness severities.[5]

Altshuler and associates[6] and Strakowski and co-workers[187] reported an increase in the size of the amygdala in patients with bipolar depression, but Pearlson and colleagues reported the converse.[144] Discrepant findings related to changes in the size of the basal ganglia in mood disorders have also been reported (see reference 182). Perhaps the most consistent findings in bipolar illness are those of increased periventricular hyper intensities in T_2-weighted MRI scans[8] and the dilation of the 3rd ventricle.[182] These changes tend to be correlated with the severity of the neuropsychological dysfunction that is also present in these patients.[5,47]

Recently, Drevets and associates[59] reported very substantial decrements in the number of glial cells in the subgenual portion of the anterior cingulate gyrus of both unipolar and bipolar depressed patients. Should these findings be replicated, they would suggest that some psychiatric illnesses may be caused by alterations in glial function, perhaps because glial dysfunction could alter neurotransmitter regulation and neuroplasticity.

Functional Brain Imaging Studies

As listed in Tables 9–1a and 9–1b, a variety of studies have reported decreased frontal metabolism in acute depression, often in proportion to the severity of depression (rated on the *Hamilton Depression Scale*). Such relations have been reported in both primary and secondary affective disorders. For example, the secondary depressions in patients with complex partial seizures,[40] Huntington's chorea,[125] parkinsonism,[126] obsessive-compulsive disorder,[21] bulimia,[11] and cocaine abuse disorders[196] have all been associated with evidence of frontal hypometabolism, often on the left side to a greater extent than that observed on the right, and usually correlated with the severity of depression.[11,21,196] Whether this is the cause or the consequence of the psychomotor retardation remains to be resolved. The majority of 36 controlled studies of blood flow or metabolism have revealed decrements not only in frontal lobes but also in temporal lobes, the anterior cingulate gyrus, and the basal ganglia.[107]

Drevets and associates[60] investigated a select subgroup of patients with familial pure depressive disorders (i.e., those patients with a family history of only bipolar or recurrent depressive illness) and found a positive correlation between the severity of the psychiatric depression and amygdaloid activity, whereas other investigators have reported a correlation in the opposite direction in other types of affective illness.[25,57,77] Amygdaloid hypoactivity has been observed at baseline in depressed patients and in response to neuropharmacological challenges with pro-

Table 9–1a Negative Correlations Between Hamilton Depression Ratings and Cerebral Blood Flow and Metabolism in Primary Depression

Study	Region*
Baxter et al., 1989[21]	L DLPF/hemisphere
	R DLPF/hemisphere
O'Connell et al., 1989[139]	FL/cerebellum
	TL/cerebellum
Schlegel et al., 1989[171]	L TL
Kanaya and Yonekawa, 1990[100]	Cerebrum/cerebellum
Kumar et al., 1991[114]	Cerebrum/cerebellum
Austin et al., 1992[14]	R FL/occipital
Cohen et al., 1992[48]	M PF
Drevets et al., 1992[61]	L PF/global
Yazici et al., 1992[204]	L PF/slice
	M PF/slice
O'Connell et al., 1995[140]	FL/cerebellum
Ketter et al., 1997[107]	PF

*L = left; R = right; M = mesial; FL = frontal lobe; TL = temporal lobe; PF = prefrontal; DLPF = dorsolateral prefrontal (data from Ketter et al. 1997).[107]

Table 9–1b Decrements in Frontal Metabolism in Depression Secondary to Other Neuropsychiatric Conditions

Study	Frontal Cortex	Condition
Bromfield et al., 1992[40]	↓ metabolism (left)	Complex partial seizures
Mayberg et al., 1992[125]	↓ metabolism (left)	Huntington's chorea
Mayberg et al., 1990[126]	↓ metabolism (left)	Parkinsonism
Baxter et al., 1989[21]	↓ metabolism (left)*	Obsessive-compulsive disorder
Andreason et al., 1992[11]	↓ metabolism (left)*	Bulimia
Buchsbaum et al., 1992[41]	↓ metabolism (right)*	Schizophrenia
Volkow et al., 1992[196]	↓ metabolism (frontal)*	Cocaine abuse in remission

*Correlated with severity of association depression.

caine, which is a relatively selective activator of the amygdala and of its efferent pathways into frontal cortex, insula, and anterior (but not posterior) cingulate gyrus (Ketter and associates[105] unpublished data, and Fig. 9–2, top).

When depressed patients are challenged with procaine, they show a relative metabolic hyporesponsivity in limbic as well as other areas of the brain while showing approximately normal degrees of emotional activation as measured by self-rating scales. Recent evidence suggests that muscarinic cholinergic receptors may mediate the selective effect of procaine on limbic and paralimbic structures,[30] raising the possibility of cholinergic overactivity yielding a downregulation of receptor

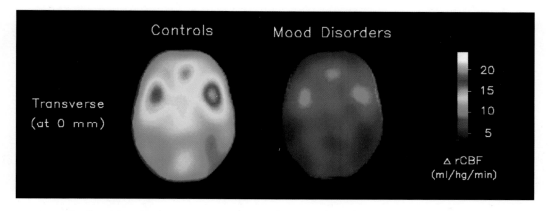

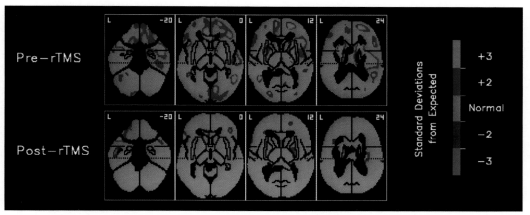

FIGURE 9–2. Top: Markedly blunted procaine-induced mean rCBF increases in 17 mood disorder patients versus 17 controls. Procaine induces striking selective activation of the amygdala, orbital frontal cortex, insula, and anterior cingulate gyrus in normal volunteers (left) in PET imaging of regional cerebral blood flow (rCBF). This activation is not obtained in mood-disordered patients (right) (Ketter et al., 1997).

Bottom: Baseline abnormalities in PET regional cerebral glucose metabolism (rCMRglu) in a 28-year-old woman with post traumatic stress disorder (PTSD) normalized after 1 month of treatment with 1 Hz rTMS over right frontal cortex. Top and bottom rows show statistical comparison of the patient's rCMRglu to an idealized healthy female control at age 28, before and after repeated transcranial magnetic stimulation (rTMS).

numbers in depression, as previously postulated.[98] This decrease could account for the hyporesponsivity evident in Figure 9–2.

In a variety of cognitive paradigms performed in the course of functional imaging, depressed patients show differential patterns of limbic and paralimbic activation compared with normal controls. For example, the *Stroop* test activates a substantial part of the midcingulate gyrus in normal volunteers, but not in depressed patients, who instead activate the left dorsolateral prefrontal cortex and visual cortex.[76] Furthermore, when asked to recognize facial emotion, patients with affective illness showed a blunted activation of blood flow in the region of the inferior frontal gyrus, although they performed as well as normals on the task.[75a] Both depressed and remitted patients, compared with normal volunteer controls, also showed decreased prefrontal and anterior limbic activation during induction of neutral and sad memories.[75] Actively depressed patients also found the mood induction task more difficult and could apparently not experience transient sadness to the same degree as remitted depressed patients or normal controls.[75] The persistence of dysfunction during remission suggests that prefrontal and limbic abnormalities may be a trait phenomenon, underlying a vulnerability to recurrence.

Much work remains to be done to elucidate which of the alterations represent trait or vulnerability markers and which are related to the state of depression itself. The potential heterogeneity and complexity of the variations in neural substrates of depression is further revealed by studies indicating that individual factors in the *Beck Depression Inventory* have different anatomical correlates and that these relationships differ in unipolar versus bipolar depressions.[63] For example, items related to depressive ideation are correlated with frontal and striatal hypometabolism in unipolar but not bipolar patients.

Prediction of Clinical Antidepressant Response

Wu and associates[203] have reported that depressed patients who had high glucose metabolism measured by 18F-fluoro-2-deoxyglucose (18FDG) in the cingulate and amygdala gave a better therapeutic response to one night of total sleep deprivation and showed relative normalization of limbic metabolism. These observations have been extended and replicated with single-photon emission computed tomography (SPECT)[64,65]

Ketter and associates have observed that patients with global cerebral hypermetabolism—particularly in the left insula—were more likely to respond to the antidepressant effects of carbamazepine, which also normalized the metabolism. In comparison, patients with relative hypometabolism, particularly in the left insula, were more likely to respond to the calcium channel blocker nimodipine.[108] Furthermore, unipolar depressed patients with high glucose metabolism in the anterior cingulate cortex (areas 24a/b) were responsive to antidepressant medications whereas those with cingulate hypometabolism were not.[124] These data are of interest in relation to other evidence suggesting that the degree of cingulate hypometabolism is highly correlated with the severity of unipolar depression.[31]

In unipolar patients carefully matched for medication status, clinical remission tended to normalize low regional cerebral blood flow (rCBF) in left dorsolateral prefrontal cortex (DLPFC), medial prefrontal cortex, and the anterior cingulate.[24] These data parallel those of Baxter and co-workers[21] and Martinot and associates[123] with FDG but not those of Drevets and colleagues.[61] Preliminary studies using O^{15} positron emission tomography (PET) showed that responders to lamotrigine and gabapentin display a trend toward baseline hypoperfusion that normalized with treatment, whereas normal flow at baseline in nonresponders was significantly reduced with these treatments.[110]

In addition, Kimbrell and co-workers[111] and Speer and associates[184] suggest that patients who show baseline *hypermetabolism* or hyperperfusion compared with normals were more likely to respond to 1 Hz rTMS whereas those with a pattern of baseline hypometabolism or hypoperfusion appear to show a better antidepressant effect to 20 Hz rTMS over left prefrontal cortex. Ten daily 1 Hz rTMS sessions decreased frontal and left amygdala blood flow, whereas 20 Hz rTMS increased activity in frontal cortex, cingulate gyrus (L> R) and in the left amygdala for up to 72 hours following the last treatment.[184] In keeping with this finding, low-frequency stimulation tends to induce neuronal long-term depression (rather than potentiation) in animal models and reduces frontal glucose utilization bilaterally in normal volunteers (Fig. 9–2).[109,184] These data raise the possibility that the classification of depression syndromes according to the distribution and direction of aberrant brain activity could lead to indications for differential treatment strategies.

Pathophysiological Integration

Many subtypes of primary and secondary unipolar depressions are associated with frontal lobe hypoactivity. Some of the abnormality is located within the limbic components of the frontal lobe such as orbital frontal cortex, the subcallesal (parolfactory) gyrus, and the anterior cingulate. These structures are tightly interconnected with the hippocampus and amygdala. Even the nonlimbic parts of the frontal lobe may influence the function of temporolimbic structures. For example, cortical inputs may increase the flexibility of learned associations in the amygdala.[116,165] Thus, in the face of frontal hypoactivity, limbic structures may be relatively disconnected from normal cortical modulatory influences and may promote more rigid stimulus–response linkages. Emotional biases driven by more primitive amygdaloid and hypothalamic processes may thus escape the modulatory cognitive influences mediated by the frontal lobe. In the presence of defective frontal modulation, early experiences of real or threatened loss or lack of social support may become embedded in the limbic system and generate fixed negative biases toward the self, the world, and the future without the possibility of modulation by a more realistic and adaptive cognitive assessment.

Patients with primary affective illness have as much difficulty in assessing facial emotional expression as patients who have had right anterior temporal lobectomies for the treatment of refractory epilepsy, suggesting that depression may also be associated with a dysfunction of the anterior temporal lobe.[168] Intravenous procaine is associated with the dose-related induction of psychosensory symptoms including illusions and hallucinations in all sensory modalities, as well as a wide range of affective responses ranging from euphoria to dysphoria. Endocrine concomitants of intravenous procaine include increased secretion of adrenocorticotropic hormone (ACTH), cortisol, and prolactin, but no significant change in growth hormone.[101,112] Procaine infusion is associated with increased fast EEG activity over temporal regions of the brain, although it is difficult to rule out the possible contributions of muscle artifact to this finding.[142] Blood flow measurements with O^{15} PET indicate that procaine induces a pattern of activation remarkably similar to the distribution of amygdaloid efferents observed in primates and confirms preclinical studies indicating that local anesthetics are relatively selective activators of limbic system structures.[9,148]

Ketter and co-workers[105] (and unpublished data) suggest that patients with affective disorders fail to show procaine-induced metabolic activation of inferior frontal cortex, anterior cingulate, and anteriomedial temporal lobes, despite the fact that they display psychosensory and endocrine activation. Although this pattern is revealed in the absolute but not normalized measures of blood flow assessed by O^{15} PET, these data suggest that the limbic and associated frontal circuits may be hyposensitive to a procaine probe in patients with affective illness.

In conjunction with the evidence of decreased blood blow and metabolism in left frontal cortex in the resting state in primary and secondary depression (Table 9–1a and b), these activation studies are beginning to define a frontotemporolimbic circuit that may provide a substrate for normal and pathological emotional modulation. Much work remains to be done to define the reliability and specificity of the preliminary findings described above and to establish the nature of the relations between putative cerebral dysfunction and the subtypes of depression.

III. ANXIETY-RELATED DISORDERS

Panic

Characteristic symptoms of a panic attack include four or more of the following symptoms emerging abruptly during a discrete period of intense fear or discomfort reaching a peak within 10 minutes: shortness of breath; dizziness; palpitations; trembling or shaking; sweating; choking; nausea or abdominal distress; numbness or tingling; hot flushing or chills; chest pain or discomfort; sense of unreality; and a fear of dying or going crazy.

For a diagnosis of Panic Disorder with or without Agoraphobia, *DSM-IV* requires:

A. Both (1) recurrent unexpected Panic Attacks, and (2) at least one of the attacks has been followed by 1 month (or more) of at least one of the following: (a) persistent concern about having additional attacks; (b) worry about the implications of the attack or its consequences (e.g., losing control, having a heart attack, "going crazy"); (c) a significant change in behavior related to the attacks

  B. The Panic Attacks are not due to the direct physiological effects of a sub-
     stance (e.g., a drug of abuse, a medication or a general medical condition
     (such as hyperthyroidism).
  C. The Panic Attacks are not better accounted for by another mental disorder,
     such as Social Phobia or Obsessive-Compulsive Disorder.

In some patients, lactate, caffeine, m-chlorophenylpiperazine (mCPP, a serotonin
receptor antagonist), yohimbine (an α_2 noradrenergic antagonist that increases the
firing of the locus coeruleus), cholecystokinin (CCK), and pentagastrin (an aden-
osine antagonist) can reproduce these symptoms. Panic patients are more vulnerable to the panicogenic effects of these agents compared to normal volunteer controls.

Reimann and associates[159] reported that those patients who were prone to
lactate-induced panic attacks (studied in a medication-free resting condition)
showed increased rCBF in the right parahippocampal area when compared to the
left. This alteration at baseline was not evident in those who were not prone to
lactate-induced panic attacks. In another study both lactate-induced panic and anticipatory anxiety in normal volunteers led to increases in rCBF in the temporal
poles.[158] However, Drevets and colleagues[62] reanalyzed these data with MRI-PET
coregistration and suggested that some of the areas of increased rCBF were actually
extracranial, perhaps related to increases in blood flow of the temporalis muscles.
These data are also of interest in relation to reports by Benkelfat and associates[28]
that CCK-induced anxiety and somatic symptoms were associated with increases
in blood flow both in bitemporal cortical as well as adjacent extra-cranial areas.

Procaine can induce panic in normal volunteers. Using MRI-PET coregistration,
Ketter and associates[104] have confirmed that procaine-induced blood flow changes
in the medial parts of the anterior temporal lobes were located within the brain.
The degree of procaine-induced anxiety in these subjects correlated with rCBF increases in the frontal lobe and left amygdala.[104]

Post-Traumatic Stress Disorder (PTSD)

The *DSM-IV* diagnosis of PTSD requires:
  A. The person has been exposed to a traumatic event in which both of the
     following were present:
     (1) The person experienced, witnessed or was confronted with an event or
         events that involved actual or threatened death or serious injury, or a
         threat to the physical integrity of others; (2) the person's response in-
         volved intense fear, helplessness, or horror.
  B. The traumatic event is persistently reexperienced in one (or more) of the
     following ways:
     (1) recurrent and intrusive distressing recollections of the event, including
         images, thoughts or perceptions; (2) recurrent distressing dreams of the
         event; (3) acting or feeling as if the traumatic event were recurring; (4)
         intense psychological distress at exposure to internal or external cues that

symbolize or resemble an aspect of the traumatic event; (5) physiological reactivity on exposure to internal or external cues that symbolize or resemble an aspect of the traumatic event.

C. Persistent avoidance of stimuli associated with the trauma and numbing of general responsiveness (not present before the trauma), as indicated by three (or more) of the following:

   (1) efforts to avoid thoughts and feelings; (2) efforts to avoid places or people that arouse recollections of the trauma; (3) inability to recall an important aspect of the trauma; (4) markedly diminished interest or participation in significant activities; (5) feeling of detachment or estrangement from others; (6) restricted range of affect; (7) sense of a foreshortened future.

D. Persistent symptoms of increased arousal as indicated by two (or more) of the following:

   (1) difficulty falling or staying asleep; (2) irritability or outbursts of anger; (3) difficulty concentrating; (4) hyper vigilance; (5) exaggerated startle response.

E. Duration of the disturbance for more than 1 month.

F. The disturbance causes clinically significant distress or impairment in social, occupational, or other important areas of functioning.

A series of recent studies based on functional imaging have begun to investigate the distribution of activation at baseline and during the induction of traumatic memories in patients with PTSD. These studies have reported frontal and medial temporal increases in activity, typically greater on the right than on the left.[157,175,180,195] Convergent with these findings, McCann and associates[127] observed that two patients with baseline right frontal hypermetabolism responded to approximately 1 month of 1 Hz rTMS with symptomatic relief and relative normalization of hypermetabolism.

Case Report

A 29-year-old right-handed woman had a history of more than 12 years of PTSD and refractory depression related to traumatic incidents experienced between the ages of 8 and 12 years. Current symptoms included depressed mood, cognitive dysfunction with poor attentional skills, irritability, chronic fatigue, decreased appetite, abnormal sleep patterns, frequent dissociative phenomena, unpleasant intrusive memories, and occasional suicidal ideation. She had been treated unsuccessfully with various medications as well as a 2-week course of left frontal 20 Hz rTMS treatment.

The patient was treated for 1 month with right frontal 1 Hz rTMS stimulation at 80% of motor threshold for 20 minutes per day. A total of 17 treatments were given three times per week for the first 2 weeks, then increased to five times weekly. During the course of treatment, the patient described an improvement in her symptoms, as measured by the modified *PTSD Symptom Scale*.[69] The improvement was most marked during the latter half of treatment when rTMS was administered more frequently. The beneficial effects of rTMS dissipated, and symptom frequency returned to baseline levels by 1 month after the last rTMS session.

Prior to treatment, the patient had a widespread pattern of metabolic hyperactivity (greater than 2 SD above the mean). Approximately 90 minutes after the final rTMS treatment, regional cerebral metabolic rates were obtained by FDG-PET scan and showed a normalization of metabolism toward the age- and sex-adjusted normative values, especially in the right hemisphere.[106,127]

These preliminary data, which require replication in controlled studies, suggest that frontal, and perhaps limbic areas, especially in the right hemisphere, may be involved in the pathophysiology of PTSD and that these regions may become suitable targets for therapeutic rTMS. It is of considerable interest that many of the physiological and endocrinological correlates of PTSD are opposite to those of depression. For example, PTSD is associated with frontal hypermetabolism and hypocortisolism, whereas depression is generally associated with frontal hypometabolism and hypercortisolism.

Southwick and colleagues[183] reported that yohimbine induced flashbacks, panic attacks, and dissociation in patients with PTSD. This occurred in the context of increased activation of brainstem areas (possibly the locus coeruleus) and decreased temporal and frontal cortical activation when compared with trauma-exposed veterans without PTSD. Forty-two percent of patients with PTSD experienced yohimbine-induced panic attacks compared to 7% in controls.[183] Thirty-one percent of patients with PTSD had panic attacks in response to mCPP and these patients tended to be resistant to yohimbine. Some patients with PTSD may thus have neural substrates that are sensitized to noradrenergic activity whereas others to serotonergic activity.

Secondary Pharmacologically-Induced Panic: Possible Limbic Kindling with the Local Anesthetic Compounds Procaine, Lidocaine, and Cocaine

Local anesthetics such as procaine, lidocaine, and cocaine cause acute limbic system activation in animals and man. Stevens and co-workers[186] have described cocaine-induced spindling and spiking in the amygdala of patients with temporal lobe epilepsy whose limbic areas were implanted with depth electrodes. Upon repeated administration to animals, these substrates can also induce a pharmacological kindling effect[148–150,201]—that is, repeated administration of subconvulsant doses may come to evoke full-blown seizures. These data parallel those observed with electrical kindling of the amygdala, wherein repeated 1-second subconvulsant stimulations eventually evoke afterdischarges of increasing amplitude and complexity, culminating in major motor seizures.[81,152,153] With sufficient numbers of repetitions, kindled seizures become autonomous; that is, they occur spontaneously in the absence of exogenous electrical stimulation. We have observed a similar progression to spontaneous seizures following repeated lidocaine administration (Weiss and colleagues, unpublished observation), but have not yet observed such a progression following cocaine-induced kindled seizures, as most of the animals succumb to the first or second cocaine seizure.[201] Pharmacological kindling may help to account for the emergence of cocaine seizures in chronic cocaine users, even at previously well-tolerated doses.[56]

Putative ictal and interictal discharges induced by cocaine may be manifested clinically in the form of panic attacks[149,150] as well as a variety of other presentations (Table 9–2). Repeated exposure to subthreshold doses of cocaine may induce full-blown panic attacks as a manifestation of pharmacological kindling. After a sufficient number of such cocaine-induced panic attacks, patients may enter a stage of spontaneity (similar to that seen in lidocaine and amygdala kindling) in which panic attacks begin to occur in the absence of pharmacological triggers.[150]

Certain doses of caffeine can also induce panic attacks and seizures. Caffeine induces dose-related increases in the transcription factor immediate early gene (IEG) c-fos (which is thought to be a marker of neural activity), predominantly in the striatum and ventral striatum,[189] including some areas of olfactory bulb and olfactory tubercle.[134] The latter structure is part of the "limbic striatum" (Chapter 1). Oral caffeine (480 mg) produces panic attacks in patients with panic disorder

TABLE 9–2 Diverse Psychiatric Manifestations Associated with Temporal Lobe Epilepsy

Syndrome or Symptom	Selected References
Affective psychosis	Dongier, 1959/60[58]; Dalby, 1971[52]; Flor-Henry, 1969[71]
Schizophreniform psychosis	Slater et al., 1963[181]; Kristensen and Sindrup, 1978[113]; Stevens, 1973[185]; Sherwin, 1982[179]; Taylor, 1975[192]
Panic-anxiety	Gloor et al., 1982[80]; McLachlan and Blume, 1980[129]; Currie et al., 1971[51]; Harper and Roth, 1962[86]
Personality changes	Bear and Fedio, 1977[22]; Bear et al., 1982[23]
Aggression	Serafetinides, 1965[176]; Ashford et al., 1980[13], Ramani and Gumnit, 1981[155]; Rodin, 1973[164]; Delgado-Escueta et al., 1981[55]
Ecstatic seizures (Dostoevsky epilepsy)	Cirignotta et al., 1980[45]
Demonic possession	Mesulam, 1981[131]
Religiosity	Waxman and Geschwind, 1975[197]
Suicidality	Pritchard et al., 1980[151]
Sexual (orgasmic)	Flor-Henry, 1976[72]; Mandell, 1980[121]; Heath, 1964[90]
Gelastic	Sackeim et al., 1982[169]
Multiple personality syndrome	Mesulam, 1981[131]; Schenk and Bear, 1981[170]
Transient global amnesia	Tharp, 1979[193]
Cognitive perceptual alteration (Psychosensory symptoms)	Dalby, 1975[53]; Penfield, 1975[145]; Gloor et al., 1982[80]
Depersonalization	Jackson and Stewart, 1899[97]

but not in normal volunteers,[194] and intravenous caffeine (3–7 mg/kg) induces a high incidence of olfactory hallucinations in normal volunteers.[137] In contrast to caffeine-induced seizures, which induce c-fos in the striatum, lidocaine and cocaine seizures increase c-fos expression, predominantly in paralimbic areas, particularly piriform cortex and the dentate gyrus of the hippocampus,[46] suggesting that different agents may induce panic through different pathways.

Obsessive-Compulsive Disorder (OCD)

Obsessions are unwanted (ego-dystonic) thoughts that relentlessly recur, whereas compulsion involves similar unwanted behavioral acts or rituals, both of which can be virtually impossible to resist, anxiety-producing when inhibited, and incapacitating. The *DSM-IV* diagnosis of obsessive-compulsive disorder requires:
    A. Either obsessions or compulsions:
        Obsessions as defined by:
           (1) recurrent and persistent thoughts, impulses, or images that are experienced, at some time during the disturbance, as intrusive and inappropriate and that cause marked anxiety or distress; and (2) the thoughts, impulses, or images are not simply excessive worries about real-life problems; (3) the person attempts to ignore or suppress such thoughts, impulses, or images, or to neutralize them with some other thought or action; (4) the person recognizes that the obsessional thoughts, impulses, or images are a product of his or her own mind (not imposed from without as in thought insertion).
        Or Compulsions as defined by:
           (1) repetitive behaviors (e.g., hand-washing, ordering, checking) or mental acts (e.g., praying, counting, repeating words silently) that the person feels driven to perform in response to an obsession, or according to rules that must be applied rigidly; (2) the behaviors or mental acts are aimed at preventing or reducing distress or preventing some dreaded event or situation.
    B. At some point during the course of the disorder, the person has recognized that the obsessions or compulsions are excessive or unreasonable.
    C. The obsessions or compulsions cause marked distress, are time consuming (take more than 1 hour a day), or significantly interfere with the person's normal routine, occupational (or academic) functioning, or usual social activities or relationships.
    D. If another Axis I disorder is present, the content of the obsessions or compulsions is not restricted to it (i.e., guilty ruminations in the presence of Major Depressive Disorder).
    E. The disturbance is not due to the direct physiological effects of a substance.
Studies by MRI in treatment-naive children with OCD show significantly decreased volume in ventral prefrontal and striatal regions but not in dorsolateral prefrontal cortex.[166] A large number of studies report abnormally high metabolism

or blood flow in orbital frontal and striatal areas of patients with OCD when compared with normal controls.[18,19,119,138,191] These abnormalities are generally attenuated following successful psychotherapy or pharmacological treatment with selective serotonin reuptake inhibitors (SSRIs).[20,29,92,156,190]

IV. SCHIZOPHRENIA

Characteristic symptoms of schizophrenia include delusions, hallucinations, thought abnormalities, disorganized speech, grossly disorganized or catatonic behavior, and negative symptoms such as affective flattening, social withdrawal, alogia, and avolition. The *DSM-IV* diagnosis of schizophrenia requires

A. Two (or more) of the following, each present for a significant portion of time during a 1-month period (or less if successfully treated):
   (1) delusions; (2) hallucinations; (3) disorganized speech (e.g., frequent derailment or incoherence); (4) grossly disorganized or catatonic behavior; (5) negative symptoms, i.e., affective flattening, alogia, or avolition.
B. Social/occupational dysfunction as a consequence of the symptoms.
C. The disturbance persists for at least 6 months.
D. Schizoaffective Disorder and Mood Disorder With Psychotic Features have been ruled out.
E. The disturbance is not due to the direct physiological effects of a substance (e.g., a drug of abuse, a medication) or a general medical condition.

Structural Studies

A large literature supports the finding of an increase in the size of the lateral ventricles in patients with schizophrenia compared with normal volunteer controls. (See reviews in references 33 and 66). Moreover, in identical twins discordant for schizophrenia, the ill twin consistently had greater ventricular volumes than the well twin, even when both sets of ventricles were within the normal range.[188] Recent evidence suggests that schizophrenic patients with a classic Kraepelinian or degenerative course show progressive bilateral increases in the size of the lateral ventricles, with the greater changes occurring in the left hemisphere.

With the use of MRI, a variety of investigators have reported reduced volume in the frontal lobes of schizophrenics.[39,87] In a number of these studies, the differences were confirmed at autopsy. A number of groups have measured N-acetyl aspartate (NAA), a putative marker of neuronal integrity, with magnetic resonance spectroscopy (MRS) and have found a consistent decrease of NAA in prefrontal areas of schizophrenics compared with controls.[34,35,43,54,135]

Akbarian and associates[1-4] have described an abnormal distribution of neurons in prefrontal cortex suggestive of a defect in neural migration during development. They also reported a decrease in the number of neurons expressing the GABAergic marker glutamic acid decarboxylase. Selemon[173,174] reported on increased density of neurons in area 46 of prefrontal cortex of schizophrenic patients compared to controls. Benes[26] reported deficits in GABAergic neurons, increases in GABA receptors and evidence of excess glutamatergic function in the anterior cingulate cortex. However, the anatomical consistency of these alterations from one patient group to another, their specificity for schizophrenia,[202] and how they relate to the clinical picture remain to be elucidated.

Decreases in the volume of the temporal lobes have also been reported.[38,144,167,206] Several studies have reported a reduced size of the hippocampus.[36,37] Neural loss in the hippocampus of schizophrenic patients has been seen in some studies[67,99] but not others.[12,91] Benes[27] reported a highly selective decrease in the number of nonpyramidal, possibly GABAergic neurons in the CA2 region of the hippocampus. Similar findings, however, were also observed in bipolar patients.

Some investigators have reported a loss of volume in the posterior superior temporal gyrus of the left hemisphere and a correlation between the size of this structure and the degree of thought disorder.[136,178] This is particularly interesting considering the prevalence of verbal auditory hallucinations in schizophrenia and the role of this area in auditory and language function.

Reports of thalamic volume reductions in schizophrenic patients have been inconsistent although Portas and co-workers (146) reported a significant inverse correlation of thalamic size with bizarre behaviors, hallucinations, and thought disorder.

Functional Brain Imaging Studies

There is substantial convergence in the findings of studies of frontal hypometabolism (hypofrontality) at rest in schizophrenia, extending from the pioneering studies of Ingvar and associates using blood flow,[73,96] to more recent, elegant studies using PET. It was observed that schizophrenic subjects, compared with controls, had deficient activation of the DLPFC while performing the *Wisconsin Card Sorting Test*, a test sensitive to frontal dysfunction (Chapter 2), but not while performing a variety of tasks that did not place as high a demand on the activity of this region.[198,200] Other tasks such as *Raven's Progressive Matrices (RPM)* and a symbols matching task did not show this degree of differential activation in schizophrenic patients compared with normals.[32] In studies of identical twins discordant for schizophrenia, deficient activation of the DLPFC during the performance of the *Wisconsin Card Sorting Test* dissociated the ill from the well twin in every instance.[199] The degree of hypofrontality in these studies was correlated with the negative symptoms of schizophrenia.

Although the DLPFC is not considered to lie within the classical boundaries of the limbic system, it has rich interconnections with the paralimbic cortices of the orbitofrontal and cingulate areas.[9,82,130] Frontal hypometabolism may account for many of the negative symptoms of schizophrenia, whereas putative limbic hyperfunction[10,85] (perhaps caused by a release from the inhibitory effects of the frontal lobes) could account for many of the positive symptoms.

V. Autism

The essential features of Autistic Disorder—sometimes referred to as early infantile autism, childhood autism, or Kanner's autism—are the presence of markedly abnormal or impaired development in social interaction and communication and a markedly restricted repertoire of activity and interests. The *DSM-IV* diagnosis of autism requires that:

  A. A total of six (or more) items from (*1*), (*2*), and (*3*), with at least two from (*1*), and one each from (*2*) and (*3*):

  (*1*) qualitative impairment in social interaction, as manifested by at least two of the following:

  (a) marked impairment in the use of multiple nonverbal behaviors such as eye-to-eye gaze, facial expression, body postures, and gestures to regulate social interaction; (b) failure to develop peer relationships appropriate to developmental level; (c) a lack of spontaneous seeking to share enjoyment, interests, or achievements with other people (e.g., by a lack of showing, bringing, or pointing out objects of interest); (d) lack of social or emotional reciprocity.

  (*2*) qualitative impairments in communication as manifested by at least one of the following:

  (a) delay in, or total lack of, the development of spoken language; (b) in individuals with adequate speech, marked impairment in the ability to initiate or sustain a conversation with others; (c) stereotyped and repetitive use of language or idiosyncratic language; (d) lack of varied, spontaneous make-believe play or social imitative play appropriate to developmental level.

  (*3*) restricted repetitive and stereotyped patterns of behavior, interests, and activities, as manifested by at least one of the following:

  (a) encompassing preoccupation with one or more stereotyped and restricted patterns of interest that is abnormal either in intensity or focus; (b) apparently inflexible adherence to specific, nonfunctional routines or rituals; (c) stereotyped and repetitive motor mannerisms (e.g., hand or finger flapping or twisting, or complex whole-body movements); (d) persistent preoccupation with parts of objects.

  B. Delays or abnormal functioning in at least one of the following areas, with onset prior to age 3 years: (1) social interaction, (2) language as used in social communication, or (3) symbolic or imaginative play.

  C. The disturbance is not better accounted for by Rett's Disorder or Childhood Disintegrative Disorder.

  D. Delays or abnormal functioning in at least one of the following areas, with onset prior to age 3 years: (1) social interaction, (2) language used in social communication.

Inroads into the neuroanatomy of autism are just beginning to emerge. The data of Bauman[17] are unique, representing one of the first systematic explorations of autopsy specimens of patients who died with autism compared with age-matched controls. These studies reported increased numbers of abnormally small neurons in many limbic structures. Anatomical and MRI findings of cerebellar abnormalities have also been reported, but have not always been replicated. (See the review in reference 50.)

Using a new PET marker, Chugani and associates[44] have found decrements of serotonin turnover in autistic patients in the left prefrontal cortex and right cerebellum, perhaps convergent with the earlier reports of structural cerebellar abnormalities. The serotonergic deficit could relate to the fact that serotonergic agents have been reported to be effective in ameliorating some of the symptoms of autism.[83] Furthermore, a number of groups have also reported genetic linkages to chromosome 15q,[42,49,172] a potential location for the serotonin transporter. Other recent functional imaging studies in autism have suggested reduced activity and volume in the right anterior cingulate,[89] an area also reported to be disordered in both schizophrenia and affective disorders.

Neonatally sustained combined lesions of the amygdala and the hippocampus produce deficits in the social behavior of rhesus monkeys that are similar to those observed in autistic individuals. Following up on these initial observations in primates, Bachevalier[15,16] has observed striking deficits in the ability of autistic individuals to recognize facial emotions, a function typically mediated by the amygdala and related parts of the temporal lobe. These findings are also consistent with the recent PET observations in autistic patients showing that emotionally expressive faces lead to the activation of areas traditionally responsive to inanimate objects rather than the more anterior, medial temporal, and frontal areas normally activated by such stimuli in control subjects (Bachevalier and colleagues, 1998, unpublished data).

Thus, the emerging neuroanatomy of autism appears to implicate a variety of limbic, cerebellar, and anterior prefrontal substrates in the profound abnormalities of cognitive function and social communication characteristic of this devastating syndrome.

VI. OVERVIEW

There appears to be a relative specificity in the patterns of cerebral alterations associated with major neuropsychiatric illnesses. Orbitofrontal hyperactivity in OCD contrasts with dorsolateral prefrontal hypoactivity in depression and schizophrenia and with the early reports of predominantly right-sided frontal hyperactivity in PTSD. The consistency of these patterns across many studies and, in some instances, the normalization of the deviance with successful therapy support the validity of these associations.

The emerging functional neuroanatomy of the major psychiatric syndromes can now begin to be interwoven with the literature on the neuropharmacology of these conditions. The dopamine antagonists are highly effective agents for treating patients with schizophrenia, mania, and psychotic depression. Clozapine, in particular, appears to exert its actions on the mesolimbic component of the dopaminergic system. Lithium and the mood stabilizing anticonvulsants carbamazepine and valproate are effective in the acute and prophylactic treatment of bipolar manic-depressive illness.

The tricyclic antidepressants, monoamine oxidase inhibitors, and a new generation of noradrenergic and serotonin-selective reuptake blockers are noteworthy for their broad utility in the treatment of depression and panic. In contrast, only the serotonin-selective agents appear to be effective in obsessive-compulsive disorders. Similarly, the high-potency benzodiazepines alprazolam, clonazepam, and lorazepam are effective antipanic agents but weak or ineffective in major depression or OCD. How are these pharmacological specificities related to the neuroanatomical patterns of dysfunction reviewed above? The next decade promises important advances in addressing this question as studies are conducted on the site-specific impacts of these pharmacological agents.

The evidence is now highly suggestive that both frontal cortex and limbic system dysfunction are implicated in many of the major psychiatric disorders. Given the intimate relation of frontal and limbic function to emotion and cognition (Chapter 1), the frontal and limbic networks are likely neural substrates for many of the signs and symptoms of the major psychiatric illnesses. This argument is further supported by the wide range of psychiatric symptomatology that can, in fact, be generated by frontal lobe lesions and by paroxysmal dysfunction of limbic structures associated with complex partial seizures (see Table 9–2 and Chapters 1, 4, and 8).

The phenomena of kindling and experience-induced plasticity show that acute events, including seizures and selective types of environmental and behavioral stressors, could induce long-lasting effects on emotion, cognition, and behavior. Depending on the neural systems involved and on the nature and temporal pattern of the stressors, different patterns of neurobiological alterations can be induced and can become associated with different psychiatric syndromes. This process is not static. The neuroanatomical substrates may change dramatically with illness evolution. Some of the lessons emerging from this field may thus help fulfill the Jacksonian and Freudian goals of establishing a neuroanatomical and neurobiological understanding of the major psychiatric disorders.

REFERENCES

1. Akbarian, S, Bunney, W E J, Potkin, S G, Wigal, S B, Hagman, J O, Sandman, C A and Jones, E G: Altered distribution of nicotinamide-adenine dinucleotide phosphate-diaphorase cells in frontal lobe of schizophrenics implies disturbances of cortical development. Arch Gen Psychiatry 50:169–177, 1993.
2. Akbarian, S, Kim, J J, Potkin, S G, Hagman, J O, Tafazzoli, A, Bunney, W E J and Jones, E G: Gene expression for glutamic acid decarboxylase is reduced without loss of neurons in prefrontal cortex of schizophrenics. Arch Gen Psychiatry 52:258–266, 1995.
3. Akbarian, S, Kim, J J, Potkin, S G, Hetrick, W P, Bunney, W E Jr and Jones, E G: Maldistribution of interstitial neurons in prefrontal white matter of the brains of schizophrenic patients. Arch Gen Psychiatry 53:425–436, 1996.

4. Akbarian, S, Vinuela, A, Kim, J J, Potkin, S G, Bunney, W E J and Jones, E G: Distorted distribution of nicotinamide-adenine dinucleotide phosphate-diaphorase neurons in temporal lobe of schizophrenics implies anomalous cortical development. Arch Gen Psychiatry 50:178–187, 1993.

5. Ali, S O, Denicoff, K D, Altshuler, L L, Hauser, P, Li, X, Conrad, A J, Mirsky, A F, Smith-Jackson, E E and Post, R M: A preliminary study of the relationship of neuropsychological performance to neuroanatomical structures in bipolar disorder. Neuropsychiatry Neuropsychol Behav Neurol, 1999, in press.

6. Altshuler, L L, Bartzokis, G, Grieder, T, Curran, J and Mintz, J: Amygdala enlargement in bipolar disorder and hippocampal reduction in schizophrenia: an MRI study demonstrating neuroanatomic specificity (letter). Arch Gen Psychiatry 55:663–664, 1998.

7. Altshuler, L L, Conrad, A, Hauser, P, Li, X M, Guze, B H, Denicoff, K, Tourtelotte, W and Post, R M: Reduction of temporal lobe volume in bipolar disorder: a preliminary report of magnetic resonance imaging (letter). Arch Gen Psychiatry 48:482–483, 1991.

8. Altshuler, L. L, Curran, J. G, Hauser, P, Mintz, J, Denicoff, K and Post, R M: T2 hyperintensities in bipolar disorder: magnetic resonance imaging comparison and literature meta-analysis. Am J Psychiatry 152:1139–1144, 1995.

9. Amaral, D G, Price, J L, Pitkanen, A and Carmichael, S T: Anatomical organization of the primate amygdaloid complex. In Aggleton, J P (Ed.): The Amygdala: Neurobiological Aspects of Emotion, Memory, and Mental Dysfunction. Wiley-Liss, New York, 1992, pp. 1–66.

10. Andreasen, N C, Flashman, L, Flaum, M, Arndt, S, Swayze, V, O'Leary, D S, Ehrhardt, J C and Yuh, W T: Regional brain abnormalities in schizophrenia measured with magnetic resonance imaging. JAMA 272:1763–1769, 1994.

11. Andreason, P J, Altemus, M, Zametkin, A J, King, A C, Lucinio, J and Cohen, R M: Regional cerebral glucose metabolism in bulimia nervosa. Am J Psychiatry 149:1506–1513, 1992.

12. Arnold, S E, Franz, B R, Gur, R C, Gur, R E, Shapiro, R M, Moberg, P J and Trojanowski, J Q: Smaller neuron size in schizophrenia in hippocampal subfields that mediate cortical-hippocampal interactions. Am J Psychiatry 152:738–748, 1995.

13. Ashford, J W, Schulz, C and Walsh, G O: Violent automatism in a partial complex seizure. Arch Neurol 37:120–122, 1980.

14. Austin, M P, Dougall, N, Ross, M, Murray, C, O'Carroll, R E, Moffoot, A, Ebmeier, K P and Goodwin, G M: Single photon emission tomography with 99mTc-exametazime in major depression and the pattern of brain activity underlying the psychotic/neurotic continuum. J Affect Disord 26:31–43, 1992.

15. Bachevalier, J: Medial temporal lobe structures and autism: a review of clinical and experimental findings. Neuropsychologia 32:627–648, 1994.

16. Bachevalier, J: Brief report: medial temporal lobe and autism: a putative animal model in primates. J Autism Dev Disord 26:217–220, 1996.

17. Bauman, M L: Microscopic neuroanatomic abnormalities in autism. Pediatrics 87:791–796, 1991.

18. Baxter, L R J: Neuroimaging studies of obsessive compulsive disorder. Psychiatr Clin North Am 15:871–884, 1992.

19. Baxter, L R J, Phelps, M E, Mazziotta, J C, Guze, B H, Schwartz, J M and Selin, C E: Local cerebral glucose metabolic rates in obsessive-compulsive disorder. A comparison with rates in unipolar depression and in normal controls. Arch Gen Psychiatry 44:211–218, 1987.

20. Baxter, L R J, Thompson, J M, Schwartz, J M, Guze, B H, Phelps, M E, Mazziotta, J C, Selin, C E and Moss, L: Trazodone treatment response in obsessive-compulsive disorder—correlated with shifts in glucose metabolism in the caudate nuclei. Psychopathology 20 (Suppl 1): 114–122, 1987.

21. Baxter, L R Jr, Schwartz, J M, Phelps, M E, Mazziotta, J C, Guze, B H, Selin, C E Gerner, R H and Sumida, R M: Reduction of prefrontal cortex glucose metabolism common to three types of depression. Arch Gen Psychiatry 46:243–250, 1989.

22. Bear, D M and Fedio, P: Quantitative analysis of interictal behavior in temporal lobe epilepsy. Arch Neurol 34:454–467, 1977.

23. Bear, D M, Leven, K, Blumer, D Chetham, D and Ryder, J: Interictal behavior in hospitalized temporal lobe epileptics: relationship to idiopathic psychiatric syndromes. J Neurol Neurosurg Psychiatry 45:481–488, 1982.

24. Bench, C J, Frackowiak, R S and Dolan, R J: Changes in regional cerebral blood flow on recovery from depression. Psychol Med 25:247–261, 1995.

25. Bench, C J, Friston, K J, Brown, R G, Frackowiak, R S J and Dolan, R J: Regional cerebral blood flow in depression measured by positron emission tomography: the relationship with clinical dimensions. Psychol Med 23:579–590, 1993.

26. Benes, F M: Altered glutamatergic and GABAergic mechanisms in the cingulate cortex of the schizophrenic brain. Arch Gen Psychiatry 52:1015–1018, 1995.

27. Benes, F M, Kwok, E W, Vincent, S L and Todtenkopf, M S: A reduction of nonpyramidal cells in sector CA2 of schizophrenics and manic depressives. Biol Psychiatry 44:88–97, 1998.

28. Benkelfat, C, Bradwejn, J, Meyer, E, Ellenbogen, M, Milot, S, Gjedde, A and Evans, A: Functional neuroanatomy of CCK4-induced anxiety in normal healthy volunteers. Am J Psychiatry 152:1180–1184, 1995.

29. Benkelfat, C, Nordahl, T E, Semple, W E, King, A C, Murphy, D L and Cohen, R M: Local cerebral glucose metabolic rates in obsessive-compulsive disorder. Patients treated with clomipramine. Arch Gen Psychiatry 47:840–848, 1990.

30. Benson, B E, Carson, R E, Sandoval, W, Linthicum, W L, Kimbrell, T A, Kieswetter, D O, Herscovitch, P, Eckelman, W C, McCann, U D, Weiss, S R B, Post, R M and Ketter, T A: A potential cholinergic mechanism of procaine's limbic activation (abstract). Biol Psychiatry 43:27S–28S, 1998.

31. Benson, B E, Kimbrell, T A, Ketter, T A, Little, J T, Dunn, R T and Post, R M: Outpatient antidepressant responders have lower paralimbic regional cerebral glucose metabolism than inpatient nonresponders (abstract). APA New Res Prog Abstr Abstr NR539:213, 1997.

32. Berman, K F, Illowsky, B P and Weinberger, D R: Physiological dysfunction of dorsolateral prefrontal cortex in schizophrenia. IV. Further evidence for regional and behavioral specificity. Arch Gen Psychiatry 45:616–622, 1988.

33. Berman, K F and Weinberger, D R: Functional localization in the brain in schizophrenia. In Tasman, A and Goldfinger, S M (Eds.): American Psychiatric Press Review of Psychiatry, Vol. 10. American Psychiatric Press, Washington, DC, 1991, pp. 24–59.

34. Bertolino, A, Callicott, J H, Nawroz, S, Mattay, V S, Duyn, J H, Tedeschi, G, Frank, J A and Weinberger, D R: Reproducibility of proton magnetic resonance spectroscopic imaging in patients with schizophrenia. Neuropsychopharmacology 18:1–9, 1998.

35. Bertolino, A, Nawroz, S, Mattay, V S, Barnett, A S, Duyn, J H, Moonen, C T, Frank, J A, Tedeschi, G and Weinberger, D R: Regionally specific pattern of neurochemical pathology in schizophrenia as assessed by multislice proton magnetic resonance spectroscopic imaging. Am J Psychiatry 153:1554–1563, 1996.

36. Bilder, R M, Bogerts, B, Ashtari, M, Wu, H, Alvir, J M, Jody, D, Reiter, G, Bell, L and Lieberman, J A: Anterior hippocampal volume reductions predict frontal lobe dysfunction in first episode schizophrenia. Schizophr Res 17:47–58, 1995.

37. Bogerts, B, Falkai, P, Haupts, M, Greve, B, Ernst, S, Tapernon-Franz, U and Heinzmann, U: Post-mortem volume measurements of limbic system and basal ganglia structures in chronic schizophrenics. Initial results from a new brain collection. Schizophr Res 3:295–301, 1990.

38. Bogerts, B, Lieberman, J A, Ashtari, M, Bilder, R M, DeGreef, G, Lerner, G, Johns, C and

Masiar, S: Hippocampus-amygdala volumes and psychopathology in chronic schizophrenia. Biol Psychiatry 33:236–246, 1993.

39. Breier, A, Buchanan, R W, Elkashef, A, Munson, R C, Kirkpatrick, B and Gellad, F: Brain morphology and schizophrenia. A magnetic resonance imaging study of limbic, prefrontal cortex, and caudate structures. Arch Gen Psychiatry 49:921–926, 1992.

40. Bromfield, E B, Altshuler, L, Leiderman, D B, Balish, M, Ketter, T A, Devinsky, O, Post, R M and Theodore, W H: Cerebral metabolism and depression in patients with complex partial seizures. Arch Neurol 49:617–623, 1992.

41. Buchsbaum, M S, Haier, R J, Potkin, S G, Nuechterlein, K, Bracha, H S, Katz, M, Lohr, J, Wu, J, Lottenberg, S and Jerabek, P A: Frontostriatal disorder of cerebral metabolism in never-medicated schizophrenics. Arch Gen Psychiatry 49:935–942, 1992.

42. Bundey, S, Hardy, C, Vickers, S, Kilpatrick, M W and Corbett, J A: Duplication of the 15q11–13 region in a patient with autism, epilepsy and ataxia. Dev Med Child Neurol 36:736–742, 1994.

43. Choe, B Y, Kim, K T, Suh, T S, Lee, C, Paik, I H, Bahk, Y W, Shinn, K S and Lenkinski, R E:¹H magnetic resonance spectroscopy characterization of neuronal dysfunction in drug-naive, chronic schizophrenia. Acad Radiol 1:211–216, 1994.

44. Chugani, D C, Muzik, O, Rothermel, R, Behen, M, Chakraborty, P, Mangner, T, da Silva, E A and Chugani, H T: Altered serotonin synthesis in the dentatothalamocortical pathway in autistic boys. Ann Neurol 42:666–669, 1997.

45. Cirignotta, F, Todesco, C V and Lugaresi, E: Temporal lobe epilepsy with ecstatic seizures (so-called Dostoevsky Epilepsy). Epilepsia 21:705–710, 1980.

46. Clark, M, Post, R M, Weiss, S R B and Nakajima, T: Expression of c-fos mRNA in acute and kindled cocaine seizures in rats. Brain Res 592:101–106, 1992.

47. Coffman, J A, Bornstein, R A, Olson, S C, Schwarzkopf, S B and Nasrallah, H A: Cognitive impairment and cerebral structure by MRI in bipolar disorder. Biol Psychiatry 27:1188–1196, 1990.

48. Cohen, R M, Gross, M, Nordahl, T E, Semple, W E, Oren, D A and Rosenthal, N: Preliminary data on the metabolic brain pattern of patients with winter seasonal affective disorder. Arch Gen Psychiatry 49:545–552, 1992.

49. Cook, E H J, Lindgren, V, Leventhal, B L, Courchesne, R, Lincoln, A, Shulman, C, Lord, C and Courchesne, E: Autism or atypical autism in maternally but not paternally derived proximal 15q duplication. Am J Hum Genet 60:928–934, 1997.

50. Courchesne, E: Neuroanatomic imaging in autism. Pediatrics 87:781–790, 1991.

51. Currie, S, Heathfield, K W, Henson, R A and Scott, D F: Clinical course and prognosis of temporal lobe epilepsy. A survey of 666 patients. Brain 94:173–190, 1971.

52. Dalby, M A: Antiepileptic and psychotropic effect of carbamazepine (Tegretol) in the treatment of psychomotor epilepsy. Epilepsia 12:325–334, 1971.

53. Dalby, M A: Behavioral effects of carbamazepine. In Penry, J K, Daly, D D (Eds.): Complex partial seizures and their treatment; Advances in neurology, Vol. 11. Raven Press, New York, 1975, pp. 331–343.

54. Deicken, R F, Zhou, L, Schuff, N, Fein, G and Weiner, M W: Hippocampal neuronal dysfunction in schizophrenia as measured by proton magnetic resonance spectroscopy. Biol Psychiatry 43:483–488, 1998.

55. Delgado-Escueta, A V, Mattson, R H, King, L, Goldensohn, E S, Spiegel, H, Madsen, J, Crandall, P, Dreifuss, F and Porter, R J: Special report. The nature of aggression during epileptic seizures. N Engl J Med 305:711–716, 1981.

56. Dhuna, A, Pascual-Leone, A and Langendorf, F: Chronic, habitual cocaine abuse and kindling-induced epilepsy: a case report. Epilepsia 32:890–894, 1991.

57. Dolan, R J, Bench, C J, Brown, R G, Scott, L C, Friston, K J and Frackowiak, R S J: Regional cerebral blood flow abnormalities in depressed patients with cognitive impairment. J Neurol Neurosurg Psychiatry 55:768–773, 1992.

58. Dongier, S: Statistical study of clinical and electroencephalographic manifestations of 536 psychotic episodes occurring in 516 epileptics between clinical seizures. Epilepsia 1:117–142, 1960.

59. Ongur, D, Drevets, W C and Price, J L: Glial reduction in the subgenual prefrontal cortex in mood disorders. Proc Natl Acad Sci USA 95:13290–13295, 1998.

60. Drevets, W C, Price, J L, Simpson, J R J, Todd, R D, Reich, T, Vannier, M and Raichle, M E: Subgenual prefrontal cortex abnormalities in mood disorders. Nature 386:824–827, 1997.

61. Drevets, W C, Videen, T O, Price, J L, Preskorn, S H, Carmichael, S T and Raichle, M E: A functional anatomical study of unipolar depression. J Neurosci 12:3628–3641, 1992.

62. Drevets, W C, Videen, T Q, MacLeod, A K, Haller, J W, and Raichle, M E: PET images of blood flow changes during anxiety: correction (letter). Science 256:16961992.

63. Dunn, R T, Kimbrell, T A, Ketter, T A, Frye, M A, Speer, A M, Osuch, E A and Post, R M: Beck Depression Inventory and regional cerebral metabolism (abstract). APA New Res Progr Abstr Abstr NR49:80–81, 1998.

64. Ebert, D, Feistel, H and Barocka, A: Effects of sleep deprivation on the limbic system and the frontal lobes in affective disorders: a study with Tc-99m-HMPAO SPECT. Psychiatry Res 40:247–251, 1991.

65. Ebert, D, Loew, T, Feistel, H, Kaschka, W P and Barocka, A: HMPAO and IBZM SPECT and sleep deprivation in major depression (abstract). Biol Psychiatry 33:78A, 1993.

66. Elkis, H, Friedman, L, Wise, A and Meltzer, H Y: Meta-analyses of studies of ventricular enlargement and cortical sulcal prominence in mood disorders. Comparisons with controls or patients with schizophrenia. Arch Gen Psychiatry 52:735–746, 1995.

67. Falkai, P and Bogerts, B: Cell loss in the hippocampus of schizophrenics. Eur Arch Psychiatry Neurol Sci 236:154–161, 1986.

68. Fallon, J H and Ciofi, P. Distribution of monoamines within the amygdala. In Aggleton, JP (Ed.): The amygdala: Neurobiological Aspects of Emotion, Memory, and Mental Dysfunction. Wiley-Liss, New York, 1992, pp. 97–114.

69. Falsetti, S A, Resnick, H S, Resick, P A and Kilpatrick, D G: The modified PTSD symptom scale: a brief self-report measure of post-traumatic stress disorder. Behav Ther 161–162, 1993.

70. Feinberg, I, Thode, H C, Chugani, H T and March, J D: Gamma distribution model maturational curves for delta wave amplitude, cortical metabolic rate and synaptic density. J Theor Biol 142:149–161, 1993.

71. Flor-Henry, P: Psychosis and temporal lobe epilepsy: a controlled investigation. Epilepsia 10:363–395, 1969.

72. Flor-Henry, P: Lateralized temporal-limbic dysfunction and psychopathology. Ann N Y Acad Sci 280:777–797, 1976.

73. Franzen, G and Ingvar, D H: Absence of activation in frontal structures during psychological testing of chronic schizophrenics. J Neurol Neurosurg Psychiatry 38:1027–1032, 1975.

74. Gage, F H, Ray, J and Fisher, L J: Isolation, characterization, and use of stem cells from the CNS. Annu Rev Neurosci 18:159–192, 1995.

75. George, M S, Kimbrell, T A, Parekh P I, Ketter T A, Pazzaglia P J, Callahan A, Frye M, Marangell L, Herscovitch P and Post, R M: Actively depressed subjects have difficulty inducing, and blunted rCBF during, transient sadness (abstract). APA New Res Progr Abstr Abstr NR167: 99, 1995.

75a. George M S, Ketter T A, Parekh P, Gill D S, Marangell L, Pazzaglia P J, Herscovitch P and Post, R M: Depressed subjects have abnormal right hemisphere activation during facial emotion recognition. CNS Spectrums 2:45–55, 1997.

76. George, M S, Ketter, T A, Parekh, P I, Rosinsky, N, Ring, H A, Pazzaglia, P J, Marangell,

L B, Callahan, A M and Post, R M: Blunted left cingulate activation in mood disorder subjects during a response interference task (the Stroop). J Neuropsychiatry Clin Neurosci 9:55–63, 1997.

77. George, M S, Ketter, T A and Post, R M: Prefrontal cortex dysfunction in clinical depression. Depression 2:59–72, 1994.

78. George, M S, Wassermann, E M, Kimbrell, T A, Little, J T, Williams, W E, Danielson, A L, Greenberg, B D, Hallett, M and Post, R M: Mood improvement following daily left prefrontal repetitive transcranial magnetic stimulation in patients with depression: a placebo-controlled crossover trial. Am J Psychiatry 154:1752–1756, 1997.

79. George, M S, Wassermann, E M, Williams, W A, Callahan, A, Ketter, T A, Basser, P, Hallett, M and Post, R M. Daily repetitive transcranial magnetic stimulation (rTMS) improves mood in depression. Neuroreport 6:1853–1856, 1995.

80. Gloor, P, Olivier, A, Quesney, L F, Andermann, F and Horowitz, S: The role of the limbic system in experiential phenomena of temporal lobe epilepsy. Ann Neurol 12:129–144, 1982.

81. Goddard, G V, McIntyre, D C and Leech, C K: A permanent change in brain function resulting from daily electrical stimulation. Exp Neurol 25:295–330, 1969.

82. Goldman-Rakic, P S, Selemon, L D and Schwartz, M L: Dual pathways connecting the dorsolateral prefrontal cortex with the hippocampal formation and the parahippocampal cortex in the rhesus monkey. Neuroscience 12:719–743, 1984.

83. Gordon, C T, State, R C, Nelson, J E, Hamburger, S D and Rapoport, J L: A double-blind comparison of clomipramine, desipramine, and placebo in the treatment of autistic disorder. Arch Gen Psychiatry 50:441–447, 1993.

84. Gould, E, Tanapat, P, McEwen, B S, Flugge, G and Fuchs, E: Proliferation of granule cell precursors in the dentate gyrus of adult monkeys is diminished by stress. Proc Natl Acad Sci USA 95:3168–3171, 1998.

85. Gur, R E, Gur, R C, Skolnick, B E, Caroff, S, Obrist, W D, Resnick, S and Reivich, M: Brain function in psychiatric disorders. III. Regional cerebral blood flow in unmedicated schizophrenics. Arch Gen Psychiatry 42:329–334, 1985.

86. Harper, M and Roth, M: Temporal lobe epilepsy and the phobic anxiety—depersonalization syndrome. Compr Psychiatry 3:129–151, 1962.

87. Harvey, I, Ron, M A, Du, B G, Wicks, D, Lewis, S W and Murray, R M: Reduction of cortical volume in schizophrenia on magnetic resonance imaging. Psychol Med 23:591–604, 1993.

88. Hauser, P, Altshuler, L L, Berrettini, W, Dauphinais, I D, Gelernter, J and Post, RM: Temporal lobe measurement in primary affective disorder by magnetic resonance imaging. J Neuropsychiatry Clin Neurosci 1:128–134, 1989.

89. Haznedar, M M, Buchsbaum, M S, Metzger, M, Solimando, A, Spiegel-Cohen, J and Hollander, E: Anterior cingulate gyrus volume and glucose metabolism in autistic disorder. Am J Psychiatry 154:1047–1050, 1997.

90. Heath, R G: Pleasure response of human subjects to direct stimulation of the brain: physiologic and psychodynamic considerations. In Heath, R G (Ed.): The Role of Pleasure in Behavior. Hoeber, New York, 1964, pp. 219–243.

91. Heckers, S, Heinsen, H, Geiger, B and Beckmann, H: Hippocampal neuron number in schizophrenia. A stereological study. Arch Gen Psychiatry 48:1002–1008, 1991.

92. Hoehn-Saric, R, Pearlson, G D, Harris, G J, Machlin, S R and Camargo, E E: Effects of fluoxetine on regional cerebral blood flow in obsessive-compulsive patients. Am J Psychiatry 148:1243–1245, 1991.

93. Hokfelt, T, Everitt, B, Holets, V R, Meister, B, Melander, T, Schalling, M, Staines, W and Lundberg, JM: Coexistence of peptides and other active molecules in neurons: diversity of chemical signaling potential. In Iversen, L L and Goodman, E (Eds.): Fast and Slow Chemical Signaling in the Nervous System. Oxford University Press, Oxford, 1986, pp. 205–231.

94. Hubel, D H and Wiesel, T N. Brain mechanisms of vision. Scientific Am 241:150–162, 1979.

95. Huttenlocher, P R: Synaptic density in human frontal cortex—developmental changes and effects of aging. Brain Res 163:195–205, 1979.

96. Ingvar, D H and Franzen, G: Abnormalities of cerebral blood flow distribution in patients with chronic schizophrenia. Acta Psychiatr Scand 50:425–462, 1974.

97. Jackson, J H and Stewart, P: Epileptic attacks with a warning of a crude sensation of smell and with the intellectual aura (dreamy state) in a patient who had symptoms pointing to gross organic disease of the right temporo-sphenoidal lobe. Brain 22:534–549, 1899.

98. Janowsky, D S, El-Yousef, M K, and D Avis, JM: Acetylcholine and depression. Psychosom Med 36:248–257, 1974.

99. Jeste, D V and Lohr, J B: Hippocampal pathologic findings in schizophrenia. A morphometric study. Arch Gen Psychiatry 46:1019–1024, 1989.

100. Kanaya, T and Yonekawa, M: Regional cerebral blood flow in depression. Jpn J Psychiatry Neurol 44:571–576, 1990.

101. Kellner, C H, Post, R M, Putnam, F, Cowdry, R W, Gardner, D, Kling, M A, Minichiello, M D, Trettau, J R and Coppola, R: Intravenous procaine as a probe of limbic system activity in psychiatric patients and normal controls. Biol Psychiatry 22:1107–1126, 1987.

102. Kellner, C H, Rubinow, D R, Gold, P W and Post, R M: Relationship of cortisol hypersecretion to brain CT scan alterations in depressed patients. Psychiatry Res. 8:191–197, 1983.

103. Kempermann, G, Kuhn, H G and Gage, F H: More hippocampal neurons in adult mice living in an enriched environment. Nature 386:493–495, 1997.

104. Ketter, T A, Andreason, P J, George, M S, Lee, C, Gill, D S, Parekh, P I, Willis, M W, Herscovitch, P and Post, R M: Anterior paralimbic mediation of procaine-induced emotional and psychosensory experiences. Arch Gen Psychiatry 53:59–69, 1996.

105. Ketter, T A, Andreason, P J, George, M S, Pazzaglia, P J, Marangell, L B and Post, R M: Blunted CBF response to procaine in mood disorders (abstract). Abstracts of the 146th Annual Meeting of the American Psychiatric Association Abstract NR297, 1993.

106. Ketter, T A, George, M S, Kimbrell, T A, Stein, R M, Willis, M W, Little, J T, Frye, M A, Cora-Locatelli, G, Benson, B E, Herscovitch, P and Post, R M: Assessment of PET data in individual patients with mood disorders (abstract). ACNP Abstracts, p. 230, 1995.

107. Ketter, T A, George, M S, Kimbrell, T A, Willis, M W, Benson, B E and Post, R M: Neuroanatomical models and brain-imaging studies. In Young, L T and Joffe, R T (Eds.): Bipolar Disorder. Marcel Dekker, New York, 1997, pp. 179–217.

108. Ketter, T A, Kimbrell, T A, George, M S, Willis, M W, Benson, B E, Danielson, A, Frye, M A, Herscovitch, P and Post, R M: Baseline cerebral hypermetabolism associated with carbamazepine response, and hypometabolism with nimodipine response in mood disorders. Biol Psychiatry, 1999, in press.

109. Kimbrell, T A, Dunn, R T, Wassermann, E M, George, M S, Danielson, A L, Benson, B E, Herscovitch, P and Post, R M: Regional decreases in glucose metabolism with 1 Hz prefrontal transcranial magnetic stimulation (TMS): A new technique for tracing functional networks in the human brain (abstract). Soc Neurosci Abstr 23:1576, 1997.

110. Kimbrell, T A, Ketter, T A, Frye, M A, Dunn, R M, Speer, A M, Osuch, E A and Post, R M: Neuroimaging of response to lamotrigine and gabapentin (abstract). Syllabus and Proceedings Summary of the 151st Annual Meeting of the American Psychiatric Association Abstract No. 77E:150, 1998.

111. Kimbrell, T A, Little, J T, Dunn, R T, Frye, M A, Greenberg, B D, Wassermann, E M, Repella, J D, Danielson, A L, Willis, M W, Benson, B E, Speer, A, Osuch, E and Post, R M: Frequency dependence of antidepressant response to left prefrontal repetitive transcranial magnetic stimulation (rTMS) as a function of baseline cerebral glucose metabolism. Biol Psychiatry, in press, 1999.

112. Kling, M A, Gardner, D L, Calogero, A E, Coppola, R, Trettau, J, Kellner, C H, Lefter, L, Hart, M J, Cowdry, R W and Post, R M: Effects of local anesthetics on experiential,

physiologic and endocrine measures in healthy humans and on rat hypothalamic corticotropin-releasing hormone release in vitro: clinical and psychobiologic implications. J Pharmacol Exp Ther 268:1548–1564, 1994.

113. Kristensen, O and Sindrup, E H: Psychomotor epilepsy and psychosis. Acta Neurol Scand 57:370–379, 1978.

114. Kumar, A, Mozley, D and Dunham, C: Semiquantitative I-123 IMP SPECT studies in late onset depression before and after treatment. Int J Geriatr Psychiatry 6:775–777, 1991.

115. LeDoux, J E: Brain mechanisms of emotion and emotional learning. Curr Opin Neurobiol 2:191–197, 1992.

116. LeDoux, J E: Emotion, memory and the brain. Sci Am 270:50–57, 1994.

117. Li, H, Weiss, S R, Chuang, D M, Post, R M and Rogawski, M A: Bidirectional synaptic plasticity in the rat basolateral amygdala: characterization of an activity-dependent switch sensitive to the presynaptic metabotropic glutamate receptor antagonist 2S-alpha-ethylglutamic acid. J Neurosci 18:1662–1670, 1998.

118. Lidow, M S, Goldman-Rakic, P S and Rakic, P: Synchronized overproduction of neurotransmitter receptors in diverse regions of the primate cerebral cortex. Proc Natl Acad Sci USA 15:10218–10221, 1991.

119. Machlin, S R, Harris, G J, Pearlson, G D, Hoehn-Saric, R, Jeffery, P and Camargo, EE: Elevated medial-frontal cerebral blood flow in obsessive-compulsive patients: a SPECT study. Am J Psychiatry 148:1240–1242, 1991.

120. MacLean, P D: The limbic system and its hippocampal formation; studies in the animals and their possible application to man. J Neurosurg 11:29–44, 1954.

121. Mandell, A J: Toward a psychobiology of transcendence: God in the brain. In Davidson, R J, Davidson, J M (Eds.): The Psychobiology of Consciousness. Plenum Press, New York, 1980, pp. 379–464.

122. Margolis, R L, Chuang, D M and Post, R M: Programmed cell death: Implications for neuropsychiatric disorders. Biol Psychiatry 35:946–956, 1994.

123. Martinot, J L, Hardy, P, Feline, A, Huret, J D, Mazoyer, B, Attar, L D, Pappata, S and Syrota, A: Left prefrontal glucose hypometabolism in the depressed state: a confirmation. Am J Psychiatry 147:1313–1317, 1990.

124. Mayberg, H S, Brannan, S K, Mahurin, R K, Jerabek, P A, Brickman, J S, Tekell, J L, Silva, J A, McGinnis, S, Glass, T G, Martin, C C and Fox, P T: Cingulate function in depression: a potential predictor of treatment response. Neuroreport 8:1057–1061, 1997.

125. Mayberg, H S, Starkstein, S E, Peyser, C E, Brandt, J, Dannals, R F and Folstein, S E: Paralimbic frontal lobe hypometabolism in depression associated with Huntington's disease. Neurology 42:1791–1797, 1992.

126. Mayberg, H S, Starkstein, S E, Sadzot, B, Preziosi, T, Andrezejewski, P L, Dannals, R F, Wagner, H N Jr and Robinson, R G: Selective hypometabolism in the inferior frontal lobe in depressed patients with Parkinson's disease. Ann Neurol 28:57–64, 1990.

127. McCann, U D, Kimbrell, T A, Morgan, C M, Anderson, T, Geraci, M, Benson, B E, Wassermann, E M, Willis, M W and Post, R M: Repetitive transcranial magnetic stimulation for posttraumatic stress disorder (letter). Arch Gen Psychiatry 55:276–279, 1998.

128. McEwen, B S: Corticosteroids and hippocampal plasticity. Ann NY Acad Sci. 746:134–142, 1994.

129. McLachlan, R S and Blume, W T: Isolated fear in complex partial status epilepticus. Ann Neurol 8:639–641, 1980.

130. Mesulam, M-M: Patterns in behavioral neuroanatomy: association areas, the limbic system, and hemispheric specializations. In Mesulam, M-M (Ed.): Principles of Behavioral Neurology. F. A. Davis Company, Philadelphia, 1985, pp. 1–70.

131. Mesulam, M-M: Dissociative states with abnormal temporal lobe EEG. Multiple personality and the illusion of possession. Arch Neurol 38:176–181, 1981.

132. Morris, P L P, Robinson, R G and Raphael, B: Lesion location and depression in hospi-

talized stroke patients. Evidence supporting a specific relationship in the left hemisphere. Neuropsych Neuropsychol Behav Neuro 5:75–82, 1992.

133. Mukherjee, S, Schnur, D B, Lo, E S, Sackeim, H A and Cooper, T B: Post-dexamethasone cortisol levels and computerized tomographic findings in manic patients. Acta Psychiatr Scand. 88:145–148, 1993.

134. Nakajima, T, Daval, J L, Morgan, P F, Post, R M and Marangos, P J: Adenosinergic modulation of caffeine-induced c-fos mRNA expression in mouse brain. Brain Res 501:307–314, 1989.

135. Nasrallah, H A, Skinner, T E, Schmalbrock, P and Robitaille, P M: Proton magnetic resonance spectroscopy (1H MRS) of the hippocampal formation in schizophrenia: a pilot study. Br J Psychiatry 165:481–485, 1994.

136. Nestor, P G, Shenton, M E, Wible, C, Hokama, H, O'Donnell, B F, Law, S and McCarley, R W: A neuropsychological analysis of schizophrenic thought disorder. Schizophr res 29: 217–225, 1998.

137. Nickell, P V and Uhde, T W: Dose-response effects of intravenous caffeine in normal volunteers. Anxiety 1:161–168, 1994.

138. Nordahl, T E, Benkelfat, C, Semple, W E, Gross, M, King, A C and Cohen, R M: Cerebral glucose metabolic rates in obsessive compulsive disorder. Neuropsychopharmacology 2: 23–28, 1989.

139. O'Connell, R A, Van Heertum, R L, Billick, S B, Holt, A R, Gonzalez, A, Notardonato, H, Luck, D and King, L N: Single photon emission computed tomography (SPECT) with [123I]IMP in the differential diagnosis of psychiatric disorders. J Neuropsychiatry.Clin Neurosci. 1:145–153, 1989.

140. O'Connell, R A, Van Heertum, R L, Luck, D, Yudd, A P, Cueva, J E, Billick, S B, Cordon, D J, Gersh, R J and Masdeu, J C: Single-photon emission computed tomography of the brain in acute mania and schizophrenia. J Neuroimaging. 5:101–104, 1995.

141. Papez, J W: A proposed mechanism of emotion. Arch Neurol Psychiatry 38:725–743, 1937.

142. Parekh, P I, Spencer, J W, George, M S, Gill, D S, Ketter, T A, Andreason, P, Herscovitch, P and Post, R M: Procaine-induced increase in limbic rCBF correlates positively with increase in occipital and temporal EEG fast activity. Brain Topography 7:209–216, 1995.

143. Pascual-Leone, A, Rubio, B, Pallardo, F and Catala, M D: Rapid-rate transcranial magnetic stimulation of left dorsolateral prefrontal cortex in drug-resistant depression. Lancet 348:233–237, 1996.

144. Pearlson, G D, Barta, P E, Powers, R E, Menon, R R, Richards, S S, Aylward, E H, Federman, E B, Chase, G A, Petty, R G and Tien, A Y: Ziskind-Somerfeld Research Award 1996. Medial and superior temporal gyral volumes and cerebral asymmetry in schizophrenia versus bipolar disorder. Biol Psychiatry 41:1–14, 1997.

145. Penfield, W: The Mystery of the Mind. A Critical Study of Consciousness and the Human Brain. Princeton University Press, Princeton, 1975.

146. Portas, C M, Goldstein, J M, Shenton, M E, Hokama, H H, Wible, C G, Fischer, I, Kikinis, R, Donnino, R, Jolesz, F A and McCarley, R W: Volumetric evaluation of the thalamus in schizophrenic male patients using magnetic resonance imaging. Biol Psychiatry 43:649–659, 1998.

147. Post, R M: Transduction of psychosocial stress into the neurobiology of recurrent affective disorder. Am J Psychiatry 149:999–1010, 1992.

148. Post, R M, Kennedy, C, Shinohara, M, Squillace, K, Miyaoka, M, Suda, S, Ingvar, D H and Sokoloff, L: Metabolic and behavioral consequences of lidocaine-kindled seizures. Brain Res 324:295–303, 1984.

149. Post, R M, Uhde, T W, Joffe, R T and Bierer, L: Psychiatric manifestations and implications of seizure disorders. In Extein, I and Gold, M (Eds.): Medical Mimics of Psychiatric Disorders. American Psychiatric Association Press, Washington, DC, 1986, pp. 35–91.

150. Post, R M, Weiss, S R B, Pert, A and Uhde, T W: Chronic cocaine administration: sensitization and kindling effects. In Raskin, A and Fisher, S (Eds.): Cocaine: Clinical and Biobehavioral Aspects. Oxford University Press, New York, 1987, pp. 109–173.

151. Pritchard, P B, Lombrose, C T and McIntyre, M: Psychological complications of temporal lobe epilepsy. Neurology 30:227–232, 1980.

152. Racine, R J: Modification of seizure activity by electrical stimulation. I. After-discharge threshold. Electroencephalogr Clin Neurophysiol 32:269–279, 1972.

153. Racine, R. J. Modification of seizure activity by electrical stimulation. II. Motor seizure. Electroencephalogr Clin Neurophysiol 32:281–294, 1972.

154. Rakic, P, Bourgeois, J P, Eckenhoff, M F, Zecevic, N and Goldman-Rakic, P S: Concurrent overproduction of synapses in diverse regions of the primate cerebral cortex. Science 232: 232–234, 1986.

155. Ramani, V and Gumnit, R J: Intensive monitoring of epileptic patients with a history of episodic aggression. Arch Neurol 38:570–571, 1981.

156. Rauch, S L, Jenike, M A, Alpert, N M, Baer, L, Breiter, H C, Savage, C R and Fischman, A J: Regional cerebral blood flow measured during symptom provocation in obsessive-compulsive disorder using oxygen 15-labeled carbon dioxide and positron emission tomography. Arch Gen Psychiatry 51:62–70, 1994.

157. Rauch, S L, Van der Kolk, B A, Fisler, R E, Alpert, N M, Orr, S P, Savage, C R, Fischman, A J, Jenike, M A and Pitman, R K: A symptom provocation study of posttraumatic stress disorder using positron emission tomography and script-driven imagery. Arch Gen Psychiatry 53:380–387, 1996.

158. Reiman, E M, Fusselman, M J, Fox, P T and Raichle, M E: Neuroanatomical correlates of anticipatory anxiety. Science 243:1071–1074, 1989.

159. Reiman, E M, Raichle, M E, Robins, E, Mintun, M A, Fusselman, M J, Fox, P T, Price, J L and Hackman, K A. Neuroanatomical correlates of a lactate-induced anxiety attack. Arch Gen Psychiatry 46:493–500, 1989.

160. Roberts, G W: Neuropeptides: Cellular morphology, major pathways, and functional considerations. In Aggleston, J P (Ed.): The Amygdala: Neurobiological Aspects of Emotion, Memory, and Mental Dysfunction. Wiley-Liss, New York, 1992, pp. 115–142.

161. Robertson, M M and Trimble, M R: Depressive illness in patients with epilepsy: a review. Epilepsia 24:S109–S116, 1983.

162. Robinson, R G: The use of an animal model to study post-stroke depression. In Koob, G F, Ehlers, C L and Kupfer, D J (Eds.): Animal Models of Depression. Birkhauser, Boston, 1989, pp. 74–98.

163. Robinson, R G and Starkstein, S E: Mood disorders following stroke: new findings and future directions. J Geriatr Psychiatry 22:1–15, 1989.

164. Rodin, E A: Psychomotor epilepsy and aggressive behavior. Arch Gen Psychiatry 28: 210–213, 1973.

165. Rolls, E T: Neurophysiology and functions of the primate amygdala. In Aggleton, J P (Ed.): The Amygdala: Neurobiological Aspects of Emotion, Memory, and Mental Dysfunction. Wiley-Liss, New York, 1992, pp. 143–165.

166. Rosenberg, D R and Keshavan, M S: A. E. Bennett Research Award. Toward a neurodevelopmental model of obsessive-compulsive disorder. Biol Psychiatry 43:623–640, 1998.

167. Rossi, A, Stratta, P, Mancini, F, Gallucci, M, Mattei, P, Core, L, DiMichele, V and Casacchia, M: Magnetic resonance imaging findings of amygdala-anterior hippocampus shrinkage in male patients with schizophrenia. Psychiatr Res 52:43–53, 1994.

168. Rubinow, D R and Post, R M: Impaired recognition of affect in facial expression in depressed patients. Biol Psychiatry 31:947–953, 1992.

169. Sackeim, H A, Greenberg, M S, Weiman, A L, Gur, R C, Hungerbuhler, J P and Geschwind, N: Hemispheric asymmetry in the expression of positive and negative emotions. Neurologic evidence. Arch Neurol 39:210–218, 1982.

170. Schenk, L and Bear, D: Multiple personality disorder and related dissociative phenomena in patients with temporal lobe epilepsy. Am J Psychiatry 138:1311–1315, 1981.

171. Schlegel, S, Aldenhoff, J B, Eissner, D, Lindner, P and Nickel, O: Regional cerebral blood flow in depression: associations with psychopathology. J Affect Disord 17:211–218, 1989.

172. Schroer, R J, Phelan, M C, Michaelis, R C, Crawford, E C, Skinner, S A, Cuccaro, M, Simensen, R J, Bishop, J, Skinner, C, Fender, D and Stevenson, R E: Autism and maternally derived aberrations of chromosome 15q. Am J Med Genet 76:327–336, 1998.

173. Selemon, L D, Rajkowska, G and Goldman-Rakic, P S: Abnormally high neuronal density in the schizophrenic cortex. A morphometric analysis of prefrontal area 9 and occipital area 17. Arch Gen Psychiatry 52:805–818, discussion 819–822, 1995.

174. Selemon, L D, Rajkowska, G and Goldman-Rakic, P S: Elevated neuronal density in prefrontal area 46 in brains from schizophrenic patients: application of a three-dimensional, stereologic counting method. J Comp Neurol 392:402–412, 1998.

175. Semple, W E, Goyer, P, McCormick, R, Morris, E, Compton, B, Muswick, G, Nelson, D, Donovan, B, Leisure, G and Berridge, M: Preliminary report: brain blood flow using PET in patients with posttraumatic stress disorder and substance-abuse histories. Biol Psychiatry 34:115–118, 1993.

176. Serafetinides, E A: Aggressiveness in temporal lobe epileptics and its relation to cerebral dysfunction and environmental factors. Epilepsia 6:33–42, 1965.

177. Sheline, Y I, Wang, P W, Gado, M H, Csernansky, J G and Vannier, M W: Hippocampal atrophy in recurrent major depression. Proc Natl Acad Sci USA 93:3908–3913, 1996.

178. Shenton, M E, Kikinis, R, Jolesz, F A, Pollak, S D, LeMay, M, Wible, C G, Hokama, H, Martin, J, Metcalf, D and Coleman, M: Abnormalities of the left temporal lobe and thought disorder in schizophrenia. A quantitative magnetic resonance imaging study. N Engl J Med 327:604–612, 1992.

179. Sherwin, I: The effect of the location of an epileptogenic lesion on the occurrence of psychosis in epilepsy. In Koella, W P and Trimble, M R (Eds.): Advances in Biological Psychiatry, Vol. 8: Temporal Lobe Epilepsy, Mania, and Schizophrenia and the Limbic System. S. Karger, Basel, 1982, pp. 81–97.

180. Shin, L M, Kosslyn, S M, McNally, R J, Alpert, N M, Thompson, W L, Rauch, S L, Macklin, M L and Pitman, R K: Visual imagery and perception in posttraumatic stress disorder. A positron emission tomographic investigation. Arch Gen Psychiatry 54:233–241, 1997.

181. Slater, E, Beard, A W, and Glithero, E: The schizophrenia-like psychosis of epilepsy. Br J Psychiatry 109:95–150, 1963.

182. Soares, J C and Mann, J J: The anatomy of mood disorders—review of structural neuroimaging studies. Biol Psychiatry 41:86–106, 1997.

183. Southwick, S M, Krystal, J H, Bremner, J D, Morgan, C A., Nicolaou, A L, Nagy, L M, Johnson, D R, Heninger, G R and Charney, D S: Noradrenergic and serotonergic function in posttraumatic stress disorder. Arch Gen Psychiatry 54:749–758, 1997.

184. Speer, A M, Kimbrell, T A, Dunn, R T, Osuch, E A, Frye, M A, Willis, M W and Wassermann, E M: Differential changes in rCBF with one versus 20 Hz rTMS in depressed patients (abstract). APA New Res Progr Abstr Abstr NR55:82, 1998.

185. Stevens, J R: Psychomotor epilepsy and schizophrenia: a common anatomy? In Brazier, M A B (Ed.): Epilepsy: Its Phenomena in Man. Academic Press, New York, 1973, pp. 190–214.

186. Stevens, J R, Mark, V H, Erwin, F, Pacheco, P and Suematsu, K: Deep temporal stimulation in man. Arch Neurol 21:157–167, 1969.

187. Strakowski, S M, DelBello, M P, Sax, K W, Zimmerman, M E, Shear, P K, Hawkins, J M and Larson, E R: Brain magnetic resonance imaging of structural abnormalities in bipolar disorder. Arch Gen Psychiatry 56:254–260, 1999.

188. Suddath, R L, Christison, G W, Torrey, E F, Casanova, M F and Weinberger, D R: Anatomical abnormalities in the brains of monozygotic twins discordant for schizophrenia. N Engl J Med 322:789–794, 1990.

189. Svenningsson, P, Strom, A, Johansson, B and Fredholm, B B: Increased expression of c-jun, junB, AP-1, and preproenkephalin mRNA in rat striatum following a single injection of caffeine. J Neurosci 15:3583–3593, 1995.
190. Swedo, S E, Pietrini, P, Leonard, H L, Schapiro, M B, Rettew, D C, Goldberger, E L, Rapoport, S I, Rapoport, J L and Grady, C L: Cerebral glucose metabolism in childhood-onset obsessive-compulsive disorder. Revisualization during pharmacotherapy. Arch Gen Psychiatry 49:690–694, 1992.
191. Swedo, S E, Schapiro, M B, Grady, C L, Cheslow, D L, Leonard, H L, Kumar, A, Friedland, R, Rapoport, S I and Rapoport, J L: Cerebral glucose metabolism in childhood-onset obsessive-compulsive disorder. Arch Gen Psychiatry 46:518–523, 1989.
192. Taylor, D C: Factors influencing the occurrence of schizophrenia-like psychosis in patients with temporal lobe epilepsy. Psychol Med 5:249–254, 1975.
193. Tharp, B R: Transient global amnesia: manifestation of medial temporal lobe epilepsy (letter). Clin Electroencephalogr 10:54–56, 1979.
194. Uhde, T W: Caffeine provocation of panic: a focus on biological mechanisms. In Ballenger, J C (Ed.): Neurobiology of Panic Disorder (Frontiers of Clinical Neuroscience). Alan Liss, New York, 1990, pp. 365–376.
195. Van der Kolk, B A, Burbridge, J A and Suzuki, J: The psychobiology of traumatic memory. Clinical implications of neuroimaging studies. Ann NY Acad Sci 821:99–113, 1997.
196. Volkow N D, Hitzemann, R, Wang, G J, Fowler, J S, Wolf, A P, Dewey, S L and Handlesman, L. Long-term frontal brain metabolic changes in cocaine abusers. Synapse 11:184–190, 1992.
197. Waxman, S G and Geshwind, N: The interictal behavior syndrome of epilepsy. Arch Gen Psychiatry 32:1580–1588, 1975.
198. Weinberger, D R, Berman, K F and Illowsky, B P: Physiological dysfunction of dorsolateral prefrontal cortex in schizophrenia. III. A new cohort and evidence for a monoaminergic mechanism. Arch Gen Psychiatry 45:609–615, 1988.
199. Weinberger, D R, Berman, K F, Suddath, R and Torrey, E F: Evidence of dysfunction of a prefrontal-limbic network in schizophrenia: a magnetic resonance imaging and regional cerebral blood flow study of discordant monozygotic twins. Am J Psychiatry 149:890–897, 1992.
200. Weinberger, D R, Berman, K F and Zec, R F: Physiologic dysfunction of dorsolateral prefrontal cortex in schizophrenia. I. Regional cerebral blood flow evidence. Arch Gen Psychiatry 43:114–124, 1986.
201. Weiss, S R B, Post, R M, Szele, F, Woodward, R and Nierenberg, J: Chronic carbamazepine inhibits the development of local anesthetic seizures kindled by cocaine and lidocaine. Brain Res 497:72–79, 1989.
202. Winsberg, M E, Sachs, N, Tate, D L, Dunai, M, Strong, C M, Spielman, D M and Ketter, T A: Decreased dorsolateral prefrontal n-acetyl aspartate in bipolar disorder (abstract). Biol Psychiatry 43:23S, 1998.
203. Wu, J C, Gillin, J C, Buchsbaum, M S, Hershey, T, Johnson, J C and Bunney, W E Jr: Effect of sleep deprivation on brain metabolism of depressed patients. Am J Psychiatry 149:538–543, 1992.
204. Yazici, K M, Kapucu, O, Erbas, B, Varoglu, E, Gulec, C and Bekdik, C F: Assessment of changes in regional cerebral blood flow in patients with major depression using the 99mTc-HMPAO single photon emission tomography method. Eur J Nucl Med 19:1038–1043, 1992.
205. Zhang, L X, Xing, G Q, Levine, S, Post, R M and Smith, M A: Maternal deprivation induces neuronal death (abstract). Soci Neurosci Abstracts 23:1113, 1997.
206. Zipursky, R B, Marsh, L, Lim, K O, DeMent, S, Shear, P K, Sullivan, E V, Murphy, G M, Csernansky, J G and Pfefferbaum, A: Volumetric MRI assessment of temporal lobe structures in schizophrenia. Biol Psychiatry 35:501–516, 1994.

10

Aging, Alzheimer's Disease, and Dementia

Clinical and Neurobiological Perspectives

M.-Marsel Mesulam

I. Introduction

Dementia is one of the most common diagnoses made by behavioral neurologists, neuropsychologists, and neuropsychiatrists. One goal of this chapter is to provide a practical approach to the diagnosis and management of dementia. Another is to explore the principles which link the patterns of neuropathology to the neurobehavioral manifestations of the major dementing diseases. The chapter starts with a discussion of aging because age is the single most important risk factor for dementia and also because the neurobiology of aging remains a challenging field where methodological hurdles often interfere with the ability to obtain clear answers to questions which initially appear to be quite straightforward. Subsequent sections review the definition, differential diagnosis, and clinical diversity of dementias. They are followed by a comprehensive description of Alzheimer's disease (AD), the most common form of dementia. Sections VI and VII provide a highly technical analysis of AD neuropathology and its relationship to the neurobehavioral features of the dementia. The tremendous accumulation of information related to AD may occasionally give the impression that this field holds no further secrets. These two sections show that this is not the case and outline a speculative hypothesis according to which a generalized perturbation of neuroplasticity may play a pivotal in the pathogenesis of AD. This detailed analysis of AD is followed by sections which briefly review the clinical features and clinicopathological correlations of non-AD dementias such as lobar atrophies, hereditary tauopathies, Pick's disease, diffuse Lewy body disease, prion diseases, and vascular dementia. The chapter ends with guidelines for patient care and a general overview.

II. Aging and the Human Brain

A major goal of the human brain is to accumulate knowledge over time so that the individual can benefit from experience. This process unfolds within two interrelated anatomical substrates. First, genetically programmed species-specific axonal connections determine which sets of neurons will be responsive to which types of information. The details of this organization have been reviewed in Chapter 1. Second, epigenetic modifications in the synaptic strengths of these connections establish a record of personal experience and enable the gradual accumulation of a knowledge base that is unique for each individual. These acquired patterns of synaptic strengths are not encoded at the level of the genome and cannot be transmitted through mitosis. Cell division in the adult CNS would thus tend to interfere with the accumulation of knowledge during the life span. This biological constraint may provide one of the many reasons why the brain is a largely postmitotic organ where the vast majority of neurons grow to be as old as their owner. As an inevitable outcome of this arrangement, each neuron in the brain becomes exposed to the cumulative effect of biological wear and tear throughout the life span. This chapter reviews the resultant vulnerability of the CNS to aging and the relevance of this vulnerability to the pathophysiology of dementing diseases.

Cognitive Components

The elderly frequently complain of declining cognitive skills, especially in the area of memory. Such complaints are so widespread that they have led to the belief that a gradual loss of intellectual ability is part of "normal" aging. It turns out that this disarmingly simple assumption is extremely difficult to substantiate or refute. Much of this difficulty is based on details of methodology and inference. It is universally accepted, for example, that the average scores obtained by groups of 80–90-year-olds in tasks that emphasize response speed, memory span, visuospatial skills, and mental flexibility are significantly worse than the average scores obtained by groups of 20–30-year-olds. Additional evidence shows that groups of older subjects may also have, on average, a smaller number of neurons, less cortical volume, fewer synapses and receptors, lower metabolic rates, and less blood flow.[84,156,201,218] The problem arises when this information is used to infer the nature, magnitude, and universality of changes within the life span of individual subjects. This challenge is based on at least five sets of factors: the nonlinearity of the relationship between the passage of time and aging, the influence of genetic backgrounds, the existence of a "cohort" effect in cross-sectional studies, the age-dependent increase in the variability of performance, and the "contamination" of older subject groups with individuals who are in the preclinical stages of dementia-causing diseases.

Aging and time overlap only in the simplest of systems. In the process of radioactive decay, for example, the aging of a nucleotide, defined as the loss of its radioactivity, is entirely dependent on the passage of time. In more complex systems, such as the brain, however, aging depends on an interaction among three major variables: *time*, the constitutional or *genetic background* of the vehicle within which time flows, and the cumulative impact of *stochastic encounters with diverse events* such as stress, hypertension, oxidation, head trauma, exposure to xenobiotics, and so on. The maturing of red wine illustrates the complex interrelationships among these variables: The passage of time may improve the quality of wine, but only wines of certain pedigrees age well, and even then only if the aging occurs in an optimal environment. Eventually, the laws of thermodynamics prevail and even the best wines spoil, but the time to maturity and the number of years that can elapse before the onset of deterioration may range from a few to a hundred years, varying greatly from wine to wine as well as from harvest to harvest.

Much of the existing literature on aging overlooks these complex relationships and assumes that the lower memory scores or synaptic densities in groups of older individuals reflect changes that are *intrinsic* to aging, that is to say, are caused by the passage of time. However, such changes could also reflect the impact of particularly common (that is, *endemic*) but theoretically preventable events. Aging may not cause these events but may increase the probability of encountering them. Differentiating the inevitable consequences of time from the cumulative but preventable impact of stochastic phenomena embedded within time is one of the most important goals of current aging research.

Another source of difficulty is based on the "cohort effect," which stems from the widespread use of the cross-sectional methodology. Cross-sectional studies use the deceptively simple strategy of recruiting subjects of different age ranges (cohorts). If the group of older subjects performs less well than the group of younger subjects, an age-related decline is inferred. Such cross-sectional studies may be quite useful for revealing the presence of a generation gap in mental function and may have profound implications for shaping public policy, targeting advertisements, and so on. The problem arises when this methodology is used to infer longitudinal changes within an individual life span. Such inferences are problematic since the octogenarian who is being tested today may have been born and raised in a physical and intellectual environment that promoted the development of different skills. It is therefore unwarranted to conclude that the lower score of the older subject indicates a decline from a previously higher level of performance.

The importance of the cohort effect was demonstrated in a meta-analysis in which several groups (cohorts) of subjects were tested longitudinally at 7-year intervals with the same battery of tasks. This analysis revealed that the differences between two same-age cohorts were at least as strong as the longitudinal test-retest differences in a single cohort.[233,274] These types of observations are consistent with the widely accepted view that cross-sectional studies may seriously exaggerate the impact of aging. In contrast, longitudinal studies may underestimate aging effects because of the selective attrition of the more impaired subjects. Despite this bias, however, many longitudinal studies tend to reveal a progressive decline of cognitive function after the age of 80, leading to the inference that such changes may represent inevitable consequences of longevity.

The alternative possibility that such late-life changes are not necessarily universal has been raised in a number of studies, including one on more than 1000 physicians ranging in age from their 30s to 80s.[271] As expected, the group of physicians above 75 years of age performed significantly worse than the group of physician under 35 years of age in all cognitive tasks. The top and bottom ten performers were then identified in both groups. The top- and bottom-performing subgroups of young physicians did not vary significantly in their scores and were therefore pooled. The situation was quite different among the older physicians. The bottom ten obtained significantly lower scores than the young physicians in all tasks. The top ten elderly physicians, however, displayed performance levels that were identical to those of the young physicians in nearly all areas of cognition that were assessed.

This study leads to two potential conclusions. First, aging appears to be characterized by increased interindividual variability, probably because each individual faces a unique set of "slings and arrows of outrageous fortune" in the course of life. Secondly, there may be a subgroup of individuals who, because of either good fortune or genetic makeup, may manage to age without major changes of mental acuity. The putative importance of genetic contributions to brain aging was demonstrated in a study which found that the concordance of cognitive state in twins at or above the age of 80 was greater in identical pairs than in fraternal pairs of the same gender.[158] These results suggest that the effects of aging upon mental state may be constrained by genetic factors and point to an additional pitfall of cross-sectional studies where genetic factors cannot be controlled.

Another potentially relevant factor is the contamination of "healthy" subject groups. Although many cross-sectional and longitudinal studies on aging have carefully eliminated clinically obvious common diseases, the group of older subjects is still likely to include a larger number of individuals who are in the prodromal stages of various degenerative central nervous system (CNS) diseases. In fact, many of the so-called age-related involutional effects reported by previous studies have been attributed to the inclusion of subjects in the pre-clinical stages of Alzheimer's disease.

This very brief and incomplete review attempts to explain why it has been so difficult to determine whether (or to what extent) aging is, by itself, a cause of cognitive decline. The answer to this question is of considerable importance since it will help to establish whether the preservation of cognitive strength during advanced senescence is a biological possibility. Everyone agrees that the score of an "average" 80 year-old in many tests of cognitive function is likely to be lower than the score of an "average" 20- or 40-year-old. What is not clear is whether this difference reflects a longitudinal decline for that individual and, if so, whether it is based on potentially preventable causes which can be decoupled from the passage of time.

Biological Components

The effects of aging on the structure, chemistry, and physiology of the brain have also attracted a great deal of research. The adult human cerebral neocortex contains approximately 20 billion neurons. Unbiased stereological methods have revealed that specimens from 90 year-old subjects have nearly 10% fewer neurons than ones from 20-year-old subjects.[201] Despite the unavoidable cross-sectional design of this study, the authors concluded that aging is associated with a 10% loss of neocortical neurons in the interval between 20 to 90 years of age, raising the possibility that this change could provide a potential substrate for age-related changes of cognition. However, other stereological studies confined to entorhinal and superior temporal cortex have failed to show any significant age-related neuronal loss in the range from 60 to 90 years.[94,95] It is interesting to note that recent studies in macaque monkeys have also failed to show any age-related loss of neurons.[212] The traditional view that aging is associated with a massive loss of neurons is therefore almost certainly incorrect.

Measures of cortical volume reflect the contributions of neuronal cell bodies and also of neuroglia, fiber pathways, dendritic trees, myelin, and vasculature. One study in 18–77-year-old subjects reported a substantial but regionally selective volumetric decline that became most pronounced in prefrontal cortex, reaching a magnitude of nearly 5% per decade.[218] However, another study based on postmortem neuropathological examination found a 2 mL/year decline in the volume of the white matter but no consistent age-related decline of cortical volume in the interval from the sixth to the ninth decade.[60] Another volumetric study found that only 25% of elderly subjects (68–86 years old) had medial temporal lobe atrophy and that those with atrophy performed less well on tests of memory function,[138] suggesting that the age-related loss of brain volume may be idiosyncratic and that it may reflect the presence of preclinical Alzheimer's disease.

A study which included a longitudinal component in a sample of cognitively normal healthy individuals found that 85–93-year-olds had a smaller brain volume than either 75–84- or 66–73-year-olds, that all three groups showed a mild and regionally selective loss of volume within a 3–8-year follow up period (of 0.01–0.06 cm³/year in the medial temporal lobe), and that the rate of volume loss did not differ from one age group to another.[188] These results suggest that healthy aging may be associated with a relatively small and perhaps regionally selective loss of volume but that the rate of this loss does not accelerate with advancing age.

Hundreds of research papers, some more sophisticated than others, have explored the influence of age upon additional parameters such as synaptic density, receptor binding, transmitter turnover, cortical blood flow, and the functional coherence of neural networks. These additional studies provide valuable data but do not substantially alter the conclusions reached by the stereological and volumetric experiments reviewed earlier. Many of these studies show a decrement in the marker under investigation, others show no decline, and nearly all suffer the limitations of the cohort effect.

Even if age-related decrements in various aspects of brain structure turned out to be the rule, they do not necessarily have to have involutional implications. For example, a set of very interesting animal studies has shown that age-related decrements of synaptic density are accompanied by an increase in the efficacy of the remaining synapses.[14,212] Furthermore, a programmed loss of neurons and synapses is a necessary aspect of early development and could conceivably serve a similar plasticity-related purpose during adulthood. This would not be the only manifestation of plasticity in the adult human brain. Cortical myelination, for example, can continue to increase into the seventh decade of life;[120] the dendritic branching of parahippocampal neurons can become enriched during the same period of life;[32] growth-associated protein 43 (GAP-43), which is a marker of axonal sprouting, continues to be expressed in association and limbic cortices during late adulthood;[17] and a special subset of pyramidal neurons with high levels of acetylcholinesterase show a preservation and perhaps increase of density in advanced senescence.[168] It appears, therefore, that the aging human brain may maintain a considerable potential for structural plasticity. As will be described in section VII, a breakdown of this neuroplasticity may play a key role in the pathogenesis of Alzheimer's disease.

The persistence of plasticity in the CNS of old individuals and its potential role in promoting cognitive stability in the course of aging may initially appear to serve no good biological purpose. In all other species, traits are selected only if they lead to more and fitter offspring. It is therefore difficult to see how it would be possible to select a trait, such as successful aging, which becomes active only after the reproductive age has come to an end. Nonetheless, reasons for promoting cognitively healthy longevity are likely to have arisen in the course of human evolution, specifically in association with the emergence of civilization.[174] Individuals who can live long and also remain intellectually sharp, for example, would stand a better chance of integrating more experiences, synthesizing them with the information derived from the past, and transmitting them to subsequent generations. This process would promote the emergence of superior civilizations which would, in turn, offer their members a greater chance of survival and more successful reproduction. The uniquely human ability to establish civilizations may thus have engendered a driving force for promoting successful aging.[174]

On average, advancing age increases the probability of losing neurons, synapses, transmitters, and cognitive acuity. However, the considerations listed in this section also suggest that successful human aging is a biological possibility, that this possibility makes good evolutionary sense, that the aging human brain displays considerable potential for plasticity, and that much of the so called age-related changes in the literature may reflect the influence of stochastic and theoretically preventable phenomena. Despite this relatively positive outlook, however, it is also necessary to realize that aging, while not a disease by itself, reflects a period of greatly enhanced vulnerability to a whole host of dementing diseases. Some of the most prominent examples of these diseases and their relationship to aging are discussed in this chapter.

III. THE DEFINITION AND DIFFERENTIAL DIAGNOSIS OF DEMENTIA

Although "dementia" is not a very precise term, it has acquired great heuristic value and is now irretrievably lodged in the medical vocabulary. We use the term dementia to designate *a chronic and usually progressive decline of intellect and/or com-*

portment which causes a gradual restriction of customary daily living activities unrelated to changes of alertness, mobility, or sensorium. To qualify for the designation of dementia, the change of mental state should not be secondary to physical discomfort, situational stress, or psychiatric symptoms such as anxiety, depression, and paranoia. Acutely acquired and subsequently static deficits, such as those that result from a single stroke, encephalitis, or head injury, do not usually fit this definition.

The intellectual decline in dementia can affect any cognitive domain, including memory, language, attention, spatial orientation, or thinking. The decline of comportment (conduct) can involve changes in judgment, insight, foresight, reality testing, and social competence. Some definitions of dementia, such as the one advocated by the fourth edition of the *Diagnostic and Statistical Manual of Mental Disorders (DSM-IV)*,[5] require the presence of memory dysfunction. This is not part of our definition since many types of dementia, including frontotemporal dementia and some forms of vascular dementia, are characterized by a relative preservation of memory.

The definition of dementia in *DSM-IV* also requires the presence of abnormalities in multiple areas of mental functioning. We prefer less restrictive criteria and would consider a progressive impairment of a single domain as sufficient, especially since the number of cognitive functions deemed affected can be influenced by the method of evaluation and the theoretical outlook of the clinician. For example, attentional impairments can lead to secondary deficits of memory; and an aphasia can interfere with the ability to comprehend instructions related to all other tasks (Chapter 2). When assessing an inattentive or aphasic patient, the clinician may choose to give equal prominence to all abnormal scores or may identify the primary deficit and seek indirect evidence to infer that the other domains are relatively intact. The former approach might lead to a *DSM-IV* diagnosis of dementia whereas the latter might not.

As in the case of renal failure or anemia, dementia is a syndrome, not a disease. Dementia and dementia-like syndromes can be caused by dozens of pathophysiological processes including infectious agents, inflammatory processes, nutritional deficiencies, neurotoxins, cerebrovascular diseases, autoimmune diseases, neoplasms, space-occupying lesions, storage diseases, and an entire family of primary CNS diseases which cause a gradual destruction of neurons (Table 10–1). A comprehensive review of the relevant entities would require an entire textbook of medicine. This chapter takes a very restrictive approach and covers only a few relatively common dementias caused mostly by primary neuronal diseases in patients who do not display other prominent psychiatric or medical abnormalities. These are the patients who look physically healthy during the clinical encounter, who do not have any major neurological findings other than the dementia, and who have a nonspecific neurodiagnostic workup which may reveal the anatomical distribution of the disease (in the form of atrophy, electroencephalographic [EEG] slowing, or hypometabolism) but not its etiology. The entities that fulfill these criteria include Alzheimer's disease, focal atrophies, Pick's disease, familial tauopathies, prion protein diseases, and diffuse Lewy body disease. A discussion of vascular dementia will

TABLE 10–1. The Differential Diagnosis of the Dementia Syndrome

DISEASE GROUPS THAT CAN PRESENT AS A PURE DEMENTIA

Space-Occupying Lesions
   Neoplasm
   Normal-pressure hydrocephalus
   Subdural hematoma
   Parasitic cysts, brain abscesses

Infectious Organisms
   HIV
   Syphilis
   Herpes simplex
   Lyme disease
   Whipple's disease

Nutritional-Metabolic-Toxic
   Wernicke-Korsakoff disease
   Chronic alcoholism
   B_{12} deficiency
   Pellagra
   Organic solvent exposure
   Heavy metal intoxication
   Hepatic encephalopathy

Immune Inflammatory
   Paraneoplastic limbic encephalitis
   Systemic lupus
   Cerebritis associated with collagen–immune diseases

Vascular Disease
   Multiple infarcts
   Binswanger's disease
   Various arteritides
   CADASIL*

(continued)

be included because of the practical dilemmas associated with the differentiation of this relatively common condition from other dementias. Alzheimer's disease will receive the most extensive coverage because of its high prevalence.

Differential Diagnosis

The diagnosis of dementia can only be made by clinical examination. No radiological, neurophysiological, or other laboratory investigation can eliminate the need to examine the mental state of the patient. Advanced dementia can be diagnosed readily whereas the diagnosis of early dementia taxes the judgment of even the most seasoned clinician (Chapter 2). Especially in highly accomplished individuals, for example, test scores that fall within the age-appropriate range may still represent

TABLE 10–1.—Continued

Storage Diseases
Metachromatic leukodystrophy
Kufs' disease

Prion Diseases
  Creutzfeld-Jacob
  Fatal insomnia

Primary (Degenerative) Neuronal Diseases
  Alzheimer's disease
  Focal atrophies (frontotemporal dementia, primary
    progressive aphasia)
  Pick's disease
  Diffuse Lewy body disease
  Hereditary tauopathies

DISEASES THAT PRESENT WITH SALIENT
SENSORY-MOTOR DEFICITS IN ADDITION TO
THE DEMENTIA

Parkinson's disease
Progressive supranuclear palsy
Cortico-basalganglionic degeneration
Huntington's disease
Wilson's disease
Hallervorden-Spatz disease
Spinocerebellar ataxias
Amyotrophic lateral sclerosis
Multiple sclerosis
Gerstmann-Sträussler-Scheinker disease
Kuru

*CADASIL = cerebral autosomal dominant arteriopathy with subcortical infarcts and leukoencephalopathy.

a major decline from former levels of performance. In such individuals, the first sign of dementia may be an increase in the effort and time needed to carry out customary activities. For example, a university professor with an incipient dementing disease complained that the preparation of lectures took substantially more time. In some cases, the diagnosis cannot be reached in the first visit and the magnitude of change from one test period to another becomes the most important confirmatory evidence.

The diagnosis of dementia becomes supported by the presence of one or more of the following three factors: (*1*) history of a persistent and progressive decline of cognition, comportment, personality, or daily living activities, preferably corroborated by an independent observer; (*2*) scores that fall beyond 2 SD from age- and education-matched ranges in one or more neuropsychological tests or in standardized screening instruments such as the *Mini Mental State Examination (MMSE), Blessed Dementia Scale*, or *Clinical Dementia Rating Scale (CDR);*[159] (*3*) a change of scores in any domain that exceeds 1 SD within a 6–12 month test-retest period, even if the initial scores are within the normal range. Cogent arguments have been made for basing the diagnosis of early dementia on clinical impression or collateral sources of information, either one of which can be more sensitive to mild cognitive changes than standardized neuropsychological tests and batteries.[181] The MMSE is used quite frequently by non-neuropsychologists. A score below 26 (out of 30) is usually considered abnormal but the cutoff scores vary by age, education, and race (Chapter 2). It is important to point out that the MMSE and similar brief cognitive tests are very insensitive and miss many cases of mild dementia.

When a clinical diagnosis of dementia becomes entertained, three realms of possible causes need to be considered: idiopathic psychiatric diseases, toxic–metabolic encephalopathies, and intrinsic CNS diseases. The first two entities are major causes of potentially reversible dementias.

Depression and Dementia

Depression enters the differential diagnosis of dementia in several settings. First, the self-deprecation associated with major depression can lead to complaints of deteriorating cognitive function, especially memory, even when no such deterioration can be documented by objective testing. Secondly, the preoccupation with the mental pain of depression may disrupt the patient's ability to concentrate on the examination and may lead to abnormal scores in tests of cognitive function. Thirdly, the physiological processes associated with depression (perhaps an abnormality in monoamine neurotransmission or cortical metabolism) can directly interfere with mental function, especially in the areas of attention and memory.

The memory impairment of depression is usually characterized by difficulties at the level of registration and depth of encoding. Repeated practice trials tend to overcome the memory deficit whereas similar maneuvers are usually not effective in the memory loss associated with Alzheimer's disease. Depressed patients tend to exaggerate their difficulties, tend to give up quickly, and err on the side of false-negative answers (such as, "I can't remember.") In contrast, patients with Alzheimer's disease tend to minimize deficits and tend to err on the side of false-positive confabulations, especially in the more advanced stages. Aphasic deficits such as paraphasias or misspelling are almost never seen as a result of depression whereas they are frequent in Alzheimer's disease.

In the elderly, the diagnosis of an underlying major depression may be challenging because the expression of dysphoria, hopelessness, and helplessness may be muted and because the traditional vegetative signs may be substituted by nonspecific somatic symptoms such as forgetfulness, pain, constipation, or itching. A personal or family history of depression should increase the index of suspicion. Unfortunately, the expectation that a substantial number of patients with the clinical picture of dementia would turn out to have a primary depression and show cognitive improvement in response to antidepressants has not materialized. Despite the very small number of such patients, however, this possibility needs to be considered in every case of dementia because of the potential for treatment. Whenever in doubt, the clinician would be justified in starting a medication trial, preferably with an antidepressant that has few anticholinergic effects. The following patient provides an example of a dementia-like clinical picture caused by depression.

Case Report

(S. T.)   A 58-year-old designer reported a gradually worsening memory problem over the course of 3 years. He forgot instructions at work and misplaced important files to the point where he was asked to consider early retirement. During the neuropsychological examination, he was able to recall only four of ten words after 10 minutes and recalled 14 of 50 details from a short story after a delay of 10 minutes. These scores were 2 SD below the normative values for his age. The patient was dysphoric during the interview and reported a family history of depression. He was placed on 150 mg of bupropion. Seven months later, he reported that his memory had improved. He recalled six of ten words after 10 minutes (performance within the normal range) and 17 of 50 details of a story (one detail short of the normal range). Retesting after an additional 6 months of antidepressant treatment showed that he recalled all ten words after 10 minutes and 35 of the 50 details in the short story. His initial presentation and testing were consistent with a diagnosis of dementia. Depression turned out to be a major factor, and its treatment was associated with a gradual improvement of cognitive performance over the period of a year.

In contrast to the very small number of patients who develop a dementia-like picture exclusively on the basis of a primary depression, a large number of demented patients also happen to be depressed. These patients are very susceptible to toxic side effects of medications and need to be started on very low doses of antidepressants. Such treatment may improve the mood of such patients but does not reverse their cognitive deficits. Depression may be particularly common in diffuse Lewy body disease. In many patients with frontotemporal dementia or Alzheimer's disease, the neuropathological lesions may lead to an amotivational state known as abulia. This condition may be misinterpreted as depression but does not respond to antidepressants.

Toxic–Metabolic Encephalopathies and Dementia

The efficiency of neuronal function depends on the glucose content, oxygenation level, hormonal state, and electrolyte balance of the extracellular environment. Systemic diseases that interfere with cardiac, renal, hematological, hepatic, endocrine, or pulmonary function can disrupt this balance and can trigger a metabolic encephalopathy. Furthermore, many analgesics, hypnotics, sedatives, antihypertensives, antiarrythmics, antiepileptics, antidepressants and antipsychotics can directly interfere with neuronal function and cause a toxic encephalopathy. Most toxic–

metabolic encephalopathies have an acute onset and do not fit the clinical picture of dementia. Others, however, may have a chronic course and may lead to a clinical picture that has many characteristics of dementia.

The most common clinical state associated with a toxic–metabolic encephalopathy is designated a confusional state (also known as delirium) and is reviewed in Chapter 3. Attention and "executive" functions are almost always the most severely affected cognitive domains. These impairments give rise to secondary deficits in most other realms of cognition and comportment. Patients with preexisting brain disease are exquisitely sensitive to toxic–metabolic encephalopathy. A toxic–metabolic encephalopathy superimposed upon a preexisting dementia can give rise to a severe (usually agitated, hallucinatory and delusional) confusional state which is also known as a "beclouded" dementia.

As noted in Chapter 3, elderly individuals are more vulnerable to toxic–metabolic encephalopathy, perhaps because they have less neural reserve. In the elderly, toxic–metabolic encephalopathies usually reflect the interaction of multiple factors; thus no single laboratory value may be strikingly abnormal. In a young individual with hypoglycemia, an acute confusional state may emerge only after glucose levels drop to 30–40 mg/dL whereas an elderly individual may start to display substantial changes in response to only borderline hypoglycemia. In the young patient, the correction of the abnormality with a bolus of glucose may normalize the mental state within minutes, whereas this may take days to months in the elderly, as if the encephalopathy had caused some damage that needed to be repaired.

Patients in confusional states are unable to give a coherent history and are usually difficult to examine at the bedside. We have seen patients who have been admitted to the hospital with a dementia-like picture, without any specific findings on the physical examination, and who have subsequently been found to have ascending cholangitis, subphrenic abscess, or epidural spinal abscess as the cause of the encephalopathy. The most important step in the diagnosis is a thorough medical and laboratory examination, including a lumbar puncture. An EEG is useful since a background of 8 cps or higher is usually incompatible with a significant toxic–metabolic encephalopathy. In a general hospital, toxic–metabolic encephalopathy constitutes the single most common cause of a reversible dementia-like clinical picture.

CNS Diseases Causing Dementia

After depression and toxic–metabolic encephalopathy have been ruled out in a patient with the clinical picture of dementia, the possibility of structural CNS diseases needs to be entertained. Almost all progressive extrapyramidal diseases, including Parkinson's disease, Huntington's disease, progressive supranuclear palsy, corticobasalganglionic degeneration, Hallervorden-Spatz disease, and Wilson's disease are associated with a dementia. Furthermore, many patients with spinocerebellar ataxia, amyotrophic lateral sclerosis (ALS), and multiple sclerosis (MS) may develop dementia. Many of these dementias present with salient attentional and comportmental impairments reminiscent of a frontal network syndrome (Chapter 1). This clinicopathological correlation reflects the existence of damage in the subcortical components of the frontal network in extrapyramidal diseases, the potential extension of neuropathology from primary motor cortex to adjacent prefrontal areas in ALS, and the existence of demyelinating plaques in the white matter of the frontal lobes in MS. These dementias (some of which are also known as "subcortical" dementias) will not be reviewed here because the diagnosis of the underlying condition and its treatment revolve around the much more salient sensory–motor deficits.

The group of CNS diseases that can lead to an isolated or "pure" dementia include space occupying lesions (neoplasm, subdural hematoma, normal-pressure hydrocephalus, cyst, abscess), diseases caused by infectious organisms (HIV, syphilis, herpes simplex, Lyme disease, Whipple's disease), nutritional–metabolic–toxic diseases (Wernicke-Korsakoff disease, B_{12} deficiency, pellagra, alcohol, organic solvents, heavy metals, hepatic encephalopathy), immune-inflammatory conditions (paraneoplastic limbic encephalitis, systemic lupus erythematosus, cerebritis associated with scleroderma or Hashimoto's thyroiditis), cerebrovascular diseases (multiple strokes, arteritis, Binswanger's disease, and cerebral autosomal dominant arteriopathy with subcortical infarcts and leukoencephalopathy [CADASIL]), storage diseases (metachromatic leukodystrophy, Kufs' disease), prion diseases (Creutzfeldt-Jacob disease, fatal insomnia), and an entire family of primary degenerative neuronal diseases (Alzheimer's disease, focal atrophies, Pick's disease, diffuse Lewy body disease, and hereditary tauopathies) (Table 10–1).

A detailed history and appropriate laboratory tests can lead to the accurate diagnosis of each of the dementia-causing conditions listed in Table 10–1 except for the prionopathies and primary neuronal diseases. The primary neuronal degenerations account for the vast majority of patients with an indolent dementia who outwardly appear healthy, who have no other neurological or medical findings, and whose laboratory tests are essentially negative except for the demonstration of atrophy and neuronal dysfunction. One feature common to these diseases is that definitive diagnosis can only be made after death by a postmortem examination of the brain.

The Workup

The workup begins with a detailed history and physical examination. The mental state assessment and brief screening tests such as the *MMSE* help to confirm the initial impression of dementia. Formal neuropsychological evaluation becomes important for quantitating and characterizing the dementia, for determining change over time, and especially for detecting early and questionable cases. Every patient should have serological tests for syphilis, B_{12} and folate levels, sedimentation rate, and thyroid function tests. A computed tomography (CT), or preferably magnetic resonance imaging (MRI), should be obtained to look for intracerebral lesions. Depending on the specific details of individual patients, the investigation may include chest X-ray, EEG, lumbar puncture, single photon emission computed tomography (SPECT), position emission tomography (PET), electromyogram (EMG), electrocardiogram (EKG), complete blood count, liver function tests, HIV tests, electrolytes, antiphospholipid, antinuclear or paraneoplastic antibodies, heavy metal levels, and other specialized tests dictated by the diagnostic possibilities that are raised. The workup can become particularly intense in patients suspected of having toxic-metabolic encephalopathies of unknown cause.

IV. SOME CLINICAL PROFILES OF BEHAVIORALLY FOCAL PRIMARY DEMENTIAS

Dementias are clinically and neuropathologically very heterogeneous. Any cognitive or comportmental domain can be affected, either in isolation or as part of a distinctive cluster. However, each dementia-causing primary degenerative disease listed in Table 10–1 is also characterized by a preferred (though not invariable) anatomical predilection pattern and a corresponding profile of clinical manifestations. The conceptualization of dementia as a "global" dysfunction arising from "diffuse" disease is therefore quite inaccurate.

Since there are no specific laboratory tests for identifying the etiology of a primary degenerative dementia and since the clinical symptoms are presently the only diagnostic indicators, we have attempted to define several clinical profiles, each of which has a different probability of being associated with specific disease entities. Each of the four clinical profiles we identified is characterized by one cognitive deficit which is distinctly more salient than the others during at least the first 2 years after symptom onset.[269] A classification based on the first 2 years emphasizes the period during which the anatomical predilection patterns are most conspicuous. These four profiles do not accommodate all possible dementia cases. Some patients will not fit any of these profiles, either because the pattern of deficits is different or because the 2-year rule cannot be satisfied. In cases where the patient is seen before the end of the initial 2-year period, a provisional classification can be made with the understanding that confirmation will require further stability of the behavioral profile. Despite these limitations, the identification of the behavioral profiles described in this section may be of practical value not only for differential diagnosis but also for helping to educate the patient and family about the nature of the impairment and for generating specific (rather than generic) recommendations concerning remedial interventions.

Progressive Comportmental/Executive Dysfunction (PC/ED) (Progressive Frontal Network Syndrome)

Patients are included in this group when the insidious onset and gradual progression of abnormalities in comportment, attention, motivation, and other executive functions constitute the only significant areas of primary impairment for at least 2 years after disease onset. The interpretation of the neuropsychological testing can be quite challenging because the attentional and motivational deficits may induce secondary impairments in other cognitive domains. The deficits in comportment include social inappropriateness, excessive docility or irritability, disinhibited behaviors, impaired judgment and foresight, diminished concern about failing competence, carelessness with respect to social and personal responsibilities, and a loss of empathy. Socially inappropriate, puerile, reckless behaviors may dominate the clinical picture. The relative sparing of language, visuospatial skills, and especially memory is a central feature of this syndrome.

On occasion, the diagnosis may need to rely on informant-based data since the patient tends to deny shortcomings and since many neuropsychological tests of cognitive function may detect no abnormality at a time when comportment may be dramatically abnormal. Alterations of dietary habits, usually increased food intake, can be quite pronounced. Patients with this profile of dementia may be divided into two groups: those with prominent apathy, and those with prominent disinhibited behaviors. The absence of major sensory–motor deficits, aphasia, or amnesia occasionally leads to psychiatric diagnoses where the apathy may be misdiagnosed as depression and the disinhibition as mania. The following is an example of a patient with the this profile of dementia:

Case Report

(Z. T.)   At the age of 58, a right-handed electronics technician became less willing to follow instructions at work and to perform her usual household chores. She spent money frivolously and, when in company, would tend to expose more of her body than her customary modesty had previously allowed. On one occasion, she neglected to pick up her grandson from school and later appeared unperturbed by the mishap. These changes became increasingly more accentuated during the subsequent 2 years and she started to show difficulties in handling money and shopping. Her problems had initially been attributed to depression. A neurological examination showed abulia mixed with restlessness, inability to maintain a coherent stream of thought, poor insight, impaired concentration span, and defective mental flexibility. Memory, language, and visuospatial skills were preserved. Sensory–motor function, CT scans, and EEGs were unremarkable. Within 4 years after onset, she progressed to the point where the only task she could accomplish was to write her name. She had assumed a stooped posture and would giggle continuously. She died during the fifth year of her disease. The brain weighed 1010 g and showed a remarkably focal atrophy of the prefrontal cortex bilaterally (Fig. 10–1a). The microscopic examination showed a severe loss of neurons and gliosis in prefrontal cortex with some spongioform changes in the superficial layers. There were no neurofibrillary tangles, neuritic plaques, Lewy bodies, or Pick bodies. Her mother had died of a similar presenile dementia with prominent behavioral abnormalities but no autopsy had been performed.

This clinical profile is identical to the "frontal network syndrome" described in Chapter 1. When it arises in the context of a degenerative neuronal disease, symp-

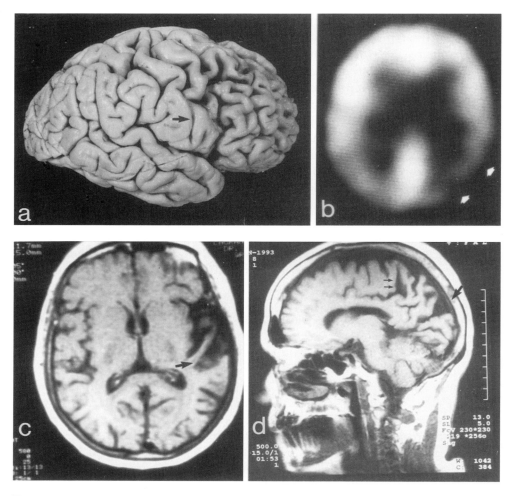

FIGURE 10–1. a. Autopsy specimen from Z. T. who died at 63 years of age after a 5-year history of a dementia with the clinical profile of progressive comportmental/executive dysfunction (PC/ED). The arrow points to the central sulcus. The cortex behind the central sulcus (including the parietal, occipital, and temporal lobes) and the precentral gyrus look relatively well preserved. The gyri of prefrontal cortex give a vermicular appearance indicative of severe and anatomically very restricted atrophy. b. Two-deoxyglucose positron emission tomography (PET) scan of patient N. F. 5 years after onset of primary progressive aphasia (PPA). The arrows point to a left hemisphere perisylvian region of hypometabolism.[41] The contralateral right hemisphere had normal metabolism. c. Horizontal magnetic resonance (MR) scan of a 63-year-old right-handed former secretary with a 3-year history of PPA. The arrow points to Heschl's gyrus, which is the only recognizable structure of the perisylvian temporal neocortex of the left hemisphere. In contrast to the severe atrophy of the lateral temporal lobe of the left, the prefrontal, parital, and occipital cortices of the left hemisphere and the entire right hemisphere look relatively well preserved. d. Parasagittal MR scan of a 65-year-old right-handed woman with a 2-year history of dementia with the clinical profile of progressive visuosputial dysfunction (PVD), characterized by a prominent simultanagnosia. The two parallel arrows point to the cingulate sulcus and the larger single arrow points to the gaping parito-occipital sulcus. The frontal cortex anterior to (to the left of) the cingulate sulcus is relatively intact. The dorsal parieto-occipital areas, including the precuneus, which is located between the cingulate and parito-occipital sulci, are selectively atrophied.

tom onset is usually before the age of 65. This syndrome is also known as frontal lobe dementia (FLD), dementia of the frontal type (DFT), and frontotemporal dementia (FTD). The majority of patients do not show a pattern of either autosomal dominant or recessive inheritance, but their first-degree relatives may have an increased prevalence of relatively early onset dementia.[247] In a minority of patients, the disease can be caused by an autosomal dominant tauopathy, in which case it tends to be associated with additional motor symptoms.[207]

Neuroimaging studies frequently show atrophy, hypoperfusion, and decreased metabolism of the frontal lobes. On occasion, there may also be hypometabolism in the posterior parietal cortex, probably reflecting the phenomenon of diaschisis. These neurodiagnostic findings may be quite subtle until the clinical condition becomes very severe. The literature and our own experience show that approximately 75%–80% of patients with this clinical profile have an underlying nonspecific lobar atrophy, also known as dementia without distinctive histopathology, whereas the other 20%–25% have Pick's disease.[30,270] The few patients who have the autosomal dominant form of this syndrome show neuronal and glial tauopathy in the brain.[207] Some patients with diffuse Lewy body dementia may also show a dementia that fits this clinical profile. We have not seen this clinical pattern in association with the neuropathology of AD.

Primary Progressive Aphasia (PPA) (Progressive Language Network Syndrome)

Primary progressive aphasia (PPA) is characterized by the gradual and relatively isolated dissolution of language function.[173,175,272] A diagnosis of PPA is made when other mental faculties such as memory, visuospatial skills, reasoning, and comportment are relatively free of primary deficits and when the language impairment is the only factor that compromises daily living activities for at least the first 2 years of the disease.[172] Although the language disorder in PPA may interfere with the ability to memorize word lists or to solve verbal reasoning tasks, the patient characteristically has no difficulty recalling daily events or behaving with sound judgment, indicating that declarative/episodic memory and executive functions remain intact. Primary deficits in other cognitive domains may emerge after the first 2 years of the disease but many patients show no impairment other than the aphasia for as many as 5 to 10 years. The only nonaphasic primary impairments that are part of the PPA syndrome include acalculia and ideomotor apraxia, deficits that are usually associated with damage to the language network of the brain.

There is no single pattern of language disorder that is pathognomonic of primary progressive aphasia.[257,272,273] Fluent and nonfluent aphasias, comprehension abilities ranging from very poor to intact, and isolated deficits such as pure word deafness have been described.[173,200] The aphasias may not necessarily fit the syndromes identified on the basis of focal strokes. In contrast to the aphasias of AD, which are almost always of the fluent type, the aphasias in PPA are frequently nonfluent.[216] The term "semantic dementia" has been used to designate PPA patients with fluent aphasias and impaired comprehension.[244] The remarkable clinical specificity of PPA is demonstrated by longitudinal studies which show that tasks related to language display a much greater proportional decline than those related to memory, visuospatial skills, and executive functions (Fig. 10–2). When PPA also compromises language comprehension, other cognitive domains become exceedingly difficult to assess. The disease tends to be indolent and may last for 15–20 years. Onset is usually before the age of 65 and there may be a slight predominance of males over females.[172] The following patient illustrates the clinical picture of this syndrome.

Case Report

(N. F.)   A 47-year-old executive noticed difficulties in finding words while speaking in public. These were initially attributed to stress. However, the symptoms increased in intensity and new difficulties emerged in reading and writing. He was seen 5 years later, at which time he reported problems in composing letters. During the examination, he displayed minor errors of syntax and a few phonemic paraphasias. All other domains of cognition and daily professional and social activities were intact. A 2-deoxyglucose PET scan showed left parietotemporal hypometabolism in the absence of any abnormality in the right hemisphere (Fig. 10–1b). During the subsequent 5 years his language difficulty progressed from an anomic aphasia to a nonfluent aphasia with dissolution of articulation, fluency, syntax, and grammar. Comprehension and other cognitive and comportmental domains remained unchanged. Twenty years after onset he had advanced to the stage of a global aphasia where he could only comprehend commands directed to axial musculature and where other domains of cognition were not testable. Even at that stage however, family members related anecdotal evidence showing that his memory for events and locations had remained intact.

More than 100 patients with PPA have now been reported in the literature and many hundreds of additional patients with this diagnosis are being followed at clinical centers with an interest in dementia and behavioral neurology. Many of these patients show relatively subtle neurological signs on the right side of the body and also asymmetrical EEG slowing, gyral atrophy, and hypometabolism in the frontal, temporal and perisylvian regions of the left hemisphere.[172] These neurodiagnostic abnormalities progress in parallel with the clinical deterioration. In several PPA patients with marked left hemisphere hypometabolism, the metabolic state of the contralateral right hemisphere remains within the normal range.[41,263] The clinical focality of PPA is thus matched by the anatomical selectivity of the underlying pathological process for the frontotemporoperisylvian components of the language network in the left hemisphere (Figs. 10–1b, 10–1c, and 10–2).

Although postmortem examinations tend to occur at the end stage of the disease, at a time when the behavioral focality may no longer be conspicuous, the reported neuropathological changes have tended to be more pronounced in frontal, perisyl-

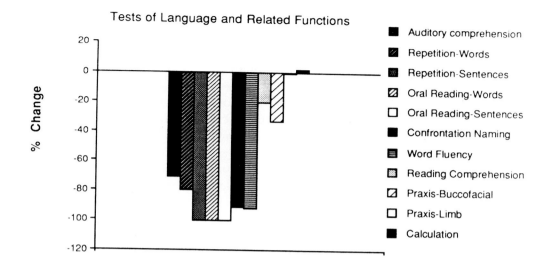

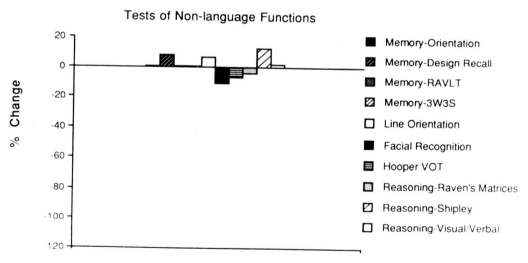

FIGURE 10–2. Performance in various neuropsychological tests in a right-handed woman who started to develop a nonfluent primary progressive aphasia (PPA) at the age of 40. The size of the bars indicates change in a 3-year interval from 6 to 9 years after onset. There is substantial deterioration of almost all language tasks in contrast to a relative preservation of all nonlanguage tasks.[272] Postmortem examination revealed Pick's disease.

vian, and temporal cortex than in the hippocampus, and usually more severe in the left hemisphere.[103,262] In one patient, the disease was centered in the thalamus.[42] At least 33 patients with the clinical syndrome of PPA have yielded information related to the underlying microscopic pathology.[42,103,172,262] Not more than approximately 20% of these cases have shown the pathology of AD and this frequency may be even lower among patients with the nonfluent type of PPA.[172,216,262] The distinction from AD is further shown by the fact that patients with PPA have different patterns of apolipoprotein E allele frequencies.[170]

The single most common pathological process associated with PPA is a focal degeneration characterized by a nonspecific neuronal loss with gliosis and mild spongioform changes within superficial cortical layers. This pattern is encountered in approximately 60% of patients with PPA. Pick's disease with Pick bodies occurs in an additional 20% of patients with PPA. Some patients with hereditary tauopathy and neuronal τ inclusions may develop a clinical syndrome similar to PPA, but usually with additional cognitive and motor deficits.[141] Indolent forms of Creutzfeldt-Jacob disease may present with a progressive aphasia which may remain quite isolated for as long as 12 months.[87]

Progressive Visuospatial Dysfunction (PVD)

The insidious onset and relentless progression of prominent deficits in visuospatial processing (as manifested by components of Bálint's syndrome, spatial disorientation, dressing apraxia, hemispatial neglect) characterizes this group of patients. According to the criteria that we have proposed, amnesia must be absent for at least the first 2 years but other cognitive deficits of lesser severity in language and executive functions may be present, reflecting the close functional relationship between the regions of parietal cortex involved in spatial orientation and those involved in language and executive functions.[270] Some patients display a combination of Bálint's syndrome with Gerstmann's syndrome, reflecting the biparietal distribution of the disease. A failure to locate objects that are in full view, spatial disorientation, and dressing and reading difficulties are some of the initial symptoms that interfere with daily living activities. A poorly defined "visual blurring" may be the initial complaint but ophthalmological investigations and multiple prescriptions for corrective lenses prove ineffective. The following patient illustrates some features of this clinical profile.

Case Report

(B. L.)   A right-handed 61-year-old prominent scholar started to experience problems with penmanship. He could not master the use of new household appliances and had difficulty staying in the lane while driving. These symptoms progressed and he subsequently found it exceedingly difficult to follow the lines of text while reading. He nonetheless continued to teach seminars and dictate papers which were well received internationally. There were initially no abnormalities of language, comportment, or memory. The examination, 6 years after onset, revealed a mild left facial paresis, decreased concentration span, inability to inhibit responses in no-go tasks, left spatial neglect, and a combination of Bálint's syndrome and Gerstmann's syndrome (Fig. 10–3). When he was last examined, 9 years after onset, all symptoms had continued to worsen and he was unable to find objects or get dressed. However, he continued to lecture and produce papers based on original thinking. The MR scan did not reveal definite abnormalities but a 2-deoxyglucose PET scan showed biparietal hypometabolism, more pronounced in the right hemisphere.

In keeping with the deficits of visuospatial processing, neuroimaging in these patients shows focal atrophy or hypometabolism in parieto-occipital cortex along the dorsal visuofugal processing pathways (Fig. 10–2d).[46] The handful of cases that have come to autopsy have shown the neuropathology of nonspecific focal degen-

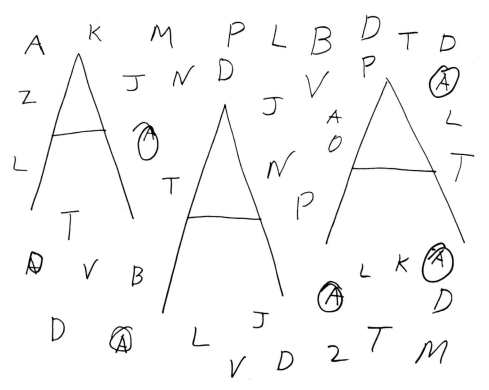

FIGURE 10–3. Patient B. L., who had a dementia with the clinical profile of progressive visuospatial dysfunction (PVD) was asked to circle "all the A's." He does well with the small ones but misses the larger ones. The information needed to identify the small A's can be acquired by single foveations whereas the identification of the larger A's necessitates the integration of visual information across multiple fixations and the filtering out of distracting information. These latter two aspects of visual processing are severely impaired in patients with the simultanagnosia of Bálint's syndrome.

eration, AD (with an unusual concentration of neurofibrillary tangles in the superior colliculus and parietal neocortex), adult-onset glycogen storage disease (in one of our unpublished cases), and indolent forms of Creutzfeldt-Jacob disease.[39,110,225,269] More rarely, some patients will develop a relatively isolated impairment of visual recognition as manifested by prosopagnosia, object agnosia, and alexia. Such patients tend to show a selective hypometabolism of occipitotemporal cortex along the ventral visuofugal processing pathways.[264]

Progressive Amnestic Dysfunction (PAD)

A progressive amnesia which eventually interferes with daily living activities is the defining feature of this clinical profile. In order to fit this diagnostic category, the amnesia must not be secondary to attentional, affective, motivational, linguistic, or visuospatial disturbances. The amnesia can remain isolated or it can be accompanied, even within the first 2 years, by other cognitive deficits. The latter pattern fulfills the criteria for the diagnosis of probable Alzheimer's disease (PRAD) or dementia of the Alzheimer type (DAT), which will be described in the following section. The quintessential feature of this profile is the presence of a primary deficit in declarative memory, as shown in the case of the following patient.

Case Report

(T. P.)   A 68-year-old salesman reported a 2-year history of progressive memory difficulties, especially for remembering names and places. He resented being bested by a younger colleague at work and the symptoms were initially attributed to stress, especially since they did not interfere with his professional and recreational activities. Examination revealed an isolated and mild memory impairment. During the subsequent 2 years, he displayed a detachment from customary social and recreational interests and experienced a pronounced worsening of memory to the point where he was unaware of the date or current news. He also started to show spelling errors although there was no aphasia during spontaneous speech. His clinical course was exacerbated by lung cancer and he died 4 years after the onset of the symptoms. The neuropathological examination revealed findings of AD with a characteristic limbic concentration of neurofibrillary tangles.

This is the single most common clinical profile of dementia and accounts for at least 80% of all late-onset dementias. Onset is usually after the age of 65 and there is a slight preponderance of females over males. Hippocampal and parahippocampal atrophy are the most prominent initial findings in neuroimaging.[43,54] The vast majority of cases show the pathology of AD which, as will be shown below, has a preferential affinity for the hippocampo-entorhinal components of the limbic system. In a smaller number of cases, the neuropathology can be one of focal nonspecific degeneration, Pick's disease, or diffuse Lewy body dementia with a concentration of lesions within the limbic system.[63,130,258]

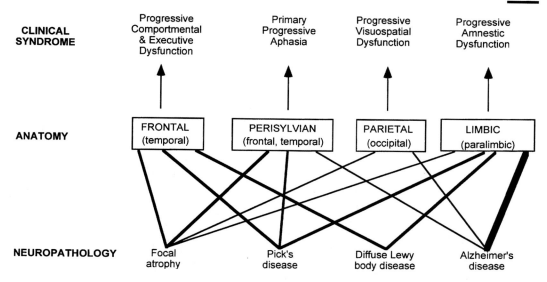

FIGURE 10–4. Relationships among neuropathological entities, anatomical distribution of the most prominent lesions, and the clinical syndrome. The thickness of the lines is proportional to the strength of the relationship. Anatomical areas at the core of a syndrome are capitalized, whereas areas of lesser but common additional involvement are placed in parentheses.

The Clinicopathological Correlations of Clinically Focal Dementias

The first three clinical profiles, PC/ED, PPA, PVD, are dementias in the sense that they involve a gradual dissolution of cognition and comportment. They are also unusual dementias because they are based on the relatively isolated impairment of a single domain and the relative preservation of memory. The four profiles outlined in this section show that the clinical picture of a dementing disease reflects the anatomical distribution of the lesions rather than the nature of the disease (Fig. 10–4). The same neuropathological entity may have several clinical manifestations, each reflecting a different anatomical distribution of the lesions. In turn, the same clinical profile may be caused by different diseases sharing similar patterns of anatomical distribution. However, each neuropathological entity also has preferred patterns of distribution, so the identification of the clinical profile helps to improve the accuracy with which the underlying pathology can be predicted. The likelihood of AD, for example, is very low in patients with PC/ED or the nonfluent forms of PPA, whereas it is very high in a patient with the clinical profile of PAD.

V. ALZHEIMER'S DISEASE—GENETICS, CLINICAL PICTURE, AND DIAGNOSIS

In 1901 Alois Alzheimer, then in Frankfurt, examined a 51-year-old demented woman, Auguste D. Several years later, following Alzheimer's move to Munich, the patient died and was autopsied. In the course of the microscopic examination,

Alzheimer detected two types of pathological lesions which are now known as neurofibrillary tangles (NFT) and senile amyloid plaques. These findings were reported in 1906 at a meeting in Tübingen and published in 1907. By 1908, Kraepelin had started to refer to this condition as Alzheimer's disease (*morbus Alzheimer*) in the eighth edition of his monumental textbook on psychiatry.[4,111,133] Nearly 100 years later, dementia, NFT, and amyloid plaques continue to provide the core diagnostic triad for AD (Fig. 10–5).

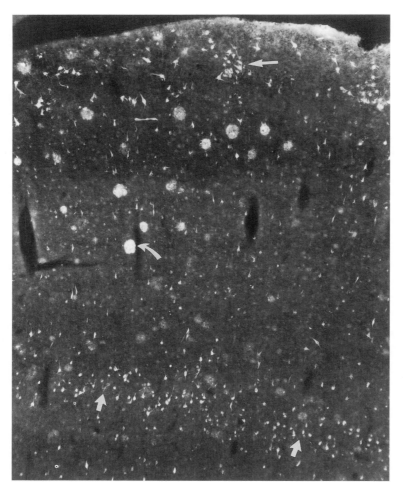

FIGURE 10–5. Entorhinal cortex in a 78-year-old man who died with severe dementia. The bright objects are the sites of thioflavin S histofluorescence. Positive staining occurs in plaques where the amyloid has a β-pleated or compact structure and in neurons that contain neurofibrillary tangles (NFT). The curved arrow points to a characteristic plaque. Under higher magnification, most of these plaques turn out to be neuritic. The horizontal arrow on top points to a layer II island of cells most of which contain NFTs. The two arrows in the bottom point to NFT in layer V. Magnification 40×.

As recently as the early 1970s, AD was considered rare, mostly because it was used to designate only "presenile" cases with onset before the age of 65 years. The subsequent acceptance that the same neuropathology was also associated with late-life dementias led to the realization that AD is one of the most common diseases of the human brain.[121,255] There is no evidence for a recent increase in the incidence of AD. This disease was probably just as widespread in Alzheimer's time as it is now, but its symptoms in old age were being attributed to aging, hardening of the arteries, or senility. Despite the nearly 100 years that have elapsed since its identification, AD continues to pose formidable challenges: Its ultimate cause remains unknown; no single theory of pathogenesis can account for all of its major features; it is not entirely clear if it represents a traditional "disease" or an exaggeration of physiological aging; there are no tests for its definitive diagnosis while the patient is alive; and there are no proven means for preventing or curing it. Perhaps because of these challenges, AD has also become one of the most intensely investigated diseases in the clinical neurosciences. Thus, while AD was included as a keyword for only 36 papers published in 1975–1977, this number increased to 1269 in 1995–1997.

Genetics, Prevalence, Incidence, Risk Factors

In approximately 5% of all patients with AD, the disease is transmitted in an autosomal dominant fashion as a result of mutations in chromosomes 21, 14, and 1. The chromosome 14 mutations are the most common. The known mutations do not account for all families with dominantly inherited disease, so new mutations are likely to be discovered. The dementia in patients with autosomal dominant disease may emerge as early as in the 30s and 40s. The chromosome 21 mutations occur within the gene that encodes the amyloid precursor protein (AβPP) whereas the chromosome 14 and 1 mutations are located in the genes that encode two closely related proteins known as presenilin 1 (PS1) and presenilin 2 (PS2).

The AβPP as well as the presenilins are transmembrane proteins of unknown function although there are indications that they may be involved in neuronal plasticity.[104,250] All three types of mutations promote the production of a longer form of Aβ amyloid which is known to be more insoluble and probably more neurotoxic, at least in vitro. Another association with chromosome 21 occurs in the population of patients with Down's syndrome (trisomy 21). These patients have three copies of the gene for AβPP. They overproduce AβPP and almost invariably develop all the neuropathological manifestations of AD by the time they are 30–40 years old.[104,143]

In over 95% of patients, AD does not show an autosomal dominant transmission. Some patients with this nondominant form of the disease come from families where the prevalence of AD is higher than that of the general population, and these patients are said to have a nondominant but familial form of AD. Other patients in this group come from families where the prevalence of AD is similar to that of the general population. These patients are said to have a sporadic form of AD. This is the type of AD that starts late in life, usually after the age of 65. Although no causative mutations are associated with this type of AD, several risk factors have been identified.

Some (but not all) epidemiological studies show that stroke and head injury may increase the vulnerability to AD and that the disease is more common among women than men. Another very important risk factor is family history. The presence of AD in a first-degree relative increases total lifetime risk from 23% to 48%.[143] The single most important risk factor is age. Prevalence doubles every 5 years after 65. It is over 10% among those above 65 and over 40% among those older than 85.[66] However, the increase of prevalence appears to slow down over the age of 80 and shows no further increase beyond the age of 95,[219] suggesting that the passage of time is only one of several relevant risk factors.

Additional risk factors have been linked to chromosomes 19 and 12.[210,224] Thus, the e4 allele of apolipoprotein E (ApoE), a cholesterol-transporting enzyme encoded by a gene on chromosome 19, has emerged as a major risk factor. ApoE exists in the e2, e3, and e4 allelic forms. The e4 allele frequency is 20% in the general population and 40% in AD. Individuals with even a single e4 allele may have a threefold increase in the risk of developing AD.[224] There is considerable specificity to this relationship, so the e4 frequency is increased in AD but not in PPA or in the nonspecific lobar degenerations of the frontotemporal type.[83,170] The e4 allele appears to increase the risk of developing the sporadic form of AD by decreasing the age at which the dementia becomes clinically detectable.[224] It is important to realize, however, that the e4 allele is a risk factor, not a cause, of AD. Thus e4 homozygotes may live to a ripe old age without AD, while some individuals with no e4 alleles may develop severe AD. In fact, Alzheimer's first patient, Auguste D., had an e3/e3 genotype.[96] All of the genetic backgrounds listed above lead to clinical and pathological features that are nearly identical, indicating that AD represents the common phenotypic expression of diverse genotypes.

Clinical Picture of AD

Age of onset varies greatly. One of our patients developed AD in his 20s. However, the vast majority of patients become symptomatic after the age of 65. The disease usually displays a very indolent course and the interval from diagnosis to death may be as long as 15–20 years. The clinical presentation of AD is usually consistent with the profile of progressive amnestic dementia described in the previous section. The memory loss tends to constitute the most salient component of the clinical picture throughout the course of the disease.

The *initial stages* of AD are characterized by the various manifestations of memory impairment.[184,216] The patient repeats her- or himself, forgets names, and misplaces personal objects. The memory impairment selectively affects the declarative recall of recent events and experiences. In comparison, remote events related to childhood and recent events with high emotional impact can be recalled relatively well. Initially, the major difficulty is confined to voluntary recall. Clues and multiple choices usually help the retrieval and recognition of the pertinent information. Although forgetfulness may initially be the only deficit that interferes with daily living activities, the neuropsychological examination reveals additional but lesser deficits in complex attention, naming, reasoning, and visuospatial skills. The presence of such additional deficits is necessary in order to fulfill the currently accepted criteria for the clinical diagnosis of AD.

Initially, the deficits may fluctuate in intensity and the patient may appear healthy, vigorous, and in full control of social graces. Self-awareness of the impairments may elicit a reactive depression. A certain sense of detachment from professional, social, and recreational activities may be a characteristic component of the early phase. Driven, meticulous, intense individuals become lax and complacent, occasionally to the short-lived delight of a spouse who interprets this change as an improvement in personality. The patient also appears less interested in appetitive behaviors related to eating, drinking, and libido. In fact, weight gain and increased sexual activity are almost never seen in AD and should raise the possibility of an alternative diagnosis. The initial stages of AD are compatible with considerable independence: the patient can keep house, drive, play bridge or golf, participate in nearly all forms of social activity, pay bills, and even conduct complex professional activities, especially if protected by an understanding professional staff in the office. In the course of these functions, however, the patient appears more superficial, less decisive, ineffective, and in need of increasingly more assistance.

In the *intermediate stage* of the disease, deficits in other domains such as language, reasoning, spatial orientation, and executive functions become fully established and erect additional obstacles to the conduct of daily living activities. The forgetfulness continues to increase in severity and starts to interfere with recognition memory, eventually reaching a stage where the patient cannot store any new information for more than a few minutes. Attentional deficits interfere with the ability to maintain a coherent stream of thought and to sequence goal-directed activities. Language deficits (aphasia) emerge in the form of word-finding and spelling deficits and interfere with the ability to communicate. The aphasias of AD are almost always fluent; nonfluent aphasias are extremely rare and should raise the possibility of an alternate diagnosis.[216] Judgment and insight falter to the point where the patient loses awareness of the impairments and becomes indifferent if not jocular. Independence in cooking, housekeeping, paying bills, and driving is gradually lost. This intermediate stage usually includes a disruption of the sleep–wake cycle; a worsening of cognitive and behavioral symptoms toward the end of the day (sundowning); an erosion of decorum and hygiene; and the emergence of psychiatric symptomatology including delusions (mostly of spousal infidelity and of misplaced objects being stolen), hallucinations, agitation, rituals, belligerence, and hoarding behaviors. An increasingly more intense dependency on the healthy spouse (or other significant person) is quite typical at this stage of the disease.

The *final stage* of the disease is characterized by incontinence, inability to recognize family members, and difficulties with mobility and feeding. Hardly any cognitive, comportmental, or psychiatric function escapes the ravages of end-stage

AD. Primary sensory and motor functions may remain relatively intact until late in the course of the disease but extrapyramidal deficits such as myoclonus, rigidity, cogwheeling, hypomimia, and gait instability become increasingly more frequent. Death is usually caused by cardiopulmonary arrest or complications of infection.

In addition to this "usual" form, other less typical clinical patterns have also been reported in patients with neuropathologically confirmed AD. In early onset forms of the disease associated with chromosome 14 mutations, for example, motor deficits and personality changes may emerge early.[143] In other patients, sensory deficits in the olfactory, visual, and auditory modalities may appear in the initial stages of the disease.[78,196,228] In a very small number of patients the typical neuropathology of AD may be associated with progressive hemispatial neglect, progressive aphasia, and even myoclonic epilepsy.[47,97,164] Rarely, AD leads to an isolated memory disorder that may progress insidiously for up to two decades without any other cognitive deficits of significant magnitude.[59] These unusual clinical patterns may represent equally unusual anatomical distributions of the AD neuropathology. Alternatively, the diagnosis of AD may have been unwarranted in some of these patients and may have reflected the coincidental occurrence of age-related plaques and tangles in patients whose basic symptomatologies might have been caused by another disease process undetected by the conventional microscopic examination.

Clinical and Laboratory Diagnosis of AD

The only unequivocal diagnosis of AD can be reached by a postmortem examination of the brain. There are currently no laboratory tests for the definitive diagnosis of AD in a living patient. However, a provisional clinical diagnosis can be made if the patient fulfills the criteria for dementia, if the profile of the dementia fits the "usual" pattern of AD described above, and if other identifiable causes of dementia have been ruled out. This clinical diagnosis is codified as PRAD (probable Alzheimer's disease) according to the nomenclature of the National Institutes of Neurological and Communicative Disorders and Stroke and the Alzheimer's Disease and Related Disorders Association (NINCDS–ADRDA) and as DAT (dementia of the Alzheimer's type) according to the nomenclature of the American Psychiatric Association (APA).[5,162] *In essence, PRAD (or DAT) is used to designate a clinical state where progressive impairments of memory and at least one other cognitive domain induce a chronic decline from previous levels of social, professional, and domestic functioning in the absence of other identifiable causes for dementia.* The diagnostic assessment of cognitive functions and daily living activities can be accomplished through the use of numerous standardized tests (Chapter 2). The Consortium to Establish a Registry for AD (CERAD) has bundled some of these tests into a battery designed for the clinical diagnosis of PRAD.[183]

Although these criteria have had an extremely positive influence in standardizing diagnostic practices throughout the world, they have also introduced some ambiguities. The minimal time that must elapse before the condition is determined to be "progressive" has not been specified and the possibility that an impairment in one domain (such as attention, motivation, or language) can interfere with the function of another (such as memory) has not been considered. Most importantly, the recommended deductive process gives the false impression that AD is the only primary degenerative dementia. In fact, the criteria for PRAD are as suitable for AD as they are for Pick's disease and some forms of focal atrophies. A practical problem associated with the PRAD designation is the need to explain to the patient, caregivers, and referring physician that the diagnosis does not have the *weak* connotation that "the patient probably has Alzheimer's disease," but, rather, the *strong* meaning that "the clinical features are typical of Alzheimer's disease." With respect to wording, the diagnosis of DAT creates fewer such difficulties.

If a patient with dementia fails to fulfill the criteria for PRAD because memory is relatively preserved in the initial stages, because there is an isolated memory deficit without the involvement of other domains, because the clinical course displays transient improvements, or because there are other identifiable diseases that might contribute to the emergence of the dementia, the diagnostic designation becomes more consistent with POAD (possible Alzheimer's disease), indicating that the certainty with which the dementia can be attributed to AD is diminished. The POAD diagnosis is consistent with the PPA, PVD, and PC/ED profiles described in the previous section of this chapter. Several scales have been developed for staging the severity of AD. The *Clinical Dementia Rating (CDR)* scale, based on collateral information and subjective clinical assessment, is quite effective for staging mild to moderate impairments whereas the *Functional Assessment Staging (FAST)* or *Global Deterioration Scale (GDS)* is more appropriate for staging severe impairments.[23,159]

In specialty clinics, the concordance between the diagnosis of PRAD and the postmortem confirmation of AD is close to 90% and often much higher.[216,217,251] This success rate may have more to do with the extremely high prevalence of AD than the virtues of the diagnostic criteria or the acumen of the clinician. Although the concordance between PRAD and AD is excellent in large *groups* of patients, one can never be completely sure that an *individual* patient has AD until the postmortem examination has been concluded. Even in research centers, approximately 10% of the patients with the clinical diagnosis of PRAD turn out to have a disease other than AD.

The wish to eliminate this inherent uncertainty has fueled the search for biological markers which can definitively diagnose AD in the living patient. Ideally, a test based on such markers might also allow the identification of patients at the very early stages of the disease, perhaps even before any of the clinical signs became noticeable. Candidate markers that have been suggested include parietotemporal hypometabolism on PET or SPECT,[118] loss of hippocampal volume in MRI,[117] exaggerated pupillary responses to a tropicamide challenge,[238] the presence of apolipoprotein e4 alleles,[232] decreased cerebroscinal fluid (CSF) levels of certain Aβ amyloid fragments,[186] and elevated CSF levels of τ[76] or neuronal thread proteins.[51] None of these tests provides a one-to-one relationship with AD: parietotemporal hypometabolism and hippocampal atrophy may have other causes, nondemented patients may give an abnormal pupillary response to tropicamide, AD may develop in the absence of e4 alleles, and there is considerable overlap of CSF τ, Aβ, and neuronal thread protein levels between demented and nondemented individuals. Despite the absence of reliable diagnostic tests for the sporadic forms of AD, it is now possible to test for the dominantly inherited AD-causing mutations of the PS1 gene on chromosome 14 in patients with a strong family history of dementia. A positive test is diagnostic of AD since the penetrance of such mutations is nearly complete.

In some settings, laboratory tests may be used as adjuncts to the diagnosis. For example, the presence of an apoE e4 allele in a patient with the clinical diagnosis of PRAD may increase the positive predictive value of this diagnosis to better than 90%. However, the absence of the e4 allele cannot rule out AD since the negative predictive value of this test is in the order of 40%. Reliance on the e4 allele alone greatly decreases sensitivity and slightly increases specificity in the diagnosis of AD.[157]

With the possible exception of PS1 sequencing, we have never seen an instance where it has been possible to definitively "rule in" or "rule out" AD as the underlying pathological entity with the help of any of these tests. None of these tests is yet at a stage where it can improve the diagnostic accuracy of a good clinician or help an inexperienced clinician make good diagnoses. Nonetheless, some of these tests may be useful for identifying biologically more uniform subtypes of PRAD patients, such as those who have an apoE e4 allele versus those who do not, or those who have more hippocampal atrophy than others.

The Continuum of AD, Mild Cognitive Impairment, and Age-Related Cognitive Changes

A diagnosis of PRAD is made when impairments of memory and at least one additional cognitive domain interfere with customary daily living activities. How does the patient get to that stage? Is there an abrupt conversion from normalcy to dementia? Longitudinal studies addressing these questions show that PRAD is preceded by a transitional "preclinical" phase which may last for several years and which is characterized by relatively isolated impairments of memory.[72,145] Complaints of forgetfulness are extremely common among the elderly, even among those who are in full control of all daily living activities. Some of these individuals may not experience further cognitive deterioration and may qualify for the diagnosis of benign senescent forgetfulness,[134] whereas others may be in a preclinical phase which will eventually progress to the full-blown dementia of PRAD. Subjects in this intermediate stage between complete normalcy and PRAD are said to be in a state of "mild cognitive impairment" (MCI).

The state of normalcy may itself need to be qualified further. As noted in section II, cross-sectional studies have shown that groups of older individuals score less well on cognitive tests than groups of younger subjects. These studies have led to the establishment of age-adjusted normative scores. Raw scores that are "normal" may therefore vary from one age to another and the degree of the variation may change from one cognitive domain to another. In the vocabulary subtest of the Wechsler

Adult Intelligence Scale-Revised (*WAIS-R*), for example, performance at the 50th percentile corresponds to a raw score of 49–52 at 25–34 years and to a nearly identical raw score of 41–45 at 70–74 years of age. In a delayed recall subtest of the Wechsler Memory Scale-Revised (*WMS-R*) (*Visual Reproduction 2*), however, performance at the 50th percentile corresponds to a raw score of 31 at 25–34 years but to a raw score of only 15 at 70–74 years of age. Thus, elderly individuals with considerable loss of memory function from a previous baseline could be labeled as neuropsychologically "normal" if age-adjusted values were used in reaching a diagnostic assessment.

These considerations suggest that four different levels of memory function can be identified during the life span of an individual. (*1*) A stage of peak performance is reached at some point in adulthood. It may be maintained during senescence by rare individuals who are said to enjoy *superior aging*. (*2*) Many individuals experience a loss of function from this hypothetical peak but are said to show an *age-appropriate cognitive performance* because their scores remain within a range that is average for that population. (*3*) Some individuals show a level of performance which falls significantly below the age-adjusted averages without, however, experiencing impairments of daily living activities. They are said to have *mild cognitive impairment (MCI)*.[213] (*4*) In still other individuals, the deterioration reaches a level of severity which interferes with daily living activities and which fulfills the diagnostic criteria for *dementia*. The relative proportion of individuals displaying peak performance, age-appropriate function, mild cognitive impairment, and dementia varies from one age group to another. As will be shown below, the neuropathology of AD may have implication for each of these four stages of cognitive performance.

VI. THE NEUROPATHOLOGY OF AD

Alzheimer's disease can be defined as a predominantly amnestic dementia associated with multiple neuropathological markers, the most conspicuous of which are the amyloid plaques and neurofibrillary tangles (Fig. 10–5). A definitive diagnosis of AD is reached at postmortem by the microscopic identification of neurofibrillary tangles (NFT) and senile amyloid plaques in a certain density and distribution. Diagnosis in AIDS, Pick's disease, or Wilson's disease is greatly helped by pathognomonic markers such as a positive HIV titer, the detection of Pick bodies, or the identification of a Kayser-Fleischer ring. There is, in comparison, nothing pathognomonic about either the cognitive or neuropathological features of AD: Memory disorders (with or without other deficits) can arise in dozens of diseases, and at least some plaques and tangles (and all other known components of the AD neuropathology) can be seen in elderly individuals with no known symptoms of dementia. These are some of the reasons why the definitive neuropathological diagnosis of AD is still challenging despite the great ease with which the two cardinal markers, plaques and tangles, can be detected.

The probability that AD is the correct diagnosis increases as the pattern of the dementia approaches the clinical pattern described above, as the density and distribution of plaques and tangles increase according to the anatomical pattern that will be described later, and as the prominence of alternative substrates of dementia (such as cerebrovascular disease or Lewy bodies) decreases. Prior to the current resurgence of interest in AD, neuropathologists tended to give equal prominence to plaques and tangles in reaching a diagnosis. However, the first two sets of diagnostic criteria described during the modern era of AD research, the Khachaturian[126] and CERAD[178] criteria, provided guidelines based exclusively on the distribution of plaques. Although plaques are very heterogeneous, and only certain forms of plaques, known as "senile" or "neuritic," are consistently associated with dementia, neither the Khachaturian nor the CERAD system clearly articulated how to identify individual plaque subtypes. In general, these criteria tended to promote false-positive diagnostic errors.

The 1997 criteria proposed by the National Institute on Aging and the Reagan Institute of the Alzheimer's Association are more consistent with the classical approach, which emphasized tangles as well as plaques in the diagnosis of AD. According to these criteria, the likelihood that the clinical dementia is caused by AD is *high* if numerous (20–30 per 10× field) NFT and neuritic plaques are present not only in the hippocampal–entorhinal complex but also in neocortex; *intermediate* if the density of neocortical neuritic plaques and limbic NFT is moderate (5–10 per 10× field) ; and *low* if both lesions display a relatively sparse density and remain confined to the limbic system.[114] The virtues of this system include simplicity, the descriptive and probabilistic approach, the anatomical specification of limbic versus neocortical pathology, and the emphasis on tangles as well as plaques.

In addition to the plaques and tangles, the neuropathology of AD also includes a loss of neurons, loss of synapses, depletion of cortical cholinergic innervation, and gliosis. The interactions among these components are being investigated intensively in an attempt to identify a "prime mover" in the pathogenesis of AD. Numerous clinicopathological investigations have attempted to isolate the one aspect of the neuropathology which is most closely associated with the clinical dementia. Such claims have been made for the amyloid plaques,[49] neurofibrillary tangles,[9] neuronal loss,[94] synaptic loss,[256] and cholinergic depletion.[74]

Four Stages of NFT—A Continuum From Aging to AD

Phosphorylated τ proteins are the major constituents of NFT in AD. Tau is a low-molecular-weight microtubule-associated protein encoded by a gene on chromosome 17. It plays a major role in stabilizing microtubules, maintaining cytoskeletal integrity, and sustaining axoplasmic transport. In AD, hyperactive kinases or hypoactive phosphatases lead to a net increase in the phosphorylation of τ and interfere with its ability to bind microtubules.[55,92,261] The unbound phosphorylated τ polymerizes into insoluble paired helical filaments (PHFs) which eventually condense into characteristic flame-shaped or globose NFT. Axonal and dendritic PHFs give rise to "neuropil threads" and to the neuritic component of amyloid plaques. PHF-positive neuritic plaques therefore represent a conjunction of amyloid with neurofibrillary pathology and are almost exclusively seen in NFT-containing regions of the brain. This is why diagnostic criteria and clinicopathological correlations based on NFT are identical to those based on neuritic plaques in studies where neuritic is defined as "PHF-positive."

In some specimens from old but nondemented subjects, neurons containing phosphorylated τ may be substantially more numerous than neurons which have fully formed NFT,[10] suggesting that the transformation of phosphorylated τ into PHF and NFT is not instantaneous and that the underlying process may take a considerable amount of time, perhaps years. The NFT eventually lead to the distortion of the cytoskeleton, impairment of axonal transport, and perturbation of neuronal function. Many (but not all) NFT appear to trigger neuronal death through a poorly understood process which may also take many years.[24,33] The death of the neuron leaves behind an insoluble extracellular NFT which is known as a "ghost tangle." In situ hybridization studies show that NFT-bearing neurons express less mRNA for markers of mitochondrial energy metabolism.[106] Furthermore, the extrapyramidal deficits in AD are correlated with the number of substantia nigra NFT even in the absence of any detectable neuronal loss.[147] The NFT may thus contribute to neural dysfunction directly, without the obligatory mediation of neuronal death.

The number of NFT is positively correlated with chronological age in demented as well as nondemented individuals. Nearly everyone above the age of 60, whether demented or not, will develop NFT in the brain. However, the density of NFT is also much higher in patients with AD than in nondemented age-matched individuals. Whenever a brain contains very few tangles, these are *always* confined to components of the limbic system. Neocortical NFT emerge only after the limbic NFT burden becomes very high, and the appearance of NFT clusters in neocortex is almost always associated with clinical dementia. The invariance of these patterns has led to an inferential reconstruction of temporal and spatial stages of NFT distribution (Fig. 10–6). Braak and Braak have provided the most systematic documentation of such stages but they have confined their detailed observations prin-

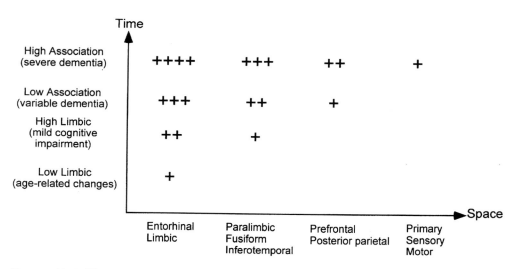

FIGURE 10–6. The progression of neurofibrillary tangles in time and in space.

TABLE 10–2 NFT Distributions in Six Subjects*

				COMPONENTS OF THE LIMBIC SYSTEM									INFEROTEMPORAL CORTICES		OTHER ASSOCIATION NEOCORTEX				PRIMARY SENSORY MOTOR			
Subject	Age/Sex/Educ	Clinical State	NFT Stage	Nucleus Basalis	Entorhinal and Transentorhinal BA28, 35	Hippocampus	Amygdala	Temporal Pole BA38	Insula	Orbito Frontal BA12, 25	Olfactory Cortex	Cingulate BA23, 24	Fusiform Gyrus BA36	Inferior Temporal Gyrus BA20	Middle Temporal Gyrus BA21	Superior Temporal Gyrus BA22	Prefrontal Cortex BA9, 10, 46	Posterior Parietal Cortex BA39, 40	1° Visual BA17	1° Auditory BA41, 42	1° Somatosensory BA3b	1° Motor BA4
1	61 / F / NA	Died suddenly of MI, detailed chart review shows no evidence of cognitive change	Low limbic	4	2	2	0	2	0	1	0	0	0	0	0	0	0	0	0	0	0	0
2	89 / F / 16	No dementia, memory normal if age-adjusted. Word fluency normal for any age	Low limbic	3	20	8	25	5	2	0	0	0	2	3	4	0	0	1	0	0	0	0
3	86 / M / 10	No dementia, memory mildly impaired for age. Word fluency normal for any age	High limbic	25	120	39	5	27	4	6	NA	1	30	2	0	0	0	0	0	0	0	0
4	90 / M / 16	No dementia, memory mildly impaired for age. Word fluency normal for any age	High limbic	81	850	143	46	158	10	16	33	1	97	5	0	0	0	0	0	0	0	0
5	99 / F / 16	No dementia, memory normal if age-adjusted. Word fluency mildly abnormal for age	Low neocortical	167 / *6/20x*	2000 / *35/20x*	200 / *13/20x*	200 / *7/20x*	100 / *7/20x*	66 / *3/20x*	40 / *3/20x*	NA / *NA*	29 / *2/20x*	300 / *7/20x*	200 / *4/20x*	200 / *3/20x*	100 / *3/20x*	12 / *1/20x*	30 / *1/20x*	5 / *1/20x*	0 / *0/20x*	2 / *1/20x*	4 / *1/20x*
6	84 (6 years before death) / F / NA	Severe dementia	High neocortical	*50/20x*	*90/20x*	*75/20x*	*90/20x*	*45/20x*	*25/20x*	*20/20x*	*20/20x*	*30/20x*	*70/20x*	*70/20x*	*60/20x*	*40/20x*	*30/20x*	*40/20x*	*10/20x*	*10/20x*	*4/20x*	*1/20x*

*The whole numbers indicate total NFT counts in a 0.04 mm-thick whole-hemisphere section that contained the most NFT in the area of interest. In subjects 1–4 there were too few tangles to obtain meaningful densities per microscopic field. In subject 5, NFT are expressed as total number per section (on top) and also as a number per microscopic field with a 20× objective (in italics). This number reflects the most characteristic maximum density within the area of interest. In case 6, there were too many NFT to give total counts and only densities are given. There is no simple relationship between the total numbers and densities since the distribution of NFT is not uniform. In general, however, the total NFT count in subject 6 was at least one order of magnitude higher than that of subject 5. NFT = neurofibrillary tangle; MI = myocardial infarction.

cipally to the medial temporal lobe.[26,27] The following account incorporates their experience and also draws upon unpublished observations in our laboratory based on the examination of whole brain sections in over 100 subjects, many with known cognitive status (Table 10–2 and Fig. 10–7).

LOW LIMBIC STAGE (SIMILAR TO THE BRAAK+BRAAK STAGES I AND II)
This is the stage where the NFT are the least numerous (subjects 1 and 2 in Table 10–2). In relatively young individuals (such as subject 1 who died at the age of 61), a coronally cut 0.04 mm-thick whole-hemisphere section may contain no more than a total of five or six NFT at this stage. In older individuals (such as subject 2 who died at the age of 89) the number of NFT increases but not their distribution. Clusters of three or more NFT occur only in limbic areas such as the nucleus basalis, entorhinal–transentorhinal cortex, the hippocampus, the amygdala and the temporopolar cortex. Isolated tangles can also be seen in other components of the limbic system such as the hypothalamus, insula, orbitofrontal cortex, and the parolfactory gyrus. Tangles in the nucleus locus coeruleus appear at around this stage.[33]

In some specimens the NFT are most numerous in the entorhinal–transentorhinal area of the parahippocampal gyrus as described by Braak and Braak; in others they are just as numerous in the amygdala, hippocampus, or nucleus basalis. In the parahippocampal gyrus, the tangles are found almost exclusively in layer II of entorhinal cortex and the transverse layer of transentorhinal pyramidal neurons lining the collateral sulcus. In the hippocampus, the few tangles are invariably located in CA1 and spare the immediately adjacent subiculum, CA 2–4, and the dentate gyrus. Rare NFT are also seen in the fusiform, inferior temporal, and middle temporal gyri.

This stage of NFT distribution is seen in nearly all nondemented subjects above the age of 60 and is not compatible with a diagnosis of AD.[26] There is a tendency to consider these NFT benign, normal, or "physiological" outcomes of aging. We prefer the alternative interpretation that all NFT are abnormal but that they may be *endemic* to aging. The NFT at this stage could conceivably be responsible, at least in part, for the so called age-related (or age-appropriate) changes in mental function. Thus subject 2 in Table 10–2 had a *WMS-R* logical memory retention score of 11, which is within the normative range (8–15) for her age and education level but distinctly below the normative range (21–30) for young adults. Age-related adjustments to normative scores for the WMS-R must have been computed by testing healthy elderly individuals with this pattern of NFT distribution. The use of these age-adjusted ranges would thus promote the potentially misleading conclusion that NFT have no effect on cognitive performance.

HIGH LIMBIC STAGE (SIMILAR TO BRAAK+BRAAK STAGES III AND IV)
This stage represents a sharp increase in the concentration of NFT within limbic and paralimbic cortices (subjects 3 and 4 in Table 10–2). No part of the limbic system is free of NFT at this stage (Fig. 10–7). Isolated NFT also emerge in the thalamus and substantia nigra. Despite the many thousands of NFT that are present in the limbic system, prefrontal, posterior parietal, and occipital cortex remain virtually

free of NFT. The only conspicuous clusters of neocortical NFT at this stage are seen in the fusiform gyrus and, to a much lesser extent, in the inferior and medial temporal gyri, as if representing a spread of the vulnerability to NFT formation from the adjacent parahippocampal areas.

In the elderly, this stage of NFT distribution can be compatible with normal daily living activities although neuropsychological test scores, especially of memory function, can be abnormal even when compared to age-adjusted ranges. Subjective cognitive difficulties and subtle personality changes may emerge but not with a severity that would be consistent with the diagnosis of dementia.[26] This level of NFT distribution may therefore become associated with what has been referred to as "benign senescent forgetfulness," "mild cognitive impairment," or "the preclinical stage of AD."

Thus, although subjects 3 and 4 were not demented (on the basis of the *MMSE* scores and daily living activities), their *WMS-R* logical memory scores (6 and 7) were below the age-adjusted normative ranges (8–15). However, their performances on a nonmemory task such as word fluency (which depends on the integrity of frontal, parietal, and lateral temporal association areas) were within the normative range even for young adults. Considering the continuity between mild cognitive impairment and very early AD, this stage of NFT distribution could be associated with mild dementia in some subjects.

LOW NEOCORTICAL STAGE (SIMILAR TO BRAAK AND BRAAK STAGE V)

At this stage, the density of NFT increases further in all components of the limbic system (subject 5 in Table 10–2). The entorhinal–transentorhinal area contains thousands of NFT per section and hippocampal NFT appear in the CA3 and subicular sectors as well. The fusiform and inferior temporal gyri contain hundreds of NFT per section. Scores of NFT appear in the middle and superior temporal gyri, and smaller clusters emerge within prefrontal and posterior parietal association cortices. Primary sensory and motor cortices contain only rare NFT.

The most common clinical correlate of this stage of NFT distribution is probably an early dementia where memory deficits are prominent and other domains start to show initial impairments. This stage of NFT distribution and a "frequent" plaque score in neocortex in a demented subject lead to a reasonably high probability that the dementia is caused by AD. However, in the very old, this stage may be com-

---

FIGURE 10–7. The four stages of neurofibrillary tangle (NFT) distribution. Each red dot represents one NFT in the two columns on the left and one to three NFT in the two columns on the right. The sections of the "low limbic" stage are from case 2 in Table 10–2, the "high limbic" stage from case 4, the "low neocortical" stage from case 5, and the "high neocortical" stage from case 6. Abbreviations: amy=amgdala; cg=cingulate gyrus; cs=central sulcus; dlpfc=dorsolateral prefrontal cortex; ento=entorhinal cortex; fg=fusiform gyrus; h=hippocampus; hy=hypothalamus; in=insula; itg=inferior temporal gyrus; mtg=mddle temporal gyrus; nbm=nucleus basalis of Meynert; ofc=orbitofrontal cortex; p=putamen; ppc=posterior parietal cortex; sf=sylvian fissure; stg=superior temporal gyrus; t=thalamus; tp=temporopolar cortex.

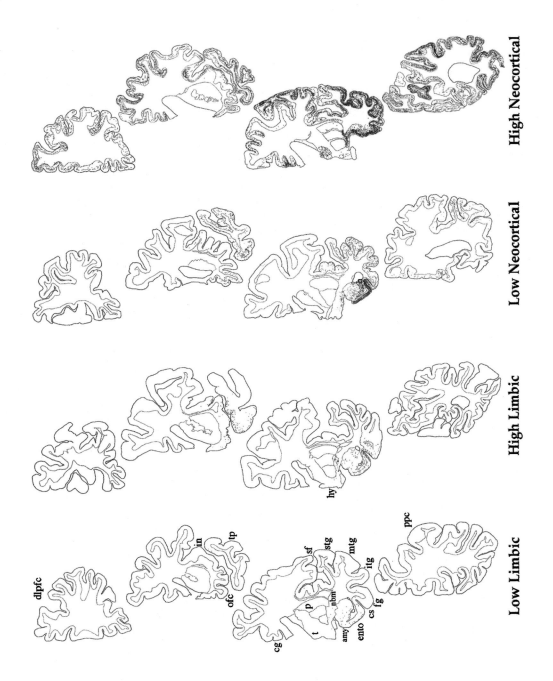

Low Limbic High Limbic Low Neocortical High Neocortical

patible with age-appropriate daily living activities. For example, subject 5 who died at the age of 99 (Table 10–2) could not be classified as demented because of an *MMSE* score of 27 and intact daily living activities. Her memory was within the age-adjusted normative range but some nonmemory tests such as verbal fluency were abnormal even by age-adjusted normative values.

HIGH NEOCORTICAL STAGE (SIMILAR TO BRAAK+BRAAK STAGE VI)

This is the stage where all areas of association neocortex show a high density of NFT (subject 6 in Table 10–2). At this stage, the striatum also contains NFT. It is interesting to note, however, that the highest densities of striatal NFT are usually found in the nucleus accumbens and olfactory tubercle, two sectors that are part of the limbic striatum.[239] The neuropathological identification of this NFT stage, in the presence of neocortical plaques of equivalent density, leads to the extremely high likelihood that the dementia is caused by AD. In keeping with the high NFT density in association neocortices, this is the stage where substantial impairments encompass almost all cognitive and behavioral domains, including language, visuospatial skills, reasoning, and social graces. This may also be the stage at which extrapyramidal disorders begin to appear, probably as a consequence of NFT in the substantia nigra and striatum. Even at this stage, primary sensory and motor cortices contain very few NFT. This is in keeping with the usual picture of AD where primary sensory–motor deficits are usually not prominent, even in the terminal stages of the disease.

Vulnerability to NFT and Impact upon Cognitive Networks

The foregoing account suggests that the vulnerability of a neuron to neurofibrillary degeneration is determined by its age and synaptic proximity to the limbic system. At around the age of 60, NFT emerge within the nucleus basalis of Meynert and within limbic components of the temporal lobe such as the entorhinal–transentorhinal cortices, the amygdala, and the hippocampus. The vulnerability to NFT formation then seems to spread, as if along axonal connection pathways, first to other paralimbic and adjacent temporal areas, then to more distant neocortical association areas, and finally to primary sensory and motor areas.

The spread of this vulnerability cannot be explained on the basis of spatial contiguity alone since the subicular cortices which are immediately adjacent to the entorhinal cortex contain less NFT than the more distant CA1 sector. Furthermore, distant subcortical nuclei which are interconnected with NFT-prone limbic and paralimbic cortical areas are themselves vulnerable to NFT formation. These subcortical structures include the hypothalamus; intralaminar, anterior, midline, and medial nuclei of the thalamus; the substantia nigra; the raphe nuclei; parts of the nucleus locus coeruleus; and the limbic striatum. In contrast, subcortical structures such as the globus pallidus which have few, if any, monosynaptic connections with the cerebral cortex have a very low vulnerability to NFT formation. Furthermore, areas with predominantly efferent projections to the cerebral cortex (such as the nucleus locus coeruleus) seem to have a greater vulnerability to NFT formation than areas with predominantly afferent projections from the cerebral cortex (such as the striatum or subthalamic nucleus), suggesting that the vulnerability to NFT formation may spread predominantly in the retrograde direction, from synapse to cell body.

The low and high limbic stages (Braak+Braak stages I–IV), during which NFT are almost entirely confined to the limbic system and immediately adjacent parts of temporal neocortex, appear compatible with the preservation of daily living activities but may nonetheless contribute to the onset of memory deficits associated first with "normal aging" and then with "mild cognitive impairment" and the "preclinical" stage of AD.[25,145] Dementia appears to emerge after certain thresholds of NFT density and distribution have been exceeded, especially when the NFT become established in superior temporal, parietal, and frontal association neocortices. Throughout the course of AD, the core limbic areas continue to display the highest numbers of NFT, in keeping with the fact that the memory disorder remains prominent throughout the course of the disease. The progression from the clinically silent low-limbic stage to the terminal dementia at the high neocortical stage may take as long as 50 years.[26]

The universality of this tight correspondence between NFT distribution and mental state has been challenged by reports of rare patients who were not demented despite the presence of advanced neurofibrillary degeneration at the "high neocortical" stage.[49a] One possible explanation is that these patients might have experienced a considerable decline of mental function from an exceptionally high former level without necessarily fulfilling the criteria for dementia. Alternatively, they may have had an unusual neuronal reserve capacity which may have compensated for the impact of the NFT-related neurodegeneration.

Considerable emphasis has been placed on the early emergence and high concentration of NFT in layer II of entorhinal cortex.[113] The entorhinal cortex is the most important neural relay between association neocortex and the hippocampus. Its layer II gives rise to the perforant pathway, the major projection system linking entorhinal cortex to the hippocampus. The NFT-related neural dysfunction in layer II of entorhinal cortex could thus create a state of corticohippocampal disconnection which would interfere with the memory-related functions of the hippocampo-entorhinal complex (Chapters 1 and 4). Most of the NFT in association neocortex are located within large pyramidal neurons that give rise to long corticocortical connections.[185] The neurofibrillary pathology in these neurons may lead to extensive corticocortical disconnections. One outcome of such a process would be to interfere with the function of the NFT-free neurons in the disconnected cortical areas.

Neuronal and Synaptic Loss

While it is possible to detect the existence of a handful of plaques or tangles, tens of thousands of neurons and synapses must die before their loss becomes detectable. Even then, neuronal and synaptic loss in an individual specimen can only be inferred on the basis of comparisons to age-matched control groups. Exploring the early phases of neuronal and synaptic death has therefore been much more challenging than exploring the early phases of plaque and tangle formation. Investigations based on unbiased stereology show that the earliest detectable stage of dementia is already associated with a 50% reduction in the layer II neurons of entorhinal cortex but a relative preservation of neocortical neurons in the banks of the superior temporal sulcus.[95] As the dementia progresses and additional deficits arise in language and other cognitive domains, neuronal loss becomes detectable also in the cortex of the superior temporal sulcus.[94] These results suggest that the gradual anatomical spread of the vulnerability to NFT formation may be mirrored by a similar spread of a vulnerability to neuronal death.

There are significant negative correlations between NFT density and neuronal counts, suggesting that neurofibrillary degeneration may induce neuronal death.[33] However, some types of subcortical NFT may not lead to neuronal death and neuronal loss may greatly exceed the number of NFT in some cortical areas.[24,94] One possible explanation for the latter observation is that NFT are resorbed following the death of the host neurons. Alternatively, AD may be associated with several processes that kill neurons, some of which, such as amyloid neurotoxicity or trans-synaptic degeneration, may not be mediated by NFT. For example, a subset of nicotinamide adenine dinucleotide phosphate-diaphorase (NADPHd)-reactive cortical neurons show extensive axonal and dendritic pathology in AD although they do not contain NFT.[132] Depression of perikaryal acetylcholinesterase (AChE) enzyme activity and nicotinic receptors also displays a distribution which exceeds the distribution of NFT-bearing neurons.[108,237] In the entorhinal and hippocampal regions, even neurons without detectable tangles show a reduction in protein synthesis and mitochondrial energy metabolism.[106,229] Furthermore, parietotemporal hypometabolism can be seen relatively early in the disease although the extension of substantial neurofibrillary pathology and cell loss to parietal association cortex occurs relatively late in the disease. These considerations indicate that neurofibrillary degeneration is unlikely to be the only mechanism that compromises neuronal function in AD.

Another important factor that contributes to the emergence of the dementia in AD is the loss of cortical synapses.[52,256] There is relatively little information on the anatomical distribution of synaptic loss. Neuronal death and NFT may both lead to the secondary loss of synapses through the process of Wallerian degeneration. However, the direction of causation may also be reversed and there may be a primary injury to synapses, with the subsequent induction of retrograde abnormalities in the neuronal cell body, some of which may eventually lead to NFT formation and/or cell death.

The definitive documentation of neuronal and synaptic loss requires a careful microscopic examination of the brain following the death of the patient, usually at a time when clinical deficits have reached their maximal severity. It is possible to obtain an earlier in vivo approximation of neuronal mass by the quantitative examination of CT and MR scans. Many textbooks use a dramatically shrunken brain to illustrate AD and therefore promote the mistaken impression that severe and global atrophy is a characteristic component of the disease. In fact, global atrophy occurs only at the end stages of the disease, and a CT or MR "consistent with stated age" is the rule during the many years of mild-to-moderate dementia.

However, recent morphometric investigations are also showing that focal atrophy in the medial temporal lobe may turn out to be one of the most specific and early markers for the processes that lead first to "mild cognitive impairment" and then to AD. For example, selective hippocampal atrophy has been noted in nondemented elderly subjects who display deficits of delayed recall but not in those who are free of such symptoms.[43] Furthermore, a longitudinal study in nondemented subjects at risk for developing hereditary AD reported hippocampal atrophy only in those who had memory deficits and who, during the subsequent 3 years, developed a full-blown dementia.[71] The progression from the stage of "mild cognitive impairment" to full-blown AD appears to be associated with the further intensification of hippocampal atrophy, spread of the atrophy to the temporal cortex, and the emergence of hypoperfusion in mediotemporal limbic areas.[43,71,119] A more specific in vivo assessment of neuronal mass can be achieved by the MR spectroscopic measurement of the neuronal marker N-acetyl aspartate (NAA). In early and moderate stages of PRAD, hippocampal volumes were reduced by about 20% while the spectroscopically determined levels of NAA were reduced by 15%, showing that the degree of hippocampal atrophy accurately reflects the extent of neuronal loss.[179] These morphemetric and spectroscopic studies suggest that neuronal loss within the medial temporal lobe may provide a crucial substrate for the memory deficits related to "mild cognitive impairment" and AD.

Cholinergic Loss

The cholinergic innervation of the cerebral cortex arises from the nucleus basalis of Meynert, a major component of the limbic system. As reviewed in Chapters 1 and 3, this pathway plays an important role in the neural regulation of memory and attention.[166] The nucleus basalis is one of the first areas in the entire brain to show τ hyperphosphorylation and isolated NFT formation in the course of aging. A modest age-related decline of cortical cholinergic innervation has been reported and may contribute to the emergence of age-related memory deficits.[86] Alzheimer's disease is associated with extensive NFT formation in the nucleus basalis and a profound loss of cholinergic axons in the cerebral cortex.[84] This depletion of cholinergic innervation appears to be more severe and to occur earlier than the depletion of other transmitter-specific systems in the cerebral cortex.[84] The cholinergic depletion in AD is most accentuated within the limbic system and temporal lobe and least prominent in primary sensory–motor areas (Fig. 10–8).

The finding that the biochemically determined level of the cholinergic marker choline acetyltransferase (ChAT) is significantly decreased only in advanced AD has been used to question the early involvement of cortical cholinergic pathways.[49] However, the interpretation of cortical ChAT activity is quite problematic. In the monkey, for example, nearly total destruction of the basal forebrain cholinergic neurons gives rise to a cortical ChAT depletion of only 48%–74%, and substantial but partial lesions induce depletions that do not exceed 12%–62%.[268a] Cortical ChAT levels are therefore not very sensitive indicators of cortical cholinergic depletion. The accurate assessment of cortical cholinergic denervation requires a microscopic quantitation of cholinergic axons. Studies based on this approach show that cortical cholinergic depletion may start even before the onset of clinical dementia and that it becomes exceedingly severe in advanced AD.[86]

In contrast to the profound loss of cholinergic axons in the cerebral cortex, the cholinergic innervation of the striatum (which is derived mostly from intrinsic sources) and thalamus (which is derived mostly from brainstem sources) remains relatively intact. There is therefore no evidence for a generalized cholinergic deficiency in AD. Instead, the cholinergic depletion is based on a selective vulnerability of the pathway from the nucleus basalis to the cerebral cortex. The mechanisms which contribute to this selective vulnerability are poorly understood. Amyloid is unlikely to be the culprit since the nucleus basalis is not particularly prone to amyloid deposition and since there is no evidence that amyloid exerts a selective neurotoxic effect upon cortical cholinergic axons.[64]

The cerebral cortex in AD also shows a loss of cholinergic receptors. The nicotinic and m2-subtype muscarinic receptors are depleted whereas the m1-subtype muscarinic receptors are relatively preserved. In vitro experiments have shown that cholinergic neurotransmission mediated through the m1 and m3 receptor subtypes can shunt AβPP metabolism away from the pathway that produces the plaque-forming Aβ fragment, leading to the inference that the cholinergic depletion in AD could potentially increase the production of Aβ.[195] Additional in vitro experiments have shown that the loss of nicotinic receptors may accentuate the neurotoxicity of Aβ and that Aβ may interfere with the release, synthesis, and postsynaptic effectiveness of acetylcholine.[11,123,127,209] It appears, therefore, that AD may be associated with a vicious cycle wherein the impairment of cholinergic neurotransmission intensifies the toxicity and production of amyloid at the same time that the amyloid further depresses cholinergic neurotransmission.[167] This self-reinforcing and potentially pathogenic process could conceivably be interrupted by the use of agonists directed to m1, m3, and nicotinic receptors. In contrast to these putative interactions with amyloid metabolism, there is currently no evidence that cholinergic transmission influences τ phosphorylation, NFT formation, or neuronal death.

Ovarian hormones play an important role in promoting the synthesis of acetylcholine by the nucleus basalis.[90] The precipitous estrogen deficiency triggered by menopause may thus perturb cortical cholinergic neurotransmission. This relationship could conceivably help to explain why women are at higher risk of developing AD and also why this risk appears to be lowered by postmenopausal estrogen replacement.[122] In nondemented subjects, neurons of the nucleus basalis display a selective age-related loss of the calcium-binding protein calbindin D28K. The resultant disruption in the ability to buffer intracellular calcium may increase the susceptibility of these neurons to age-related involutional changes such as those that lead to AD.[276] These observations raise the possibility that calcium channel blockers could be useful for preventing age-related degenerative changes in the

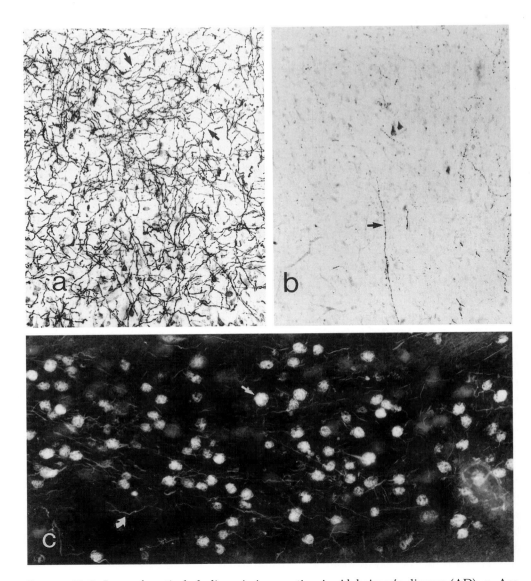

FIGURE 10–8. Loss of cortical cholinergic innervation in Alzheimer's disease (AD). a. Acetylcholinesterase histochemistry was used to stain cholinergic axons (arrows) in the middle temporal gyrus of subject 2 in Table 10–1. She died at the age of 89 with no dementia. Her nucleus basalis contained very few neurofibrillary tangles (NFT). The density of cholinergic fibers is high. b. Same staining procedure and same part of the brain in subject 6 of Table 10–1. She died at the age of 84 with a severe dementia and the neuropathology of AD. The cortex of the middle temporal gyrus has lost almost all of its cholinergic axons. Only a few isolated axons (arrow) remain. c. Same subject as in b. The intermediate sector of the nucleus basalis has been stained with thioflavin S. This is the part of the nucleus basalis that is the most likely source of projections to the middle temporal gyrus.[171] The majority of nucleus basalis neurons contained tangles (arrow). There are also neuropil threads in the background (curved arrow). Magnification in all three photomicrographs is 100×.

nucleus basalis. The cholinergic depletion is the only aspect of AD that can be addressed by currently available pharmacological interventions (section X).

The Amyloid Plaques and Gliosis: Oxidation, Inflammation, and Molecular Chaperones

The senile plaque is one of the two principal neuropathological markers of AD. Although the existence of Aβ-negative plaques has been reported,[236] Aβ amyloid provides the principal constituent for the vast majority of plaques in AD. The Aβ peptide is a relatively insoluble fragment of a much larger, membrane-spanning amyloid β precursor protein (AβPP). AβPP is expressed by almost all cells, inside as well as outside of the CNS, and is encoded by a single gene on chromosome 21. Through a process of differential splicing, AβPP can be produced in several molecular forms containing 695, 751 and 770 amino acids. The longer forms contain a Kunitz protease inhibitor domain but the dominant CNS form is AβPP-695, which lacks the Kunitz domain.

The metabolism of AβPP has been investigated in great detail.[56,104,240,278,279] AβPP is processed by three proteases designated as α, β and γ secretases (Fig. 10–9). Bleomycin hydrolase is a candidate for the β-secretase[67] and PS1 for the γ-secretase.[274a] The α-secretase splits the AβPP in the middle of the Aβ domain and therefore precludes the formation of the full Aβ moiety whereas the β and γ secretases exert their action just outside of the Aβ domain, at the N- and C-terminal regions, respectively, and yield split products that contain intact Aβ (Fig. 10–9). Depending on the exact site of γ-secretase activity, the Aβ fragment may be short (39–40 amino acids) or long (42–43 amino acids). The long form (long Aβ) is more likely to form insoluble fibrils and, by inference, may have a greater potential for neurotoxicity.[241] Another potentially insoluble AβPP fragment that can precipitate in plaques is the Aβ17–42 fragment, which results from the combined action of α and γ secretases.[56]

The processing of AβPP and the production of Aβ-containing moieties occur everywhere in the brain and throughout life. During most of the life span, however, no plaques are deposited, even in individuals who will later develop AD, either because there are factors which maintain the solubility of Aβ or because the deposited Aβ is rapidly cleared. At some point in the life span, Aβ starts to precipitate in the form of plaques so that brains of nearly all individuals above the age of 60, whether destined to develop the dementia of AD or not, show some Aβ-containing plaques. In contrast to neurofibrillary degeneration, which is an intracellular event, amyloid deposition occurs extracellularly in the neuropil, mostly in the cerebral cortex, to a lesser extent in the subcortical gray matter, and only rarely in the white matter. The walls of a few cortical vessels may also contain Aβ, but prominent amyloid angiopathy occurs infrequently in AD. Neurons and neuroglia are both potential sources for the Aβ that accumulates in plaques.

The quantitation of Aβ plaques is more challenging than the quantitation of NFT. Methods differ greatly in their relative sensitivities for detecting Aβ. For example, Congo red birefringence is extremely insensitive whereas immunolabeling methods that call for formic acid pretreatment may lead to false positives. The

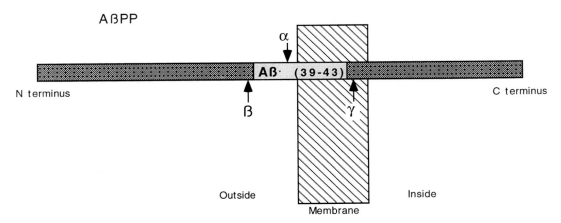

FIGURE 10–9. A cartoon of β-amyloid precursor protein (AβPP). "Outside" and "inside" refer to the extracellular and intracellular compartments.

counting of plaques may also be misleading since large and small plaques, displaying thousandfold differences in surface area, may receive equal weight. This difficulty can be addressed by measuring the proportional cortical area covered by Aβ deposits in order to compute a regional "amyloid burden."[169] In contrast to NFT, which spread according to consistent temporal and spatial patterns that have been reviewed above, Aβ plaque deposits do not necessarily increase with age and display somewhat idiosyncratic patterns of distribution that may vary greatly from one individual to another. For example, the entorhinal cortex may have very little Aβ in one specimen and may become the site of the heaviest Aβ burden in another.[98]

When there is very little Aβ in the brain, it tends to be preferentially located in the cerebral neocortex rather than in limbic areas. Subcortical structures that receive cortical projections (such as thalamic nuclei, the striatum, and the subthalamic nucleus) eventually display plaques, but without any preferential concentrations within their limbic sectors. Thus, in contrast to the NFT, which are usually confined to the limbic part of the striatum (nucleus accumbens), Aβ plaques are as numerous in the nonlimbic parts of the striatum (caudate and putamen) as they are in its limbic part. Plaques are more prominent than NFT in subcortical nuclei such as the caudate, putamen, and subthalamic nucleus which receive cortical projections but which do not project back to the cerebral cortex. In contrast, plaques are much less prominent than NFT in subcortical nuclei such as the nucleus basalis, substantia nigra, the brainstem raphe, and the nucleus locus coeruleus, which have much stronger corticofugal outputs than corticopetal inputs. It seems, therefore, that the vulnerability to Aβ deposition arises in the cerebral neocortex and tends to be exported mostly in an anterograde direction whereas the vulnerability to NFT formation arises from a temporolimbic source and tends to be exported mostly in a retrograde direction.

Plaques display a bewildering heterogeneity of shape, composition, and size: They can be diffuse or compact, they can develop with or without a central core, their amyloid can be β-pleated or not, and they can incorporate variable amounts of degenerated synapses, axons, and dendrites. The recent literature contains more than a dozen distinct terms for designating different plaque subtypes.[48] The term "neuritic" has been used as a qualifier for plaques that contain degenerated axons or dendrites. Some investigators use the term "senile plaque" as a synonym for "neuritic plaque" whereas others also use it to designate plaques containing any fibrillar material, including amyloid, as identified by nonspecific silver stains. The neuritic components of plaques generally contain τ-PHF, indicating that they originate from NFT-positive neurons. Such plaques are only seen in NFT-containing regions of the brain. However, PHF-negative neuritic plaques containing synaptic debris and neurofilament-positive dystrophic neurites have also been described.[56,266]

We will use the term "neuritic plaque" to designate Aβ plaques that contain degenerated neurites (mostly PHF-positive), and the term "Aβ plaque" to designate all Aβ-immunopositive plaques, whether neuritic or not. The presence of thioflavin S histofluorescence indicates that the Aβ has assumed a β-pleated configuration. Plaques that are Aβ-immunoreactive but thioflavin S–negative are said to be "diffuse" (also known as preamyloid plaques) whereas those that are also thioflavin S–positive are said to be "compact." Virtually all neuritic plaques are also compact. The only setting where diffuse plaques predominate is in the brains of nondemented subjects, whereas neuritic plaques become prominent only in demented subjects. Compact, non-neuritic plaques are seen in both demented and nondemented subjects. The diffuse Aβ plaque appears to induce no local tissue injury whereas the β-pleated form of amyloid in compact and neuritic plaques seems to exert considerable local neurotoxic effects.[241,277] The definitive diagnosis of AD requires the presence of frequent or moderate densities of neuritic plaques in the cerebral neocortex.[194]

The diffuse plaques of nondemented subjects could conceivably contain a kind of amyloid (perhaps Aβ17–42) which does not undergo further transformation into neuritic forms.[56] An alternative possibility is that all diffuse plaques are similarly constituted at the time of initial deposition and that they all have the potential to mature into neuritic plaques. According to this second scenario, diffuse amyloid may provide an initially benign deposit which undergoes pathogenic transformation into a β-pleated (compact) and eventually neuritic plaque associated with tissue injury and dementia. Observations in trisomy 21 support this sequence of events and suggest that this transformation may take several decades.[227]

Multiple factors may participate in the gradual transformation of an initially benign Aβ deposit into a pathogenic neuritic plaque. One possibility is that the initial Aβ deposits lead to the generation of free radicals and other reactive oxygen species which, in turn, induce a physical transformation of the plaque into a neurotoxic one.[36] This putative role of oxidative stress provides a rationale for the numerous reports suggesting that antioxidants such as vitamin E, deprenyl, melatonin, and ginko biloba may have beneficial effects in AD.[139,204,231]

Gliosis is a characteristic component of AD. The initial Aβ deposits may activate microglia and astroglia in a way that leads them to release cytokines, to express acute phase reactants, and to activate complement.[56] These processes can collectively lead to the transformation of diffuse Aβ into a β-pleated form and may mediate local events of cell death and neuritic degeneration.[220a] The participation of these processes in plaque maturation provides a rationale for reports suggesting that nonsteroidal antiinflammatory agents (NSAIDs) may decrease the risk of AD.[248] In a retrospective study, NSAIDs intake did not seem to influence the total number of Aβ plaques but did seem to be associated with a reduced number of activated microglia in the brain.[152]

Astrocytes are also potential sources of additional molecules that are associated with plaques and that could potentially influence their maturation into pathogenic structures. These molecular chaperones include apolipoproteins E and J, α1-antichymotrypsin, heparan sulfate proteoglycan, protease nexin–1, serum amyloid P, acetylcholinesterase, and butyrylcholinesterase (BChE). Each of these molecules has a different pattern of association with Aβ. For example, BChE is not present in the diffuse plaque and makes its appearance when the plaque assumes a compact and neuritic form, leading to the assumption that it may be playing a role in the transition of the plaque from a diffuse to a compact form.[99] Polymorphisms of BChE and α1-antichymotrypsin have been shown to increase the risk of late-onset sporadic AD in some populations but not in others.[116,140,242]

The Case for and Against the Amyloid Cascade as the Prime Mover of AD

The genetics of AD, briefly reviewed in section V, have focused a great deal of attention on AβPP and Aβ in the pathogenesis of AD. The arguments in favor of this emphasis are quite overwhelming: (1) Deposition of Aβ in the neuropil is the *sine qua non* for the diagnosis of AD. (2) Point mutations in the AβPP gene are sufficient to cause an early and particularly virulent form of AD. (3) A triplication of the genetic message for AβPP in trisomy 21 leads to the invariable appearance of AD pathology early in life. (4) The AD-causing mutations of PS1, PS2, and AβPP have a common denominator: They all shift the processing of AβPP toward the more insoluble and potentially more neurotoxic "long" form of Aβ.[104] (5) A major risk factor for AD, apoE4, promotes the aggregation of Aβ.[198] (6) At least in vitro, Aβ appears to be neurotoxic and to induce apoptotic neuronal death as well as τ phosphorylation.[278] (7) Transgenic mice made to overexpress AD-causing mutants of AβPP show neuropil plaques, local dystrophic degeneration, τ phosphorylation, glial activation, hippocampal neuronal loss, and behavioral abnormalities in old age.[38,62,252]

These facts would initially appear to endorse the contention that Aβ represents the prime mover of AD pathogenesis. According to such a scenario, also known as the amyloid cascade hypothesis, the initial deposits of diffuse Aβ would induce gliosis, inflammatory responses, and oxidative stress as they undergo a transformation into compact plaques which would, in turn, trigger neuritic dystrophy, synaptic loss, neurofibrillary degeneration, cell death, cholinergic depletion, and dementia. There are, however, two major considerations which challenge this scenario.

1. *There is relatively little convincing evidence that Aβ plaques are linked to the other aspects of the neuropathology in AD.* There are no significant correlations between local Aβ plaque burdens and NFT density, neuronal loss, or depletion of cholinergic innervation.[85,94] Although the suggestion has been made that neurofibrillary degeneration could result from the local compression of axons by plaques,[266] this is unlikely in view of the poor anatomical correlation between Aβ deposits and NFT. In AD, many plaques do contain degenerated PHF-positive neurites. However, such plaques are only seen in areas that contain NFT and are more likely to represent the spatial conjunction of the two types of pathologies rather than the causation of neurofibrillary pathology by Aβ plaques. In fact, none of the transgenic mice experiments has yet provided any evidence that overexpression of AD-causing mutant AβPP can trigger NFT formation. A key experiment for addressing this question would be to prepare transgenic mice which express not only the AD-causing AβPP mutations but also human τ.

   2. *There is relatively little correspondence between Aβ plaques and the clinical symptoms.* The Aβ burden does not increase with increasing duration and severity of the dementia in AD.[94] In contrast to the NFT, which display a consistent pattern of distribution, the distribution of Aβ plaques displays interindividual variations and these variations have no known relationship to the clinical deficits of the patient. The initial Aβ deposits also tend to emerge in neocortex and show no preference for the limbic system although the prominence of memory deficits in AD strongly suggests the presence of a predominantly limbic dysfunction at the initial stages of the disease. In patients with atypical clinical presentations of AD, the expected anatomical distribution of the pathology (as inferred by neuropsychological examination) is closely correlated with the distribution of NFT but not of amyloid plaques.[88] Furthermore, large numbers of diffuse and compact neocortical plaques can be seen in nondemented elderly individuals.[89,94,98,107] Thus, subject 2 in Table 10–2 (an 89-year-old woman who had three neuropsychological evaluations over 3 years without any evidence of dementia or cognitive impairment, even during her last assessment 9 months before death) had widespread compact Aβ plaques in almost all parts of the neocortex. In another study addressing the pathogenicity of Aβ, senile plaques were detected in the surgically removed temporal lobes of 11 patients who had no evidence of significant neuropsychological deficit either preoperatively or during the 2–7 years of follow-up.[151]

   Counter arguments have been provided by a study which showed a significant correlation between dementia and Aβ burden.[49] However, these results were reported only for the entorhinal cortex and did not resolve the discrepancies that are so commonly seen between the anatomical distribution of amyloid and the overall clinical picture of the dementia. The possibility has also been raised that the neurotoxic effects of amyloid may be exerted through diffusible oligomers of Aβ rather than the fibrillar deposits in the plaque.[136] According to such a scenario, the exact anatomical distribution of the amyloid plaques would not have to be correlated with the other neuropathological markers. However, such a hypothesis has not yet been able to explain how a diffusible Aβ species can induce the specific pattern of clinical impairment and NFT distribution characteristic of AD.

VII. PLASTICITY FAILURE—A HYPOTHESIS FOR UNIFYING THE PATHOGENESIS OF PLAQUES AND TANGLES

As shown in the previous section, the genetics of AD favor a pathogenic mechanism revolving around amyloid deposition whereas the clinicopathological correlations favor a disease based on NFT. Although numerous mechanisms have been proposed for reconciling these two aspects of AD, none has adequately linked the amyloid deposits to the spatial and temporal patterns of neurofibrillary degeneration. If plaques cause dementia, why is there such a discrepancy between their anatomical distribution and the anatomical distribution of the areas implicated in the dementia? If plaques cause NFT, why do the regions with highest plaque densities not have the highest NFT densities, and why do NFT occasionally emerge in brains without any plaques? One solution to this dilemma is based on the assumption that these two markers of AD are independent manifestations of a common underlying phenomenon. This section outlines a speculative course of events according to which a prolonged perturbation of neural plasticity may represent such a common denominator.[175a]

Plasticity of the Adult Brain and its Differential Distribution

Neuroplasticity is a lifelong process that mediates the structural and functional reaction of dendrites, axons, and synapses to new experience, attrition, and injury. The manifestations of neuroplasticity in the adult CNS include alterations of dendritic ramifications, synaptic remodeling, long-term potentiation (LTP), axonal sprouting, neurite extension, synaptogenesis, and neurogenesis. In the adult rodent, for example, contact with toys and conspecifics induces synaptogenesis and neurogenesis, whereas[21,124] perforant pathway stimulation increases the relative number of perforated synapses in the molecular layer of the dentate gyrus.[81]

Plasticity plays a particularly important role in response to injury. Lesions of the entorhino-hippocampal (perforant) pathway induce intact neurons to sprout collateral branches so that they can occupy the denuded synaptic targets in the molecular layer of the dentate gyrus.[44] In the adult monkey, trauma to a forelimb causes a large-scale axonal sprouting and lateral expansion of connections within neocortical somatosensory areas, presumably in response to the loss of the afferent input from the injured limb.[70] Neuronal death may also induce a compensatory increase of dendritic branching among residual neurons at that site, presumably so that the synaptic inputs that have lost their original targets can be accommodated.[1]

The process of reactive synaptogenesis may be of vital importance for replacing terminals that succumb to physiological attrition. The presence of such attrition was demonstrated in the ciliary muscle of the monkey, where the half-life of synapse turnover was estimated to be around 18 days.[44] There are approximately $7-8 \times 10^8$ synapses in the dentate gyrus of the rat alone.[37] The number of synapses in the human cerebral cortex is undoubtedly many orders of magnitude higher and these synapses are probably also subject to turnover and structural upkeep. Even if the recycling rate is much slower in the human CNS than in the ciliary muscle of the monkey, the immense number of synapses suggests that synapse turnover and up-keep are likely to constitute major activities of the brain.

Conceptually, these plasticity-related phenomena can be divided into *down-stream* processes at the level of axons, synapses and dendrites, and *upstream* regulatory processes at the level of the neuronal perikaryon. The regulation of neuroplasticity is likely to involve signals (such as growth factors) transmitted anterogradely from the perikaryon (in the downstream direction), and also retrogradely from dendrites, axons, and postsynaptic targets to the perikaryon (in the upstream direction).[44] Some of these effects are exerted transsynaptically and many are likely to be mediated by neuroglia.[44,192]

Multiple lines of evidence indicate that the potential for neuroplasticity is distributed unevenly in the adult brain so that the propensity for LTP, axonal sprouting, dendritic remodeling, and perhaps reactive synaptogenesis is higher in the limbic system that in other parts of the cerebral cortex.[6,7,22,32,193] Thus, GAP-43, which is a marker for axonal sprouting, is most intensely expressed in parts of limbic cortex, especially along the entorhino-hippocampal pathway, suggesting that experience-dependent remodeling and synaptic turnover may be highest in this part of the brain.[144,193] Furhermore, plasticity-related increases in the length and branching of the dendritic tree during adulthood appear to be most extensive in limbic–paralimbic regions such as transentorhinal, entorhinal, and hippocampal cortex; somewhat less pronounced in the association neocortex of posterior parietal and prefrontal areas; and undetectable in primary sensory-motor areas.[7] It appears, therefore, that neurons which are more vulnerable to NFT formation in AD also have a higher baseline level of plasticity.

Causes and Risk Factors of AD Interfere with Plasticity

In view of this overlap between areas with a high vulnerability to NFT formation and those with a high basal level of neuroplasticity, it is interesting that all genetic backgrounds and risk factors associated with AD appear to impair neuroplasticity.

AMYLOID AND PLASTICITY

Transgenic experiments suggest that AβPP plays a critical role in maintaining neuroplasticity in the adult brain. Thus, AβPP-null mice display greater age-dependent cognitive deficits, LTP impairments, and synapse loss than wild-type animals.[50] The molecular basis of this relationship is unknown but full-length AβPP has been shown to influence cell–substrate interactions during neurite extension and to promote the formation and maintenance of synapses in the CNS.[187,243,250] In keeping with these findings, exposure to enriched environments that promote experience-induced synaptogenesis causes a fourfold increase of AβPP in the rat CNS.[112] The soluble/secreted AβPP product of α-secretase processing, known as sAPP, also displays plasticity-promoting properties. Thus, sAPP has been shown to induce neurite outgrowth, experience-related synaptogenesis, and LTP.[112,115,220] Furthermore, infusion of sAPP in adult rodents increases memory performance and the number of cortical synaptic terminals.[176,220]

In contrast to AβPP and sAPP, the Aβ fragment of amyloid, especially its "long" form, is neurotoxic and inhibits axonal sprouting as well as LTP.[136,222] Trisomy 21 (Down's syndrome) and the AD-causing genetic mutations of AβPP may interfere with neural plasticity because they shift the balance of AβPP processing toward the longer and more neurotoxic forms of Aβ.[3,104] The dendritic atrophy and synaptic rarefaction reported in trisomy 21 may thus reflect an impairment of neuroplasticity.[253] Furthermore, transgenic mice overexpressing AD-causing mutations of AβPP show decreased synaptic and dendritic density in the dentate gyrus of the hippocampal formation and a reduced ability for compensatory synaptogenesis in response to injury.[77,153]

PRESENILINS AND PLASTICITY

Presenilin genes are homologous to the *Caenorhabditis elegans* sel-12 gene which facilitates the activity of lin-12, a member of the Notch family. Notch is a critical protein involved in neurogenesis and cell-fate decisions in the developing nervous system. Immunohistochemical experiments show that Notch 1 and PS1 are coexpressed in the hippocampal neurons of the adult human brain, suggesting that interactions of PS1 and Notch-type receptors could continue to influence neuroplasticity even in the postmitotic neurons of the adult human brain.[18] In fact, after ischemic injury to the CA1 sector of the hippocampus in the adult rat, mRNA for PS1 is increased in the dentate and CA3 neurons, as if in response to the increased demand for reactive dendritic remodeling and synaptogenesis that the death of CA1 neurons is likely to have induced within these two resistant sectors of the hippocampus.[254] The sel-12 mutant phenotype in *C. elegans* can be rescued by normal human PS1 but not by AD-causing mutants of PS1, showing that this mutation interferes with a Notch-related function of PS1.[142] Furthermore, the expression of an AD-causing mutant of PS1 in PC12 cells causes a depression of NGF-induced neurite outgrowth.[75] The AD-causing PS1 and PS2 mutations can thus suppress plasticity for two reasons: They interfere with putative plasticity-promoting effects of PS1 and they favor the processing of AβPP into the longer, more neurotoxic Aβ moieties.

ApoE AND PLASTICITY

The e4 allele of apolipoprotein E (ApoE) is one of the most intensely investigated risk factors of AD.[224] ApoE, encoded by a gene on chromosome 19, promotes axonal growth and synaptogenesis, probably because it regulates the transcellular transport of cholesterol and phospholipids. Following entorhinal cortex lesions, for example, the phase of compensatory synaptogenesis is characterized by a rapid increase of ApoE expression by astrocytes within the denervated molecular layer of the dentate gyrus.[215] The importance of ApoE for plasticity is supported by transgene experiments which show that ApoE-deficient mice display a distinct impairment of reactive synaptogenesis.[154] Individual ApoE alleles have differential impacts on plasticity. Thus, the e4 allele which is a major risk factor for AD inhibits neurite growth and dendritic plasticity whereas the e3 allele promotes these processes.[8,189]

ESTROGEN AND PLASTICITY

Estrogen replacement in postmenopausal women descreases the risk of developing AD.[122] Estrogens promote axonal and dendritic plasticity in the limbic neurons of male as well as female brains.[68,148,160,275] In female mice, ovariectomy severely impairs the reactive hippocampal synaptogenesis which follows entorhinal damage. This effect is reversed by estrogen replacement.[249] Postmenopausal estrogen deficiency may thus suppress the potential for neuroplasticity.

AGE AND PLASTICITY

The single most important risk factor for AD is age. Age influences both reactive and experience-dependent plasticity. Thus, reactive synaptogenesis in response to complex experience, compensatory synaptogenesis following injury, and the ability to sustain the effects of LTP are all diminished or slowed as a consequence of age.[137,180,234] Indirect evidence based on the examination of the cerebrospinal fluid (CSF) suggests that aging may also shift the complex balance of AβPP metabolism away from the potentially neurotrophic products of α secretase processing and toward the production of neurotoxic moieties containing the intact Aβ fragment.[202,265] Age interacts with other variables that influence neuroplasticity. For example, the age-related loss of synaptic and dendritic density becomes substantially more intensified in ApoE-deficient mice.[154]

Speculations on the Linkage Between Plasticity Burden and AD Neuropathology

The foregoing review shows that all AD-promoting factors share a common feature. They interfere with mechanisms that normally facilitate neuroplasticity. The hypothesis in this section is based on the assumption that the resultant barrier to neuroplasticity occurs at downstream dendritic and synaptic sites and that it triggers a reactive (or compensatory) upstream intensification of plasticity-related perikaryal activity. In other words, AD-promoting factors create a setting where neurons must work harder to meet neuroplasticity needs at their axonal and dendritic terminals. Over many years, such compensatory processes would lead to chronically high and eventually unsustainable levels of plasticity-related cellular activity, some of which could trigger the neuropathological events related to AD.

In fact animal experiments show that a high level of neuroplasticity tends to be associated with the increased production and phosphorylation of τ.[28,34,149,261,267] Chronically high levels of plasticity-related activity could thus upregulate the phosphorylation of τ, decrease its ability to bind microtubules, and eventually promote the polymerization of unbound τ into NFT. The NFT produced by such a sequence of events would initially appear within limbic–paralimbic neurons because these neurons have the highest baseline levels of plasticity and would therefore have the highest exposure to compensatory upregulations of plasticity-related cellular activity.

The resultant NFT-induced cytoskeletal dysfunction in these limbic–paralimbic neurons would lead to a degeneration of their dendrites and a loss of their synapses at axonal projection targets. The adjacent limbic and paralimbic neurons (many of which share the same connectivity patterns) would then face at least two additional plasticity demands: (1) more reactive synaptogenesis at their projection targets in order to replace the synapses originally provided by the degenerated axons of adjacent NFT-containing neurons and (2) more local dendritic remodeling to receive the synapses which can no longer be accommodated by the degenerated dendrites of adjacent NFT-containing neurons. Because of the downstream barriers to plasticity, these attempts at reactive remodeling would be relatively ineffective and would induce an excessive upstream intensification of plasticity-related neuronal activity, leading to the formation of NFT in these additional neurons. This sequence of events would promote the "horizontal" spread of NFT within the tightly interconnected components of limbic–paralimbic cortices and would initiate the relatively slow "limbic" phase of disease progression.

The loss of dendrites and synapses belonging to limbic–paralimbic neurons would increase the plasticity burden of the association cortices with which they are reciprocally interconnected. These association areas would need to accelerate dendritic remodeling to cope with the loss of inputs from limbic–paralimbic neurons and would also need to remodel axonal endings to cope with the loss of synaptic sites at their limbic targets. This would cause a "vertical" expansion of the disease during which the neurofibrillary degeneration (and eventually cellular death) would spread centrifugally from limbic–paralimbic areas to other parts of the brain along axonal connection pathways, in keeeping with the pattern shown in Figure 10–6.

Animal experiments show that plasticity-related activity can also lead to an overexpression of AβPP.[13] The resultant AβPP would be processed into the neurotrophic sAPP and the neurotoxic Aβ moieties, in a ratio influenced by age and genetic background. The overexpression of AβPP would initially occur at sites of maximal plasticity burden, namely in limbic–paralimbic areas and their axonal projection targets. The released Aβ would first have a soluble form and would diffuse within the extracellular fluid in the form of 10–100 kDa monomers and oligomers.[135] Upon exceeding local concentration thresholds, this Aβ could form fibrils and condense into initially inert diffuse plaques which would eventually mature into neurotoxic structures. The formation of plaques by local condensation after the diffusion of the amyloid from production sites, the fact that the production sites can overlap with NFT-prone limbic–paralimbic neurons or their widespread projection targets, and the initial inertness of the deposited amyloid may explain why plaques display a variable distribution from patient to patient, why they do not mirror the distribution of the NFT, and why they do not necessarily display a spatial and temporal distribution that fits the clinical features of the dementia.

According to this hypothesis, the neuropathology of AD reflects the consequences of excessive but ineffective neuroplasticity. In keeping with this formulation, tangle-bearing hippocampal neurons show more extensive dendritic trees than immediately adjacent tangle-free neurons, suggesting that NFT formation may be accompanied (or preceded) by increased plasticity.[82] The NFT and NFT-prone areas in AD are associated with greater PS1 and Notch 1 expression,[18,35] providing additional evidence that neurofibrillary degeneration is accompanied by an upregulation of plasticity-related mechanisms. The initial stages of AD are also associated with increased τ in the CSF,[76] suggesting that an increased expression of this plasticity-related protein occurs at a time when the NFT are undergoing a steep increase in density and distribution.

The premature development of NFT and Aβ deposits in the brains of ex-boxers provides further circumstantial support for the contention that a heightened state of reactive neuroplasticity (in this case, injury-induced) can trigger the neuropathological changes of AD.[79,259] This relationship may also explain why head injury and stroke have both been implicated as risk factors for AD.[230,245] However, the relationships between brain injury and AD-like neuropathology may only emerge when the injury is widespread and when it occurs on a background of additional factors which erect downstream barriers to neuroplasticity. Otherwise, this hypothesis would predict that all brain injury should eventually lead to AD pathology.

As noted above, a severe depletion of cortical cholinergic innervation is a consistent feature of AD.[84] Numerous experiments have shown that cholinergic neurotransmission plays an essential role in supporting reactive and experience-induced synaptic reorganization in the cerebral cortex.[15,128,281] Furthermore, cortical cholinergic innervation also promotes the α-secretase pathway and therefore the release of the neurotrophic sAPP moieties.[195] The loss of cholinergic innervation would therefore further jeopardize neuroplasticity in the cerebral cortex and lead to an acceleration of the neuropathological process related to AD.

Neuroplasticity and Pathogenesis in AD: Decades of Interacting Causes, Risks, Modulators

Plasticity-related approaches to AD pathogenesis have surfaced before but have not received the attention they deserve.[1,7,32,155,192,214,235,243] The evidence summarized above shows that all genetic causes and risk factors of AD increase the physiological burden of neuroplasticity. This evidence has been used to generate a hypothesis according to which the resultant compensatory upregulation of neuroplasticity leads to an initially adaptive increase of τ phosphorylation and AβPP turnover, to the subsequent formation of NFT and Aβ plaques as independent manifestations of excessive (but ineffective) plasticity-related cellular activity, and to the eventual loss of neurons, dendrites, and synapses as ultimate expressions of plasticity failure. The two pathological markers of AD are therefore independent manifestations of a more fundamental underlying process which also provides a common denominator through which the different genotypes of AD cause an identical clinical and neuropathological phenotype.

The biological capacity for plasticity decreases with age, explaining why age is the single most important and universal risk factor for AD. According to this formulation, the AD of old age may not be a disease at all but the inevitable manifestation of a failure to keep up with the increasingly more burdensome demands of reactive and experience-induced plasticity. The advanced cognitive and mnemonic activities of the human brain impose a very high plasticity load. The combination of this property with a long life span may endow the human brain with its unique susceptibility to AD. Factors such as trisomy 21, the e4 allele of ApoE, estrogen deficiency, head trauma, and the AD-related mutations of AβPP, PS1, and PS2 accelerate the time course of the events leading to AD by increasing the burden of neuroplasticity (Fig. 10–10). Genetic mutations do not really cause AD; they simply accelerate the temporal course of events that lead to plasticity failure and therefore lower the age at which the pathological process begins to gather momentum.

For those with the autosomal dominant forms of AD, the production of mutant forms of AβPP and presenilins starts at birth. In these individuals, as well as in everyone else, Aβ is constantly produced as a byproduct of AβPP processing throughout life, but it does not precipitate for many years. At some point during adulthood, the genetic background interacts with epigenetic factors to trigger an uncompensated plasticity gap, leading to the emergence of NFT in the limbic system and diffuse plaques in the cerebral neocortex. Every individual above the age of 60 will have these kinds of lesions in the brain. They are not sufficient to cause detectable symptoms, but they may be responsible for the so-called "age-related" changes of cognitive function.

As the plasticity gap widens, the neuropathology progresses in several directions: Mobile Aβ moieties exert neurotoxic effects; diffuse Aβ deposits attract chaperone molecules as they become compact and eventually neuritic; NFT formation, cell death, and synaptic loss spread beyond the temporolimbic areas and invade association cortices; a depletion of cortical cholinergic innervation becomes estab-

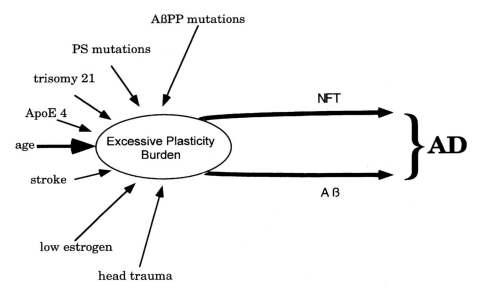

FIGURE 10–10. The convergence of genetic and environmental risk factors. The excessive plasticity burden induces neurofibrillary tangle (NFT) formation as well as the release of mobile forms of β-amyloid (Aβ) which eventually condense into plaques. The conjunction of NFT and plaques causes Alzheimer's disease (AD).

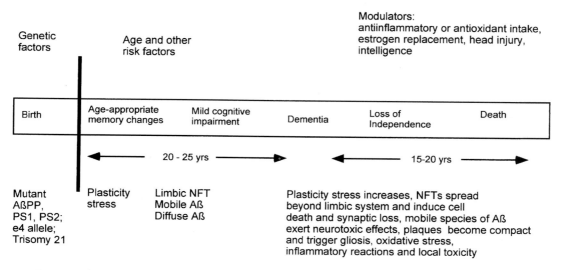

FIGURE 10-11. The temporal evolution of phenomena leading to Alzheimer's disease (AD).

lished; gliosis, oxidative stress, and inflammatory reactions become increasingly more prominent at sites of plaque deposition. This escalation of the neuropathology leads to the emergence of mild cognitive impairments followed by dementia, loss of independence, and death. The interval between the appearance of the AD-related pathological changes and the emergence of the first symptoms may be as long as 20–25 years and the interval between the appearance of these symptoms and death may be 15–20 years (Fig. 10–11).

Several modulatory factors may influence the temporal course of these events. For example, the intake of antiinflammatory agents or antioxidants and postmenopausal estrogen replacement may have protective influences for reasons that have already been discussed.[160,231,248] A high premorbid intelligence may have a protective effect as well, probably because it indicates the presence of a greater potential for experience-induced neuroplasticity.[2] Even red wine has been reported to have a protective effect,[199] perhaps because it contains a substance that acts as an estrogen receptor agonist.[80] A thorough understanding of modulatory factors is of crucial importance since they can potentially slow down the course of events shown in Figure 10.11. It has been estimated that delaying the disease milestones by about 5 years may decrease the number of individuals with a diagnosis of AD by 50%, presumably because natural death would intervene before the NFT, cell death, and synaptic loss can invade association neocortex.[125]

VIII. Some Non-AD Dementias

Alzheimer's disease accounts for more than 80% of the late-onset primary dementias. Most of the remaining 20% can be attributed to diverse clinicopathological entities, the most common of which are the focal (lobar) atrophies, diffuse Lewy body disease and Pick's disease. As in the case of AD definitive diagnosis can only be reached at postmortem examination. There is no known specific pharmacological treatment for any of these conditions. Although the dementias in this group can occur at anytime during adulthood and can present with any one of the clinical profiles described in section IV, the index of suspicion for a non-AD primary dementia increases if onset is before 65 and if memory loss is not a prominent feature of the clinical picture.

Sporadic Focal (Lobar) Atrophy

This generic term designates a family of relatively common primary dementias the only common feature of which is a sharply delineated loss of neurons in a gyral, lobar, or regional distribution accompanied by gliosis and spongioform changes. This entity has also received designations such as "dementia without distinctive histology," "focal atrophy," or "nonspecific atrophy."[65,130,172,270] The atrophic region is quite sharply demarcated. It can be as small as part of a single gyrus in one hemisphere (as in case No. 24949 of Critchley) or as large as both frontal and temporal lobes.[31,45] The microscopic examination fails to detect identifiable histopathological lesions such as Pick bodies, cortical Lewy bodies, or argyrophilic grains. Occasional ballooned neurons containing phosphorylated neurofilament protein can be present. Rare NFT and neuritic plaques may be found but not in a density and distribution consistent with the diagnosis of AD.

The site of atrophy displays a severe loss of neurons and synapses, especially in layers II and III. The same layers also show spongioform changes. There is widespread gliosis and occasional pallor of myelin in the underlying white matter.[31,146,280] Axons and dendrites in the affected areas may contain ubiquitin but no abnormal τ inclusions unless the condition is hereditary (see later). The apical dendrites of layer III neurons may show abnormal tortuosities and a loss of spines. The cholinergic innervation tends to be preserved but somatostatin and calbindin D28K-containing interneurons may be diminished.[69,73,163,260]

The anatomical distribution of the atrophy defines the clinical picture. Several patterns have attracted more attention than others.

1. Atrophy centered in *prefrontal cortex bilaterally and occasionally extending to the anterior temporal lobes and caudate nucleus* has received designations such as "frontal lobe dementia" (FLD), "dementia of frontal lobe type" (DFT), or "frontotemporal dementia" (FTD).[31] The exvacuo enlargement of the ventricles is prominent and these patients may inappropriately receive a ventricular shunt. The clinical manifestations of this pattern of atrophy corresponds to the profile of progressive comportmental/executive dysfunction (PC/ED) that has been described above and also fulfills the research criteria for POAD rather than PRAD because memory tends to be preserved (see Fig. 10–1a and case Z. T. in section IV). When the atrophy is predominantly in the right hemisphere, psychiatric symptomatology such as psychosis, compulsions, and disinhibition may be quite prominent.[177] Criteria have been published for reaching a clinical diagnosis of probable FTD.[190] The first-degree relatives of these patients have a higher risk of dementia, suggesting the influence of genetic factors in this condition.[247]

2. Atrophy centered in the *perisylvian cortex of the language-dominant (usually left) hemisphere and extending into the adjacent parts of the frontal and temporal lobes* is the most common cause of primary progressive aphasia (PPA) and also fulfills the research criteria for POAD.[172] The clinical picture of PPA has been reviewed above (see section IV). One group of investigators has suggested that the designation "frontotemporal lobar degeneration" should be used as an umbrella term for both frontal lobe dementia and primary progressive aphasia.[191] Although neither gene mutations nor observable tauopathies have been linked to these sporadic focal atrophies, the discovery that mutations of the τ gene on chromosome 17q21 can give rise to prominent frontal lobe dementia in some patients with hereditary tauopathy and progressive aphasia in others has been used to support this approach. In our experience, many patients with sporadic frontal lobe dementia have had no aphasia even late in the disease whereas many patients with primary progressive aphasia have shown no signs of prefrontal dysfunction even when the aphasia is very severe. We therefore prefer the generic term "focal atrophy" to designate the pathological entity in these conditions. We then use the appropriate qualifier to indicate the anatomical distribution of the process and its corresponding clinical picture, maintaining the distinction between frontal lobe dementia and primary progressive aphasia. However, after 8–10 years of "pure" PPA, several of our patients have shown abnormalities of comportment and atrophy of prefrontal cortex. Determining whether FLD and PPA are two different phenotypes of the same fundamental pathological entity will be an interesting subject for future research.

3. Atrophy involving *the hippocampus to a greater extent than other parts of the cerebral cortex* (as in patient 6 of Knopman and associates.[131]) can present with the profile of a progressive amnestic dysfunction and, upon the emergence of other cognitive deficits, can fit the research criteria for PRAD.

4. Atrophy in the *parietooccipital cortices bilaterally* gives rise to a profile of progressive visuospatial dysfunction and fulfills the research criteria for POAD.[39,225]

5. Atrophy of the *frontal and temporal lobes can be accompanied by motor neuron disease*, giving rise to a combination of a frontal network syndrome together with predominantly lower motor neuron abnormalities.[208] Nigral depigmentation is common but extrapyramidal signs are not conspicuous. In some of these patients, the motor deficits evolve in conjunction with a severe hyperphagia and hypersexuality of the Klüver-Bucy type.[58] The motor symptoms vary greatly. Sometimes they dominate the clinical picture, in which case the complex can be described as "amyotrophic lateral sclerosis with dementia." In other cases, as in the patient described next, the dementia becomes the dominant feature and the condition is usually described as "dementia–motor neuron disease."

Case Report

(V. S.)   A 38-year-old administrator developed the insidious onset of personality changes characterized by apathy, irritability, and decreased libido. She started making careless errors in routine activities and had great difficulty shifting perspectives when analyzing situations of everyday life. She was seen 2 years after onset at which time she displayed dysarthria, abulia, poor insight, and an impairment of lexical fluency with a severity beyond what would have been expected on the basis of the dysarthria. No aphasia or amnesia of visuospatial dysfunction was noted. Rare fasciculations were noted in the tongue but the MR, EEG, and EMG were reported as normal. Four months later (during the third year of the disease) the EMG started to show widespread denervation potentials. The examination revealed hyperreflexia, weakness of bulbar musculature, and pseudobulbar affect. She died during the fourth year of the disease. The neuropathological examination showed very severe atrophy of the frontal lobes, extending into motor cortex, with neuronal loss, gliosis, and spongioform changes in the superficial layers of the cerebral cortex. The cholinergic innervation of the cerebral cortex was preserved. There were no Pick bodies, NFT, amyloid plaques or Lewy bodies.

Hereditary Tauopathies

Some patients with clinical pictures reminiscent of frontal dementia and progressive aphasia have displayed an autosomally dominant mode of inheritance linked to chromosome 17 in several families and chromosome 3 in at least one family.[20,29,109] The chromosome 17 mutations have been mapped to the τ gene on 17q21. Some of these are exonic missense mutations; others are intronic mutations which alter the splicing of exon 10, leading to a change in the ratio of three-repeat to four-repeat τ isoforms.[91] All mutations disrupt microtubule binding and result in abnormal τ accumulations in neurons as well as in glia, but not necessarily in anatomical distributions that fit the details of the clinical picture. Mutations that affect the alternate splicing of exon 10 tend to increase the amount of τ with four microtubule-binding repeats and lead to ribbon-like neuronal and glial accumulations of τ. Some exonic missense mutations give rise to AD-like NFT accumulations, but with an anatomical distribution distinctly different from what is seen in AD.[91,105] All familial tauopathies also display some of the neuropathological features of the focal atrophies described above. Nigral depigmentation is frequent.

   The clinical pictures of the hereditary tauopathies are extremely heterogeneous. Even within single families, there can be major variations in the clinical presentation and, presumably, also in the distribution of the neuropathology.[16] In addition to clinical pictures reminiscent of frontal lobe dementia and progressive aphasia, the syndromes caused by hereditary tauopathies include hereditary dysphasic disinhibition dementia (HDDD), frontotemporal dementia with parkinsonism (FTDP-17), disinhibition–dementia–parkinsonism–amyotrophy complex

(DDPAC), pallidopontonigral degeneration, progressive subcortical gliosis, familial multisystem tauopathy, and schizophrenia-like behavior with amygdala degeneration.[19,141]

In general, motor findings are usually much more prominent in the hereditary tauopathies than in the sporadic focal degenerations. Furthermore, the hereditary tauopathies do not usually give rise to the "pure" forms of frontal dementia or primary progressive aphasia. For example, in the pedigree with hereditary dysphasic disinhibition dementia, 22 of the 23 patients had initial memory deficits and the one patient who presented with a relatively isolated language deficit had memory problems within a year.[141]

Pick's Disease

The diagnosis of Pick's disease can be made with varying degrees of strictness. In the most permissive sense, the term can be used to designate any lobar or focal atrophy and can therefore apply to all the focal atrophies described above. In the strictest sense, which will be followed here, the diagnosis is made only when Pick bodies are identified. This type of Pick's disease is relatively rare and is seen in less than 2% of dementia cases.[65] As in the focal degenerations, the majority of cases are sporadic but an autosomal dominant inheritance is seen in about 20% of the cases. Age of onset peaks in the range of 45 to 65 years. The onset is insidious and progression may be somewhat more rapid than AD, leading to death within 5–10 years.

Pick bodies are intraneuronal spherical inclusions. They are argentophilic, ubiquitin-positive and contain phosphorylated neurofilament and τ proteins. The τ in the Pick bodies contains only the three-repeat isoforms.[53] In many instances, ballooned and hypochromic "Pick cells" containing phosphorylated neurofilament proteins will also be present.[65] As in the case of the focal atrophies, and in contrast to AD, the cortical pathology is mostly in the superficial cortical layers. The regions that contain Pick bodies and Pick cells display severe neuronal loss and gliosis. The cholinergic innervation of the cerebral cortex is generally preserved. The following patient provides an example of Pick's disease.

Case Report

(L. B.)   A 44-year-old right handed prominent attorney experienced difficulties remembering names and preparing his tax returns. He also appeared less willing to participate in customary social activities. Over the subsequent 4 years there was a progression of these problems and the emergence of new difficulties in calculations, word finding, and memory. He had to take a leave of absence from work but continued to sing in choir and play tennis. The MRI and SPECT scans showed subtle atrophy and decreased blood flow in the left frontotemporal areas of the brain. Examination 4 years after onset revealed a shallow insight, poor verbal memory, and a fluent paraphasic aphasia characterized by frequent "lexical lacunes." When asked to point to the telephone or his wrist, for example, he looked puzzled, and wondered aloud what "wrist" or "point" might mean although his comprehension of most conversational speech was adequate. Visuospatial skills were preserved. The disease progressed rapidly and he died at the age of 50, 6 years after onset. The neuropathological examination showed numerous ubiquitin-positive Pick bodies and intense neuronal loss in the superficial cortical layers of limbic, temporal, and prefrontal cortex but not in parietal or occipital cortex. There were no NFT or amyloid plaques. This anatomical distribution of the pathology fits the combination of comportmental abnormalities, aphasia, and amnesia. The patient fulfills the clinical criteria for PRAD although he does not have AD.

The distribution of the pathology in Pick's disease varies from case to case but the prefrontal cortex and the anterior temporal lobes, including the mediotemporal limbic structures, are the most frequent sites of maximum pathology. Different anatomical patterns of neuropathology give rise to different clinical presentations.[65,258] Several clinicopathological patterns can be identified.

1. Neuropathology centered in the *prefrontal cortex, occasionally extending to anterior temporal cortex,* can give rise to a frontal network syndrome (the progressive comportmental/executive dysfunction profile) and fits the research criteria for POAD. In some of these patients the behavioral abnormalities may be quite dramatic and may involve hypersexuality, hyperorality, and dramatic disinhibition.

2. Neuropathology centered in the *perisylvian cortex of the language-dominant (usually left) hemisphere, and extending into the adjacent parts of the frontal and temporal lobes,* can give rise to the clinical profile of primary progressive aphasia and also fulfills the research criteria for POAD.

3. Neuropathology involving the *mediotemporal limbic structures to a greater extent than other parts of the cerebral cortex* can present with the profile of a progressive amnestic dysfunction and/or severe behavioral abnormalities.

4. Combinations of these three patterns give rise to mixtures of a frontal network syndrome, progressive aphasia and amnesia, as in the case of the patient described above.

Pick's disease shares many features with the focal atrophies and has, on occasion, been considered as a subtype of focal atrophy, but one which happens to have a specific histopathological marker. The possibility that sporadic focal atrophies as well as Pick's disease represent different manifestations of a primary tauopathy has been raised and is under intense scrutiny.

Diffuse (Cortical) Lewy Body Disease (DLBD)

Lewy bodies are intracellular, ubiquitin-positive, hyaline inclusions composed of phosphorylated neurofilaments rather than τ. They contain α-synuclein, a presynaptic protein of unknown function which is mutated in some familial forms of

Parkinson's disease.[246] Lewy bodies are seen in the substantia nigra of patients with idiopathic Parkinson's disease with or without dementia. They can also be seen in the cerebral cortex, especially in the parahippocampal gyrus, amygdala, insula, and cingulate cortex. These cortical Lewy bodies are less conspicuous than those seen in the substantia nigra, lack a halo, and usually require ubiquitin or α-synuclein immunocytochemistry for detection. They tend to be found in the small to medium-sized pyramidal neurons of deeper cortical layers, but almost always in low densities. When found in the cerebral cortex, they also tend to exist in additional subcortical regions such as the nucleus basalis of Meynert, the nucleus locus coeruleus, the midbrain raphe nuclei, and the hypothalamus.

Occasionally, cortical Lewy bodies are seen in demented patients who also have the pathology of AD, and this leads to a diagnosis of "AD with DLBD." In other demented patients, cortical Lewy bodies are seen in the presence of numerous Aβ plaques but without NFT, and this has been called the "Lewy body variant of AD."[102] In a third and relatively small group of demented patients, cortical and subcortical Lewy bodies are seen without other conspicuous histopathological lesions or significant focal atrophy. The term DLBD most appropriately applies to this third group of patients The depletion of cortical cholinergic innervation in DLBD can be even more severe than the one seen in AD.[57,65]

As in the case of all other primary degenerative dementias, the definitive diagnosis can only be made at autopsy. Age of onset is variable but is usually between 50 and 70. Onset can be slightly more abrupt than in AD and the rate of progression may be more rapid[197] or, in some patients, more indolent. When amnesia is salient, the initial clinical picture may fit the criteria for PRAD. In other patients, the most salient cognitive deficits tend to involve attention and executive functions rather than memory, giving rise to a picture that is reminiscent of a frontal network syndrome.

Three clinical features increase the likelihood that a patient has DLBD: (1) considerable fluctuations which may include days or even longer periods of apparent improvement or even normalcy, (2) prominent depression, hallucinations, and delusions at the initial stages of the disease, and (3) extrapyramidal deficits, ranging from mild hypomimia to frank parkinsonism, which become prominent early in the course of the disease The presence of these three features in a patient with primary dementia leads to a diagnosis of probable DLBD.[161] The following patient illustrates the clinical picture of a patient with the Lewy body variant of AD.

Case Reprot

(R. K.)   A 73-year-old businessman developed progressive memory difficulties, unstable gait, loss of facial expressiveness, visual hallucinations, and delusions. The problems fluctuated in intensity so that he would have some good days interspersed with bad days. Within 2 years of onset, he lost the ability to handle his business. Examination 3 years after onset revealed very poor insight and judgment, impaired concentration, an inability to maintain a coherent stream of thought, and an inability to inhibit premature responses. There was no aphasia or visuospatial deficit and only a mild problem with memory. He also displayed prominent hypomimia, hypophonia, shuffling gait, cogwheeling, and bilateral hyperreflexia. He died 3 years after disease onset at which time the neuropathological examination revealed Lewy bodies in the substantia nigra but also in the cerebral cortex, especially in the cingulate gyrus. The density of NFT was not at a level that warranted the additional diagnosis of AD but there were frequent neocortical plaques, consistent with the diagnosis of the Lewy body variant of AD.

The visual hallucinations may be associated with a monoaminergic–cholinergic imbalance in temporal neocortex.[211] The particularly severe cholinergic depletion suggests that cholinomimetic therapies may be particularly effective, but this has not yet been corroborated. The possibility that cholinomimetics can exacerbate the extrapyramidal symptoms of the patient needs to be entertained. The parkinsonian features do not respond well to dopaminergic therapies. The psychiatric symptoms may require treatment with antidepressants and sometimes with major tranquilizers. However, these patients are also unusually sensitive to typical as well as atypical neuroleptics. Such drugs may give rise to a prolonged worsening of the dementia and sometimes even to components of the neuroleptic malignant syndrome.[12]

Prion Diseases

Human prion diseases include Creutzfeldt-Jacob disease (CJD), Gerstmann-Sträussler-Scheinker syndrome (GSS), fatal familial insomnia (FFI), and kuru. They are all largely transmissible diseases characterized by the cerebral deposition of an abnormal protease-resistant isoform of a membrane-bound glycoprotein known as prion protein (PrP).[205] The GSS and FFI are predominantly hereditary syndromes linked to a PrP mutation, kuru is acquired by transmission, and CJD includes sporadic, familial, and transmitted (usually iatrogenic) forms.[205] Although familial CJD and FFI can both be linked to the same mutation at codon 178 of the PrP gene, the nature of a polymorphism at codon 129 determines whether the patients develop CJD or FFI, two syndromes with very different clinical pictures and neuropathologies.[206] Different polymorphisms at codon 129 are also associated with different clinical forms of sporadic CJD, such as the myoclonic, Heidenhain, and ataxic variants. Prion diseases such as CJD are usually associated with a precipitous course and tend to display prominent motor findings (such as myoclonus, ataxia, and startle) which help to distinguish them from other causes of primary dementia. However, some forms of CJD lead to relatively pure dementias which unfold over 1 or more years and which can have clinical similarities to PRAD, primary progressive aphasia, or progressive visuospatial dysfunction.[87,205,270] Definitive diagnosis can only be reached by biopsy or autopsy. Periodic complexes in the

EEG, occasionally considered diagnostic of CJD, may be absent in many of these patients.

IX. Vascular Dementia [Also Known As Multiinfarct Dementia (MID)]

Existing diagnostic criteria for vascular dementia (VaD) are both too restrictive and too permissive.[61,93,100,101,223] They are too restrictive because they require the presence of primary sensory–motor deficits to make a clinical diagnosis of "probable VaD." This would tend to eliminate patients who have strokes that do not involve sensory or motor function, a serious limitation since more than 90% of the cerebral hemispheres deal with mental rather than sensory–motor functions. Existing criteria are also too permissive because they would include patients with cognitive deficits caused by single "strategically located" strokes.

We prefer to use the term VaD in a more liberal and also more limited sense. We reserve the term for patients in whom cerebrovascular events (such as occlusive infarcts, intermittent ischemia, arteritis, abnormal vascular permeability, hypertensive vasculopathy, and perfusion deficits) constitute the predominant cause of a dementia-like clinical picture. A clinically identifiable stroke-like sensory–motor episode is not a necessary for the diagnosis of VaD since some cerebrovascular lesions, especially when small and confined to association areas or their white matter pathways, may remain "silent" with respect to consciously identifiable symptoms. We require a clinical state that approximates the definition of dementia in section III, except that periods of stability or transient improvement may be reported. We do not ordinarily use the diagnosis of VaD for single strokes even if they induce multiple cognitive impairments.

In some patients, the clinical picture of VaD can be identical to that of the other primary dementias reviewed earlier. The details of the clinical picture always reflect the anatomical distribution of the lesions. Involvement of mediotemporal limbic structures or nuclei of the limbic thalamus, for example, can give rise to salient memory deficits whereas bilateral subcortical lesions tend to impair comportment and executive functions because such lesions interfere with the coordinating functions of the prefrontal network. In fact, a "frontal network syndrome" is probably the single most common clinical picture of VaD even when there is no direct involvement of prefrontal cortex.

The clinical diagnosis of VaD becomes unlikely if sensitive neuroimaging modalities such as MRI with diffusion-weighted or fluid-attenuated inversion-recovery (FLAIR) sequences fail to show relevant lesions. The clinical diagnosis of VaD becomes increasingly more compelling if the distribution of the lesions fits the clinical picture, if there is a temporal relationship between the onset of the lesions and the clinical deficits, and if there is a stepwise pattern of worsening interspersed with periods of partial improvement. The definitive diagnosis can only be made at autopsy by establishing the presence of vascular lesions with an appropriate anatomical distribution and by excluding the presence of other dementia-causing pathological processes. Many elderly patients with features of VaD also have the microscopic lesions of AD. These patients fit the diagnosis of mixed AD with VaD. The following patient illustrates the clinical picture of VaD.

Case Report

(T. R.)   A 55-year old, nonhypertensive, right-handed salesperson successfully managed multimillion dollar accounts. His wife was caught by total surprise when she learned that he had been dismissed from work because of poor performance. It turned out that he had been warned (but did not tell his wife) about slipping performance and that he had squandered a small fortune gambling. The behavioral changes were attributed to psychological factors. Three months later he experienced a sudden and transient slurring of speech and left-sided weakness. An MRI showed bilateral "lacunar" infarcts in the basal ganglia and periventricular white matter, more on the right (Fig. 10–12). Six months later he had another event during which he felt "strange." A second MRI at that time revealed an additional subacute infarction in the left putamen. An extensive investigation did not reveal evidence for vascular occlusion, arteritis, or coagulopathy. His wife reported a gradual worsening of difficulties with cognition and comportment. He had not been able to organize a search for a new position, lost interest in golfing, started to soil his clothes, and was occasionally incontinent. Upon questioning, the patient showed no concern about his predicament and felt no remorse about his gambling. His performance was impaired in tests of working memory and cognitive flexibility (as assessed by the *Wisconsin Card Sorting Test*). Memory, language, and visuospatial skills were relatively preserved. Sensory and motor functions were nearly intact except for bilateral posturing during stressed gait. Although there is no postmortem examination, the young age of the patient makes it unlikely that he has the additional findings of AD. The bilateral multifocal distribution of the lesions and the involvement of the basal ganglia are consistent with the emergence of a frontal network syndrome.

Numerous cerebrovascular pathologies can be associated with VaD.[65] The most common setting is one of multiple cortical and subcortical occlusive infarcts associated with hypertension, heart disease, atherosclerosis, or diabetes. Amyloid angiopathy can lead to dementia, usually because it is associated with infarctions and bleeds. Myocardial disease, hypoglycemia, and hypoperfusion states may lead to a severe ischemia of the CA1 sector of the hippocampus and can cause a dementia-like picture with a prominent amnesia even when no specific episodes of arrest or hypotension can be documented.[268]

Binswanger's disease is another cause of VaD. This syndrome is associated with the hyalinization and thickening of arterioles, giving rise to ischemic and demyelinating lesions of the white matter. Contributing factors include hypertension, polycythemia, hyperlipedemia, and hyperviscosity.[40] Similar risk factors may also cause relatively isolated periventricular white matter lucencies, designated leu-

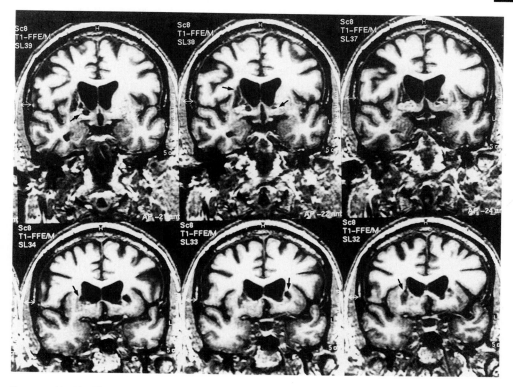

FIGURE 10–12. The magnetic resonance (MR) image of patient T. R. Arrows point to multiple bilateral infarctions which involve the putamen, caudate, basal forebrain, and anterior commissure. Some of these were clinically "silent" since the dementia predated any stroke-like episode. Even after all of these infarcts, the sensory–motor findings were minimal.

koaraiosis, which are being detected with increasing frequency in CT and MR scans of elderly subjects. These lucencies may influence cognitive function but are unlikely, by themselves, to be the primary cause of dementia.[203]

A genetic Binswanger-like vasculopathy that can lead to multiple white matter and basal ganglia lesions is the "cerebral autosomal dominant arteriopathy with subcortical infarcts and leukoencephalopathy" (CADASIL), caused by a mutation of the Notch 3 gene on chromosome 19.[226] The clinical spectrum of CADASIL is broad but includes isolated dementias with prominent comportmental, attentional, and executive dysfunction.[165] Neuroimaging with CT or MRI always shows abnormalities. In some patients, the clinical picture of CADASIL may be indistinguishable from any of the other primary dementias, including AD. In these patients, CADASIL represents the purest form of vascular dementia. The cerebral dysfunction in this syndrome may be caused by perfusion abnormalities which then cause neuronal and axonal dysfunction.[165] Research on this syndrome may be extremely productive for understanding the principles of vascular dementias. The full spectrum of VaD is in the process of being clarified. This is one type of dementia where a prevention of further progression can become a realistic goal.

X. Patient Care and Treatment in AD and Other Dementias

Dementias are not curable but they are treatable. The first goal is to reach a diagnosis according to the principles that were summarized earlier. A next step is to find substitutes for drugs that may have a deleterious effect on mental state. For example, β-blockers may be replaced with angiotensin-converting enzyme inhibitors for the control of hypertension, and drugs with anticholinergic effects (such as those used for Parkinson's disease or depression) may be substituted by those with less anticholinergic effects. If the clinical diagnosis favors AD, a subsequent step is to prescribe substances that may slow its progression. In patients where there are no contraindications, we recommend 1200–2000 units of vitamin E, 500 mg of vitamin C, ibuprofen (or naproxen), and estrogen replacement in postmenopausal women.

For patients who are thought to have AD or DLBD, we also recommend at least an initial trial on one of the existing cholinergic therapies at the highest recommended dose that can be tolerated. Tetrahydroaminoacridine (tacrine or Cognex) and donepezil (Aricept) are the first two cholinomimetic drugs that have been approved by the Food and Drug Administration (FDA) for the treatment of AD. Others that may soon become available include metrifonate, ENA 713 and galantamine. Each of these drugs works by inhibiting the hydrolysis of ACh by acetylcholinesterase so as to make more ACh available to the cerebral cortex. Relatively large clinical trials based on tacrine, donepezil, and metrifonate have been conducted for periods of up to 7 months. At the end of such trials the patients on the drugs had significantly better cognitive and behavioral scores than patients who were on placebo.[129,182,221] The differences, however, have been so modest (in the order of less than 2 points in the *MMSE*) that they would probably not be noticed by the family or the physician during a routine office visit. It is unclear whether these drugs offer only transient symptomatic relief, if they also influence the rate of disease progression, and if they can delay the transition from the stage of mild cognitive impairment to AD.

Donepezil is more convenient to administer than tacrine because it can be given in a single dose and because it does not require monitoring for hepatic toxicity. Side effects are usually confined to reversible nausea and diarrhea. Occasionally, adverse effects may include depression, tearfulness, rhinorrhea, and bradycardia. Despite the absence of dramatic (or even noticeable) benefits on these cholinergic agents, the decision to withdraw them is a difficult one to make since it is necessary to consider the possibility that the drug may be slowing disease progression. For reasons that have been described, it is extremely unlikely that cholinergic therapies will, by themselves, have a major impact on the course and symptomatology of AD. However, they may continue to play important adjunctive roles as part of more comprehensive therapeutic approaches that are likely to emerge in the future.

Patients with dementia may also develop insomnia, depression, hallucinations, delusions, agitation, and a number of additional disruptive behaviors. These symptoms can be treated very effectively with the appropriate hypnotic, antidepressant, anxiolytic, or tranquilizer drug. The patient with dementia is usually very sensitive to these drugs. They should therefore be initiated in very low doses. We prefer to use antidepressants with very low anticholinergic effects (such as desipramine or SSRIs), and to select major tranquilizers with relatively low extrapyramidal side effects (such as risperidone or olanzapine). For reasons that have been mentioned above, neuroleptics should not be given in DLBD unless absolutely necessary.

Circadian rhythm abnormalities are particularly common in dementia. Many patients experience excessive daytime sleepiness, take frequent naps, and remain awake for most of the night. Stimulants such as methylphenidate, pemoline, and modafinil may be very useful for keeping the patient awake during the day in order to promote more regular sleep during the night.

The approach to the patient with dementia should also address the devastating psychosocial impact of these diseases. Questions related to driving safety arise almost invariably. In early stages, driving to familiar places need not be curtailed. As the dementia progresses, however, it may no longer be safe to drive. Family members often request the physician to impose the restrictions in order to exonerate themselves from the difficult task of depriving the patient of an important source of independence. A formal road test may sometimes help the physician and family take a firm stand by introducing a greater measure of objectivity. When financial decisions can no longer be made or when the patient becomes vulnerable to predatory pressures with respect to finances, the issues of mental competence and durable power of attorney need to be raised.

The care of patients with dementia imposes formidable burdens on caregivers. Spouses who have been shielded from practical responsibility may have to assume the role of head of the household and children may take on the role of parenting. The clinical course may extend over many years. Each stage brings new limitations and new challenges. The patient's behavior may be misinterpreted as a deliberate display of hostility and may trigger a vicious cycle of anger and guilt on the part of the caregiver. The expertise of a clinical social worker can be called upon to help families deal with the required emotional adjustment, plan for current and future care, and identify resources that fit each stage of the disease, including adult day health programs, hired companions, homemaker services, hot meal programs, respite care, and assisted living. Genetic counseling is crucial for families with autosomal dominant dementias and should be offered prior to performing potentially definitive diagnostic tests.

When care at home is no longer feasible, the family needs to be assisted in the complex and emotionally demanding task of nursing home placement. Depression is endemic in the population of caregivers and should be treated. Support groups for caregivers may be very helpful for providing advice, dispelling the sense of uniqueness, and dealing with the anxiety. Helpful books have been written on how to face these problems.[150] The local chapters of the Alzheimer's Association have useful literature and can provide important advice which is also applicable to other less frequent forms of dementia.

XI. OVERVIEW AND CONCLUSIONS

Dementia is one of the most common syndromes encountered in the practice of behavioral neurology, neuropsychiatry, and neuropsychology. The behavioral deficits in dementia are subject to the same principles of anatomical correlation and neuropsychological assessment that govern all the other syndromes reviewed in this book. However, clinicopathological correlations are also more complex because of the partial nature of the lesions, their multifocal distribution, and their gradual progression. A cortical area targeted by a dementing disease is never destroyed completely but sustains damage to only some of its neurons, usually with some degree of selectivity for those of a certain type or in a certain layer. The effects of multiple lesions in dementia are not just additive but also include complex interactions. The slow temporal evolution may allow a greater degree of functional reorganization than is customary after acute lesions. These may be some of the reasons why the language deficits in PPA do not always fit the aphasia subtypes that are seen after cerebrovascular disease and why the memory disorders in AD do not necessarily display all the characteristic features of the amnestic syndrome seen after acute hippocampal lesions.

Dementias induce partial dysfunctions of individual neurocognitive networks and undermine their ability to interact coherently. A patient with a dementing disease may intermittently perform the basic functions of naming, object identification, and recall, but these fragments of cognition cannot be integrated with any degree of coherence, and the patient becomes lost and puzzled when the task requires more than a simple response. There is no such thing as a "typical" dementia. The deficits vary greatly from one type of dementia to another and reflect the past personality of the patient and the anatomical distribution of the underlying lesions to a greater degree than the identity of the causative disease. Thus, AD and Pick's disease may have nearly identical clinical manifestations if the NFT and Pick bodies have identical anatomical distributions, and very different clinical manifestations if the anatomical distribution of the two lesions are different. However, each dementia-causing disease also displays preferred anatomical predilection patterns so that the clinical profile of the patient tends to provide important clues concerning the identity of the underlying disease.

The dementia-causing diseases reviewed in this chapter are unique in that they selectively target the large-scale neural networks related to cognition and comportment. The NFT of AD, for example, have a predilection for the limbic system whereas Pick's disease and the focal abiotrophies can selectively invade the language, prefrontal, or visuospatial networks. The selectivities are remarkable: The spread and accumulation of NFT in AD can remain confined to the limbic system for many years, during which the clinical impact may be limited to memory dysfunction, and a focal degeneration can remain confined to the language network for an equally long period of time, during which the patient experiences a progressive deterioration almost entirely limited to language function. In some instances, such as the predilection of the limbic system for the NFT of AD, the determinant of selectivity may be the high burden of neuroplasticity characteristic of limbic neurons. In other cases, the nature of the factors that anchor the disease process to a single neurocognitive network remains to be elucidated.

There is a sense that Pick or Lewy bodies arise outside the normal flow of events and that they are markers of avoidable "diseases." Even this small comfort becomes uncertain in the case of AD. Is late-onset AD really a disease if its lesions are present in all aging brains? When does AD begin if its lesions appear decades before the onset of symptoms and what does this say about the likelihood of developing diagnostic or predictive tests?

Few prospects are as frightening as the gradual dissolution of mental faculties. The affectionate ties to family and friends, a lifetime's accumulation of passionate likes and dislikes, the complex fabric of individual remembrances are all gradually blurred and distorted as the patient is left with a body that appears healthy but a consciousness that is gradually stripped of its content. The toll that this process takes on the patient and family members is incalculable. Although the diseases that cause dementia are not yet curable or preventable, they are treatable in ways that can substantially improve the quality of life for the patient and caregivers. Early diagnosis, prevention, slowing of progression, and the development of more effective symptomatic treatments remain the principal goals of this field. Further advances toward the fulfillment of these goals will require rigorous integrative approaches that can successfully link the neurobiological bases of these diseases with their distinctive clinical manifestations.

This work was supported in part by AG 13854 from the National Institute on Aging (NIA) and NS 20285 from the National Institute for Neurological Disorders and Stroke (NINDS).

I thank my patients and their families, who willingly served the research enterprise even when they knew they were facing an incurable disease, and my colleagues, who contributed to the clinical care and diagnostic investigations. I also thank Sandra Weintraub, PhD, for a critical reading of this chapter and Angie Guillozet and Karen Hoyne for assistance with illustrations.

REFERENCES

1. Agnati, L F, Zoli, M, Biagini, G and Fuxe, K: Neuronal plasticity and ageing processes in the frame of the 'Red Queen Theory'. Acta Physiol Scand 145:301–309, 1992.
2. Alexander, G E, Furey, M L, Grady, C L, Pietrini, P, Brady, D R, Mentis, M J and Schapiro, M B: Association of premorbid intellectual function with cerebral metabolism in Alzheimer's disease: implications for a cognitive reserve hypothesis. Am J Psychiatry 154:165–172, 1997.
3. Almkvist, O, Basun, H, Wagner, S L, Rowe, B A, Wahlund, L-O and Lannfelt, L: Cerebrospinal fluid levels of a-secretase-cleaved soluble amyloid precursor protein mirror cognition in a Swedish family with Alzheimer disease and a gene mutation. Arch Neurol 54:641–644, 1997.
4. Alzheimer, A: Über einen eigenartigen schweren Erkrankungsprozess der Hirnrinde. Neurol Zbl 25:1134, 1906.
5. American Psychiatric Association: Diagnostic and Statistical Manual of Mental Disorders, DSM-IV. American Psychiatric Association, Washington, DC, 1994.

6. Arendt, T, Brückner, M K, Bigl, V and Marcova, L: Dendritic reorganization in the basal forebrain under degenerative conditions and its defects in Alzheimer's disease. III. The basal forebrain compared with other subcortical areas. J Comp Neurol 351:223–246, 1995.

7. Arendt, T, Brückner, M K, Gertz, H-J and Marcova, L: Cortical distribution of neurofibrillary tangles in Alzheimer's disease matches the pattern of neurons that retain their capacity of plastic remodeling in the adult brain. Neuroscience 83:991–1002, 1998.

8. Arendt, T, Schindler, C, Brückner, M K, Eschrich, K, Bigl, V, Zedlick, D and Marcova, L: Plastic neuronal remodeling is impaired in patients with Alzheimer's disease carrying apolipoprotein e4 allele. J Neurosci 17:516–529, 1997.

9. Arriagada, P V, Growdon, J H, Hedley-Whyte, E T and Hyman, B T: Neurofibrillary tangles but not senile plaques parallel duration and severity of Alzheimer's disease. Neurology 42:631–639, 1992.

10. Arriagada, P V, Marzloff, K and Hyman, B T: Distribution of Alzheimer-type pathologic changes in nondemented elderly individuals matches the pattern in Alheimer's disease. Neurology 42:1681–1688, 1992.

11. Auld, D S, Kar, S and Quirion, R: β-Amyloid peptides as direct cholinergic neuromodulators: a missing link? Trends Neurosci 21:43–49, 1998.

12. Ballard, C, Grace, J, McKeith, I and Holmes, C: Neuroleptic sensitivity in dementia with Lewy bodies and Alzheimer's disease. Lancet 351:1032–1033, 1998.

13. Banati, R B, Gehrmann, J, Czech, C, Monning, U, Jones, L L, Konig, G, Beyreuther, K and Kreutzberg, G W: Early and de novo synthesis of Alzheimer beta A4-amyloid precursor protein (APP) in activated microglia. Glia 9:199–210, 1993.

14. Barnes, C A and McNaughton, B L: Physiological compensation for loss of afferent synapses in rat hippocampal granule cells during senescence. J Physiol 309:473–485, 1980.

15. Baskerville, K A, Schweitzer, J B and Herron, P: Effects of cholinergic depletion on experience-dependent plasticity in the cortex of the rat. Neuroscience 80:1159–1169, 1997.

16. Basun, H, Almkvist, O, Axelman, K, Brun, A, Campbell, T A, Collinge, J, Forsell, C, Froelich, S, Wahlund, L-O, Wetterberg, L and Lannfelt, L: Clinical characteristics of a chromosome 17-linked rapidly progressive familial frontotemporal dementia. Arch Neurol 54:539–544, 1997.

17. Benowitz, L I, Perrone-Bizzozero, N I, Filkelstein, S P and Bird, E D: Localization of the growth-associated phosphoprotein GAP-43 (B-50, F1) in the human cerebral cortex. J Neurosci 9:990–995, 1989.

18. Berezovska, O, Xia, M Q and Hyman, B T: Notch is expressed in adult brain, is coexpressed with presenilin-1, and is altered in Alzheimer disease. J Neuropathol Exp Neurol 57:738–795, 1998.

19. Bird, T D: Genotypes, phenotypes, and frontotemporal dementia. Take your pick. Neurology 50:1526–1527, 1998.

20. Bird, T D, Wijsman, E M, Nochlin, D, Leehy, M, Sumi, S M, Payami, H, Poorkaj, P, Nemens, E, Rafkind, M and Schellenberg, G: Chromosome and hereditary dementia: linkage studies in three non-Alzheimer families and kindreds with late onset FAD. Neurology 48:949–954, 1997.

21. Black, J E, Polinsky, M and Greenough, W T: Progressive failure of cerebral angiogenesis supporting neural plasticity in aging rats. Neurobiol Age 10:353–358, 1989.

22. Bliss, T V and Collinridge, G L: A synaptic model of memory: long-term potentiation in the hippocampus. Nature 361:31–39, 1993.

23. Bobinski, M, Wegiel, J, Wisniewski, H M, Tarnawski, M, Reisberg, B, Mlodzik, B, De Leon, M J and Miller, D C: Atrophy of hippocampal formation subdivisions correlates with stage and duration of Alzheimer disease. Dementia 6:205–210, 1995.

24. Bondareff, W, Mountjoy, C Q, Roth, M and Hauser, D L: Neurofibrillary degeneration and neuronal loss in Alzheimer's disease. Neurobiol Age 10:709–715, 1989.

25. Braak, H and Braak, E: The human entorhinal cortex: normal morphology and lamina-specific pathology in various diseases. Neurosci Res 15:6–31, 1992.

26. Braak, H and Braak, E: Evolution of the neuropathology of Alzheimer's disease. Act Neurol Scand 165 (Suppl):3–12, 1996.

27. Braak, H and Braak, E: Frequency of stages of Alzheimer-related lesions in different age categories. Neurobiol Aging 18:351–357, 1997.

28. Brion, J-P, Octave, J N and Couck, A M: Distribution of the phosphorylated microtubule-associated protein tau in developing cortical neurons. Neuroscience 63:895–909, 1994.

29. Brown, J, Ashworth, A, Gydesen, S, Sorensen, A, Rossor, M, Hardy, J and Collinge, J: Familial non-specific dementia maps to chromosome 3. Hum Mol Genet 4:1625–1628, 1995.

30. Brun, A: Frontal lobe degeneration of non-Alzheimer type. I. Neuropathology. Arch of Gerontol and Geriatr 6:193–208, 1987.

31. Brun, A: Frontal lobe degeneration of non-Alzheimer type revisited. Dementia 4:126–131, 1993.

32. Buell, S J and Coleman, P D: Dendritic growth in the aged human brain and failure of growth in senile dementia. Science 206:854–856, 1979.

33. Busch, C, Bohl, J and Ohm, T G: Spatial, temporal and numeric analysis of Alzheimer changes in the nucleus coeruleus. Neurobiol Age 18:401–406, 1997.

34. Busciglio, J, Ferreira, A, Steward, O and Caceres, A: An immunocytochemical and biochemical study of the microtubule-associated protein tau during post-lesion afferent reorganization in the hippocampus of adult rats. Brain Res 419:244–252, 1987.

35. Busciglio, J, Hartmann, H, Lorenzo, A, Wong, C, Baumann, K, Sommer, B, Staufenbiel, M and Yankner, B A: Neuronal localization of presenilin-1 and association with amyloid plaques and neurofibrillary tangles in Alzheimer's disease. J Neurosci 17:5101–5107, 1997.

36. Butterfield, D A, Hansley, K, Hall, N, Subramaniam, R, Howard, B J, Cole, P, Yatin, S, Lafontaine, M, Harris, M E, Aksenova, M, Aksenov, M and Carney, J M: β-amyloid-derived free radical oxidation: a fundamental process in Alzheimer's disease. In Wasco, W and Tanzi, R E (Eds.): Molecular Mechanisms of Dementia. Humana Press, Totowa, NJ, pp. 145–167.

37. Calhoun, M E, Jucker, M, Martin, L J, Thinakaran, G, Price, D L and Mouton, P R: Comparative evaluation of synaptophysin-based methods for quantification of synapses. J Neurocytol 25:821–828, 1996.

38. Calhoun, M E, Wiederhold, K H, Abramowski, D, Phinney, A L, Probst, A, Sturchler-Pierrat, C, Staufenbiel, M, Sommer, B and Jucker, M: Neuron loss in APP transgenic mice. Nature 395:755–756, 1998.

39. Cambier, J, Masson, M, Dairou, R and Henin, D: A parietal form of Pick's disease: clinical and pathological study. Rev Neurol (Paris) 137:33–38, 1981.

40. Caplan, L: Binswanger's disease. Neurology 45:626–633, 1995.

41. Chawluk, J B, Mesulam, M M, Hurtig, H, Kushner, M, Weintraub, S, Saykin, A, Rubin, N, Alavi, A and Reivich, M: Slowly progressive aphasia without generalized dementia: studies with positron emission tomography. Ann Neurol 19:68–74, 1986.

42. Chin, S S-M, Goldman, J E, Devenand, D R, Mesulam, M-M and Weintraub, S: Thalamic degeneration presenting as primary progressive aphasia. Brain Pathol 4:515, 1994.

43. Convit, A, DeLeon, M J, Tarshish, C, DeSanti, S, Tsui, W, Rusinek, H and George, A: Specific hippocampal volume reductions in individuals at risk for Alzheimer's disease. Neurobiol Age 18:131–138, 1997.

44. Cotman, C W and Nieto-Sampedro, M: Cell biology of synaptic plasticity. Science 225: 1287–1294, 1984.

45. Critchley, M: The Parietal Lobes. Edward Arnold, London, 1953.

46. Croisile, B, Trillet, M, Hibert, O, Cinotti, L, Maugiere, F and Aimand, G: Désordres visuoconstructifs et alexie-agraphie associés à une atrophie corticale postérieure. Rev Neurol (Paris) 147:138–143, 1991.

47. Crystal, H A, Haroupian, D S, Katzman, R and Jotkowitz, S: Biopsy-proved Alzheimer's disease presenting as a parietal lobe syndrome. Ann Neurol 12:186–188, 1982.

48. Cummings, B J: Plaques and tangles: searching for primary events in a forest of data. Neurobiol Age 18:358–362, 1997.

49. Cummings, B J, Pike, C J, Shankle, R and Cotman, C W: β-amyloid deposition and other measures of neuropathology predict cognitive status in Alzheimer's disease. Neurobiol Age 17:921–933, 1996.

49a. Davis, D G, Schmitt, F A, Wekstein, D R, and Markesbery, W R: Alzheimer neupathologic alterations in aged cognitively normal subjects. J Neuropath Exper Neurol 58: 376–388, 1999.

49b. Davis, K L, Mohs, R C, Marin, D, Purohit, D P, Perl, D P, Lantz, M, Austin, G, and Haroutunian, V: Cholinergic markers in elderly patients with early signs of Alzheimer's disease. JAMA 281: 1401–1406, 1999.

50. Dawson, G R, Seabrook, G R, Zheng, H, Smith, D W, Grahan, S, O'Dowd, G, Bowery, B J, Boyce, S, Trumbauer, M E, Chen, H Y, Van Der Ploeg, L H T and Sirinathsinghji, DJS: Age-related cognitive deficits, impaired long-term potentiation and reduction in synaptic marker density in mice lacking the β-amyloid precursor protein. Neuroscience 90:1–13, 1999.

51. de la Monte, S M, Ghanbari, K, Frey, W H, Beheshti, I, Averback, P, Hauser, S L and Wands, J R: Characterization of the AD7C-NTP cDNA expression in Alzheimer's disease and measurement of a 41-kD protein in cerebrospinal fluid. J Clin Invest 100:3093–3104, 1997.

52. DeKosky, S T and Scheff, S W: Synapse loss in frontal cortex biopsies in Alzheimer's disease: correlation with cognitive severity. Ann Neurol 27:457–464, 1990.

53. Delacourte, A and Bueé, L: Normal and pathological tau proteins as factors for microtubule assembly. Int Rev Cytol 171:167–224, 1997.

54. Detoledo-Morrell, L, Sullivan, M P, Morrell, F, Wilson, R S, Bennett, D A and Spencer, S: Alzheimer's disease: in vivo detection of differential vulnerability of brain regions. Neurobiol Age 18:463–468, 1997.

55. Dickson, D W: Neurodegenerative diseases with cytoskeletal pathology: a biochemical classification. Ann Neurol 42:541–544, 1997.

56. Dickson, D W: The pathogenesis of senile plaques. J Neuropathol Exp Neurol 56:321–339, 1997.

57. Dickson, D W, Davies, P, Mayeux, R, Crystal, H, Horoupian, D S, Thompson, A and Goldman, J E: Diffuse Lewy body disease. Acta Neuropathol 75:8–15, 1987.

58. Dickson, D W, Horoupian, D S, Thal, L J, Davies, P, Walkley, S and Terry, R D: Kluver-Bucy syndrome and amyotrophic lateral sclerosis: a case report with biochemistry, morphometrics, and Golgi study. Neurology 36:1323–1329, 1986.

59. Didic, M, Chérif, A A, Gambarelli, D, Poncet, M and Boudouresques, J: A permanent pure amnestic syndrome of insidious onset related to Alzheimer's disease. Ann Neurol 43:526–530, 1998.

60. Double, K L, Halliday, G M, Kril, J J, Harasty, J A, Cullen, K, Brooks, W S, Creasey, H and Broe, G A: Topography of brain atrophy during normal aging and Alheimer's disease. Neurobiol Age 17:513–521, 1996.

61. Drachman, D A: New criteria for the diagnosis of vascular dementia: do we know enough yet? Neurology 43:243–245, 1993.

62. Duff, K: Alzheimer transgenic mouse models come of age. Trends Neurosci 20:279–280, 1997.

63. Eggerston, D E and Sima, A A F: Dementia with cerebral Lewy bodies: a meso-cortical dopaminergic deficit? Arch Neurol 43:524–527, 1896.

64. Emre, M, Geula, C, Ransil, B J and Mesulam, M-M: The acute neurotoxicity and effects upon cholinergic axons of intracerebrally injected beta-amyloid in the rat brain. Neurobiol Aging 13:553–559, 1992.

65. Esiri, M M, Hyman, B T, Beyreuther, K and Masters, C L: Ageing and dementia. In Graham, D I and Lantos, P L, (Eds.): Greenfield's Neuropathology, Vol. 2. Arnold, London, 1997, pp. 153–233.

66. Evans, D A, Funkenstein, H H, Albert, M S, Scherr, P A, Cook, N R, Chown, M J, Hebert, L E, Hennekens, C H and Taylor, J O: Prevalence of Alzheimer's disease in a community population of older persons. J Am Med Assoc 262:2551–2556, 1989.

67. Farrer, L A, Abraham, C R, Haines, J L, Rogaeva, E A, Song, Y, McGraw, W T, Brindle, N, Premkumar, S, Scott, W K, Yamaoka, L H, Saunders, A M, Roses, A D, Auerbach, S A, Sorbi, S, Duara, R, Pericak-Vance, M A and St. George-Hyslop, P H: Association between bleomycin hydrolase and Alzheimer's disease in Caucasians. Ann Neurol 44:808–811, 1998.

68. Ferreira, A and Caceres, A: Estrogen-enhanced neurite growth: evidence for a selective induction of tau and stable microtubules. J Neurosci 11:392–400, 1991.

69. Ferrer, I: Dementia of frontal type and amyotrophy. Behav Neurol 5:87–96, 1992.

70. Florence, S L, Taub, H B and Kaas, J H: Large-scale sprouting of cortical connections after peripheral injury in adult macaque monkeys. Science 282:1117–1121, 1998.

71. Fox, N C, Warrington, E K, Freeborough, P A, Hartikainen, P, Kennedy, A M, Stevens, J M and Rossor, M N: Presymptomatic hippocampal atrophy in Alzheimer's disease. A longitudinal MRI study. Brain 119:2001–2007, 1996.

72. Fox, N C, Warrington, E K, Seiffer, A L, Agnew, S K and Rossor, M N: Presymptomatic cognitive deficits in individuals at risk of familial Alzheimer's disease: A longitudinal prospective study. Brain 121:1631–1639, 1998.

73. Francis, P T, Holmes, C, Webster, M-T, Stratmann, G C, Procter, A W and Bowen, D M: Preliminary neurochemical findings in non-Alzheimer type revisited. Dementia 4:126–131, 1993.

74. Francis, P T, Palmer, A M, Sims, N R, Bowen, D M, Davison, A N, Esiri, M M, Neary, D, Snowden, J S and Wilcock, G K: Neurochemical studies of early-onset Alzheimer's disease. Possible influence on treatment. N Engl J Med 313:7–11, 1985.

75. Furukawa, K, Guo, Q, Schellenberg, G D and Mattson, M P: Presenilin-1 mutation alters NGF-induced neurite outgrowth, calcium homeostasis, and transcription factor (AP-1) activation in PC12 cells. J Neurosci Res 52:618–624, 1998.

76. Galasko, D, Clark, C, Chang, L, Miller, B, Green, R C, Motter, R and Seubert, P: Assessment of CSF levels of tau protein in mildly demented patients with Alzheimer's disease. Neurology 48:632–635, 1997.

77. Games, D, Adams, D, Alessandrini, R, Barbour, R, Berthelette, P, Blackwell, C, Carr, T, Clemens, J, Donaldson, T, Gillespie, F, Guido, T, Hagopian, S, Johnson-Wood, K, Khan, K, Lee, M, Leibowitz, P, Lieburg, I, Little, S, Masliah, E, McConlogue, L, Montoya-Zavala, M, Mucke, L, Paganini, L, Penniman, E, Power, M, Schenk, D, Seubert, P, Snyder, B, Soriano, F, Tan, H, Vitale, J, Wadsworth, S, Wolozin, B and Zhao, J: Alzheimer-type neuropathology in transgenic mice overexpressing V717F β-amyloid precursor protein. Nature 373:523–527, 1995.

78. Gates, G A, Karzon, R K, Garcia, P, Peterein, J, Storandt, M, Morris, J C and Miller, J P: Auditory dysfunction in aging and senile dementia of the Alzheimer type. Arch Neurol 52:626–634, 1995.

79. Geddes, J F, Vowles, G H, Robinson, S F and Sutcliffe, J C: Neurofibrillary tangles, but not Alzheimer-type pathology, in a young boxer. Neuropathol Appl Neurobiol 22:12–16, 1996.

80. Gehm, B D, McAndrews, J M, Chien, P-Y and Jameson, J L: Resveratrol, a polyphenolic compound found in grapes and wine, is an agonist for the estrogen receptor. Proc Natl Acad Sci USA 94:14138–14143, 1997.

81. Geinisman, Y, Morrell, F and deToledo-Morrell, L: Perforated synapses on double-headed dendritic spines: a possible structural substrate of synaptic plasticity. Brain Res 1988.

82. Gertz, H-J, Krüger, H, Patt, S and Cervos-Navarro, J: Tangle-bearing neurons show more extensive dendritic trees than tangle-free neurons in area CA1 of the hippocampus in Alzheimer's disease. Brain Res 548:260–266, 1990.

83. Geschwind, D, Karrim, J, Nelson, S F and Miller, B: The apolipoprotein E epsilon4 allele is not a significant risk factor for frontotemporal dementia. Ann Neurol 44:134–138, 1998.

84. Geula, C and Mesulam, M-M: Cholinergic systems and related neuropathological predilection patterns in Alzheimer disease. In Terry, R D, Katzman, R and Bick, K L (Eds.): Alzheimer Disease. Raven Press, New York, 1994, pp. 263–294.

85. Geula, C, Mesulam, M-M, Saroff, D M and Wu, C-K: Relationship between plaques, tangles, and loss of central cholinergic fibers in Alzheimer's disease. J Neuropathol Exp Neurol 57:63–75, 1998.

86. Geula, C and Mesulam, M-M: Cortical cholinergic fibers in aging and Alzheimer's disease: a morphometric study. Neuroscience 33:469–481, 1989.

87. Ghorayeb, I, Series, C, Parchi, P, Sawan, B, Guez, S, Laplanche, J L, Capellari, S, Gambetti, P and Vital, C: Creutzfeldt-Jakob disease with long duration and panencephalopathic lesions: Molecular analysis of one case. Neurology 51:271–274, 1998.

88. Giannakopoulos, P, Gold, G, Duc, M, Michel, J-P, Hof, P R and Bouras, C: Neuroanatomical correlates of visual agnosia in Alzheimer's disease. A clinicopathologic study. Neurology 52:71–77, 1999.

89. Giannakopoulos, P, Hof, P R, Michel, J-P, Guimon, J and Bouras, C: Cerebral cortex pathology in aging and Alzheimer's disease: a quantitative survey of large hospital-based geriatric and psychiatric cohorts. Brain Res Rev 25:217–245, 1998.

90. Gibbs, R B: Impairment of basal forebrain cholinergic neurons associated with aging and long-term loss of ovarian function. Exp Neurol 151:289–302, 1998.

91. Goedert, M, Crowther, R A and Spillantini, M G: Tau mutations cause frontotemporal dementias. Neuron 21:955–958, 1998.

92. Goedert, M, Trojanowski, J Q and Lee, V M Y: τ protein and the neurofibrillary pathology of Alzheimer's disease. In Wasco, W and Tanzi, R E (Eds.): Molecular Mechanisms of Dementia. Humana Press, Totowa, NJ, pp. 199–217.

93. Gold, G, Giannakopoulos, P, Montes-Paixao C, Jr, Hermann, F R, Mulligan, R, Michel, J P and Bouras, C: Sensitivity and specificity of newly proposed clinical criteria for possible vascular dementia. Neurology 49:690–694, 1997.

94. Gómez-Isla, T, Hollister, R, West, H, Mui, S, Growdon, J H, Petersen, R C, Parisi, J E and Hyman, B T: Neuronal loss correlates with but exceeds neurofibrillary tangles in Alzheimer's disease. Ann Neurol 41:17–24, 1997.

95. Gómez-Isla, T, Price, J L, McKeel Jr, D W and Morris, J C: Profound loss of layer II entorhinal cortex neurons occurs in very mild Alzheimer's disease. J Neurosci 16:4491–4500, 1996.

96. Graeber, M B, Kösel, S, Grasbon-Frodl, E, Möller, H J and Mehraein, P: Histopathology and APOE genotype of the first Alzheimer disease patient, Auguste D. Neurogenetics 1:223–228, 1998.

97. Greene, J D W, Patterson, K, Xuereb, J and Hodges, J R: Alzheimer disease and nonfluent progressive aphasia. Arch Neurol 53:1072–1079, 1996.

98. Guillozet, A, Smiley, J F, Mash, D C and Mesulam, M-M: The amyloid burden of the cerebral cortex in non-demented old age. Soc Neurosci Abstratcts 21:1478, 1995.

99. Guillozet, A L, Smiley, J F, Mash, D C and Mesulam, M-M: Butyrylcholinesterase in the life cycle of amyloid plaques. Ann Neurol 42:909–918, 1997.

100. Hachinski, V and Norris, J W: Vascular dementia: an obsolete concept. Curr Opin Neurol 7:3–4, 1994.

101. Hachinski, V C, Lassen, N A and Marshall, J: Multi-infarct dementia. A cause of mental deterioration in the elderly. Lancet ii:207–210, 1974.

102. Hansen, L A, Masliah, E, Galasko, D and Terry, R D: Plaque-only Alzheimer disease is usually the Lewy body variant and vice versa. J Neuropathol Exp Neurol 52:648–654, 1993.

103. Harasty, J A, Halliday, G M, Code, C and Brooks, W S: Quantification of cortical atrophy in a case of progressive fluent aphasia. Brain 119:181–190, 1996.

104. Hardy, J: Amyloid, the presenilins and Alzheimer's disease. Trends Neurosci 20:154–159, 1997.

105. Hardy, J, Duff, K, Hardy, K G, Periz-Tur, J and Hutton, M: Alzheimer's disease and related dementias: amyloid and its relationship to tau. Nat Neurosci 1:355–358, 1998.

106. Hatanpää, K, Brady, D R, Stoll, J, Rapoport, S I and Chandrasekaran, K: Neuronal activity and early neurofibrillary tangles in Alzheimer's disease. Ann Neurol 40:411–420, 1996.

107. Hauw, J-J, Uchihara, T, He, Y, Seilhean, D, Piette, F and Duyckaerts, C: The time course of lesions in the neocortex in ageing and Alzheimer's disease. In Iqbal, K, Winblad, B, Nishimura, T, Takeda, M and Wisniewski, H M, (Eds.): Alzheimer's Disease: Biology, Diagnosis and Therapeutics. John Wiley, New York 1997, pp. 239–246.

108. Heckers, S, Geula, C and Mesulam, M-M: Acetylcholinesterase-rich pyramidal neurons in Alzheimer's disease. Neurobiol Age 13:455–460, 1992.

109. Heutink, P, Stevens, M, Rizzu, P, Bakker, E, Kros, J M, Tibben, A, Niermeijer, M F, van Duijn, C M, Oostra, B A and van Swieten, J C: Hereditary frontotemporal dementia is linked to chromosome 17q21-q22: a genetic and clinicopathological study of three Dutch families. Ann Neurol 41:150–159, 1997.

110. Hof, P R, Bouras, C, Constantinidis, J and Morrison, J H: Selective disconnection of specific visual association pathways in cases of Alzheimer's disease presenting with Balint's syndrome. J Neuropathol Exp Neurol 49:168–194, 1990.

111. Hoff, P: Alzheimer and his time. In Berrios, G E and Freeman, H L (Eds.): Alzheimer and the Dementias. Royal Society of Medicine Services Limited, London, 1991, pp. 29–55.

112. Huber, G, Bailly, Y, Martin, J R, Mariani, J and Brugg, B: Synaptic β-amyloid precursor proteins increase with learning capacity in rats. Neuroscience 80:313–320, 1997.

113. Hyman, B T, Damasio, A R, Van Hoesen, G W and Barnes, C L: Alzheimer's disease: cell specific pathology isolates the hippocampal formation. Science 298:83–95, 1984.

114. Hyman, B T and Trojanowski, J Q: Editorial on consensus recommendations for the postmortem diagnosis of Alzheimer's disease from the National Institute on Aging and the Reagan Institute Working Group on Diagnostic Criteria for the Neuropathological Assessment of Alzheimer's Disease. J Neuropathol Exp Neurol 56:1095–1097, 1997.

115. Ishida, A, Furukawa, K, Keller, J N and Mattson, M P: Secreted form of β-amyloid precursor protein shifts the frequency dependency for induction of LTD, and enhances LTP in hippocampal slices. Neuroreport 8:2133–2137, 1997.

116. Itabashi, S, Arai, H, Matsui, T, Matsushita, S, Muramatsu, T, Higuchi, S, Trojanowski, J Q and Sasaki, H: Absence of association of α1-antichymotrypsin polymorphisms with Alzheimer's disease: a report on autopsy-confirmed cases Exp Neurol 151:237–240, 1998.

117. Jack, C R, Petersen, R C, X u, Y C, Waring, S C, O'Brien, P C, Tangalos, E G, Smith, G E, Ivnik, R J and Kokmen, E: Medial temporal atrophy on MRI in normal aging and very mild Alzheimer's disease Neurology 49:786–794, 1997.

118. Jobst, K A, Hindley, N J, King, E and Smith, A D: The diagnosis of Alzheimer's disease: a question of image? Journal of Clinical Psychiatry 55(Suppl):22–31, 1994.

119. Johnson, K A, Jones, K, Holman, B L, Becker, J A, Spiers, P A, Satlin, A and Albert, M S: Preclinical prediction of Alzheimer's disease using SPECT. Neurology 50:1563–1571, 1998.

120. Kaes, T: Die Grosshirnrinde des Menschen in ihren Massen und ihren Fasergehalt. Gustav Fischer, Jena, 1907.

121. Katzman, R: The prevalence and malignancy of Alzheimer disease. Arch Neurol 33:217–218, 1976.

122. Kawas, C, Resnick, S, Morrison, A, Brookmeyer, R, Corrada, M, Zonderman, A, Bacal, C, Lingle, D D and Metter, E: A prospective study of estrogen replacement therapy and the risk of developing Alzheimer's disease: the Baltimore longitudinal study of aging. Neurology 48:1517–1521, 1997.

123. Kelly, J F, Furukawa, K, Barger, S W, Rengen, M R, Mark, R J, Blanc, E M, Roth, G S and Mattson, M P: Amyloid β-peptide disrupts carbachol-induced muscarinic cholinergic signal transduction in cortical neurons. Proc Natl Acad Sci USA 93:6753–6758, 1996.

124. Kempermann, G, Brandon, E P and Gage, F H: Environmental stimulation of 129/SvJ mice causes increased cell proliferation and neurogenesis in the adult dentate gyrus. Curr Biol 8:939–942, 1998.

125. Khachaturian: The five-five, ten-ten plan for defeating Alzheimer's disease. Neurobiol Age 13:197–198, 1992.

126. Khachaturian, Z: Diagnosis of Alzheimer's disease. Arch Neurol 42:1097–1105, 1985.

127. Kihara, T, Shimohama, S, Sawaa, H, Kimura, J, Kume, T, Kochiyama, H, Maeda, T and Akaike, A: Nicotinic receptor stimulation protects neurons against β-amyloid toxicity. Ann Neurol 42:159–163, 1997.

128. Kilgard, M P and Merzenich, M M: Cortical map reorganization enabled by nucleus basalis activity. Science 279:1714–1718, 1998.

129. Knapp, M J, Knopman, D S, Solomon, P R, Pendlebury, W W, Davis, C S and Gracon, S I: A 30-week randomized controlled trial of high-dose tacrine in patients with Alzheimer's disease. J Am Med Assoc 271:985–991, 1994.

130. Knopman, D S: Overview of demetia lacking distinctive histology: pathological designation of a progressive dementia. Dementia 4:132–136, 1993.

131. Knopman, D S, Mastri, A R, Frey I I, W H, Sung, J H and Rustan, T: Dementia lacking distinctive histologic features: a common non-Alzheimer degenerative dementia. Neurology 40:251–256, 1990.

132. Kowall, N W and Beal, M F: Cortical somatostatin, neuropeptide Y, and NADPH diaphorase neurons: Normal anatomy and alterations in Alzheimer's disease. Ann Neurol 23:105–114, 1988.

133. Kraepelin, E: Lehrbuch der Psychiatrie. Barth, Leipzig, 1910.

134. Kral, V A: Senescent forgetfullness: benign and malignant. Can Med Assoc J 86:257–260, 1962.

135. Kuo, Y M, Emmerling, M R, Vigo-Pelfrey, C, Kasunic, T C, Kirkpatrick, J B, Murdoch, G H, Ball, M J and Roher, A E: Water-soluble abeta (N-40, N-42) oligomers in normal and Alzheimer disease brains. J Biol Chem 271:4077–4081, 1996.

136. Lambert, M P, Barlow, A K, Chromy, B, Edwards, C, Freed, R, Liosatos, M, Morgan, T E, Rozovsky, I, Trommer, B, Viola, K A, Wals, P, Zhang, C, Finch, C E, Krafft, G A and Klein, W L: Diffusible, nonfibrillar ligands derived from Aβ 1–42 are potent central nervous system neurotoxins. PNAS 95:6448–6453, 1998.

137. Lanahan, A, Lyford, G, Stevenson, G S, Worley, P F and Barnes, C A: Selective alteration of long-term potentiation-induced transcriptional response in hippocampus of aged, memory-impaired rats. J Neurosci 17:2876–2885, 1997.

138. Launer, L J, Scheltens, P, Lindeboom, J, Barkhof, F, Weinstein, H C and Jonker, C: Medial temporal lobe atrophy in an open population of very old persons: cognitive, brain atrophy, and sociomedical correlates. Neurology 45:747–752, 1995.

139. LeBars, P L, Katz, M M, Berman, N, Itil, T M, Freedman, A M and Schatzberg, A F: A placebo-controlled, double-blind, randomized trial of an extract of ginko biloba for dementia. J Am Med Assoc 278:1327–1332, 1997.

140. Lehmann, D J, Johnston, C and Smith, A: Synergy between the genes for butyrylcholinesterase K variant and apolipoprotein E4 in late-onset confirmed Alzheimer's disease. Hum Mol Genet 6:1933–1936, 1997.

141. Lendon, C L, Lynch, T, Norten, J, McKeel, D W, Busfield, F, Craddock, N, Chakraverty, S, Gopalakrishnan, G, Shears, S D, Grimmett, W, Wilhelmsen, K C, Hansen, L, Morris, J C and Goate, A M: Hereditary dysphasia disinhibition dementia. A frontotemporal dementia linked to 17q 21–22. Neurology 50:1546–1555, 1998.

142. Levitan, D, Doyle, T G, Brousseau, D, Lee, M K, Thinakaran, G, Slunt, H H, Sisodia, S S and Greenwald, I: Assessment of normal and mutant human presenilin function in *Caenorhabditis*. Proc Natl Acad Sci USA 93:14940–14944, 1996.

143. Levy-Lahad, E and Bird, T D: Genetic factors in Alzheimer's disease: a review of recent advances. Ann Neurol 40:829–840, 1996.

144. Lin, L-H, Bock, S, Carpenter, K, Rose, M and Norden, J J: Synthesis and transport of GAP-43 in entorhinal cortex of neurons and perforant pathway during lesion-induced sprouting and reactive synaptogenesis. Mol Brain Res 14:147–153, 1992.

145. Linn, R T, Wolf, P A, Bachman, D L, Knoefel, J E, Cobb, J L, Belanger, A J, Kaplan, E F and D'Agostino, R B: The 'preclinical phase' of probable Alzheimer's disease. A 13-year prospective study of the Framingham cohort. Arch Neurol 52:485–490, 1995.

146. Liu, X, Erikson, C and Brun, A: Cortical synaptic changes and gliosis in normal aging, Alzheimer's disease and frontal lobe degeneration. Dementia 7:128–134, 1996.

147. Liu, Y, Stern, Y, Chun, M R, Jacobs, D M, Yau, P and Goldman, J E: Pathological correlates of extrapyramidal signs in Alzheimer's disease. Ann Neurol 41:368–374, 1997.

148. Lorenzo, A, Diaz, H, Carrer, H and Caceres, A: Amygdala neurons in vitro: neurite growth and effects of estradiol. J Neurosci Res 33:418–435, 1992.

149. Lovestone, S and Reynolds, C H: The phosphorylation of tau: a critical stage in neuro-development and neurodegenerative processes. Neuroscience 78:309–324, 1997.

150. Mace, N L and Rabins, P V: The 36-Hour Day. The Johns Hopkins University Press, Baltimore, 1981.

151. Mackenzie, I R A, McLachlan, R S, Kubu, C S and Miller, L A: Prospective neuropsychological assessment of nondemented patients with biopsy proven senile plaques. Neurology 46:425–429, 1996.

152. Mackenzie, I R A and Munoz, D G: Nonsteroidal anti-inflammatory drug use and Alzheimer-type pathology in aging. Neurology 50:986–990, 1998.

153. Masliah, E, Mallory, M, Alford, M, Ge, N and Mucke, L: Abnormal synaptic regeneration in hAPP695 transgenic and APOE knockout mice. In Iqbal, K, Mortimer, J A, Winblad, B and Wisniewski, H M, (Eds.): Research Advances in Alzheimer's Disease and Related Disorders. John Wiley, New York, 1995, pp. 405–414.

154. Masliah, E, Mallory, M, Alford, M, Veinbergs, I and Roses, A D: Apolipoprotein E role in maintaining the integrity of the aging central nervous system. In Roses, A D Weisgraber, K. H. and Y. Christen (Eds.): Apolipoprotein E and Alzheimer's Disease. Springer-Verlag, Berlin, 1996, pp. 59–73.

155. Masliah, E, Mallory, M, Hansen, L, Alford, M, Albright, T, DeTeresa, R, Terry, R, Baudier, J and Saitoh, T: Patterns of aberrant sprouting in Alzheimer's disease. Neuron 6: 729–739, 1991.

156. Masliah, E, Mallory, M, Hansen, L, DeTeresa, R and Terry, R D: Quantitative synaptic alterations in the human neocortex during normal aging. Neurology 43:192–197, 1993.

157. Mayeux, R, Saunders, A M, Shea, S, Mirra, S, Evans, D, Roses, A D, Hyman, B T, Crain, B, Tang, M-X and Phelps, C H: Utility of the apolipoprotein E genotype in the diagnosis of Alzheimer's disease. N Engl J Med 338:506–511, 1998.

158. McClearn, G E, Johansson, B, Berg, S, Pedersen, N L, Ahern, F, Petrill, S A and Plomin, R: Sunstantial genetic influence on cognitive abilities in twins 80 or more years old. Science 276:1560–1563, 1997.

159. McDougall, G J: A review of screening instruments for assessing cognition and mental status in older adults. Nurse Practit 15:18–28, 1990.

160. McEwen, B S, Alves, S E, Bulloch, K and Weilan, N G: Ovarian steroids and the brain: implications for cognition and aging. Neurology 48(Suppl 7):S8-S15, 1997.

161. McKeith, L G, Galasko, D, Kosaka, K, Perry, E K, Dickson, D W, Hansen, L A, Salmon, P, Lowe, J, Mirra, S S, Byrne, E J, Lennox, G, Quinn, N P, Edwardson, J A, Ince, P G, Bergeron, C, Burns, A, Miller, B L, Lovestone, S, Collerton, D, Jansen, E N, Ballard, C, De Vos, R A, Wilcock, G K, Jellinger, K A and Perry, R H: Consensus guidelines for the clinical and pathological diagnosis of dementia with Lewy bodies (DLB): report of the consortium on DLB international workshop. Neurology 47:1113–1124, 1996.

162. McKhann, G, Drachman, D A, Folstein, M, Katzman, R, Price, D and Stadlan, E M: Clinical diagnosis of Alzheimer's disease. Neurology 34:939–944, 1984.

163. Mehler, M F, Horoupian, D S, Davies, P and Dickson, D W: Reduced somatostatin-like immuoreactivity in cerebral cortex in nonfamilial dysphasic dementia. Neurology 37: 1448–1453, 1987.

164. Melanson, M, Nalbantoglu, J, Berkovic, S, Melmed, C, Andermann, E, Roberts, L J, Carpenter, S, Snipes, G J and Andermann, F: Progressive myoclonus epilepsy in young adults with neuropathologic features of Alzheimer's disease. Neurology 49:1732–1733, 1997.

165. Mellies, J K, Bäumer, T, Müller, J A, Tournier-Lasserve, E, Chabriat, H, Knobloch, O, H. J., H, Goebel, H H, Wetzig, L and Haller, P: SPECT study of a German CADASIL family: a phenotype with migraine and progressive dementia only. Neurology 50:1715–1721, 1998.

166. Mesulam, M-M: The systems-level organization of cholinergic innervation in the cerebral cortex and its alterations in Alzheimer's disease. Prog Brain Res 109:285–298, 1996.

167. Mesulam, M-M: Some cholinergic themes related to Alzheimer's disease: synaptology of the nucleus basalis, location of m2 receptors, interactions with amyloid metabolism, and perturbatiuons of cortical plasticity J Physiol (Paris) 92:293–298, 1998.

168. Mesulam, M-M and Geula, C: Acetylcholinesterase-rich neurons of the human cerebral cortex: cytoarchitectonic and ontogenetic patterns of distribution. J Comp Neurol 306:193–220, 1991.

169. Mesulam, M-M and Geula, C: Butyrylcholinesterase reactivity differentiates the amyloid plaques of aging from those of dementia. Ann Neurol 36:722–727, 1994.

170. Mesulam, M-M, Johnson, N, Grujic, Z and Weintraub, S: Apolipoprotein E genotypes in primary progressive aphasia. Neurology 49:51–55, 1997.

171. Mesulam, M-M, Mufson, E J, Levey, A I and Wainer, B H: Cholinergic innervation of cortex by the basal forebrain: cytochemistry and cortical connections of the septal area, diagonal band nuclei, nucleus basalis (substantia innominata), and hypothalamus in the rhesus monkey. J Comp Neurol 214:170–197, 1983.

172. Mesulam, M-M and Weintraub, S: Spectrum of primary progressive aphasia. In Rossor, M N (Ed.): Unusual Dementias. Baillière Tindall, London, 1992, pp. 583–609.

173. Mesulam, M-M: Slowly progressive aphasia without generalized dementia. Ann Neurol 11:592–598, 1982.

174. Mesulam, M-M: Involutional and developmental implications of age-related neuronal changes: in search of an engram for wisdom. Neurobiol Aging 8:581–583, 1987.

175. Mesulam, M-M: Primary progressive aphasia—differentiation from Alzheimer's disease (editorial). Ann Neurol 22:533–534, 1987.

175a. Mesulam, M-M: Neuroplasticity failure in Alzheimer's disease: Bridging the gap between plaques and tangles. Neuron, in press, 1999.

176. Meziane, H, Dodart, J-C, Mathis, C, Little, S, Clemens, J, Paul, S M and Ungerer, A: Memory-enhancing effects of secreted forms of the β-amyloid precursor protein in normal and amnestic mice. Proc Natl Acad Sci USA 95:12683–12688, 1998.

177. Miller, B L, Chang, L, Mena, I, Boone, K and Lesser, I M: Progressive right frontotemporal degeneration: clinical, neuropsychological and SPECT characteristics. Dementia 4: 204–213, 1993.

178. Mirra, S S, Heyman, A, McKeel, D, Sumi, S M, Crain, B J, Brownlee, L M, Vogel, F S, Hughes, J P, van Belle, G and Berg, L: The Consortium to Establish a Registry for Alzheimer's Disease (CERAD). Part III. Standardization of the neuropathologic assessment of Alzheimer's disease. Neurology 41:479–486, 1991.

179. Mizutani, T and Kasahara, M: Hippocampal atrophy secondary to entorhinal cortical degeneration in Alzheimer-type dementia. Neurosci Lett 222:119–122, 1997.

180. Mori, N: Toward understanding of the molecular basis of loss of neuronal plasticity in ageing. Age Ageing 22:S5–18, 1993.

181. Morris, J C: Relationship of plaques and tangles to Alzheimer's disease phenotype. In Goate, A M and Ashall, F (Eds.): Pathobiology of Alzheimer's Disease. Academic Press, London, 1995, pp. 193–223.

182. Morris, J C, Cyrus, P A, Orazem, J, Mas, J, Bieber, F, Ruzicka, B B and Gulanski, B: Metrifonate benefits cognitive, behavioral, and global function in patients with Alzheimer's disease. Neurology 50:1222–1230, 1998.

183. Morris, J C, Heyman, A, Mohs, R C, Hughes, J P, van Belle, G, Fillenbaum, G, Mellits, E D and Clark, C: The consortium to establish a registry for Alzheimer's disease (CERAD). Part I. Clinical and neuropsychological assessment of Alzheimer's disease. Neurology 39: 1159–1165, 1989.

184. Morris, J C, Storandt, M, McKeel Jr., D W, Rubin, E H, Price, J L, Grant, E A and Berg, L: Cerebral amyloid deposition and diffuse plaques in "normal" aging: evidence for presymptomatic and very mild Alzheimer's disease. Neurology 46:707–719, 1996.

185. Morrison, J H and Hof, P R: Life and death of neurons in the aging brain. Science 278: 412–419, 1997.

186. Motter, R, Vigo-Pelfrey, C, Kholodenko, D, Barbour, R, Johnson-Wood, K, Galasko, D, Chang, L, Miller, B, Clark, C, Green, R, Olson, D, Southwick, P, Wolfert, R, Munroe, B, Lieberburg, I, Seubert, P and Schenk, D: Reduction of β-amyloid peptide42 in the cerebrospinal fluid of patients with Alzheimer's disease. Ann Neurol 38:643–648, 1995.

187. Mucke, L, Masliah, E, Johnson, W B, Ruppe, M D, Alford, M, Rockenstein, E M, Forss-Petter, S, Pietropaolo, M, Mallory, M and Abraham, C R: Synaptotrophic effects of human amyloid β protein precursors in the cortex of transgenic mice. Brain Res 666:151–167, 1994.

188. Mueller, E A, Moore, M M, Kerr, D C R, Sexton, G, Camicioli, R M, Howieson, D B, Quinn, J F and Kaye, J A: Brain volume preserved in healthy elderly through the eleventh decade. Neurology 51:1555–1562, 1998.

189. Nathan, B P, Bellosta, S, Sanan, D A, Weisgraber, K H, Mahley, R W and Pitas, R E: Differential effects of apolipoproteins E3 and E4 on neuronal growth in vitro. Science 264: 850–852, 1994.

190. Neary, D, Brun, A, Englund, B, Gustafson, L, Passant, U, Mann, D M A and Snowden, J S: Clinical and neuropathological criteria for frontotemporal dementia. J Neurol Neurosurg Psychiatry 57:416–418, 1994.

191. Neary, D, Snowden, J S, Gustafson, L, Passant, U, Stuss, D, Black, S, Freedman, M, Kertesz, A, Robert, P H, Albert, M, Boone, K, Miller, B L, Cummings, J and Benson, D F: Frontotemporal lobar degeneration. A consensus on clinical diagnostic criteria. Neurology 51:1546–1554, 1998.

192. Neill, D: Alzheimer's disease: maladaptive synaptoplasticity hypothesis. Neurodegeneration 4:217–232, 1995.

193. Neve, R L, Finch, E A, Bird, E D and Benowitz, L I: Growth-associated protein GAP-43 is expressed selectively in associative regions of the adult human brain. Proc Natl Acad Sci USA 85:3638–3642, 1988.

194. NIA: Consensus recommendations for the postmortem diagnosis of Alzheimer's disease. Neurobiol Age 18:S1-S2, 1997.

195. Nitsch, R M, Slack, B E, Wurtman, R J and Growdon, J H: Release of Alzheimer amyloid precursor derivatives stimulated by activation of muscarinic acetylcholine receptors. Science 258:304–307, 1992.

196. Nordin, S, Almkvist, O, Berglund, B and Wahlund, L-O: Olfactory dysfunction for pyridine and dementia progression in Alzheimer's disease. Arch Neurol 54:993–998, 1997.

197. Olichney, J M, Galasko, D, Salmon, D P, Hofstetter, C R, Hansen, L A, Katzman, R and Zhal, L J: Cognitive decline is faster in Leny body variant than in Alzheimer's disease. Neurology 51:351–357, 1998.

198. Olichney, J M, Hansen, L A, Galasko, D, Saitoh, T, Hofstetter, C R, Katzman, R and Thal, L J: The apolipoprotein E ε4 allele is associated with increased neuritic plaques and ce-

rebral amyloid angiopathy in Alzheimer's disease and Lewy body variant. Neurology 47: 190–196, 1996.

199. Orgogozo, J-M, Dartigues, J-F, Lafont, S, Letenneur, L, Commenges, D, Salamon, R, Renaud, S and Breteler, M B: Wine consumption and dementia in the elderly: a prospective community study in the Bordeaux area. Rev Neurol (Paris) 153:185–192, 1997.

200. Otsuki, M, Soma, Y, Sato, M, Homma, A and Tsuji, S: Slowly progressive pure word deafness. Eur Neurol 39:135–140, 1998.

201. Pakkenberg, B and Gundersen, H J G: Neocortical neuron number in humans: effect of sex and age. J Comp Neurol 384:312–320, 1997.

202. Palmert, M R, Usiak, M, Mayeux, R, Raskind, M, Tourtelotte, W W and Younkin, S G: Soluble derivatives of the beta amyloid protein precursor in cerebrospinal fluid: alterations in normal aging and in Alzheimer's disease. Neurology 40:1028–1034, 1990.

203. Pantoni, L and Garcia, J H: Pathogenesis of leukoaraiosis: a review. Stroke 28:652–659, 1997.

204. Pappolla, M A, Sos, M, Omar, R A, Bick, R J, Hickson-Bick, D L M, Reiter, R J, Efthimiopoulos, S and Robakis, N K: Melatonin prevents death of neuroblastoma cells exposed to the Alzheimer amyloid peptide. J Neurosci 17:1683–1690, 1997.

205. Parchi, P, Castellani, R, Capellari, S, Ghetti, B, Young, K, Chen, S G, Farlow, M, Dickson, D W, Sima, A A F, Trojanowski, J Q, Petersen, R B and Gambetti, P: Molecular basis of phenotypic variability in sporadic Creutzfeldt-Jakob disease. Ann Neurol 39:767–778, 1996.

206. Parchi, P, Petersen, R B, Chen, S G, Autilio-Gambetti, L, Capellari, S, Monari, L, Cortelli, P, Lugaresi, E and Gambetti, P: Molecular pathology of fatal familial insomnia. Brain Pathol 8:539–548, 1998.

207. Pasquier, F and Delacourte, A: Non-Alzheimer degenerative dementias. Current Opin Neurol 11:417–427, 1998.

208. Peavy, G M, Herzog, A G, Rubin, N P and Mesulam, M-M: Neuropsychological aspects of dementia of motor neuron disease: a report of two cases. Neurology 42:1004–1008, 1992.

209. Pedersen, W A, Kloczewiak, M A and Blusztajn, J K: Amyloid β-protein reduces acetylcholine synthesis in a cell line derived from cholinergic neurons of the basal forebrain. Proc Natl Acad Sci USA 93:8068–8071, 1996.

210. Pericek-Vance, M A, Bass, M P, Yamaoka, L H, Gaskell, P C, Scott, W K, Terwedow, H A, Menold, M M, Conneally, P M, Small, G W, Vance, J M, Saunders, A M, Roses, A D and Haines, J L: Complete genomic screen in late-onset familial Alzheimer's disease. Evidence for a new locus on chromosome 12. J Am Med Assoc 278:1282–1283, 1997.

211. Perry, E K, Marshall, E, Kerwin, J, Smith, C J, Jabeen, S, Cheng, A V and Perry, R H: Evidence of a monoaminergic-cholinergic imbalance related to visual hallucinations in Lewy body dementia. J Neurochem 55:1454–1456, 1990.

212. Peters, A, Morrison, J H, Rosene, D and Hyman, B T: Are neurons lost from the primate cerebral cortex during normal aging? Cereb Cortex 8:295–300, 1998.

213. Petersen, R C, Smith, G E, Waring, S C, Ivnik, R J, Tangalos, E G and Kokmen, E: Mild cognitive impairment. Clinical characterization and outcome. Arch Neurol 56:303–308, 1999.

214. Phelps, C H: Neural plasticity in aging and Alzheimer's disease: some selected comments. Prog Brain Res 86:3–9, 1990.

215. Poirier, J: Apolipoprotein E in animal models of CNS injury and in Alzheimer's disease. Trends Neuroscience 17:525–530, 1994.

216. Price, B H, Gurvit, H, Weintraub, S, Geula, C, Leimkuhler, E and Mesulam, M-M: Neuropsychological patterns and language deficits in 20 consecutive cases of autopsy-confirmed Alzheimer's disease. Arch Neurol 50:931–937, 1993.

217. Rasmusson, D X, Brandt, J, Steele, C, Hedreen, J C, Troncoso, J C and Folstein, M F: Accuracy of clinical diagnosis of Alzheimer disease and clinical features of patients with non-Alzheimer disease neuropathology. Alzheimer Dis Related Disord 10:180–188, 1996.

218. Raz, N, Gunning, F M, Head, D, Dupuis, J H, McQuain, J, Briggs, S D, Loken, W J,

Thornton, A E and Acker, J D: Selective aging of the human cerebral cortex observed in vivo: differential vulnerability of the prefrontal gray matter. Cereb Cortex 7:268–282, 1997.

219. Ritchie, K: Establishing the limits of normal cerebral aging and senile dementias. Br J Psychiatry 172:40–44, 1998.

220. Roch, J-M, Masliah, E, Roch-Levecq, A-C, Sundsmo, M P, Otero, D A C, Veinbergs, I and Saitoh, T: Increase of synaptic density and memory retention by a peptide representing the trophic domain of the amyloid β/A4 protein precursor. Proc Natl Acad Sci (USA) 91:7450–7454, 1994.

220a. Rogers, J, and O'Burr, S: O'Barr, S and Rogers, J: Inflammatory mediators in Alzheimer's disease. In Wasco, W and Tanzi, R E (Eds.): Molecular Mechanisms of Dementia. Humana Press, Totowa, NJ, 1997, pp. 177–198.

221. Rogers, S L, Farlow, M R, Doody, R S, Mohs, R and Friedhoff, L T: A 24-week, double-blind, placebo-controlled trial of donepezil in patients with Alzheimer's disease. Neurology 50:136–145, 1998.

222. Roher, A E, Ball, M J, Bhave, S V and Wakade, A R: β-amyloid from Alzheimer disease brains inhibit sprouting and survival of sympathetic neurons. Biochem Biophys Res Commun 174:572–579, 1991.

223. Roman, G C, Tatemichi, T K, Erkinjuntti, T, Cummings, J L, Masdeu, J C, Garcia, J H, Amaducci, L, Orgogozo, J-M, Brun, A, Hofman, A, Moody, D M, O'Brien, M D, Yamaguchi, T, Grafman, J, Drayer, B P, Bennett, D A, Fisher, M, Ogata, J, Kokmen, E, Bermejo, F, Wolf, P A, Gorelick, P B, Bick, K L, Pajeau, A K, Bell, M A, DeCarli, C, Culebras, A, Korczyn, A D, Bogousslavsky, J, Hartmann, A and Scheinberg, P: Vascular dementia: diagnostic criteria for research studies. Report of the NINDS-AIREN international workshop. Neurology 43:250–260, 1993.

224. Roses, A D: The predictive value of APOE genotyping in the early diagnosis of dementia of the Alzheimer type: data from three independent series. In Iqbal, K, Winblad, B, Nishimura, T, Takeda, M and Wisniewski, H M (Eds.): Alzheimer's Disease: Biology, Diagnosis and Therapeutics. John Wiley, New York, 1997, pp. 85–91.

225. Ross, G W, Benson, D F, Verity, A M and Victoroff, J I: Posterior cortical atrophy: neuropathological correlations. Neurology 40(Suppl 1):200, 1990.

226. Ruchoux, M-M and Maurage, C-A: CADASIL: cerebral autosomal dominant arteriopathy with subcortical infarcts and leukoencephalopathy. J Neuroathol Exp Neurol 56:947–964, 1997.

227. Rumble, B, Retallack, R, Hilbich, C, Simms, G, Multhaup, G, Martins, R, Hockey, A, Montgomery, P, Beyreuther, K and Masters, C L: Amyloid A4 protein and its precursor in Down's syndrome and Alzheimer's disease. N Engl J Med 320:1446–1452, 1989.

228. Sadun, A A, Borchert, M, DeVita, E, Hinton, D R and Bassi, C J: Assessment of visual impairment in patients with Alzheimer's disease. Am J Ophthalmol 104:113–120, 1987.

229. Salehi, A, Ravid, R, Gonatas, N K and Swaab, D F: Decreased activity of hippocampal neurons in Alzheimer's disease is not related to the presence of neurofibrillary tangles. J Neuropathol Exp Neurol 54:704–709, 1995.

230. Salib, E and Hillier, V: Head injury and the risk of Alzheimer's disease: a case control study. Int J Geriatr Psychiatry 12:363–368, 1997.

231. Sano, M, Ernesto, C, Thomas, R G, Klauber, M R, Schafer, K, Grundman, M, Woodbury, P, Growdon, J, Cotman, C W, Pfeiffer, E, Schneider, L S and Thal, L J: A controlled trial of selegiline, alpha-tocopherol, or both as treatment for Alzheimer's disease. The Alzheimer's Disease Cooperative Study. N Engl J Med 336:1216–1222, 1997.

232. Saunders, A M, Hulette, C, Welsh-Bohmer, K A, Schmechel, D E, Crain, B, Burke, J R, Alberts, M J, Strittmatter, W J, Breitner, J C R, Rosenberg, C, Scott, S V, Gaskell, P C J, Pericak-Vance, M A and Roses, A D: Specificity, sensitivity, and predictive value of apolipoprotein-E genotyping for sporadic Alzheimer's disease. Lancet 348:90–93, 1996.

233. Schaie, K W and Willis, S L: Adult personality and psychomotor performance: cross-sectional and longitudinal analyses. J Gerontol 46:275–284, 1991.

234. Scheff, S W, Bernardo, L S and Cotman, C W: Decline in reactive fiber growth in the dentate gyrus of aged rats as compared to young adult rats following entorhinal cortex removal. Brain Res 199:21–38, 1980.

235. Scheibel, A B and Tomiyasu, U: Dendritic sprouting in Alzheimer's presenile dementia. Exp Neurol 60:1–8, 1978.

236. Schmidt, M L, Lee, VM-Y, Forman, M, Chiu, T-S and Trojanowski, J Q: Monoclonal antibodies to a 100-kd protein reveal abumdant Aβ-negative plaques throughout gray matter of Alzheimer's disease. Am J Pathol 151:69–80, 1997.

237. Schröder, H, Giacobini, E, Struble, R G, Luiten, P G M, VanDerZee, E A, Zilles, K and Strosberg, A D: Muscarinic cholinoceptive neurons in the frontal cortex in Alzheimer's disease. Brain Res Bull 27:631–636, 1991.

238. Scinto, L, Daffner, K, Dressler, D, Ransil, B, Rentz, D, Weintraub, S, Mesulam, M-M and Potter, H: A potential non-invasive neurobiological test for Alzheimer's disease. Science 266:1051–1054, 1994.

239. Selden, N, Geula, C and Mesulam, M-M: Distribution of neurofibrillary tangles in Alzheimer's disease striatum. Soc Neurosci Abstr 19:1041, 1993.

240. Selkoe, D J: Alzheimer's disease: a central role for amyloid. J Neuropathol Exp Neurol 53:438–447, 1994.

241. Simmons, L K, May, P C, Tomaselli, K J, Rydel, R E, Fuson, K S, Brigham, E F, Wright, S, Lieberburg, I, Becker, G W and Brems, D N: Secondary structure of amyloid beta peptide correlates with neurotoxic activity in vitro. Mol Pharmacol 45:373–379, 1994.

242. Singleton, A B, Smith, G, Gibson, A M, Woodward, R, Perry, R H, Ince, P G, Edwardson, J A and Morris, C M: No association between the K variant of the butyrylcholinesterase gene and pathologically confirmed Alzheimer's disease. Hum Mol Genet 7:937–939, 1998.

243. Small, D H: The role of the amyloid precursor (APP) in Alzheimer's disease: does the normal function of APP explain the topography of neurodegeneration? Neurochem Res 23:795–806, 1998.

244. Snowden, J S, Goulding, P J and Neary, D: Semantic dementia: a form of circumscribed atrophy. Behav Neurol 2:167–182, 1989.

245. Snowdon, D A, Greiner, L H, Mortimer, J A, Riley, K P, Greiner, P A and Markesbery, W R: Brain infarction and the clinical expression of Alzheimer's disease. The nun study. J Am Med Assoc 277:813–817, 1997.

246. Spilantini, M G, Schmdit, M L, Lee, VM-Y, Trojanowski, J Q, Jakes, R and Goedert, M: α-Synuclein in Lewy bodies. Nature 388:839–840, 1997.

247. Stevens, M, van Duijn, C M, Kamphorst, W, de Knijff, P, Heutink, P, van Gool, W A, Scheltens, P, Ravid, R, Oostra, B A, Niermeijer, M F and van Swieten, J C: Familial aggregation in frontotemporal dementia. Neurology 50:1541–1545, 1998.

248. Stewart, W F, Kawas, C, Corrada, M and Metter, E J: Risk of Alzheimer's disease and duration of NSAID use. Neurology 48:626–632, 1997.

249. Stone, D J, Rozovsky, I, Morgan, T E, Anderson, C P and Finch, C E: Increased synaptic sprouting in response to estrogen via an apolipoprotein E-dependent mechanism: implications for Alzheimer's disease. J Neurosci 18:3180–3185, 1998.

250. Storey, E, Beyreuther, K and Masters, C L: Alzheimer's disease amyloid precursor protein on the surface of cortical neurons in primary culture co-localizes with adhesion patch components. Brain Res 735:217–231, 1996.

251. Strittmatter, W J and Roses, A D: Apoliproprotein E and Alzheimer's disease. Ann Rev Neurosci 19:53–77, 1996.

252. Sturchler-Pierrat, C, Abramowski, D, Duke, M, Wiederhold, K-H, Mistl, C, Rothacher, S, Liedermann, B, Bürki, K, Frey, P, Paganetti, P A, Waridel, C, Calhoun, M E, Jucker, M, Probst, A, Staufenbiel, M and Sommer, B: Two amyloid precursor protein transgenic mouse models with Alzheimer disease-like pathology. Proc Natl Acad Sci USA 94:13287–13292, 1997.

253. Takashima, S, Ieshima, A, Nakamura, H and Becker, L E: Dendrites, dementia and the Down syndrome. Brain Dev 11:131–133, 1989.

254. Tanimukai, H, Imaizumi, K, Kudo, T., Katayama, T, Tsuda, M, Takagi, T, Tohyama, M and Takada, M: Alzheimer-associated presenilin-1 gene is induced in gerbil hippocampus after transient ischemia. Molecular Brain Research 54:212–218, 1998.

255. Terry, R D: Dementia: a brief and selective review. Arch Neurol 33:1–4, 1976.

256. Terry, R D, Masliah, E, Salmon, D P, Butters, N, DeTeresa, R, Hill, R, Hansen, L A and Katzman, R: Physical basis of cognitive alterations in Alzheimer's disease: synapse loss is the major correlate of cognitive impairment. Ann Neurol 30:572–580, 1991.

257. Thompson, C K, Ballard, K J, Tait, M E, Weintraub, S and Mesulam, M-M: Patterns of language decline in non-fluent primary progressive aphasia. Aphasiology 11:297–321, 1997.

258. Tissot, R, Constantinidis, J and Richard, J: La Maladie de Pick. Masson, Paris, 1975.

259. Tokuda, T, Ikeda, S, Yanagisawa, N, Ihara, Y and Glenner, G G: Re-examination of ex-boxer's brains using immunohistochemistry with antibodies to amyloid beta-protein and tau protein. Acta Neuropathol 82:280–285, 1991.

260. Tolnay, M and Probst, A: Frotal lobe degeneration: novel ubiquitin-immunoreactive neurites within frontotemporal cortex. Neuropathol Appl Neurobiol 21:492–497, 1995.

261. Trojanowski, J Q, Schmidt, M L, Shin, R-W, Bramblett, G T, Goedert, M and Lee, V M-Y: From pathological marker to potential mediator of neuronal dysfunction and degeneration in Alzheimer's disease. Clin Neurosci 1:184–191, 1993.

262. Turner, R S, Kenyon, L C, Trojanowski, J Q, Gonatas, N and Grossman, M: Clinical, neuroimaging, and pathologic features of progressive nonfluent aphasia. Ann Neurol 39: 166–173, 1996.

263. Tyrrell, P J, Warrington, E K, Frackowiak, R S and Rossor, M N: Heterogeneity in progressive aphasia due to focal cortical atrophy. A clinical and PET study. Brain 113:1321–1336, 1990.

264. Tyrrell, P J, Warrington, E K, Frackowiak, R S J and Rossor, M N: Progressive degeneration of the right temporal lobe studied with positron emission tomography. J Neurol, Neurosurg Psychiatry 53:1046–1050, 1990.

265. van Gool, W A, Schenk, D B and Bolhuis, P A: Concentrations of beta-amyloid protein in cerebrospinal fluid increase with age in patients free from neurodegenerative disease. Neurosci Lett 172:122–124, 1994.

266. Vickers, J C: A cellular mechanism for the neuronal changes underlying Alzheimer's disease. Neuroscience 78:629–639, 1997.

267. Viereck, C, Tucker, R P and Matus, A: The adult rat olfactory system expresses microtubule-associated proteins found in the developing brain. J Neurosci 9:3547–3557, 1989.

268. Volpe, B T and Petito, C K: Dementia with bilateral medial temporal lobe ischemia. Neurology 35:1793–1797, 1985.

268a. Voytko, M L, Olton, D S, Richardson, R T, Gorman, L K, Tobin, J R and Price, D L: Basal prebrain lesions in monkeys disrupt attention but not learning and memory. J. Neurosci. 14: 167–186, 1994.

269. Weintraub, S and Mesulam, M-M: Four neuropsychological profiles in dementia. In Boller, F and Grafman, J (Eds.): Handbook of Neuropsychology, Vol. 8. Elsevier, Amsterdam, 1993, pp. 253–281.

270. Weintraub, S and Mesulam, M-M: From neuronal networks to dementia: four clinical profiles. In Fôret, F, Christen, Y and Boller, F (Eds.): *La Demence: Pourquoi?* Foundation Nationale de Gerontologie, Paris, 1996, pp. 75–97.

271. Weintraub, S, Powell, D H and Whitla, D K: Successful cognitive aging: individual differences among physicians on a computerized test ofmental state. J Geriatr Psychiatry 28: 15–34, 1994.

272. Weintraub, S, Rubin, N P and Mesulam, M-M: Primary progressive aphasia. Longitudinal course, neuropsychological profile, and language features. Arch Neurol 47:1329–1335, 1990.

273. Westbury, C and Bub, D: Primary progressive aphasia: a review of 112 cases. Brain Language 60:381–406, 1997.

274. Williams, J D and Klug, M G: Aging and cognition: methodological differences in outcome. Exp Aging Res 22:219–244, 1996.

274a. Wolfe, M S, Xia, W, Ostaszewski, B L, Diehl, T S, Kimberly, W T, and Selkoe, D J: Two transmembrane aspartases in presenilin-1 required for presenilin endoproteolysis and gamma-secretase activity. Nature 398: 513–517, 1999.

275. Woolley, C S, Wenzel, H J and Schwartzkroin, P A: Estradiol increases the frequency of multiple synapse boutons in the hippocampal CA1 region of the adult female rat. J Comp Neurol 373:108–117, 1996.

276. Wu, C-K, Mesulam, M-M and Geula, C: Age-related loss of calbindin from basal forebrain cholinergic neurons. Neuroreport 8:2209–2213, 1997.

277. Yamaguchi, H, Nakazato, Y, Hirai, S, Shoji, M and Harigaya, Y: Electron micrograph of diffuse plaques. Initial stages of senile plaque formation in the Alzheimer brain. Am J Pathol 135:593–597, 1989.

278. Yankner, B A: Mechanisms of neuronal degeneration in Alzheimer's disease. Neuron 16:921–932, 1996.

279. Yankner, B A and Mesulam, M-M: β-amyloid and the pathogenesis of Alzheimer's disease. N Engl J Med 325:1849–1856, 1991.

280. Zhou, L, Miller, B L, McDaniel, C H, Kelly, L, Kim, O J and Miller, C A: Frontotemporal dementia: Neuropil spheroids and presynaptic terminal degeneration. Ann Neurol 44:99–109, 1998.

281. Zhu, X O and Waite, P M E: Cholinergic depletion reduces plasticity of barrel field cortex. Cereb Cortex 8:63–72, 1998.

Index